编

2021
中国肿瘤登记年报
CHINA CANCER REGISTRY ANNUAL REPORT

主　编　赫　捷　魏文强

副主编　张思维　郑荣寿

人民卫生出版社
·北　京·

图书在版编目（CIP）数据

2021 中国肿瘤登记年报：汉、英/国家癌症中心编
. —北京：人民卫生出版社，2023.6
ISBN 978-7-117-34878-2

Ⅰ.①2… Ⅱ.①国… Ⅲ.①肿瘤-卫生统计-中国
-2021-年报-汉、英 Ⅳ.①R73-54

中国国家版本馆 CIP 数据核字（2023）第 103260 号

| 人卫智网 | www. ipmph. com | 医学教育、学术、考试、健康，购书智慧智能综合服务平台 |
| 人卫官网 | www. pmph. com | 人卫官方资讯发布平台 |

2021 中国肿瘤登记年报

2021 Zhongguo Zhongliu Dengji Nianbao

编　　写：国家癌症中心
出版发行：人民卫生出版社（中继线 010-59780011）
地　　址：北京市朝阳区潘家园南里 19 号
邮　　编：100021
E - mail：pmph @ pmph. com
购书热线：010-59787592　010-59787584　010-65264830
印　　刷：人卫印务（北京）有限公司
经　　销：新华书店
开　　本：889×1194　1/16　印张：21
字　　数：607 千字
版　　次：2023 年 6 月第 1 版
印　　次：2023 年 7 月第 1 次印刷
标准书号：ISBN 978-7-117-34878-2
定　　价：180.00 元

打击盗版举报电话：010-59787491　E-mail：WQ @ pmph. com
质量问题联系电话：010-59787234　E-mail：zhiliang @ pmph. com
数字融合服务电话：4001118166　E-mail：zengzhi @ pmph. com

编　委　会

主　　编　赫　捷　魏文强
副主编　张思维　郑荣寿
专家委员会（以姓氏笔画为序）

丁高恒　马　芳　马晶昱　王　宁　王　晔　王少明　王华东　王艳平　王德征　扎西宗吉　文洪梅
邓　颖　付振涛　吕晓燕　华　婧　刘　杰　刘　硕　刘玉琴　许可葵　孙可欣　杜灵彬　李　荔
李秋林　李辉章　李道娟　吴春晓　余　敏　余家华　沈成凤　宋冰冰　张　荣　张　敏　张永贞
张思维　张韶凯　陈　茹　陈　琼　周　衍　周　婕　周金意　周素霞　郑荣寿　姚　霜　贺宇彤
顾　凯　席云峰　韩仁强　曾红梅　赫　捷　颜仕鹏　穆慧娟　戴　丹　魏文强

编　　委（以姓氏笔画为序）

丁丽平　丁贤彬　丁高恒　丁梦秋　于光平　于英红　于绍轶　于鑫刚　马　龙　马　进　马　芳
马　萍　马友田　马方伟　马坤容　马周俊　马振卫　马晓彦　马朝阳　马晶昱　马新颜　王　云
王　丹　王　平　王　宁（北京）　王　宁（莲湖区）　王　宇　王　驰　王　芳　王　丽　王　英
王　春　王　剑（安福县）　王　剑（建湖县）　王　亭　王　艳　王　晔　王　彬　王　鸿　王　维
王　雯　王　裕　王　新　王小庆　王天军　王少明　王正英　王发辉　王光秀　王伟仁　王华东
王全新　王红艳　王红梅　王秀瑛　王灵珍　王现玲　王金金　王金荣　王学会　王学军　王建宁
王建新　王绍梅　王树革　王昱云　王秋婷　王修华　王洪丽　王艳平　王晓锋　王爱民　王烨菁
王浩武　王培贤　王梦元　王谋涛　王维霞　王登琪　王路思　王鹏飞　王新正　王静艳　王嘉玉
王德征　王穗湘　韦冬玲　韦汉泽　韦坚峥　韦政兴　扎西宗吉　贝晶利　牛永霞　毛　鹏　文　杰
文洪梅　文章军　文婧唯　亢连科　方吉贤　方学哲　方嘉列　尹　炜　尹　勇　孔　屏　孔　超
孔程程　邓　颖　邓海名　甘晓琴　古彩红　古错悦　左存锐　左廷杰　左顺彦　石保英　石朝晖
龙　云　卢　斌　卢玉强　卢志玲　叶开友　叶永利　叶鹏华　叶新华　申立琼　田　侠　田　燕
田凤梅　田玉平　田绍进　田密格　冉悦函　付　晨　付　敏　付振涛　代　鹏　代晓泽　白　杉
白国霞　包雨晴　包新元　冯　伟　冯　羽　冯　艳　冯　翠　冯云洪　冯华强　冯金洪　兰宏旺
兰泽龙　宁　栈　宁　锋　宁伯福　司媛媛　邢　丽　邢念增　邢婷婷　权巧玲　吕利成　吕建峰
吕晓燕　吕家爱　朱　丽　朱　健　朱云峰　朱从喜　朱庆荣　朱君君　朱晓庆　朱晓梅　朱海深
朱彩虹　朱景红　乔丽颖　乔健健　伍轩民　伍啸青　仲丽红　任　涛　任礼飞　任永彪　华　婧
华召来　华国梁　向　嫱　庄建林　刘　扬　刘　伟　刘　华　刘　会　刘　军　刘　芳　刘　宏
刘　杰（江西省）　刘　杰（邳州市）　刘　政　刘　洋　刘　彧　刘　积　刘　涛（贵州省）
刘　涛（巢湖市）　刘　娣　刘　硕　刘　森　刘　磊　刘　毅　刘韦淞　刘丹丹　刘凤香　刘凤容
刘玉琴　刘冬秀　刘庆皆　刘兴莉　刘安阜　刘纪红　刘志荣　刘轩岐　刘建平　刘树生　刘秋爽
刘勇言　刘艳玲　刘素谦　刘晓丽　刘晓玲　刘爱坡　刘家早　刘淑梅　刘婷婷　刘登湘　刘曙正
闫　萍　闫云燕　闫永峰　闫阿妮　关　勇　江　珊　江　超　江国虹　汤　成　汤丽珍　汤剑峰
汤海霞　安水玲　祁少华　许　欣　许　琴　许可葵　许瑞瑞　许慧琳　农梁伟　阮红海　孙　忠
孙　颖　孙于茹　孙正义　孙可欣　孙仕丽　孙花荣　孙青青　阳　立　严传富　严春华　严莉丽
苏　明　苏　燕　苏中婷　苏升灿　苏福康　杜　艳　杜小菊　杜月清　杜灵彬　杜国明　杜晓芳
杜海国　李　力　李　凤　李　宁　李　光　李　刚　李　军　李　宏　李　荔　李　奕　李　莹
李　倩　李　锋　李　谦　李万忠　李凡卡　李云西　李文华　李世艳　李东芝　李生芳　李白鸟
李汉福　李永刚　李永伟　李亚波　李伟生　李志霞　李林容　李忠平　李佳佳　李朋林　李育清
李诗童　李秋林　李顺翠　李保瑞　李祚成　李振东　李桂芬　李晓琴　李晓燕　李爱会　李益球
李菁玲　李彬明　李雪芳　李琰琰　李辉章　李晶晶　李道娟　李意晨　李慎榜　杨　凤　杨　竹
杨　劲　杨　俊　杨　涛　杨　娟　杨　琴　杨　琳　杨　晶　杨　媚　杨　瑞　杨　静
杨　慧（武安市）　杨　慧（梅县区）　杨可珍　杨岁旭　杨红梅　杨志杰　杨利国　杨茂敏　杨尚波
杨佳娟　杨念念　杨俊杰　杨艳蕾　杨晓光　杨璐竹　肖亚洲　肖红军　肖丽梅　肖拥军　肖幸平

肖艳玲	吴丹	吴刚	吴欢	吴畅	吴波	吴王剑	吴玉福	吴英俊	吴泽宁	吴春晓
吴美秀	吴艳伟	吴海燕	吴逸平	吴景瑜	吴新会	吴德明	邱红	邱林	邱琳	何飞
何礼	何阳	何羽	何丽	何洁	何磊	何少松	何丽明	何秀玲	何保华	何道逢
余军	余敏	余斌	余汉春	余美帆	余家华	邹红	邹晓琳	邹跃威	应洪琰	汪乃源
汪有库	沈莉	沈成凤	沈嘉航	宋冰冰	宋国慧	张旭	张邻	张劲	张英	张迪
张荣	张标	张莹	张桃	张涛	张敏	张雁	张策	张婷	张瑜	张楠
张静	张燕	张乙中	张丁丁	张小林	张元友	张艺杰	张凤鸣	张玉伟	张平稳	张冬梅
张永贞	张亚莹	张志娟	张秀芬	张武武	张坤平	张宝桐	张建安	张建鲁	张春英	张思维
张美莲	张艳艳	张晓峰	张爱红	张恋恋	张海虹	张淑萍	张瑞欣	张韶凯	张慧玲	张露新
陆艳	陆玉培	陆素颖	阿迪拉·苏力旦	陈节	陈英	陈茹	陈洁	陈琳	陈琼
陈燕	陈几文	陈小芳	陈小娜	陈小慧	陈仁忠	陈文君	陈兰芬	陈志虹	陈妙嫦	陈玥华
陈国荣	陈明丹	陈金武	陈建顺	陈珍连	陈思红	陈洪森	陈娇娇	陈艳萍	陈晓明	陈雪筠
陈清彦	陈道勇	武鸣	武霞	拉毛才让	范光	范颖	范建强	范美霞	林利	林玲
林涛	林玉成	林超兰	欧阳乐	尚明风	帖映伟	罗娜	罗源	罗睿	罗文云	罗冰贤
罗国良	罗忠芳	罗艳丽	和臣慧	和丽娜	季莹	季加孚	金锋	金泽彬	周丽	周衍
周倩	周浩	周娟	周健	周琦	周锐	周鑫	周川楠	周文群	周丽萍	周金意
周建容	周建湘	周素霞	周晓凤	周婷婷	周新玉	周福新	周静静	郑伟	郑方金	郑冬柏
郑永萍	郑亚文	郑荣寿	郑益强	郑鸿庆	郑裕明	单保恩	孟杨	陕国清	项霞霞	赵丹
赵辉	赵占峰	赵仲刚	赵寿桃	赵孝华	赵劲良	赵金永	赵宗和	赵建华	赵秋萍	赵海洲
赵朝强	赵雅芳	赵媛丽	郝士卿	郝功轩	郝青青	郝真强	胡东	胡莹	胡彪	胡燕
胡小玲	胡艳红	胡素华	胡倩华	胡燕琳	茹夏丽	南艳	柯金练	钞利娜	钟钰	钟玉美
钟伟文	钟彦丰	钮登	段叠	段乐永	段红梅	保红莉	侯亮	俞亮	俞敏	施长苗
姜帆	姜欣	姜永根	姜旭红	姜金宏	姜彩霞	娄培安	洪武	宫旭志	宫舒萍	祝章美
费琳	费兴林	姚琳	姚霜	姚永红	姚信飞	贺宇彤	贺军宏	贺绍琼	骆文书	骆秀美
秦舒	秦延锦	袁英	袁东娅	袁伟贤	袁明强	袁晓宇	袁聪玲	耿文飞	聂炜	莫兆波
贾志永	贾玲玲	贾艳芳	贾爱华	贾源瑶	夏冰	夏云磊	夏湘莲	顾凯	顾小平	顾淑君
党丽琴	晏荧	钱赟	倪志华	徐仙	徐伟	徐旭	徐薇	徐玉銮	徐绍和	徐海霞
徐媛锋	徐新红	徐蔚静	殷文学	殷建湘	凌平	高霞	高生丽	高彩云	高鸿军	高鸿敏
高瑞芳	郭伟	郭梅	郭超	郭小兰	郭天骅	郭秀连	郭昌融	郭贵周	郭秋献	郭晓雷
郭晏强	郭颖贞	席云峰	唐明	唐秀仙	陶小红	陶武明	黄艳	黄静	黄一峰	黄飞平
黄永杰	黄充盈	黄远田	黄杰周	黄佳玲	黄炯媚	黄素勤	黄海浪	黄惠玲	黄道靖	黄锦航
曹珊	曹凌	曹智	曹秋菊	曹慷慷	龚建华	龚新洪	龚巍巍	盛振海	盛根英	常蓉
符三乃	符地宝	符芳敏	符美艳	庹吉好	章文华	章有健	淳志明	梁辉	梁广忠	梁树军
梁鹏涛	彭绩	彭红伟	彭旻微	董芳	董玲	董永年	董建梅	蒋素红	韩雪	韩小玉
韩仁强	韩湘意	韩瑞贞	韩颖颖	覃宁	覃明江	覃忠书	覃燕红	程锋	程谧	程麟
程立平	程向东	程志芳	税智群	曾平	曾红梅	曾串连	曾映竹	游宁	谢平	谢淑雯
婷婷	靳万春	靳双红	蒲泓兵	蒙怡	楚淑英	雷方	雷云云	雷芸华	雷若倩	雷宝琼
虞吉寅	虞宝颖	简琳	鲍月月	赫捷	蔡伟	裴振义	管小琴	管元平	管丽娟	廖羽
廖顺连	廖倩	廖涛	廖柳艳	廖凌玲	谭家伟	颜仕鹏	颜克梅	翟玉庭	熊炜	熊维	熊斌
熊薇	熊润红	缪伟刚	樊学琼	颜仕鹏	颜克梅	潘熙	潘中伟	潘盛林	霍军荣	穆慧娟
戴丹	戴姮	戴招文	戴春云	魏丹	魏九丹	魏文强	魏矿荣	藤萝	瞿媛

Editorial Board

Li Ning, Li Guang, Li Gang, Li Jun, Li Hong, Li Li, Li Yi, Li Ying, Li Qian, Li Feng, Li Qian, Li Wanzhong, Li Fanka, Li Yunxi, Li Wenhua, Li Shiyan, Li Dongzhi, Li Shengfang, Li Bainiao, Li Hanfu, Li Yonggang, Li Yongwei, Li Yabo, Li Weisheng, Li Zhixia, Li Linrong, Li Zhongping, Li Jiajia, Li Penglin, Li Yuqing, Li Shitong, Li Qiulin, Li Shuncui, Li Baorui, Li Zuocheng, Li Zhendong, Li Guifen, Li Xiaoqin, Li Xiaoyan, Li Aihui, Li Yiqiu, Li Jingling, Li Binming, Li Xuefang, Li Yanyan, Li Huizhang, Li Jingjing, Li Daojuan, Li Yichen, Li Shenbang, Yang Feng, Yang Zhu, Yang Jin, Yang Jun, Yang Tao, Yang Juan, Yang Qin, Yang Lin, Yang Jing, Yang Mei, Yang Rui, Yang Jing, Yang Hui(Wu'an Shi), Yang Hui(Meixian Qu), Yang Kezhen, Yang Suixu, Yang Hongmei, Yang Zhijie, Yang Liguo, Yang Maomin, Yang Shangbo, Yang Jiajuan, Yang Niannian, Yang Junjie, Yang Yanlei, Yang Xiaoguang, Yang Luzhu, Xiao Yazhou, Xiao Hongjun, Xiao Limei, Xiao Yongjun, Xiao Xingping, Xiao Yanling, Wu Dan, Wu Gang, Wu Huan, Wu Chang, Wu Bo, Wu Wangjian, Wu Yufu, Wu Yingjun, Wu Zening, Wu Chunxiao, Wu Meixiu, Wu Yanwei, Wu Haiyan, Wu Yiping, Wu Jingyu, Wu Xinhui, Wu Deming, Qiu Hong, Qiu Lin, Qiu Lin, He Fei, He Li, He Yang, He Yu, He Li, He Jie, He Lei, He Shaosong, He Liming, He Xiuling, He Baohua, He Daofeng, Yu Jun, Yu Min, Yu Bin, Yu Hanchun, Yu Meifan, Yu Jiahua, Zou Hong, Zou Xiaolin, Zou Yuewei, Ying Hongyan, Wang Naiyuan, Wang Youku, Shen Li, Shen Chengfeng, Shen Jiahang, Song Bingbing, Song Guohui, Zhang Xu, Zhang Lin, Zhang Jin, Zhang Ying, Zhang Di, Zhang Rong, Zhang Biao, Zhang Ying, Zhang Tao, Zhang Tao, Zhang Min, Zhang Yan, Zhang Ce, Zhang Ting, Zhang Yu, Zhang Nan, Zhang Jing, Zhang Yan, Zhang Yizhong, Zhang Dingding, Zhang Xiaolin, Zhang Yuanyou, Zhang Yijie, Zhang Fengming, Zhang Yuwei, Zhang Pingwen, Zhang Dongmei, Zhang Yongzhen, Zhang Yaying, Zhang Zhijuan, Zhang Xiufen, Zhang Wuwu, Zhang Kunping, Zhang Baotong, Zhang Jianan, Zhang Jianlu, Zhang Chunying, Zhang Siwei, Zhang Meilian, Zhang Yanyan, Zhang Xiaofeng, Zhang Aihong, Zhang Lianlian, Zhang Haihong, Zhang Shuping, Zhang Ruixin, Zhang Shaokai, Zhang Huiling, Zhang Luxin, Lu Yan, Lu Yupei, Lu Suying, Adila Sulidan, Chen Jie, Chen Ying, Chen Ru, Chen Jie, Chen Lin, Chen Qiong, Chen Yan, Chen Jiwen, Chen Xiaofang, Chen Xiaona, Chen Xiaohui, Chen Renzhong, Chen Wenjun, Chen Lanfen, Chen Zhihong, Chen Miaochang, Chen Yuehua, Chen Guorong, Chen Mingdan, Chen Jinwu, Chen Jianshun, Chen Zhenlian, Chen Sihong, Chen Hongsen, Chen Jiaojiao, Chen Yanping, Chen Xiaoming, Chen Xuejun, Chen Qingyan, Chen Daoyong, Wu Ming, Wu Xia, Lamao Cairang, Fan Guang, Fan Ying, Fan Jianqiang, Fan Meixia, Lin Li, Lin Ling, Lin Tao, Lin Yucheng, Lin Chaolan, Ouyang Le, Shang Mingfeng, Tie Yingwei, Luo Na, Luo Yuan, Luo Rui, Luo Wenyun, Luo Bingxian, Luo Guoliang, Luo Zhongfang, Luo Yanli, He Chenhui, He Lina, Ji Ying, Ji Jiafu, Jin Feng, Jin Zebin, Zhou Li, Zhou Yan, Zhou Qian, Zhou Hao, Zhou Juan, Zhou Jie, Zhou Qi, Zhou Rui, Zhou Xin, Zhou Chuannan, Zhou Wenqun, Zhou Liping, Zhou Jinyi, Zhou Jianrong, Zhou Jianxiang, Zhou Suxia, Zhou Xiaofeng, Zhou Tingting, Zhou Xinyu, Zhou Fuxin, Zhou Jingjing, Zheng Wei, Zheng Fangjin, Zheng Dongbai, Zheng Yongping, Zheng Yawen, Zheng Rongshou, Zheng Yiqiang, Zheng Hongqing, Zheng Yuming, Shan Baoen, Meng Yang, Shan Guoqing, Xiang Xiaxia, Zhao Dan, Zhao Hui, Zhao Zhanfeng, Zhao Zhonggang, Zhao Shoutao, Zhao Xiaohua, Zhao Jinliang, Zhao Jinyong, Zhao Zonghe, Zhao Jianhua, Zhao Qiuping, Zhao Haizhou, Zhao Chaoqiang, Zhao Yafang, Zhao Yuanli, Hao Shiqing, Hao Gongxuan, Hao Qingqing, Hao Zhenqiang, Hu Dong, Hu Ying, Hu Biao, Hu Yan, Hu Xiaoling, Hu Yanhong, Hu Suhua, Hu Qianhua, Hu Yanlin, Ru Xiali, Nan Yan, Ke Jinlian, Chao Lina, Zhong Yu, Zhong Yumei, Zhong Weiwen, Zhong Yanfeng, Niu Deng, Duan Die, Duan Leyong, Duan Hongmei, Bao Hongli, Hou Liang, Yu Liang, Yu Min, Shi Changmiao, Jiang Fan, Jiang Xin, Jiang Yonggen, Jiang Xuhong, Jiang Jinhong, Jiang Caixia, Lou Peian, Hong Wu, Gong Xuzhi, Gong Shuping, Zhu Zhangmei, Fei Lin, Fei Xinglin, Yao Lin, Yao Shuang, Yao Yonghong, Yao Xinfei, He Yutong, He Junhong, He Shaoqiong, Luo Wenshu, Luo Xiumei, Qin Shu, Qin Yanjin, Yuan Ying, Yuan Dongya, Yuan Weixian, Yuan Mingqiang, Yuan Xiaoyu, Yuan Congling, Geng Wenfei, Nie Wei, Mo Zhaobo, Jia Zhiyong, Jia Lingling, Jia Yanfang, Jia Aihua, Jia Yuanyao, Xia Bing, Xia Yunlei, Xia Xianglian, Gu Kai, Gu Xiaoping, Gu Shujun, Dang Liqin, Yan Ying, Qian Yun, Ni Zhihua, Xu Xian, Xu Wei, Xu Xu, Xu Wei, Xu Yuluan, Xu Shaohe, Xu Haixia, Xu Yuanfeng, Xu Xinhong, Xu Weijing, Yin Wenxue, Yin Jianxiang, Ling Ping, Gao Xia, Gao Shengli, Gao Caiyun, Gao Hongjun, Gao Hongmin, Gao Ruifang, Guo Wei, Guo Mei, Guo Chao, Guo Xiaolan, Guo Tianhua, Guo Xiulian, Guo Changrong, Guo Guizhou, Guo Qiuxian, Guo Xiaolei, Guo Yanqiang, Guo Yingzhen, Xi Yunfeng, Tang Ming, Tang Xiuxian, Tao Xiaohong, Tao Wuming, Huang Yan, Huang Jing, Huang Yifeng, Huang Feiping, Huang Yongjie,

Huang Chongying, Huang Yuantian, Huang Jiezhou, Huang Jialing, Huang Jiongmei, Huang Suqin, Huang Hailang, Huang Huiling, Huang Daojing, Huang Jinhang, Cao Shan, Cao Ling, Cao Zhi, Cao Qiuju, Cao Kangkang, Gong Jianhua, Gong Xinhong, Gong Weiwei, Sheng Zhenhai, Sheng Genying, Chang Rong, Fu Sannai, Fu Dibao, Fu Fangmin, Fu Meiyan, Tuo Jiyu, Zhang Wenhua, Zhang Youjian, Chun Zhiming, Liang Hui, Liang Guangzhong, Liang Shujun, Liang Pengtao, Peng Ji, Peng Hongwei, Peng Minwei, Dong Fang, Dong Ling, Dong Yongnian, Dong Jianmei, Jiang Suhong, Han Xue, Han Xiaoyu, Han Renqiang, Han Xiangyi, Han Ruizhen, Han Yingying, Qin Ning, Qin Mingjiang, Qin Zhongshu, Qin Yanhong, Cheng Feng, Cheng Mi, Cheng Lin, Cheng Liping, Cheng Xiangdong, Cheng Zhifang, Shui Zhiqun, Zeng Ping, Zeng Hongmei, Zeng Chuanlian, Zeng Yingzhu, You Ningjing, Xie Ping, Xie Shuwen, Ting Ting, Jin Wanchun, Jin Shuanghong, Pu Hongbing, Meng Yi, Chu Shuying, Lei Fang, Lei Yunyun, Lei Yunhua, Lei Ruoqian, Lei Baoqiong, Yu Jiyin, Yu Baoying, Jian Lin, Bao Yueyue, He Jie, Cai Wei, Pei Zhenyi, Guan Xiaoqin, Guan Yuanping, Guan Lijuan, Liao Yu, Liao Shun, Liao Qian, Liao Tao, Liao Liuyan, Liao Lingling, Tan Jiawei, Ji Limin, Zhai Yuting, Xiong Wei, Xiong Wei, Xiong Bin, Xiong Wei, Xiong Runhong, Miao Weigang, Fan Xueqiong, Yan Shipeng, Yan Kemei, Pan Xi, Pan Zhongwei, Pan Shenglin, Huo Junrong, Mu Huijuan, Dai Dan, Dai Heng, Dai Zhaowen, Dai Chunyun, Wei Dan, Wei Jiudan, Wei Wenqiang, Wei Kuangrong, Teng Luo, Qu Yuan

前　言

　　肿瘤登记是对肿瘤流行情况、趋势变化和影响因素进行长期、连续、动态的系统性监测，是制定癌症预防控制策略、开展综合防控研究、评价防控效果的重要基础性工作。这项工作的标志性成果之一就是，每年以年报的形式及时发布全国肿瘤登记监测数据。中国肿瘤登记年报已成为我国癌症预防与控制不可或缺的宝贵资料，在不同历史时期均发挥了极其重要的作用。我国的肿瘤登记，自20世纪50年代起步至今，已走过60多年的发展历程，从无到有，从小到大，风雨兼程，愈挫弥坚，离不开几辈专业人士的拓荒与坚守，更离不开党和国家的高度重视，肿瘤登记工作已经探索出了符合我国实际的发展道路，成为我国癌症防控工作的重要组成部分。

　　目前，我国已建成覆盖全国的肿瘤登记随访监测系统，连续动态发布肿瘤登记年报，持续推进肿瘤生存随访。截至2021年底，肿瘤登记已覆盖全国2 085个县区，覆盖人口10.45亿，全国肿瘤登记中心也完成了《中国肿瘤登记数据集》团体标准立项及制定工作，完成了全国肿瘤登记信息平台建设工作，我国的肿瘤登记工作国际影响逐步扩大，国际评价我国为肿瘤登记数据质量一类地区，中国的肿瘤登记主动承担国际及区域肿瘤登记责任，不断为世界肿瘤登记工作贡献中国智慧。

　　肿瘤防控再出发，肿瘤登记先行，随着肿瘤等慢性非传染性疾病在世界公共卫生问题中的比重逐步加重，癌症负担等慢病基础数据的必要性、连续性、重要性必将日益凸显，进一步提升肿瘤登记数据质量，促进登记数据与死因监测数据、临床诊疗信息数据以及人口数据、医保数据等其他信息的对接交换、互联互通，促进信息资源共享利用，是肿瘤登记工作的重中之重，也是大势所趋。

　　《2021中国肿瘤登记年报》是自2008年首次出版以来的第15卷。本年报汇总了2018年我国肿瘤登记地区癌症监测数据。国家癌症中心收到来自中国31个省（自治区、直辖市）及新疆生产建设兵团（未包括香港特别行政区、澳门特别行政区

Foreword

Cancer Registration is a long-term, continuous, dynamic and systematic monitoring system. It monitors the epidemic state, trend changes, and influence factors of cancer. Cancer Registration is the fundamental work of formulating cancer prevention and control strategies, launching comprehensive prevention and control research, and evaluating prevention and control results. One prominent achievement of cancer registration in China is to publish the *China Cancer Registry Annual Report*, which has been a great value for cancer prevention and control in different periods of the country. Since the primary stage in the 1950s, China cancer registration has gone through 60 years of development. In the past 60 years, it has developed from scratch, from small to large, and has experienced tremendous hardships. It is inseparable from the pioneering spirit and persistence of several generations of professionals, and also inseparable from the guidance and care of the Party and the State. China cancer registration has explored a way in line with the reality of our country, and has become an important part of cancer prevention and control in China.

At present, China has established a nationwide cancer registration and follow-up monitoring system, which can continuously and dynamically release Cancer Registry Annual Report, and constantly promotes follow-up of cancer survival. By the end of 2021, cancer registration has covered 2 085 counties and districts with population coverage of 1.045 billion. The National Cancer Center has also completed the establishment and formulation of the association standard of *China Cancer Registration Data Set* and the construction of the National Cancer Registration Information Platform. The international influence of China cancer registration is gradually expanding. China has been evaluated as the first-class region in terms of the quality of cancer registration data. China actively takes the responsibility of international and regional cancer registration work, and constantly contributes China wisdom to the world.

Cancer prevention and control are having an unprecedented development opportunity, and cancer registration needs to start before the others to lead cancer prevention and control. With the increasing proportion of chronic non-infectious diseases such as cancer in the public health problem worldwide, the necessity, the continuity, and the importance of basic data of cancer and other chronic diseases will become increasingly prominent. Enhancing the quality of cancer registration data, promoting the exchange and interconnection of registration data and death causing data, the clinical diagnosis and treatment information data, population data, medical insurance data, and other information, and the sharing and utilization of information resources are the essential part and the general trend of cancer registration.

Since the first volume of *China Cancer Registry Annual Report* published in 2008, this book is the 15th Annual Report. In this volume, cancer surveillance data of China cancer registration areas in 2018 was

和台湾省)947 个肿瘤登记处上报数据。通过对数据审核和质量控制,有 700 个肿瘤登记处数据入选本年报。此次年报对所有癌症合计及 22 类癌症的发病和死亡数据进行了详细分析,并分地区、年龄别和性别比较了癌症分布差异。考虑到各省已经开始发布本地区的肿瘤负担数据,本次全国年报不再展示各省区县级的肿瘤登记数据。

60 多年转瞬即逝,肿瘤登记工作是中国人民防癌抗癌历程中浓墨重彩的一笔,但中国肿瘤登记的过去并未远去,我们仍在前辈开拓出的路上坚定前行。回顾中国肿瘤登记从小到大、从弱到强的发展历程,我们能够体会前辈的艰辛与坚守,我们更心存感激,我们更骄傲自豪,我们几辈人薪火相传,已经探索出了符合中国实际的肿瘤登记道路!我们感恩前辈的筚路蓝缕,砥砺付出,最好的回报是传承和发展,我们深信,在党和国家"健康中国"战略的指引下,我国肿瘤登记工作必将会成绩斐然,再创辉煌!

在全国新型冠状病毒感染疫情防控新常态环境下,肿瘤登记工作者在积极落实防控措施的前提下,不忘本职,无怨无悔地及时完成了年报数据上报清理、统计分析、编撰出版工作。《2021 中国肿瘤登记年报》的顺利出版凝结着全国各肿瘤登记处全体工作人员的辛苦付出和 35 位编写、审校人员的辛勤劳动,年报的出版也得到了国家疾病预防控制局、国家卫生健康委员会宣传司一如既往的具体指导和大力支持,我们在此表示最衷心的感谢!

编者从登记点选择、数据清理、统计分析、图表呈现、文字描述等方面反复核实,力求做到数字真实、描述准确,竭力避免不必要的失误,然而由于水平和知识有限,加之入选年报的登记点数量剧增,数据体量巨大,工作中难免出现纰漏,敬请国内外同行和广大读者批评指正。

国家癌症中心
2022 年 6 月

reported. A total of 947 cancer registries submitted data to National Cancer Center (NCC) in China, including 31 provinces (autonomous regions and municipalities) and Xinjiang Production and Construction Corps (not including Hongkong Tebiexingzhengqu, Macau Tebiexingzhengqu and Taiwan Sheng). After data quality control, a total of 700 cancer registries were included in the present *China Cancer Registry Annual Report*. In this volume, we summarized and analyzed data of the incidence and mortality for all cancers combined and 22 cancer sites by including overall analysis and analysis by age, sex and area. Considering that all provinces have begun to release the cancer burden data of their own regions, this national annual report will no longer show the cancer registration data at the county level.

Cancer registration is an important part of the anticancer process in China in the last 60 years. However, the history of China cancer registration has not passed away, and we are still proceeding on the way of our predecessors. We are grateful and proud of the hard work and persistence of our predecessors when looking back the development from small to large, from weak to strong of China cancer registration. Through the efforts of several generations, China cancer registration has explored a way in line with the reality of our country. We are grateful to the contribution of our predecessors and will continue the inheritance and development in return. We are convinced that China cancer registration will make brilliant achievements under the guidance of "Healthy China" Strategy of the Party and the State.

In the new period of regular prevention and control of COVID-19, all faculties of cancer registries did not forget their duties and complete the reporting, cleaning, analyzing and publishing works of the annual report without complaint while actively implementing epidemic prevention and control measures. The successful publication of the *2021 China Cancer Registry Annual Report* embodies the hard work of all staff members in different cancer registries across the country. It also reflects the hard work of 35 editors and reviewers. National Administration of Disease Prevention and Control, Department of Publicity in National Health Commission of the People's Republic of China have also provided guidance and support in the publication of the *2021 China Cancer Registry Annual Report*. We acknowledge all staff working for the cancer registries and the editorial board who contributed to this publication.

In order to assure the data is real, objective, accurate and without unnecessary mistakes, the authors write carefully and verify repeatedly for choosing the cancer registries, cleaning data, doing statistical analysis, rendering charts and describing data. However, due to the knowledge limitation, and the intensively increased cancer registries, the vast data volume may lead to some mistakes in the work. Colleagues and readers are welcome to criticize and correct.

National Cancer Center
June 2022

目　　录

Contents

第一章 概 述

1 中国人群肿瘤登记系统简介

肿瘤登记是对癌症流行情况、趋势变化和影响因素进行长期、连续、动态的系统性监测，是制定癌症预防控制策略、开展综合防控研究、评价防控效果的重要基础性工作。我国的肿瘤登记工作已走过了60多年发展历程，人群肿瘤登记工作在不同时期，都为国家癌症防控提供了科学翔实的肿瘤负担和流行情况，有力支撑了我国癌症防控政策策略制定和实施。

近几十年我国人群肿瘤登记工作进展迅速，成绩举世瞩目。2008年，国家卫生部设立"肿瘤登记随访项目"并纳入"国家重大公共卫生专项中央财政转移支付项目"，在全国31个省（自治区、直辖市）及新疆生产建设兵团（未包括香港特别行政区、澳门特别行政区和台湾省）逐步建立了覆盖全国的人群肿瘤登记和监测随访网络，逐步开展人群为基础的肿瘤发病、死亡和生存的信息收集工作。2015年国家卫生和计划生育委员会、国家中医药管理局联合下发《肿瘤登记管理办法》，从制度上保证了全国肿瘤登记工作的顺利开展。多年来，在上级主管部门的领导和大力支持下，全国肿瘤登记处数量和质量逐年提升。截至2022年底，开展人群肿瘤登记工作的登记处为2 806个，覆盖全国人口99.8%，目前收集到的肿瘤负担数据，能够较为全面地反映我国癌症发病、死亡、生存状况及变化趋势。

Chapter 1　Introduction

1　Population-based cancer registration system in China

Cancer Registration is a long-term, continuous, dynamic, systematic monitoring system. It monitors cancer's epidemic state, trend change and influence factor. Cancer Registration is the fundamental work of formulating cancer prevention and control strategies, launching comprehensive prevention and control research, and evaluating prevention and control results. After 60 years' development, the cancer registry provides scientific and detailed information about cancer burden and epidemic state for national cancer prevention and control, as well as supports the formulation and implementation of the cancer prevention and control policy in the different periods.

In recent decades, our cancer registry has progressed rapidly, and its outstanding achievements have attracted worldwide attention. Since 2008, the former Ministry of Health set up the "National Cancer Registration and Follow-up Program" to support the cancer registration in China with sustainable funding. All 31 provinces (autonomous regions and municipalities) and Xinjiang Production and Construction Corps in China (not including Hongkong Tebiexingzhengqu, Macau Tebiexingzhengqu and Taiwan Sheng) have gradually established a cancer registration framework. Population-based cancer incidence, mortality and survival information are collected through the cancer registration system. In 2015, the National Health and Family Planning Commission and the National Administration of Traditional Chinese Medicine co-published *Chinese Cancer Registration Management Regulation*, which provides a legal protection on cancer registration in China. Under the leadership of the Chinese government, there has been a steady increase in the numbers and quality of population-based cancer registries in China. Until the end of 2022, there are a total of 2 806 population-based cancer registries, with 99.8% population coverage. Trends and updated statistics of cancer incidence, mortality and survival are comprehensively reported from the data the cancer registry collected.

但我们也应看到,随着大数据时代的到来和现代网络信息技术的发展,传统登记监测手段的不足逐步显现,逐渐无法满足国家卫生决策、人民群众不断增长的健康需求及癌症预防、临床诊治、科学研究工作的及时高效服务需求。针对现阶段存在的肿瘤登记点数量不足和分布不均衡、肿瘤登记数据深度和广度不足、信息资源交互共享利用度低等问题,《健康中国行动——癌症防治实施方案(2019—2022 年)》中,对肿瘤登记工作以制度标准、数据质量和资源共享为切入点,通过"扩面""提质""增效"三个方面的具体行动措施,全面推进肿瘤登记工作。"扩面"就是要通过修订《肿瘤登记管理办法(2015)》和《中国肿瘤登记工作指导手册(2016)》、发布肿瘤登记共识性政策文件和肿瘤登记工作实施方案、扩大登记年报覆盖面、落实省级责任制等工作进一步健全肿瘤登记报告制度。"提质"就是要通过推动国家肿瘤登记平台工程、建立多级肿瘤登记点专家团队、制定登记数据收集标准及随访监测数据质量标准等方面的工作,提升肿瘤登记数据质量。"增效"就是要通过加强肿瘤登记信息化建设、制定登记数据管理方法和数据信息安全管理方法、推进不同信息资源对接、开展大数据应用研究等,促进信息资源共享利用。

积极落实国家系列规划、计划等政策文件精神,国家癌症中心已基本完成了全国肿瘤登记信息平台的建设工作,今年年报的部分数据就是通过新的平台上报。相信在新的发展机遇下,中国的肿瘤登记工作必将实现肿瘤数据实时上报、动态监测和多维呈现,更为及时有效地为我国肿瘤防控的政策制定、工作实施、效果评估等提供坚实的科学依据,更好地服务"健康中国"战略。

However, with the advent of the big data era and the development of modern internet technology, the deficiencies of traditional registration monitoring methods gradually emerged. It cannot fully support the national health decision making, satisfy the increasing demand of people's health concerns and fulfill the requirements of cancer prevention, clinical diagnosis, treatment and scientific research. Due to the insufficient and unevenly distributed cancer registries, the insufficient data depth and breadth, and the low utilization of interactive sharing of information resources, *The Plan of Healthy China—The Implementation Plan of Cancer Prevention and Control (2019-2022)* develops three implementation strategies: "Coverage Expansion" "Quality Improvement" and "Efficiency Increment" to fully promote cancer registry from system standards, data quality and resource sharing aspects. "Coverage Expansion": by revising *Chinese Cancer Registration Management Regulation (2015)* and *Chinese Guideline for Cancer Registration (2016)*, releasing consensus policy of cancer registration and implementation proposal of cancer registration, expanding the coverage of the annual report and fulfilling provincial responsibility system to further improve the cancer registration system. "Quality improvement": by promoting the "National Cancer Registration Platform Project", establishing a multi-level cancer registration expert team and developing the standards of registration data collection and data quality monitoring to improve the data quality of cancer registration. "Efficiency Increase": by strengthening the information construction of cancer registration, developing registration data management regulation and data security management regulation, promoting the integration of different resources, and conducting big data application research, to increase the efficiency of sharing and utilization of information resources.

The National Cancer Center has mainly completed the construction of the National Cancer Registration Information Platform. Part of the data in this year's annual report was reported through the new platform. It is believed that under the new development opportunity, the cancer registration work of China will achieve real-time reporting, dynamic monitoring and multi-dimensional presentation. This work will provide solid scientific support for the policy formulation, work implementation, and effect evaluation of cancer prevention and control of China in a more timely and effective manner, so as to serve the "Healthy China" strategy better.

2 本年报数据

2.1 数据上报地区及范围

本年报数据收集截止时间为 2021 年 12 月 31 日，数据上报范围为 2018 年 1 月 1 日至 2018 年 12 月 31 日全年新发癌症发病和死亡个案数据（ICD-10 编码范围：C00-C97，D32-D33，D42-D43，D45-D47），以及各肿瘤登记处 2018 年年中人口数据。上报 2018 年肿瘤登记数据的登记处分布在全国 31 个省（自治区、直辖市）及新疆生产建设兵团（未包括香港特别行政区、澳门特别行政区和台湾省），合计登记处 947 个，覆盖人口 634 376 540 人，其中城市登记处 335 个，农村登记处 612 个。

2.2 数据质量控制及最终纳入数据

国家癌症中心根据《中国肿瘤登记工作指导手册（2016）》，参照国际癌症研究机构（IARC）/国际癌症登记协会（IACR）《五大洲癌症发病率》第 11 卷对肿瘤登记质量的有关要求，从数据可比性、有效性和完整性等方面制定中国肿瘤登记年报数据纳入排除标准。依据标准对 2018 年肿瘤登记数据进行质量控制，同时充分考虑区域覆盖面，本年报最终纳入 700 个登记处合格数据作为本年报数据。

全国 700 个肿瘤登记处 2018 年覆盖人口 523 160 249 人（男性 265 488 549 人，女性 257 671 700 人），占 2018 年中国总人口（1 405 410 000）的 37.22%。其中城市地区肿瘤登记处 267 个，覆盖人口 236 047 481 人，占入选年报中国肿瘤登记地区人口数的 45.12%；农村地区肿瘤登记处 433 个，覆盖人口 287 112 768 人，占 54.88%。

2 Data specification in this annual report

2.1 Data collection scope

NCC China required all population-based cancer registries to submit new diagnoses and deaths from cancer in 2018 (ICD-10: C00-C97, D32-D33, D42-D43, D45-D47), as well as the corresponding population data before December 31st, 2021. All those submitted data in 2018 are distributed in 31 provinces (autonomous regions and municipalities) and Xinjiang production and Construction Corps (not including Hongkong Tebiexingzhengqu, Macau Tebiexingzhengqu and Taiwan Sheng). A total of 947 cancer registries submitted data to NCC China, covering a total of 634 376 540 population. Among the 947 cancer registries, 335 were urban cancer registries and 612 were rural cancer registries.

2.2 Data quality control and qualified data

According to *Chinese guideline cancer registration (2016)* and the standards of International Agency for Research on Cancer/International Association of Cancer Registries (IARC/IACR) on *Cancer Incidence in Five Continents*, *Vol. XI*, we have published a national criterion on data quality for Chinese cancer registration data from aspects of comparability, completeness and validity. We applied strict quality control on data and consider the wide coverage of different geographic areas in China. A total of 700 cancer registries were included in the present *China Cancer Registry Annual Report*.

The 700 cancer registries covered a total of 523 160 249 population (265 488 549 males, 257 671 700 females), accounting for 37.49% of the national population in 2018. Especially, there were 267 urban cancer registries covering 236 047 481 population (45.12%) and 433 rural cancer registries with population coverage of 287 112 768 (54.88%).

2.3 年报内容简介

本年报汇总了 700 个肿瘤登记处 2018 年癌症的发病、死亡及人口数据。详细描述了合计 700 个肿瘤登记处和各肿瘤登记处数据的质量控制指标，如死亡发病比例、病理诊断比例、仅有医学死亡证明书比例等。详细报道了合计癌症和 22 类癌症的发病和死亡数据指标，包括发病率、死亡率、中国人口标化率（2000 年中国人口构成）、世界人口标化率（Segi's 世界人口构成）、累积率、分年龄组发病率/死亡率、分性别发病率/死亡率等。部分癌症按亚部位和组织学分型进行了细化描述。分城市农村、东中西地区、七大区和各省（自治区、直辖市）及新疆生产建设兵团（未包括香港特别行政区、澳门特别行政区和台湾省），比较了各地区癌症发病死亡差异。

2.3 Content of this annual report

The present annual report summarized data of the cancer incidence, mortality and demography through 700 cancer registration sites in 2018. We reported the quality control indicators including mortality incidence rate ratio (M/I), percentage of morphological verification (MV%), percentage of death certificate only (DCO%), et al, overall and by registration site. We reported data of new cases and deaths of all cancers and by site, including crude incidence, mortality, age-standardized rate (ASR) of China population in 2000, ASR of Segi's world population, cumulative rates, age and sex-specific rates. Moreover, we presented detailed distribution of subsite and morphology for some cancers. We compared cancer incidence and mortality rates by urban and rural areas, three geographic areas (eastern areas, central areas and western areas), the seven administrative districts (North China, Northeast China, East China, Central China, South China, Southwest China and Northwest China), and 31 provinces (autonomous regions and municipalities) and Xinjiang Production and Construction Corps (not including Hongkong Tebiexingzhengqu, Macau Tebiexingzhengqu and Taiwan Sheng).

第二章　质量控制和统计指标

1　质量控制

质量控制贯穿肿瘤登记工作的全过程。肿瘤登记地区应在各个环节制定工作规范和质量控制程序,并严格执行。质量控制主要包括四个方面:可比性、完整性、有效性和时效性。

1.1　可比性

数据结果真实可比的基本先决条件是采用通用的标准或定义。通常而言,可比性是指发病率间的不同不是因各登记地区之间的数据质量和标准不同而产生。可比性涉及以下几个指标:对"发病"的定义,对原发、复发和转移的诊断标准、分类与编码,死亡证明等。

1.2　完整性

完整性是指在登记地区资料库的目标人群中发现所有发病病例的程度。常用的评价指标有死亡发病比(mortality/incidence,M/I)、仅有死亡医学证明书比例(death certificate only,DCO%)、形态学诊断比例(morphological verification,MV%)、病例的来源数与报告单数、不同时间发病率的稳定性、不同人群发病率的比较、年龄别发病率曲线、儿童癌症评价,等等。俘获/再俘获方法也用来评价登记报告资料的完整性。

Chapter 2　Quality control and statistical indicators

1　Quality control

The value of cancer registration relies on the data quality. This procedure aims at providing qualified cancer registration data with comparability, completeness, validity, and timeliness.

1.1　Comparability

Comparability is the extent to which coding and classification at a registry, together with the definitions of recording and reporting specific data items, adhere to standardized international guidelines. In the evaluation of the comparability of registration data, the following standards should be identical: the definition of incidence, the identification of primary cancer and cancer recurrence or metastasis of an existing one, the identification for tumor classification and coding, the criteria of death certification.

1.2　Completeness

The completeness of cancer registry data refers to the extent of all the incident cancers occurring in the population included in the cancer registration database. It is an extremely important attribute of a cancer registry's data. The methods which provide indication of the completeness include the following: mortality/incidence (M/I) ratios, percentage of death certificate only (DCO%), percentage of morphological verification of diagnosis (MV%), reporting avenues, stability of incidence rates over time, comparison of incidence rates in different populations, shape of age-specific curves and incidence rates of childhood cancers, et al. The capture-recapture methods are also used to evaluate the completeness of registration data.

1.3 有效性

有效性是指登记病例中具有给定特征属性（例如肿瘤部位、年龄）的病例所占的比例。再摘录与再编码方法是评价有效性的最客观方法，一般由另一个观察者完成对登记地区记录与相关病例文件间仔细比较。常用的评价指标有形态学诊断比例（MV%）、仅有死亡医学证明书比例（DCO%）、部位不明百分比、年龄不明百分比等。肿瘤登记地区至少进行诸如年龄/出生日期、性别/部位、部位/组织学以及部位/组织学/年龄、基本变量有无遗漏信息等基本核对。

1.4 时效性

时效性一般指从发病日期(诊断日期)到数据被利用时(年报、研究报告、论文)的间隔。登记地区应及时报告和获取癌症信息。目前对时效性的要求无统一的国际标准。为平衡与完整性和准确性的关系，国家癌症中心要求各登记地区于诊断年份后的30个月内提交数据。

1.3 Validity

Validity is defined as the proportion of cases in a dataset with a given characteristic which truly have the attribute. Re-abstracting and re-coding are the principal methods which permit comparisons with respect to specified subsets of cases. Using diagnostic criteria (MV% and DCO%), missing information analysis and internal consistency methods, the validity of the cancer registration information can be verified.

1.4 Timeliness

Timeliness relates to the rapidity at which a registry can collect, process and report reliable and complete cancer data. It indicates the time to availability as the interval between date of diagnosis and the date the case was available in the registry for further use. The cancer registries should timely collect and report cancer statistics. Whilst there are no international guidelines for the timeliness of cancer registry data, NCC China requires the cancer registries should report cancer statistics in 30 months.

2 常用质量控制指标

2.1 形态学诊断比例

由病理学家依靠显微镜下组织学检查做出诊断具有较好准确性和可靠性,包括脱落细胞学或外周血的血液病检查。MV% 是评价有效性和完整性的指标。其绝对指标意义有限,常用的方法是与相似的区域内适当的标准进行比较。

$$病理诊断比例(MV\%)=\frac{有病理诊断患者}{全部患者}\times100\%$$

2.2 死亡发病比

死亡发病比为同一时期内死亡数与新发病例数之比。死亡数据来源于生命统计,应独立于肿瘤登记数据。M/I 相对过大,提示数据不完整,发病登记存在漏报,M/I 相对过小,提示发病数据中有重复记录可能,同时还要考虑生命统计的数据完整性和有效性问题。如果死因登记数据质量有保证,那么 M/I≈1~5 年生存率。

$$死亡发病比(M/I)=\frac{同时期内癌症死亡病例数}{同时期内癌症新发病例数}$$

2 Quality control indicators

2.1 Morphological verification, MV%

The stated diagnosis of cancer cases based on histological examination under microscope, exfoliative cytology or hematological examination of peripheral blood can be more accurate. MV% is an indicator of the validity and completeness of the diagnostic information. The absolute value of the MV% can have little meaning. It is most frequently used to make comparisons with appropriate criteria within similar areas.

$$Morphological\ verification\ percent(MV\%)=$$
$$\frac{Cases\ with\ histological\ examination\ results}{All\ cases}\times100\%$$

2.2 Mortality to incidence ratios, M/I

Mortality to incidence ratios is a comparison of the number of deaths, obtained from a source independent of the registry (usually, the vital statistics system), and the number of new cases of a specific cancer registered, in the same period of time. M/I value greater than expected lead to a suspicion of incompleteness. There might be under-reporting of cancer cases. M/I value smaller than expected lead to a suspicion of duplications of cancer cases, or under-report of cancer deaths. There might be under-reporting of cancer cases. If the quality of vital statistics system is good, the M/I ratio is approximated by 1-survival probability (5 years)

$$Mortality\ to\ incidence\ ratio(M/I)=$$
$$\frac{Cancer\ deathes\ in\ the\ same\ period\ of\ time}{Cancer\ cases\ in\ the\ same\ period\ of\ time}$$

2.3 仅有死亡医学证明书比例

来自死亡证明书的病例称为死亡补充发病（Death Certificate Notification，DCN）病例，当无法追踪到死亡前任何癌症确认信息时称为"仅有死亡医学证明书"（DCO）病例。DCO%是评价有效性和完整性的指标之一，与临床或病理诊断的病例记录相比，DCO病例的信息显然准确性差。DCO%高，提示病例发现流程存在不足。

$$仅有死亡证明书比例（DCO\%）=\frac{仅有死亡医学证明书患者}{全部患者}\times100\%$$

2.4 信息缺失所占比例

信息缺失所占比例指年龄不明、性别不明、其他或未指明部位肿瘤、诊断依据不明等所占的比例，是评价有效性的指标。其他或未指明部位肿瘤的ICD-10编码包括：C26、C39、C48、C75、C76-C80。信息缺失所占比例在一个适当的范围内，且比例不能过低。

2.3 Death certificate only, DCO%

Cancer cases notified to registries via death certificates is death certificate notified (DCN) cases. Cancers cases for which no other information other than a death certificate mentioning cancer can be obtained are death certificate only registrations (DCOs). DCO% is an indicator of the validity and completeness of the diagnostic information. Compared with cancer cases with clinical or histological diagnosis, the information of DCO cases is less accurate. A high DCO% reflects flaws in case tracing procedures.

$$Death\ certificate\ only\ percent（DCO\%）=\frac{DCO\ cases}{All\ cases}\times100\%$$

2.4 Proportion of missing information

Proportion of missing information is the proportion of cases with unknown age, unknown sex, other and unspecified cancer sites or unknown diagnosis basis. It is an indicator of the validity of the diagnostic information. The ICD-10 codes for cases with other and unspecified cancer sites are: C26, C39, C48, C75, C76-C80. Proportion of missing information should be within an appropriate scope. It shouldn't be too low.

3 统计分类

3.1 癌症分类

参照国际上常用的癌症 ICD-10 分类统计表，根据 ICD-10 前三位"C"类编码，将癌症细分类为 59 个部位、25 个大类，其中脑和神经系统包括良性及良恶性未定肿瘤（D32-D33、D42-D43）。真性红细胞增多症（D45）、骨髓增生异常综合征（D46）、淋巴造血和有关组织动态未定肿瘤（D47）归入髓系白血病（C92）。原位癌暂未纳入统计分析。详见表 2-1、表 2-2。

3 Classification and coding

3.1 Cancer classification

Taken from the WHO cancer classification publications of ICD-10 version, cancers were classified into 59 types and 25 categories with different anatomic sites. The neoplasms of cerebral and central nervous system (D32-33, D42-43) are included in the ICD-10 cancer dictionary. For polycythemia vera (D45), myelodysplastic syndrome (D46), and other neoplasms of uncertain or unknown behavior of lymphoid, hematopoietic and related tissue (D47), they are coded as Myeloid leukemia (C92). Carcinoma in situ was not included in the analyses (Table 2-1, Table 2-2).

表 2-1　常用癌症分类统计表（细分类）
Table 2-1　Cancer classification of ICD-10

部位 Site	ICD-10
唇 Lip	C00
舌 Tongue	C01-C02
口 Mouth	C03-C06
唾液腺 Salivary glands	C07-C08
扁桃体 Tonsil	C09
其他口咽 Other oropharynx	C10
鼻咽 Nasopharynx	C11
下咽 Hypopharynx	C12-C13
咽,部位不明 Pharynx, unspecified	C14
食管 Esophagus	C15
胃 Stomach	C16
小肠 Small intestine	C17
结肠 Colon	C18
直肠 Rectum	C19-C20
肛门 Anus	C21
肝脏 Liver	C22
胆囊及其他 Gallbladder etc.	C23-C24
胰腺 Pancreas	C25
鼻、鼻窦及其他 Nose, sinuses etc.	C30-C31
喉 Larynx	C32
气管、支气管、肺 Trachea, bronchus & lung	C33-C34
其他胸腔器官 Other thoracic organs	C37-C38
骨 Bone	C40-C41

部位 Site	ICD-10
皮肤黑色素瘤 Melanoma of skin	C43
皮肤其他 Other skin	C44
间皮瘤 Mesothelioma	C45
卡波西肉瘤 Kaposi sarcoma	C46
周围神经、其他结缔组织、软组织 Peripheral nerve, other connective & soft tissue	C47, C49
乳腺 Breast	C50
外阴 Vulva	C51
阴道 Vagina	C52
子宫颈 Cervix uteri	C53
子宫体 Corpus uteri	C54
子宫,部位不明 Uterus, unspecified	C55
卵巢 Ovary	C56
其他女性生殖器 Other female genital organs	C57
胎盘 Placenta	C58
阴茎 Penis	C60
前列腺 Prostate	C61
睾丸 Testis	C62
其他男性生殖器 Other male genital organs	C63
肾 Kidney	C64
肾盂 Renal pelvis	C65
输尿管 Ureter	C66
膀胱 Bladder	C67
其他泌尿器官 Other urinary organs	C68
眼 Eye	C69
脑、神经系统 Brain, nervous system	C70-C72, D32-D33, D42-D43
甲状腺 Thyroid	C73
肾上腺 Adrenal gland	C74
其他内分泌腺 Other endocrine	C75
霍奇金淋巴瘤 Hodgkin lymphoma	C81
非霍奇金淋巴瘤 Non-Hodgkin lymphoma	C82-C86, C96
免疫增生性疾病 Immunoproliferative diseases	C88
多发性骨髓瘤 Multiple myeloma	C90
淋巴样白血病 Lymphoid leukemia	C91
髓系白血病 Myeloid leukemia	C92-C94, D45-D47
白血病,未特指 Leukemia, unspecified	C95
其他或未指明部位 Other and unspecified	O&U
所有部位合计 All sites	C00-C97, D32-D33, D42-D43, D45-D47
所有部位除外 C44 All sites except C44	C00-C97, D32-D33, D42-D43, D45-D47 exc. C44

表 2-2　常用癌症分类统计表（大分类）
Table 2-2　Broad cancer classification of ICD-10

部位全称 Full title of site	部位缩写 Short title of site	ICD-10
口腔和咽喉（除外鼻咽）Oral cavity & pharynx except nasopharynx	口腔 Oral cavity & pharynx	C00-C10, C12-C14
鼻咽 Nasopharynx	鼻咽 Nasopharynx	C11
食管 Esophagus	食管 Esophagus	C15
胃 Stomach	胃 Stomach	C16
结直肠肛门 Colon, rectum & anus	结直肠 Colon-rectum	C18-C21
肝脏 Liver	肝 Liver	C22
胆囊及其他 Gallbladder etc.	胆囊 Gallbladder	C23-C24
胰腺 Pancreas	胰腺 Pancreas	C25
喉 Larynx	喉 Larynx	C32
气管、支气管、肺 Trachea, bronchus & lung	肺 Lung	C33-C34
其他胸腔器官 Other thoracic organs	其他胸腔器官 Other thoracic organs	C37-C38
骨 Bone	骨 Bone	C40-C41
皮肤黑色素瘤 Melanoma of skin	皮肤黑色素瘤 Melanoma of skin	C43
乳房 Breast	乳房 Breast	C50
子宫颈 Cervix uteri	子宫颈 Cervix	C53
子宫体及子宫部位不明 Uterus & unspecified	子宫体 Uterus	C54-C55
卵巢 Ovary	卵巢 Ovary	C56
前列腺 Prostate	前列腺 Prostate	C61
睾丸 Testis	睾丸 Testis	C62
肾及泌尿系统不明 Kidney & unspecified urinary organs	肾 Kidney	C64-C66, C68
膀胱 Bladder	膀胱 Bladder	C67
脑、神经系统 Brain, nervous system	脑 Brain	C70-C72, D32-D33, D42-D43
甲状腺 Thyroid	甲状腺 Thyroid	C73
淋巴瘤 Lymphoma	淋巴瘤 Lymphoma	C81-C86, C88, C90, C96
白血病 Leukemia	白血病 Leukemia	C91-C95, D45-D47
其他或未指明部位 Other and unspecified	其他 Other	O&U
所有部位合计 All sites	合计 All sites	C00-C97, D32-D33, D42-D43, D45-D47

3.2 自然地区分类

城、乡分类根据《中华人民共和国行政区划代码》(GB/T 2260—2007),将地级以上城市归于城市地区,县及县级市归于农村地区,同时综合考虑地区经济及生活方式等因素。

东、中、西部地区的划分采用国家统计局标准。

东部地区包括:北京市、天津市、河北省、辽宁省、上海市、江苏省、浙江省、福建省、山东省、广东省、海南省、香港特别行政区、澳门特别行政区、台湾省。

中部地区包括:黑龙江省、吉林省、山西省、安徽省、江西省、河南省、湖北省、湖南省。

西部地区包括:内蒙古自治区、广西壮族自治区、重庆市、四川省、贵州省、云南省、西藏自治区、陕西省、甘肃省、青海省、宁夏回族自治区、新疆维吾尔自治区。

七大区划分根据民政部区划分类(未包括香港特别行政区、澳门特别行政区和台湾省)。

华北地区:北京市、天津市、河北省、山西省、内蒙古自治区。

东北地区:辽宁省、吉林省、黑龙江省。

华东地区:上海市、江苏省、浙江省、安徽省、福建省、江西省、山东省。

华中地区:河南省、湖北省、湖南省。

华南地区:广东省、广西壮族自治区、海南省。

西南地区:重庆市、四川省、贵州省、云南省、西藏自治区。

西北地区:陕西省、甘肃省、青海省、宁夏回族自治区、新疆维吾尔自治区。

3.2 Area classification

According to *Codes for the administrative divisions of the People's Republic of China* (GB/T 2260—2007), prefecture-level cities are classified into urban areas, whereas counties and county-level cities are classified into rural areas. And the socio-economic status of the areas are considered.

The classification of eastern areas, central areas and western areas is based on the standard of National Statistics Bureau.

The eastern areas consists of Beijing Shi, Tianjin Shi, Hebei Sheng, Liaoning Sheng, Shanghai Shi, Jiangsu Sheng, Zhejiang Sheng, Fujian Sheng, Shandong Sheng, Guangdong Sheng, Hainan Sheng, Hong Kong Tebiexingzhengqu, Macau Tebiexingzhengqu, Taiwan Sheng.

The central areas consists of Heilongjiang Sheng, Jilin Sheng, Shanxi Sheng, Anhui Sheng, Jiangxi Sheng, Henan Sheng, Hubei Sheng and Hunan Sheng.

The western areas consist of Nei Mongol Zizhiqu, Guangxi Zhuangzu Zizhiqu, Chongqing Shi, Sichuan Sheng, Guizhou Sheng, Yunnan Sheng, Xizang Zizhiqu, Shaanxi Sheng, Gansu Sheng, Qinghai Sheng, Ningxia Huizu Zizhiqu and Xinjiang Uygur Zizhiqu.

According to the standard from Ministry of Civil Affairs of the People's Repulic of China, the classification of these seven areas is shown as following (not including Hongkong Tebiexingzhengqu, Macau Tebiexingzhengqu and Taiwan Sheng).

North China: Beijing Shi, Tianjin Shi, Hebei Sheng, Shanxi Sheng, Nei Mongol Zizhiqu.

Northeast China: Liaoning Sheng, Jilin Sheng, Heilongjiang Sheng.

East China: Shanghai Shi, Jiangsu Sheng, Zhejiang Sheng, Anhui Sheng, Fujian Sheng, Jiangxi Sheng, Shandong Sheng.

Central China: Henan Sheng, Hubei Sheng, Hunan Sheng.

South China: Guangdong Sheng, Guangxi Zhuangzu Zizhiqu, Hainan Sheng.

Southwest China: Chongqing Shi, Sichuan Sheng, Guizhou Sheng, Yunnan Sheng, Xizang Zizhiqu.

Northwest China: Shaanxi Sheng, Gansu Sheng, Qinghai Sheng, Ningxia Huizu Zizhiqu, Xinjiang Uygur Zizhiqu.

4 常用统计指标

4.1 年平均人口数

年平均人口数是计算发病（死亡）率指标的分母，精确算法是一年内每一天暴露于发病（死亡）危险的生存人数之和除以年内天数，但实际上很难掌握每一天的生存人数，因而常用年初和年末人口数的算术平均数作为年平均人口数的近似值。

$$年平均人口数（人）= \frac{年初（上年末）人口数+年末人口数}{2}$$

年中人口数指 7 月 1 日零时人口数，如果人口数变化均匀，年中人口数等于年平均人口数，可以用年中人口数代替年平均人口数。

4.2 性别、年龄别人口数

性别、年龄别人口数是指按男、女性别和不同年龄分组的人口数，建议用"内插法"推算。年龄的分组，规定以 5 岁划分年龄别：0~岁、1~4 岁、5~9 岁、10~14 岁……80~84 岁、85 岁及以上。

4.3 发病（死亡）率

发病（死亡）率又称为粗发病（死亡）率，是反映人口发病（死亡）情况最基本的指标，是指某年该地登记的每 10 万人口癌症新病例（死亡）数，反映人口发病（死亡）水平。

$$发病（死亡）率（1/10 万）= \frac{某时期恶性肿瘤新病例（死亡）数}{某时期年平均人口数} \times 100\,000$$

4.4 年龄别发病（死亡）率

人口的年龄结构是影响癌症发病（死亡）水平的重要因素，年龄别发病（死亡）率是统计研究的重要指标。

$$某年龄组发病（死亡）率（1/10 万）= \frac{某年龄组发病（死亡）人数}{同年龄组人口数} \times 100\,000$$

4 Statistical indicators

4.1 Average annual population

Average annual population is the denominator of the incidence（mortality）rates. The exact method to calculate is the average of persons at risk of incidence（mortality）each day in a specific year. Considering the complexity of the calculation, we often use the estimated calculation to quantify the population effectively. The formula is：

$$Average\ annual\ population = \frac{population\ at\ the\ end\ of\ the\ year + population\ in\ the\ early\ of\ the\ year}{2}$$

The mid-year population is the number of populations in 1st July at 0 AM. If the population is relatively stable, the mid-year population can be used to represent average annual population.

4.2 Sex-and age-specific population

Sex-specific population is the population by sex. Age-specific population is the population by different age groups and it is can be calculated by interpolation. The ages may be grouped into classes of up to five years, for example, 0, 1-4, 5-9, 10-14... 80-84, 85+.

4.3 Incidence（mortality）rate

The incidence（mortality）rate is a measure of the frequency with which an event, such as a new case of cancer（cancer death）occurs in a population over a period.

$$Incidence（mortality）rate\ per\ 100\,000 = \frac{new\ cases（new\ cancer\ death）occurring\ during\ a\ given\ time\ period}{population\ at\ risk\ during\ the\ same\ time\ period} \times 100\,000$$

4.4 Age-specific incidence（mortality）rate

Age is an important factor influencing the cancer incidence and mortality. Age-specific rate is important statistical indicator.

$$Age\text{-}specific\ incidence（mortality）rate\ per\ 100\,000 = \frac{cases（cancer\ death）in\ a\ specific\ age\ group}{population\ in\ the\ age\ group} \times 100\,000$$

4.5 年龄调整率(标准化率)

由于粗发病(死亡)率受人口年龄构成的影响较大,因此在对比分析不同地区的发病(死亡)率或同一地区人群不同时期的发病(死亡)水平时,为消除人口年龄结构对发病(死亡)水平的影响,需要计算按年龄标准化的发病(死亡)率,即指按照某一标准人口的年龄结构所计算的发病(死亡)率。本年报使用中国标准人口是 2000 年全国第五次人口普查的人口构成(简称"中标率"),世界标准人口采用 Segi's 标准人口构成(简称"世标率")。表 2-3 为中国人口和世界人口年龄构成,可供计算年龄标准化率时选用。

年龄调整发病(死亡)率的计算(直接法):

(1) 计算年龄组发病(死亡)率。

(2) 各年龄组发病(死亡)率乘以相应的标准人口年龄构成百分比,得到相应的理论发病(死亡)率。

(3) 将各年龄组的理论发病(死亡)率相加,即年龄标准化发病(死亡)率。

$$\text{年龄标准化发病(死亡)率(1/10 万)} = \frac{\sum \text{标准人口年龄构成} \times \text{年龄别发病(死亡)率}}{\sum \text{标准人口年龄构成}}$$

4.5 Age-standardized rate (ASR)

Standardization is necessary when comparing populations with different age structures because age has such a powerful influence on cancer incidence and mortality. ASR is a summary measure of a rate that a population would have if it had a standard age structure. In this annual cancer report, the population standards we used are the Segi's population and the fifth Chinese national census of 2000. Table 2-3 are the details of the population standards.

Direct method calculating incidence (mortality) rate:

(1) calculating the rates for subjects in a specific age category in a study population.

(2) calculating the weighted age-specific rates. The weights applied represent the relative age distribution of the standard population.

(3) adding up each weighted age-specific rate. The summary rates reflect the adjusted rates.

$$\text{ASR per 100 000} = \frac{\sum \text{standard population in corresponding age group} \times \text{age-specific rate}}{\sum \text{standard population}}$$

表 2-3 标准人口构成
Table 2-3 Standard populations

年龄组/岁 Age group/ years	中国人口构成 2000 年 China standard population (2000)	世界人口构成 Segi's population	年龄组/岁 Age group/ years	中国人口构成 2000 年 China standard population (2000)	世界人口构成 Segi's population
0~	13 793 799	2 400	45~	85 521 045	6 000
1~	55 184 575	9 600	50~	63 304 200	5 000
5~	90 152 587	10 000	55~	46 370 375	4 000
10~	125 396 633	9 000	60~	41 703 848	4 000
15~	103 031 165	9 000	65~	34 780 460	3 000
20~	94 573 174	8 000	70~	25 574 149	2 000
25~	117 602 265	8 000	75~	15 928 330	1 000
30~	127 314 298	6 000	80~	7 989 158	500
35~	109 147 295	6 000	85+	4 001 925	500
40~	81 242 945	6 000	合计	1 242 612 226	100 000

4.6 分类构成

各类癌症发病(死亡)构成比可以反映各类癌症对居民健康危害的情况。癌症发病(死亡)分类构成比的计算公式如下：

$$某癌症构成比(\%) = \frac{某癌症发病(死亡)人数}{总发病(死亡)人数} \times 100$$

4.7 累积发病(死亡)率

累积发病(死亡)率是指某病在某一年龄阶段内的按年龄(岁)的发病(死亡)率进行累积的总指标。累积发病(死亡)率消除了年龄构成不同的影响，故不需要标准化便可以与不同地区直接进行比较。癌症一般是计算 0~74 岁的累积发病(死亡)率。

$$累积发病(死亡)率(\%) =$$
$$\{\sum[年龄组发病(死亡)率 \times 年龄组距]\} \times 100$$

4.8 截缩发病(死亡)率

通常对癌症是截取 35~64 岁这一易发年龄段计算，其标准人口构成是世界人口。

$$截缩发病(死亡)率(1/10万) =$$
$$\frac{\sum 截缩段各年龄组发病(死亡)率 \times 各段标准年龄构成}{\sum 各段标准年龄构成}$$

因为癌症在 35 岁以前是少发的，而在 65 岁以后其他疾病较多，干扰较大，所以采用 35~64 岁这一阶段的截缩发病(死亡)率比较确切，便于比较。

4.6 Relative frequency

The relative frequency indicates the proportion of new site-specific cancer cases in all cancers combined. The formular is：

$$\text{Relative frequency of a certain type of cancer}(\%) =$$
$$\frac{\text{No. of cases of a particular cancer}}{\text{No. of cases of all cancers}} \times 100$$

4.7 Cumulative incidence (mortality) rate

A cumulative incidence (mortality) rate expresses the probability of the onset of cancer between birth and a specific age. The rate can be compared without age standardization as it is not affected by age structures. This is often expressed for population between 0 and 74 years.

$$\text{Cumulative incidence(mortality)rate}(\%) =$$
$$\left[\sum(\text{age-specific incidence(mortality)rate} \times \text{width of the age group})\right] \times 100$$

4.8 Truncated incidence (mortality) rate

Truncated incidence rate is the calculation of rate over the truncated age-range 35-64, using WHO world standard population. The data are presented as truncated rates mainly because the accuracy of age-specific rates in the elderly may be much less certain and the rates in the young age groups may be rare.

$$\text{Truncated incidence(mortality)rate per 100 000} =$$
$$\frac{\sum \text{trancated rate in a specific age group} \times \text{standard proportion of the age group}}{\sum \text{standard population}}$$

5 生存率

生存率是评价癌症治疗是否有效的关键指标。以人群为基础的肿瘤登记工作收集患者的生存资料,计算生存率以反映肿瘤人群的生存状况。某时间生存率,是指某一批随访对象中,生存期大于等于该时间的研究对象的比例,如五年生存率等。常用的生存率指标有观察生存率、净生存率和相对生存率。生存率实质是累积生存概率。

5.1 观察生存率

观察生存率分析中,以患者死亡为观察终点,包括死于肿瘤和其他原因。肿瘤登记资料常用寿命表法估计观察生存率。寿命表法应用定群寿命表的基本原理计算生存率,可利用截尾数据的不完全信息。

5.2 调整生存率/净生存率

观察生存率反映的是肿瘤患者的整体死亡状况。在很多情况下,人们关注于肿瘤患者死于肿瘤的信息。此时,常常需要计算调整生存率/净生存率。净生存率的关键是必须依据完整、准确的死因信息。在比较不同年龄、性别、社会经济学状况下癌症患者的生存率时,使用净生存率显得尤为重要,因为肿瘤外其他死因会影响癌症患者的生存状况。

净生存率可通过计算疾病特异性生存率获得,即以患者死于该肿瘤为观察终点。若肿瘤患者死于肿瘤之外的其他原因,将与存活状态同等处理。

5 Survival rate

Survival rate is an overall index for measuring the effectiveness of cancer care. The survival rates calculated based on data from population-based cancer registries will therefore represent the average prognosis in the population. Survival rate can be expressed in terms of the percentage of those cases who were still alive after a specified interval (i. e. 5 years). The measures for survival rate calculation include observed survival rate, net survival rate, and relative survival rate, which are the cumulative probability of survival from diagnosis to the end of each time interval.

5.1 Observed survival rate

The observed or crude survival rate is simply the estimated probability of survival at the end of the specified period. It takes no account of the cause of death. Actuarial or life-table method provides a means for using all the follow-up information to calculate survival rate, which is often applied in population-based cancer survival analysis.

5.2 Adjusted survival/net survival rate

The observed survival rate can be interpreted as the probability of survival from cancer and all other causes of deaths combined. While this is a true reflection of total mortality in the patient group, the main interest is usually in describing mortality attributable to cancer. The concept of net (or adjusted) survival rate is the survival probability in the hypothesis that the patients only die from their cancer. It is a crucial measure for survival rate comparisons among patients with different age, sex and socio-economic status.

Net survival rate can be achieved through calculating cancer-specific survival rate, which relies on reliable individual cause of death. If the cancer patients die from causes other than cancer, it will be treated as alive.

5.3 相对生存率

当缺乏完整、准确的全死因信息时,净生存率指标往往较难通过疾病特异性生存率获取。此时,净生存率可以通过相对生存率来估计。相对生存率即为特定人群的观察生存率与该人群的期望生存率的比值。根据全死因寿命表的死亡概率,可以求得一般人群的期望生存率。

$$相对生存率 = \frac{观察生存率}{期望生存率}$$

如前所述,肿瘤登记资料中观察生存率常采用寿命表法。而期望生存率的计算常常分区间估计。估计方法有 Ederer Ⅰ、Ederer Ⅱ、Hakulinen 方法等。

5.3 Relative survival rate

Where death certificate is not publicly available, or certification of the cause of death is not sufficiently reliable, net survival rate is hardly achieved through cancer-specific survival rate, which needs the exact cause of death for cancer patients. Relative survival rate does not require information on the cause of death in the cancer patients. Relative survival rates are usually expressed as a ratio of the crude survival rate in the group of cancer patients and the corresponding expected survival rate in the general population. Observed survival rate can be achieved by life-table/actual methods, while expected survival rate can be estimated with methods of Ederer Ⅰ, Ederer Ⅱ and Hakulinen.

$$Relative\ survival\ rate = \frac{observed\ survival\ rate}{expected\ survival\ rate}$$

第三章 数据质量评价

1 数据来源

2021 年国家癌症中心收到全国 947 个登记处提交的 2018 年肿瘤登记资料。登记处分布在全国 31 个省(自治区、直辖市)及新疆生产建设兵团(未包括香港特别行政区、澳门特别行政区和台湾省),其中地级以上城市 335 个,县和县级市 612 个。四川省上报资料登记处数量最多为 150 个,其次为云南省 80 个、陕西省 54 个,江苏省和安徽省各 50 个。北京市、天津市、上海市、广州市、石家庄市登记地区覆盖了全部区县,在本年报分城乡按 2 个登记处计(表 3-1)。

Chapter 3   Evaluation of data quality

1   Data sources

A total of 947 cancer registries submitted cancer registration data of 2018 to NCC China in 2021. A total of 31 provinces (autonomous regions, municipalities) and Xinjiang Production and Construction Corps (not including Hongkong Tebiexingzhengqu, Macau Tebiexingzhengqu and Taiwan Sheng) were covered by these registries, with a total of 335 prefecture-level cities and 612 counties (county-level cities). Sichuan Sheng submitted data from most cancer registries (150), followed by Yunnan sheng (80), Shaanxi Sheng (54), Jiangsu Sheng and Anhui Sheng (50). The data from Beijing Shi, Tianjin Shi, Shanghai Shi, Guangzhou Shi and Shijiazhuang Shi covered all districts and counties. They were classified as urban and rural areas separately in this report (Table 3-1).

表 3-1   2018 年全国提交肿瘤登记资料的地区

Table 3-1   The cancer registries which submitted cancer statistics of 2018

省(自治区、直辖市) Province (autonomous region, municipality)	登记处数 No. of cancer registries	登记处名单 List of cancer registries
北京 Beijing	2	北京市 Beijing Shi、北京市郊区 Rural Areas of Beijing Shi
天津 Tianjin	2	天津市 Tianjin Shi、天津市郊区 Rural Areas of Tianjin Shi
河北 Hebei	28	石家庄市 Shijiazhuang Shi、石家庄市郊区 Rural Areas of Shijiazhuang Shi、赞皇县 Zanhuang Xian、迁西县 Qianxi Xian、迁安市 Qian'an Shi、秦皇岛市 Qinhuangdao Shi、邯郸市邯山区 Hanshan Qu,Handan Shi、大名县 Daming Xian、涉县 She Xian、磁县 Ci Xian、武安市 Wu'an Shi、邢台市 Xingtai Shi、邢台县 Xingtai Xian、临城县 Lincheng Xian、内丘县 Neiqiu Xian、邢台市任泽区 Renze Qu,Xingtai Shi、保定市 Baoding Shi、望都县 Wangdu Xian、安国市 Anguo Shi、张家口市宣化区 Xuanhua Qu,Zhangjiakou Shi、张北县 Zhangbei Xian、承德市双桥区 Shuangqiao Qu,Chengde Shi、丰宁满族自治县 Fengning Manzu Zizhixian、沧州市 Cangzhou Shi、海兴县 Haixing Xian、盐山县 Yanshan Xian、衡水市冀州区 Jizhou Qu,Hengshui Shi、辛集市 Xinji Shi

省（自治区、直辖市） Province （autonomous region, municipality）	登记处数 No. of cancer registries	登记处名单 List of cancer registries
山西 Shanxi	32	太原市小店区 Xiaodian Qu，Taiyuan Shi、太原市迎泽区 Yingze Qu，Taiyuan Shi、太原市杏花岭区 Xinghualing Qu，Taiyuan Shi、清徐县 Qingxu Xian、阳泉市 Yangquan Shi、平定县 Pingding Xian、盂县 Yu Xian、长治市 Changzhi Shi、襄垣县 Xiangyuan Xian、平顺县 Pingshun Xian、沁源县 Qinyuan Xian、阳城县 Yangcheng Xian、陵川县 Lingchuan Xian、晋中市榆次区 Yuci Qu，Jizhong Shi、晋中市太谷区 Taigu Qu，Jinzhong Shi、昔阳县 Xiyang Xian、寿阳县 Shouyang Xian、稷山县 Jishan Xian、新绛县 Xinjiang Xian、绛县 Jiang Xian、垣曲县 Yuanqu Xian、芮城县 Ruicheng Xian、忻州市忻府区 Xinfu Qu，Xinzhou Shi、定襄县 Dingxiang Xian、原平市 Yuanping Shi、临汾市尧都区 Yaodu Qu，Linfen Shi、襄汾县 Xiangfen Xian、洪洞县 Hongtong Xian、交城县 Jiaocheng Xian、临县 Lin Xian、孝义市 Xiaoyi Shi、汾阳市 Fenyang Shi
内蒙古 Nei Mongol	30	托克托县 Togtoh Xian、武川县 Wuchuan Xian、土默特右旗 Tumd Youqi、赤峰市红山区 Hongshan Qu，Chifeng Shi、赤峰市元宝山区 Yuanbaoshan Qu，Chifeng Shi、赤峰市松山区 Songshan Qu，Chifeng Shi、敖汉旗 Aohan Qi、通辽市科尔沁区 Horqin Qu，Tongliao Shi、科尔沁左翼中旗 Horqin Zuoyi Zhongqi、科尔沁左翼后旗 Horqin Zuoyi Houqi、开鲁县 Kailu Xian、库伦旗 Hure Qi、奈曼旗 Naiman Qi、扎鲁特旗 Jarud Qi、霍林郭勒市 Holin Gol Shi、呼伦贝尔市海拉尔区 Hailar Qu，Hulun Buir Shi、呼伦贝尔市扎赉诺尔区 Dalai Nur Qu，Hulun Buir Shi、阿荣旗 Arun Qi、莫力达瓦达斡尔族自治旗 Morin Dawa Daurzu Zizhiqi、鄂温克族自治旗 Ewenkizu Zizhiqi、陈巴尔虎旗 Chen Barag Qi、新巴尔虎左旗 Xin Barag Zuoqi、新巴尔虎右旗 Xin Barag Youqi、满洲里市 Manzhouli Shi、牙克石市 Yakeshi Shi、扎兰屯市 Zalantun Shi、根河市 Genhe Shi、巴彦淖尔市临河区 Linhe Qu，Bayannur Shi、锡林浩特市 Xilin Hot Shi、西乌珠穆沁旗 Xi Ujimqin Qi
辽宁 Liaoning	15	沈阳市 Shenyang Shi、康平县 Kangping Xian、法库县 Faku Xian、大连市 Dalian Shi、庄河市 Zhuanghe Shi、鞍山市 Anshan Shi、本溪市 Benxi Shi、丹东市 Dandong Shi、东港市 Donggang Shi、营口市 Yingkou Shi、阜新市 Fuxin Shi、彰武县 Zhangwu Xian、辽阳县 Liaoyang Xian、盘锦市大洼区 Dawa Qu，Panjin Shi、建平县 Jianping Xian
吉林 Jilin	25	长春市绿园区 Lüyuan Qu，Changchun Shi、德惠市 Dehui Shi、吉林市 Jilin Shi、永吉县 Yongji Xian、蛟河市 Jiaohe Shi、桦甸市 Huadian Shi、舒兰市 Shulan Shi、磐石市 Panshi Shi、通化市 Tonghua Shi、梅河口市 Meihekou Shi、集安市 Ji'an Shi、抚松县 Fusong Xian、松原市宁江区 Ningjiang Qu，Songyuan Shi、前郭尔罗斯蒙古族自治县 Qian Gorlos Mongolzu Zizhixian、乾安县 Qian'an Xian、通榆县 Tongyu Xian、大安市 Da'an Shi、延吉市 Yanji Shi、图们市 Tumen Shi、敦化市 Dunhua Shi、珲春市 Hunchun Shi、龙井市 Longjing Shi、和龙市 Helong Shi、汪清县 Wangqing Xian、安图县 Antu Xian
黑龙江 Heilongjiang	11	哈尔滨市道里区 Daoli Qu，Harbin Shi、哈尔滨市南岗区 Nangang Qu，Harbin Shi、哈尔滨市香坊区 Xiangfang Qu，Harbin Shi、尚志市 Shangzhi Shi、五常市 Wuchang Shi、勃利县 Boli Xian、牡丹江市东安区 Dong'an Qu，Mudanjiang Shi、牡丹江市阳明区 Yangming Qu，Mudanjiang Shi、牡丹江市爱民区 Aimin Qu，Mudanjiang Shi、牡丹江市西安区 Xi'an Qu，Mudanjiang Shi、海林市 Hailin Shi

省（自治区、直辖市） Province （autonomous region, municipality）	登记处数 No. of cancer registries	登记处名单 List of cancer registries
上海 Shanghai	2	上海市 Shanghai Shi、上海市郊区 Rural areas of Shanghai Shi
江苏 Jiangsu	50	南京市溧水区 Lishui Qu，Nanjing Shi、南京市高淳区 Gaochun Qu，Nanjing Shi、无锡市 Wuxi Shi、江阴市 Jiangyin Shi、宜兴市 Yixing Shi、徐州市 Xuzhou Shi、邳州市 Pizhou Shi、常州市 Changzhou Shi、溧阳市 Liyang Shi、常州市金坛区 Jintan Qu，Changzhou Shi、苏州市 Suzhou Shi、常熟市 Changshu Shi、张家港市 Zhangjiagang Shi、昆山市 Kunshan Shi、太仓市 Taicang Shi、南通市 Nantong Shi、海安市 Hai'an Shi、如东县 Rudong Xian、启东市 Qidong Shi、如皋市 Rugao Shi、南通市海门区 Haimen Qu，Nantong Shi、连云港市 Lianyungang Shi、连云港市赣榆区 Ganyu Qu，Lianyungang Shi、东海县 Donghai Xian、灌云县 Guanyun Xian、灌南县 Guannan Xian、淮安市淮安区 Huai'an Qu，Huai'an Shi、淮安市淮阴区 Huaiyin Qu，Huai'an Shi、淮安市清江浦区 Qingjiangpu Qu，Huai'an Shi、涟水县 Lianshui Xian、淮安市洪泽区 Hongze Qu，Huai'an Shi、盱眙县 Xuyi Xian、金湖县 Jinhu Xian、盐城市亭湖区 Tinghu Qu，Yancheng Shi、盐城市盐都区 Yandu Qu，Yancheng Shi、响水县 Xiangshui Xian、滨海县 Binhai Xian、阜宁县 Funing Xian、射阳县 Sheyang Xian、建湖县 Jianhu Xian、东台市 Dongtai Shi、盐城市大丰区 Dafeng Qu，Yancheng Shi、扬州市广陵区 Guangling Qu，Yangzhou Shi、宝应县 Baoying Xian、仪征市 Yizheng Shi、丹阳市 Danyang Shi、扬中市 Yangzhong Shi、泰兴市 Taixing Shi、宿迁市宿城区 Sucheng Qu，Suqian Shi、泗阳县 Siyang Xian
浙江 Zhejiang	14	杭州市 Hangzhou Shi、宁波市鄞州区 Yinzhou Qu，Ningbo Shi、慈溪市 Cixi Shi、温州市鹿城区 Lucheng Qu，Wenzhou Shi、嘉兴市 Jiaxing Shi、嘉善县 Jiashan Xian、海宁市 Haining Shi、长兴县 Changxing Xian、绍兴市上虞区 Shangyu Qu，Shaoxing Shi、永康市 Yongkang Shi、开化县 Kaihua Xian、岱山县 Daishan Xian、仙居县 Xianju Xian、龙泉市 Longquan Shi
安徽 Anhui	50	合肥市 Hefei Shi、长丰县 Changfeng Xian、肥东县 Feidong Xian、肥西县 Feixi Xian、庐江县 Lujiang Xian、巢湖市 Chaohu Shi、芜湖市 Wuhu Shi、芜湖市繁昌区 Fanchang Qu，Wuhu Shi、南陵县 Nanling Xian、蚌埠市 Bengbu Shi、五河县 Wuhe Xian、淮南市大通区 Datong Qu，Huainan Shi、淮南市田家庵区 Tianjia'an Qu，Huainan Shi、淮南市谢家集区 Xiejiaji Qu，Huainan Shi、淮南市八公山区 Bagongshan Qu，Huainan Shi、淮南市潘集区 Panji Qu，Huainan Shi、凤台县 Fengtai Xian、淮南市毛集区 Maoji Qu，Huainan Shi、淮南市高新区 Gaoxin Qu，Huainan Shi、马鞍山市 Ma'anshan Shi、当涂县 Dangtu Xian、铜陵市 Tongling Shi、铜陵市义安区 Yi'an Qu，Tongling Shi、安庆市迎江区 Yingjiang Qu，Anqing Shi、安庆市大观区 Daguan Qu，Anqing Shi、安庆市宜秀区 Yixiu Qu，Anqing Shi、怀宁县 Huaining Xian、太湖县 Taihu Xian、望江县 Wangjiang Xian、岳西县 Yuexi Xian、桐城市 Tongcheng Shi、潜山市 Qianshan Shi、天长市 Tianchang Shi、阜阳市颍州区 Yingzhou Qu，Fuyang Shi、阜阳市颍东区 Yingdong Qu，Fuyang Shi、太和县 Taihe Xian、阜南县 Funan Xian、颍上县 Yingshang Xian、宿州市埇桥区 Yongqiao Qu，Suzhou Shi、灵璧县 Lingbi Xian、六安市金安区 Jin'an Qu，Lu'an Shi、六安市叶集区 Yeji Qu，Lu'an Shi、寿县 Shou Xian、舒城县 Shucheng Xian、金寨县 Jinzhai Xian、霍山县 Huoshan Xian、蒙城县 Mengcheng Xian、东至县 Dongzhi Xian、泾县 Jing Xian、宁国市 Ningguo Shi

省(自治区、直辖市) Province (autonomous region, municipality)	登记处数 No. of cancer registries	登记处名单 List of cancer registries
福建 Fujian	12	福清市 Fuqing Shi、福州市长乐区 Changle Qu,Fuzhou Shi、厦门市 Xiamen Shi、厦门市同安区 Tong'an Qu,Xiamen Shi、厦门市翔安区 Xiang'an Qu,Xiamen Shi、莆田市涵江区 Hanjiang Qu,Putian Shi、永安市 Yong'an Shi、惠安县 Hui'an Xian、漳州市长泰区 Changtai Qu,Zhangzhou Shi、建瓯市 Jian'ou Shi、龙岩市新罗区 Xinluo Qu,Longyan Shi、龙岩市永定区 Yongding Qu,Longyan Shi
江西 Jiangxi	40	南昌市青云谱区 Qingyunpu Qu,Nanchang Shi、南昌市青山湖区 Qingshanhu Qu,Nanchang Shi、南昌市新建区 Xinjian Qu,Nanchang Shi、芦溪县 Luxi Xian、九江市浔阳区 Xunyang Qu,Jiujiang Shi、武宁县 Wuning Xian、新余市渝水区 Yushui Qu,Xinyu Shi、鹰潭市余江区 Yujiang Qu,Yingtan Shi、赣州市章贡区 Zhanggong Qu,Ganzhou Shi、赣州市南康区 Nankang Qu,Ganzhou Shi、赣州市赣县区 Ganxian Qu,Ganzhou Shi、信丰县 Xinfeng Xian、大余县 Dayu Xian、上犹县 Shangyou Xian、崇义县 Chongyi Xian、龙南市 Longnan Shi、宁都县 Ningdu Xian、于都县 Yudu Xian、兴国县 Xingguo Xian、吉安市吉州区 Jizhou Qu,Ji'anShi、峡江县 Xiajiang Xian、安福县 Anfu Xian、万载县 Wanzai Xian、上高县 Shanggao Xian、靖安县 Jing'an Xian、樟树市 Zhangshu Shi、乐安县 Le'an Xian、宜黄县 Yihuang Xian、抚州市东乡区 Dongxiang Qu,Fuzhou Shi、上饶市信州区 Xinzhou Qu,Shangrao Shi、上饶市广丰区 Guangfeng Qu,Shangrao Shi、上饶市广信区 Guangxin Qu,Shangrao Shi、铅山县 Yanshan Xian、横峰县 Hengfeng Xian、弋阳县 Yiyang Xian、余干县 Yugan Xian、鄱阳县 Poyang Xian、万年县 Wannian Xian、婺源县 Wuyuan Xian、德兴市 Dexing Shi
山东 Shandong	35	济南市 Jinan Shi、济南市章丘区 Zhangqiu Qu,Jinan Shi、济南市莱芜区 Laiwu Qu,Jinan Shi、青岛市 Qingdao Shi、青岛市黄岛区 Huangdao Qu,Qingdao Shi、淄博市临淄区 Linzi Qu,Zibo Shi、沂源县 Yiyuan Xian、滕州市 Tengzhou Shi、广饶县 Guangrao Xian、烟台市 Yantai Shi、招远市 Zhaoyuan Shi、潍坊市潍城区 Weicheng Qu,Weifang Shi、临朐县 Linqu Xian、青州市 Qingzhou Shi、高密市 Gaomi Shi、济宁市任城区 Rencheng Qu,Jining Shi、汶上县 Wenshang Xian、梁山县 Liangshan Xian、曲阜市 Qufu Shi、邹城市 Zoucheng Shi、宁阳县 Ningyang Xian、肥城市 Feicheng Shi、乳山市 Rushan Shi、日照市东港区 Donggang Qu,Rizhao Shi、莒县 Ju Xian、沂南县 Yinan Xian、沂水县 Yishui Xian、莒南县 Junan Xian、德州市德城区 Decheng Qu,Dezhou Shi、聊城市东昌府区 Dongchangfu Qu,Liaocheng Shi、高唐县 Gaotang Xian、滨州市滨城区 Bincheng Qu,Binzhou Shi、菏泽市牡丹区 Mudan Qu,Heze Shi、单县 Shan Xian、巨野县 Juye Xian
河南 Henan	44	郑州市 Zhengzhou Shi、巩义市 Gongyi Shi、开封市祥符区 Xiangfu Qu,Kaifeng Shi、洛阳市 Luoyang Shi、洛阳市孟津区 Mengjin Qu,Luoyang Shi、新安县 Xin'an Xian、栾川县 Luanchuan Xian、嵩县 Song Xian、汝阳县 Ruyang Xian、宜阳县 Yiyang Xian、洛宁县 Luoning Xian、伊川县 Yichuan Xian、洛阳市偃师区 Yanshi Qu,Luoyang Shi、平顶山市 Pingdingshan Shi、鲁山县 Lushan Xian、郏县 Jia Xian、安阳市 Anyang Shi、林州市 Linzhou Shi、鹤壁市 Hebi Shi、新乡市 Xinxiang Shi、辉县市 Huixian Shi、焦作市 Jiaozuo Shi、濮阳市华龙区 Hualong Qu,Puyang Shi、濮阳县 Puyang Xian、禹州市 Yuzhou Shi、漯河市 Luohe Shi、漯河市郾城区 Yancheng Qu,Luohe Shi、舞阳县 Wuyang Xian、临颍县 Linying Xian、三门峡市湖滨区 Hubin Qu,Sanmenxia Shi、南阳市卧龙区 Wolong Qu,Nanyang Shi、南召县 Nanzhao Xian、方城县 Fangcheng Xian、内乡县 Neixiang Xian、睢县 Sui Xian、虞城县 Yucheng Xian、信阳市浉河区 Shihe Qu,Xinyang Shi、罗山县 Luoshan Xian、固始县 Gushi Xian、沈丘县 Shenqiu Xian、郸城县 Dancheng Xian、太康县 Taikang Xian、西平县 Xiping Xian、济源市 Jiyuan Shi

省（自治区、直辖市） Province （autonomous region, municipality）	登记处数 No. of cancer registries	登记处名单 List of cancer registries
湖北 Hubei	22	武汉市 Wuhan Shi、大冶市 Daye Shi、十堰市郧阳区 Yunyang Qu,Shiyan Shi、丹江口市 Danjiangkou Shi、宜昌市 Yichang Shi、秭归县 Zigui Xian、五峰土家族自治县 Wufeng Tujiazu Zizhixian、宜都市 Yidu Shi、襄阳市 Xiangyang Shi、枣阳市 Zaoyang Shi、宜城市 Yicheng Shi、京山市 Jingshan Shi、钟祥市 Zhongxiang Shi、云梦县 Yunmeng Xian、荆州市 Jingzhou Shi、公安县 Gong'an Xian、洪湖市 Honghu Shi、麻城市 Macheng Shi、嘉鱼县 Jiayu Xian、通城县 Tongcheng Xian、恩施市 Enshi Shi、天门市 Tianmen Shi
湖南 Hunan	32	长沙市芙蓉区 Furong Qu,Changsha Shi、长沙市天心区 Tianxin Qu,Changsha Shi、长沙市岳麓区 Yuelu Qu,Changsha Shi、长沙市开福区 Kaifu Qu,Changsha Shi、长沙市雨花区 Yuhua Qu,Changsha Shi、长沙市望城区 Wangcheng Qu,Changsha Shi、长沙县 Changsha Xian、浏阳市 Liuyang Shi、株洲市芦淞区 Lusong Qu,Zhuzhou Shi、株洲市石峰区 Shifeng Qu,Zhuzhou Shi、攸县 You Xian、湘潭市雨湖区 Yuhu Qu,Xiangtan Shi、衡东县 Hengdong Xian、常宁市 Changning Shi、邵东市 Shaodong Shi、新宁县 Xinning Xian、岳阳市岳阳楼区 Yueyanglou Qu,Yueyang Shi、常德市武陵区 Wuling Qu,Changde Shi、津市市 Jinshi Shi、慈利县 Cili Xian、益阳市资阳区 Ziyang Qu,Yiyang Shi、桃江县 Taojiang Xian、临武县 Linwu Xian、资兴市 Zixing Shi、道县 Dao Xian、宁远县 Ningyuan Xian、新田县 Xintian Xian、麻阳苗族自治县 Mayang Miaozu Zizhixian、洪江市 Hongjiang Shi、娄底市娄星区 Louxing Qu,Loudi Shi、冷水江市 Lengshuijiang Shi、涟源市 Lianyuan Shi
广东 Guangdong	31	广州市 Guangzhou Shi、广州市郊区 Rural Areas of Guangzhou Shi、韶关市曲江区 Qujiang Qu,Shaoguan Shi、翁源县 Wengyuan Xian、南雄市 Nanxiong Shi、深圳市 Shenzhen Shi、珠海市 Zhuhai Shi、佛山市禅城区 Chancheng Qu,Foshan Shi、佛山市南海区 Nanhai Qu,Foshan Shi、佛山市顺德区 Shunde Qu,Foshan Shi、佛山市三水区 Sanshui Qu,Foshan Shi、佛山市高明区 Gaoming Qu,Foshan Shi、江门市 Jiangmen Shi、湛江市赤坎区 Chikan Qu,Zhanjiang Shi、湛江市霞山区 Xiashan Qu,Zhanjiang Shi、徐闻县 Xuwen Xian、肇庆市端州区 Duanzhou Qu,Zhaoqing Shi、四会市 Sihui Shi、惠州市惠阳区 Huiyang Qu,Huizhou Shi、梅州市梅江区 Meijiang Qu,Meizhou Shi、梅州市梅县区 Meixian Qu,Meizhou Shi、河源市源城区 Yuancheng Qu,Heyuan Shi、阳江市阳东区 Yangdong Qu,Yangjiang Shi、清远市清城区 Qingcheng Qu,Qingyuan Shi、阳山县 Yangshan Xian、东莞市 Dongguan Shi、中山市 Zhongshan Shi、潮州市潮安区 Chaoan Qu,Chaozhou Shi、揭西县 Jiexi Xian、普宁市 Puning Shi、罗定市 Luoding Shi

省(自治区、直辖市) Province (autonomous region, municipality)	登记处数 No. of cancer registries	登记处名单 List of cancer registries
广西 Guangxi	41	南宁市兴宁区 Xingning Qu, Nanning Shi、南宁市青秀区 Qingxiu Qu, Nanning Shi、南宁市江南区 Jiangnan Qu, Nanning Shi、南宁经济技术开发区 Nanning Economic & Technological Development Zone、南宁市西乡塘区 Xixiangtang Qu, Nanning Shi、南宁市良庆区 Liangqing Qu, Nanning Shi、南宁市邕宁区 Yongning Qu, Nanning Shi、南宁东盟经济开发区 National Nanning-ASEAN Economic Development Zone、南宁市武鸣区 Wuming Qu, Nanning Shi、隆安县 Long'an Xian、马山县 Mashan Xian、上林县 Shanglin Xian、宾阳县 Binyang Xian、横州市 Hengzhou Shi、柳州市 Liuzhou Shi、鹿寨县 Luzhai Xian、桂林市 Guilin Shi、梧州市 Wuzhou Shi、苍梧县 Cangwu Xian、岑溪市 Cenxi Shi、北海市 Beihai Shi、合浦县 Hepu Xian、钦州市钦南区 Qinnan Qu, Qinzhou Shi、贵港市港北区 Gangbei Qu, Guigang Shi、贵港市港南区 Gangnan Qu, Guigang Shi、贵港市覃塘区 Qintang Qu, Guigang Shi、平南县 Pingnan Xian、桂平市 Guiping Shi、陆川县 Luchuan Xian、北流市 Beiliu Shi、百色市右江区 Youjiang Qu, Bose Shi、百色市田阳区 Tianyang Qu, Bose Shi、田东县 Tiandong Xian、凌云县 Lingyun Xian、贺州市平桂区 Pinggui Qu, Hezhou Shi、罗城仫佬族自治县 Luocheng Mulaozu Zizhixian、来宾市兴宾区 Xingbin Qu, Laibin Shi、合山市 Heshan Shi、崇左市江州区 Jiangzhou Qu, Chongzuo Shi、扶绥县 Fusui Xian、大新县 Daxin Xian
海南 Hainan	6	三亚市 Sanya Shi、五指山市 Wuzhishan Shi、琼海市 Qionghai Shi、定安县 Ding'an Xian、昌江黎族自治县 Changjiang Lizu Zizhixian、陵水黎族自治县 Lingshui Lizu Zizhixian
重庆 Chongqing	38	重庆市万州区 Wanzhou Qu, Chongqing Shi、重庆市涪陵区 Fuling Qu, Chongqing Shi、重庆市渝中区 Yuzhong Qu, Chongqing Shi、重庆市大渡口区 Dadukou Qu, Chongqing Shi、重庆市江北区 Jiangbei Qu, Chongqing Shi、重庆市沙坪坝区 Shapingba Qu, Chongqing Shi、重庆市九龙坡区 Jiulongpo Qu, Chongqing Shi、重庆市南岸区 Nan'an Qu, Chongqing Shi、重庆市北碚区 Beibei Qu, Chongqing Shi、重庆市綦江区 Qijiang Qu, Chongqing Shi、重庆市大足区 Dazu Qu, Chongqing Shi、重庆市渝北区 Yubei Qu, Chongqing Shi、重庆市巴南区 Banan Qu, Chongqing Shi、重庆市黔江区 Qianjiang Qu, Chongqing Shi、重庆市长寿区 Changshou Qu, Chongqing Shi、重庆市江津区 Jiangjin Qu, Chongqing Shi、重庆市合川区 Hechuan Qu, Chongqing Shi、重庆市永川区 Yongchuan Qu, Chongqing Shi、重庆市南川区 Nanchuan Qu, Chongqing Shi、重庆市璧山区 Bishan Qu, Chongqing Shi、重庆市潼南区 Tongnan Qu, Chongqing Shi、重庆市铜梁区 Tongliang Qu, Chongqing Shi、重庆市荣昌区 Rongchang Qu, Chongqing Shi、重庆市万盛经济开发区 Wansheng Economic Development Zone, Chongqing Shi、重庆市梁平区 Liangping Qu, Chongqing Shi、城口县 Chengkou Xian、丰都县 Fengdu Xian、垫江县 Dianjiang Xian、重庆市武隆区 Wulong Qu, Chongqing Shi、忠县 Zhong Xian、重庆市开州区 Kaizhou Qu, Chongqing Shi、云阳县 Yunyang Xian、奉节县 Fengjie Xian、巫山县 Wushan Xian、巫溪县 Wuxi Xian、石柱土家族自治县 Shizhu Tujiazu Zizhixian、秀山土家族苗族自治县 Xiushan Tujiazu Miaozu Zizhixian、酉阳土家族苗族自治县 Youyang Tujiazu Miaozu Zizhixian、彭水苗族土家族自治县 Pengshui Miaozu Tujiazu Zizhixian

省(自治区、直辖市) Province (autonomous region, municipality)	登记处数 No. of cancer registries	登记处名单 List of cancer registries
四川 Sichuan	150	成都市锦江区 Jinjiang Qu,Chengdu Shi、成都市青羊区 Qingyang Qu,Chengdu Shi、成都市金牛区 Jinniu Qu,Chengdu Shi、成都市武侯区 Wuhou Qu,Chengdu Shi、成都市成华区 Chenghua Qu,Chengdu Shi、成都市高新区 Gaoxin Qu,Chengdu Shi、成都市龙泉驿区 Longquanyi Qu,Chengdu Shi、成都市青白江区 Qingbaijiang Qu,Chengdu Shi、成都市新都区 Xindu Qu,Chengdu Shi、成都市温江区 Wenjiang Qu,Chengdu Shi、金堂县 Jintang Xian、成都市双流区 Shuangliu Qu,Chengdu Shi、成都市天府新区 Tianfu Xinqu,Chengdu Shi、成都市郫都区 Pidu Qu,Chengdu Shi、大邑县 Dayi Xian、蒲江县 Pujiang Xian、成都市新津区 Xinjin Qu,Chengdu Shi、简阳市 Jianyang Shi、都江堰市 Dujiangyan Shi、彭州市 Pengzhou Shi、邛崃市 Qionglai Shi、崇州市 Chongzhou Shi、自贡市自流井区 Ziliujing Qu,Zigong Shi、自贡市贡井区 Gongjing Qu,Zigong Shi、自贡市大安区 Da'an Qu,Zigong Shi、自贡市沿滩区 Yantan Qu,Zigong Shi、荣县 Rong Xian、富顺县 Fushun Xian、攀枝花市东区 Dong Qu,Panzhihua Shi、攀枝花市西区 Xi Qu,Panzhihua Shi、攀枝花市仁和区 Renhe Qu,Panzhihua Shi、米易县 Miyi Xian、盐边县 Yanbian Xian、泸州市江阳区 Jiangyang Qu,Luzhou Shi、泸州市纳溪区 Naxi Qu,Luzhou Shi、泸州市龙马潭 Longmatan Qu,Luzhou Shi、泸县 Lu Xian、合江县 Hejiang Xian、叙永县 Xuyong Xian、古蔺县 Gulin Xian、德阳市旌阳区 Jingyang Qu,Deyang Shi、中江县 Zhongjiang Xian、德阳市罗江区 Luojiang Qu,Deyang Shi、广汉市 Guanghan Shi、什邡市 Shifang Shi、绵竹市 Mianzhu Shi、绵阳市涪城区 Fucheng Qu,Mianyang Shi、绵阳市游仙区 Youxian Qu,Mianyang Shi、绵阳市安州区 Anzhou Qu,Mianyang Shi、三台县 Santai Xian、盐亭县 Yanting Xian、梓潼县 Zitong Xian、北川羌族自治县 Beichuan Qiangzu Zizhixian、平武县 Pingwu Xian、江油市 Jiangyou Shi、广元市利州区 Lizhou Qu,Guangyuan Shi、广元市昭化区 Zhaohua Qu,Guangyuan Shi、广元市朝天区 Chaotian Qu,Guangyuan Shi、旺苍县 Wangcang Xian、青川县 Qingchuan Xian、剑阁县 Jiange Xian、苍溪县 Cangxi Xian、遂宁市船山区 Chuanshan Qu,Suining Shi、遂宁市安居区 Anju Qu,Suining Shi、蓬溪县 Pengxi Xian、射洪市 Shehong Shi、大英县 Daying Xian、内江市市中区 Shizhong Qu,Neijiang Shi、内江市东兴区 Dongxing Qu,Neijiang Shi、威远县 Weiyuan Xian、资中县 Zizhong Xian、隆昌市 Longchang Shi、乐山市市中区 Shizhong Qu,Leshan Shi、乐山市沙湾区 Shawan Qu,Leshan Shi、乐山市五通桥区 Wutongqiao Qu,Leshan Shi、乐山市金口河区 Jinkouhe Qu,Leshan Shi、犍为县 Qianwei Xian、井研县 Jingyan Xian、夹江县 Jiajiang Xian、沐川县 Muchuan Xian、峨边彝族自治县 Ebian Yizu Zizhixian、马边彝族自治县 Mabian Yizu Zizhixian、峨眉山市 Emeishan Shi、南充市顺庆区 Shunqing Qu,Nanchong Shi、南充市高坪区 Gaoping Qu,Nanchong Shi、南充市嘉陵区 Jialing Qu,Nanchong Shi、南部县 Nanbu Xian、营山县 Yingshan Xian、蓬安县 Peng'an Xian、仪陇县 Yilong Xian、西充县 Xichong Xian、阆中市 Langzhong Shi、眉山市东坡区 Dongpo Qu,Meishan Shi、眉山市彭山区 Pengshan Qu,Meishan Shi、仁寿县 Renshou Xian、洪雅县 Hongya Xian、丹棱县 Danling Xian、青神县 Qingshen Xian、宜宾市翠屏区 Cuiping Qu,Yibin Shi、宜宾市南溪区 Nanxi Qu,Yibin Shi、宜宾市叙州区 Xuzhou Qu,Yibin Shi、江安县 Jiang'an Xian、长宁县 Changning Xian、高县 Gao Xian、珙县 Gong Xian、筠连县 Junlian Xian、兴文县 Xingwen Xian、屏山县 Pingshan Xian、广安市广安区 Guang'an Qu,Guang'an Shi、广安市前锋区 Qianfeng Qu,Guang'an Shi、岳池县 Yuechi Xian、武胜县 Wusheng Xian、邻水县 Linshui Xian、华蓥市 Huaying Shi、达州市通川区 Tongchuan Qu,Dazhou Shi、达州市达川区 Dachuan Qu,Dazhou Shi、宣汉县 Xuanhan Xian、开江县 Kaijiang Xian、大竹县 Dazhu Xian、渠县 Qu Xian、万源市 Wanyuan Shi、雅安市雨城区 Yucheng Qu,Ya'an Shi、雅安市名山区 Mingshan Qu,Ya'an Shi、荥经县 Yingjing Xian、汉源县 Hanyuan Xian、石棉县 Shimian Xian、天全县 Tianquan Xian、芦山县 Lushan Xian、宝兴县 Baoxing Xian、巴中市巴州区 Bazhou Qu,Bazhong Shi、巴中市恩阳区 Enyang Qu,Bazhong Shi、通江县 Tongjiang Xian、南江县 Nanjiang Xian、平昌县 Pingchang Xian、资阳市雁江区 Yanjiang Qu,Ziyang Shi、安岳县 Anyue Xian、乐至县 Lezhi Xian、马尔康市 Barkam Shi、汶川县 Wenchuan Xian、理县 Li Xian、茂县 Mao Xian、松潘县 Songpan Xian、九寨沟县 Jiuzhaigou Xian、金川县 Jinchuan Xian、小金县 Xiaojin Xian、阿坝县 Aba Xian、红原县 Hongyuan Xian、泸定县 Luding Xian、白玉县 Baiyu Xian、理塘县 Litang Xian

省(自治区、直辖市) Province (autonomous region, municipality)	登记处数 No. of cancer registries	登记处名单 List of cancer registries
贵州 Guizhou	36	贵阳市花溪区 Huaxi Qu,Guiyang Shi、开阳县 Kaiyang Xian、息烽县 Xifeng Xian、修文县 Xiuwen Xian、清镇市 Qingzhen Shi、六盘水市钟山区 Zhongshan Qu,Liupanshui Shi、六盘水市六枝特区 Luzhi Tequ,Lupanshui Shi、六盘水市水城区 Shuicheng Qu,Liupanshui Shi、盘州市 Panzhou Shi、遵义市红花岗区 Honghuagang Qu,Zunyi Shi、遵义市汇川区 Huichuan Qu,Zunyi Shi、习水县 Xishui Xian、赤水市 Chishui Shi、安顺市西秀区 Xixiu Qu,Anshun Shi、普定县 Puding Xian、镇宁布依族苗族自治县 Zhenning Buyeizu Miaozu ZizhiXian、毕节市七星关区 Qixingguan Qu,Bijie Shi、黔西市 Qianxi Shi、铜仁市碧江区 Bijiang Qu,Tongren Shi、玉屏侗族自治县 Yuping Dongzu Zizhixian、沿河土家族自治县 Yanhe Tujiazu Zizhixian、铜仁市万山区 Wanshan Qu,Tongren Shi、兴义市 Xingyi Shi、册亨县 Ceheng Xian、安龙县 Anlong Xian、黄平县 Huangping Xian、剑河县 Jianhe Xian、榕江县 Rongjiang Xian、雷山县 Leishan Xian、麻江县 Majiang Xian、丹寨县 Danzhai Xian、都匀市 Duyun Shi、福泉市 Fuquan Shi、荔波县 Libo Xian、瓮安县 Weng'an Xian、龙里县 Longli Xian
云南 Yunnan	80	昆明市五华区 Wuhua Qu,Kunming Shi、昆明市盘龙区 Panlong Qu,Kunming Shi、昆明市官渡区 Guandu Qu,Kunming Shi、昆明市西山区 Xishan Qu,Kunming Shi、昆明市呈贡区 Chenggong Qu,Kunming Shi、昆明市晋宁区 Jinning Qu,Kunming Shi、富民县 Fumin Xian、宜良县 Yiliang Xian、石林彝族自治县 Shilin Yizu Zizhixian、嵩明县 Songming Xian、禄劝彝族苗族自治县 Luchuan Yizu Miaozu Zizhixian、安宁市 Anning Shi、曲靖市麒麟区 Qilin Qu,Qujing Shi、曲靖市沾益区 Zhanyi Qu,Qujing Shi、曲靖市马龙区 Malong Qu,Qujing Shi、陆良县 Luliang Xian、师宗县 Shizong Xian、罗平县 Luoping Xian、富源县 Fuyuan Xian、宣威市 Xuanwei Shi、玉溪市红塔区 Hongta Qu,Yuxi Shi、玉溪市江川区 Jiangchuan Qu,Yuxi Shi、澄江市 Chengjiang Shi、通海县 Tonghai Xian、华宁县 Huaning Xian、易门县 Yimen Xian、峨山彝族自治县 Eshan Yizu Zizhixian、新平彝族傣族自治县 Xinping Yizu Daizu Zizhixian、元江哈尼族彝族傣族自治县 Yuanjiang Hanizu Yizu Daizu Zizhixian、保山市隆阳区 Longyang Qu,Baoshan Shi、施甸县 Shidian Xian、龙陵县 Longling Xian、昌宁县 Changning Xian、腾冲市 Tengchong Shi、巧家县 Qiaojia Xian、绥江县 Suijiang Xian、水富市 Shuifu Shi、丽江市古城区 Gucheng Qu,Lijiang Shi、玉龙纳西族自治县 Yulong Naxizu Zizhixian、华坪县 Huaping Xian、宁蒗彝族自治县 Ninglang Yizu Zizhixian、景东彝族自治县 Jingdong Yizu Zizhixian、景谷傣族彝族自治县 Jinggu Daizu Yizu Zizhixian、江城哈尼族彝族自治县 Jiangcheng Hanizu Yizu Zizhixian、临沧市临翔区 Linxiang Qu,Lincang Shi、凤庆县 Fengqing Xian、镇康县 Zhenkang Xian、沧源佤族自治县 Cangyuan Vazu Zizhixian、楚雄市 Chuxiong Shi、双柏县 Shuangbai Xian、牟定县 Mouding Xian、姚安县 Yao'an Xian、大姚县 Dayao Xian、永仁县 Yongren Xian、元谋县 Yuanmou Xian、武定县 Wuding Xian、禄丰市 Lufeng Shi、个旧市 Gejiu Shi、开远市 Kaiyuan Shi、蒙自市 Mengzi Shi、屏边苗族自治县 Pingbian Miaozu Zizhixian、建水县 Jianshui Xian、石屏县 Shiping Xian、弥勒市 Mile Shi、泸西县 Luxi Xian、文山市 Wenshan Shi、砚山县 Yanshan Xian、西畴县 Xichou Xian、丘北县 Qiubei Xian、富宁县 Funing Xian、景洪市 Jinghong Shi、大理市 Dali Shi、祥云县 Xiangyun Xian、宾川县 Binchuan Xian、弥渡县 Midu Xian、南涧彝族自治县 Nanjian Yizu Zizhixian、兰坪白族普米族自治县 Lanping Baizu Pumizu ZizhiXian、香格里拉市 Shangêlila Shi、德钦县 Dêqên Xian、维西傈僳族自治县 Weixi Lisuzu Zizhixian
西藏 Xizang	4	拉萨市城关区 Chengguan Qu,Lhasa Shi、林芝市巴宜区 Bayi Qu,Linzhi Shi、昌都市卡若区 Karuo Qu,Qamdo Shi、日喀则市 XigazêShi

省（自治区、直辖市） Province （autonomous region， municipality）	登记处数 No. of cancer registries	登记处名单 List of cancer registries
陕西 Shaanxi	54	西安市碑林区 Beilin Qu，Xi'an Shi、西安市莲湖区 Lianhu Qu，Xi'an Shi、西安市未央区 Weiyang Qu，Xi'an Shi、西安市雁塔区 Yanta Qu，Xi'an Shi、西安市高陵区 Gaoling Qu，Xi'an Shi、西安市鄠邑区 Huyi Qu，Xi'an Shi、铜川市耀州区 Yaozhou Qu，Tongchuan Shi、宝鸡市渭滨区 Weibin Qu，Baoji Shi、宝鸡市金台区 Jintai Qu，Baoji Shi、宝鸡市陈仓区 Chencang Qu，Baoji Shi、宝鸡市凤翔区 Fengxiang Qu，Baoji Shi、岐山县 Qishan Xian、扶风县 Fufeng Xian、眉县 Mei Xian、陇县 Long Xian、千阳县 Qianyang Xian、麟游县 Linyou Xian、凤县 Feng Xian、太白县 Taibai Xian、三原县 Sanyuan Xian、泾阳县 Jingyang Xian、武功县 Wugong Xian、渭南市临渭区 Linwei Qu，Weinan Shi、渭南市华州区 Huazhou Qu，Weinan Shi、潼关县 Tongguan Xian、大荔县 Dali Xian、合阳县 Heyang Xian、澄城县 Chengcheng Xian、蒲城县 Pucheng Xian、富平县 Fuping Xian、韩城市 Hancheng Shi、华阴市 Huayin Shi、延安市宝塔区 Baota Qu，Yan'an Shi、延安市安塞区 Ansai Qu，Yan'an Shi、延川县 Yanchuan Xian、富县 Fu Xian、黄龙县 Huanglong Xian、黄陵县 Huangling Xian、汉中市汉台区 Hantai Qu，Hanzhong Shi、城固县 Chenggu Xian、宁强县 Ningqiang Xian、绥德县 Suide Xian、安康市汉滨区 Hanbin Qu，Ankang Shi、汉阴县 Hanyin Xian、石泉县 Shiquan Xian、宁陕县 Ningshan Xian、紫阳县 Ziyang Xian、岚皋县 Langao Xian、平利县 Pingli Xian、镇坪县 Zhenping Xian、旬阳市 Xunyang Shi、商洛市商州区 Shangzhou Qu，Shangluo Shi、洛南县 Luonan Xian、镇安县 Zhen'an Xian
甘肃 Gansu	23	兰州市城关区 Chengguan Qu，Lanzhou Shi、兰州市七里河区 Qilihe Qu，Lanzhou Shi、兰州市西固区 Xigu Qu，Lanzhou Shi、兰州市安宁区 Anning Qu，Lanzhou Shi、兰州市红古区 Honggu Qu，Lanzhou Shi、白银市白银区 Baiyin Qu，Baiyin Shi、白银市平川区 Pingchuan Qu，Baiyin Shi、靖远县 Jingyuan Xian、会宁县 Huining Xian、景泰县 Jingtai Xian、天水市秦州区 Qinzhou Qu，Tianshui Shi、天水市麦积区 Maiji Qu，Tianshui Shi、武威市凉州区 Liangzhou Qu，Wuwei Shi、民勤县 Minqin Xian、古浪县 Gulang Xian、天祝藏族自治县 Tianzhu Zangzu Zizhixian、张掖市甘州区 Ganzhou Qu，Zhangye Shi、高台县 Gaotai Xian、静宁县 Jingning Xian、敦煌市 Dunhuang Shi、庆城县 Qingcheng Xian、临洮县 Lintao Xian、临潭县 Lintan Xian
青海 Qinghai	8	西宁市 Xining Shi、大通回族土族自治县 Datong Huizu Tuzu ZizhiXian、西宁市湟中区 Huangzhong Qu，Xining Shi、海东市乐都区 Ledu Qu，Haidong Shi、民和回族土族自治县 Minhe Huizu Tuzu ZizhiXian、互助土族自治县 Huzhu Tuzu Zizhixian、循化撒拉族自治县 Xunhua Salarzu Zizhixian、海南藏族自治州 Hainan Zangzu Zizhizhou
宁夏 Ningxia	11	银川市兴庆区 Xingqing Qu，Yinchuan Shi、银川市西夏区 Xixia Qu，Yinchuan Shi、银川市金凤区 Jinfeng Qu，Yinchuan Shi、贺兰县 Helan Xian、石嘴山市大武口区 Dawukou Qu，Shizuishan Shi、石嘴山市惠农区 Huinong Qu，Shizuishan Shi、平罗县 Pingluo Xian、青铜峡市 Qingtongxia Shi、固原市原州区 Yuanzhou Qu，Guyuan Shi、中卫市沙坡头区 Shapotou Qu，Zhongwei Shi、中宁县 Zhongning Xian
新疆 Xinjiang	15	乌鲁木齐市天山区 Tianshan Qu，Ürümqi Shi、乌鲁木齐市沙依巴克区 Saybag Qu，Ürümqi Shi、乌鲁木齐市新市区 Xinshi Qu，Ürümqi Shi、乌鲁木齐市水磨沟区 Shuimogou Qu，Ürümqi Shi、乌鲁木齐市头屯河区 Toutunhe Qu，Ürümqi Shi、乌鲁木齐市米东区 Midong Qu，Ürümqi Shi、克拉玛依市 Karamay Shi、阜康市 Fukang Shi、库尔勒市 Korla Shi、阿克苏市 Aksu Shi、拜城县 Baicheng Xian、和田市 Hotan Shi、和田县 Hotan Xian、霍城县 Huocheng Xian、新源县 Xinyuan Xian
新疆生产建设兵团 Xinjiang Production and Construction Corps	3	第二师 Di'ershi、第七师 Diqishi、第八师 Dibashi

2 数据纳入排除标准

国家癌症中心成立肿瘤登记专家委员会和《中国肿瘤登记年报》编委会。在既往《中国肿瘤登记年报》数据入选原则基础上，根据《肿瘤随访登记技术方案》（卫生部疾病预防控制局 2009）、《中国肿瘤登记工作指导手册（2016）》中的数据质量要求，参照国际癌症研究机构（IARC）/国际癌症登记协会（IACR）对肿瘤登记数据的质量控制规则，经充分研究与讨论，制定了《2021 中国肿瘤登记年报》纳入排除标准。

本年报入选标准，注重肿瘤登记数据的真实性、稳定性和均衡性，根据登记地区的特点，综合评估该肿瘤登记处数据质量。重点考核指标要求发病率大于 180/10 万，死亡率水平基本不低于 100/10 万，MV%、DCO%、M/I 合理。并兼顾地区差异，综合考虑肿瘤登记处各个指标在本地区的合理范围。对于新建立第一次上报数据的登记处，在上述规则的原则上，考虑社会经济发展水平、工作基础、少数民族地区等因素综合评估后择优录取，MV% 标准适当放宽。对于曾经被收录的登记处，在行政区划没有变化的情况下，一般粗率变化幅度不能超过 20%。对于曾经上报过数据，但未曾被收录的登记处，变化幅度如果不在上述范围内，根据实际情况进一步核实评估。对于连续 5 年及以上被纳入年报的登记处数据，若个别指标不符合要求，但为保持连续性适当保留。

2 Data inclusion and exclusion criteria

NCC has established a panel of cancer registry experts and the editorial committee of *China Cancer Registry Annual Report*. According to the principle of selecting data of the previous *China Cancer Registry Annual Report*, basing on *Technical Protocols of Cancer Registration and Follow Up* by Ministry of Health 2009, *Chinese Guideline for Cancer Registration (2016)* and the quality control rules of cancer registration by the International Agency for Research on Cancer (IARC)/the International Agency for Cancer Registry (IACR), the editorial committee has established a comprehensive data inclusion and exclusion criteria of *2021 Chinese Cancer Registry Annual Report* after thorough investigation and discussion.

The data inclusion criteria were focused on the authenticity, stability, and comparability of cancer registry data quality. The quality of data was evaluated based on the characteristics of the corresponding regions. To pass the data inclusion criteria, one registry data should have an incidence of more than 180 per 100 000, while the morality of the data should be greater or equal to 100 per 100 000. The MV%, DCO%, and M/I should be reasonable. Taking regional disparity into account, the proper ranges of quality control indexes of registration data differed by areas. For registries which submitted data for the first time, the quality control index MV% could be flexible. And registries were enrolled with due consideration of their social economic development level, working foundation and ethnic minority conditions. For registries which data have already been included in the report before, changes of crude rates should be less than 20% if the administrative divisions of the registries remained the same. For registries which have submitted data but have never been included in the report before, over 20% changes of crude rates should be evaluated according to the actual situation of registries. For registries which have been consecutively included in the report over 5 years, their data were included in this report even if individual indexes were not qualified, in order to guarantee data continuity.

3 肿瘤登记资料评价

3.1 覆盖人口、发病数和死亡数

提交数据的947个肿瘤登记地区2018年登记覆盖人口634 376 540人，其中城市地区为275 501 650人，占全部覆盖人口的43.43%，农村地区为358 874 890人，占56.57%。全国登记地区覆盖人口占2018年全国年末人口数的45.14%。2018年报告癌症新发病例数合计1 765 264例，其中城市地区占47.38%，农村地区占52.62%。共计报告癌症死亡病例男女合计1 007 868例，城市地区占44.62%，农村地区占55.38%（表3-2）。

3.2 数据质量评价

在提交2018年资料的947个登记处中，形态学诊断比例（MV%）在55%~95%的登记处有721个（76.14%），形态学诊断比例（MV%）小于55%和大于95%的分别为206个和20个，占23.86%。仅有死亡证明书比例（DCO%）在0~5%的登记处有631个（66.63%），DCO%为0的登记处有223个（23.55%），大于5%的登记处有93个（9.82%）。死亡发病比（M/I）为0.55~0.85的登记处有634个（66.95%），M/I小于0.55和大于0.85的登记处分别为283个和30个，占33.05%。

2018年第一次提交数据的登记处有170个，占17.95%。与提交过2017年数据的778个登记处癌症发病率相比，变化幅度在10%以内的登记处有578个，占提交过数据登记处总数的74.29%。

3 Evaluation of cancer registration data

3.1 Population coverage, new cancer cases and cancer deaths

Among 947 cancer registries which submitted cancer statistics, the population coverage was 634 376 540, with 275 501 650 in urban areas（43.43%）and 358 874 890 in rural areas（56.57%）. The covering population accounted for 45.14% of the overall national population of 2018. A total of 1 765 264 new cancer cases were reported in 2018. Among them, 47.38% were from urban areas and 52.62% were from rural areas. There were 1 007 868 new cancer deaths in 2018. The urban cancer deaths accounted for 44.62% of overall cancer deaths and rural cancer deaths accounted for 55.38%（Table 3-2）.

3.2 Evaluation of data quality

Among the 947 registries which submitted the data of 2018, 721 registries（76.14%）had MV% between 55% and 95%. A total of 206 registries had MV% less than 55%, and 20 had MV% more than 95%, accounting for 23.86% of all registries. There were 631 registries having DCO% between 0 and 5%, accounting for 66.63% of all registries. A total of 223 registries（23.55%）reported no DCO cases, and 93 registries（9.82%）reported more than 5% of DCO cases. Among all registries, there were 634 registries（66.95%）having M/I between 0.55 and 0.85. 283 registries had M/I less than 0.55, 30 registries had M/I more than 0.85, accounting for 33.05%.

There were 170 registries（17.95%）submitted data to NCC for the first time. Compared with all cancer incidence rates in 2017, 578 registries reported a change of rate in 2018 less than 10%, accounting for 74.29% of all registries.

表 3-2　2018 年全国肿瘤登记地区覆盖人口、发病数、死亡数及主要质控指标

Table 3-2　The population coverage, new cancer cases, cancer deaths and major indicators for data quality of 2018 in cancer registration areas

序号 No.	肿瘤登记处 Cancer registries	人口数 Population	发病数 New cases	死亡数 Deaths	MV%	DCO%	M/I	发病率变化 Change for CR%	接受 Accepted
1	北京市 Beijing Shi	8 434 510	34 743	17 564	82.05	0.03	0.51	3.95	Y
2	北京市郊区 Rural Areas of Beijing Shi	5 240 592	18 162	9 403	78.22	0.02	0.52	3.31	Y
3	天津市 Tianjin Shi	5 441 094	23 058	12 235	53.20	0.43	0.53	2.66	Y
4	天津市郊区 Rural Areas of Tianjin Shi	5 375 169	15 614	8 081	53.39	0.24	0.52	−0.49	Y
5	石家庄市 Shijiazhuang Shi	2 305 914	6 210	3 524	86.47	0.45	0.57	−3.15	Y
6	石家庄市郊区 Rural Areas of Shijiazhuang Shi	2 408 170	5 526	3 449	76.46	1.10	0.62	1.06	Y
7	赞皇县 Zanhuang Xian	272 656	617	458	72.77	0.49	0.74	−2.25	Y
8	迁西县 Qianxi Xian	407 963	909	637	83.17	1.21	0.70	−1.65	Y
9	迁安市 Qian'an Shi	776 711	1 538	1 262	69.05	0.20	0.82	−0.63	Y
10	秦皇岛市 Qinhuangdao Shi	1 467 658	3 223	2 002	84.92	0.16	0.62	−3.63	Y
11	邯郸市邯山区 Hanshan Qu, Handan Shi	521 761	975	674	78.05	0.10	0.69	−5.10	Y
12	大名县 Daming Xian	795 610	1 678	1 006	64.30	0.60	0.60	2.31	Y
13	涉县 She Xian	431 146	1 397	1 033	77.09	0.14	0.74	1.23	Y
14	磁县 Ci Xian	659 466	1 890	1 409	84.81	1.16	0.75	−3.70	Y
15	武安市 Wu'an Shi	849 046	1 808	1 193	60.12	0.17	0.66	4.67	Y
16	邢台市 Xingtai Shi	878 538	1 686	1 161	67.26	0.12	0.69	4.21	Y
17	邢台县 Xingtai Xian	361 711	753	584	71.85	0.27	0.78	0.62	Y
18	临城县 Lincheng Xian	211 215	440	296	76.82	0.23	0.67	2.71	Y
19	内丘县 Neiqiu Xian	258 260	550	361	71.64	0.18	0.66	−4.49	Y
20	邢台市任泽区 Renze Qu, Xingtai Shi	339 474	700	533	84.29	1.71	0.76	−6.12	Y
21	保定市 Baoding Shi	1 180 118	2 562	1 833	75.10	1.17	0.72	−2.23	Y
22	望都县 Wangdu Xian	260 314	522	311	67.82	0.96	0.60	−0.10	Y
23	安国市 Anguo Shi	386 459	853	559	67.64	3.40	0.66	−10.73	Y
24	张家口市宣化区 Xuanhua Qu, Zhangjiakou Shi	533 240	1 308	849	79.89	0.38	0.65	12.77	Y
25	张北县 Zhangbei Xian	364 774	1 233	750	73.64	0.65	0.61	−0.26	Y
26	承德市双桥区 Shuangqiao Qu, Chengde Shi	315 235	638	388	71.79	0.47	0.61	−1.14	Y

序号 No.	肿瘤登记处 Cancer registries	人口数 Population	发病数 New cases	死亡数 Deaths	MV%	DCO%	M/I	发病率变化 Change for CR%	接受 Accepted
27	丰宁满族自治县 Fengning Manzu Zizhixian	408 470	824	521	76.94	0.12	0.63	-3.03	Y
28	沧州市 Cangzhou Shi	515 578	1 073	639	80.34	0.09	0.60	-10.71	Y
29	海兴县 Haixing Xian	223 117	467	283	77.52	0.21	0.61	-3.63	Y
30	盐山县 Yanshan Xian	464 284	921	566	70.25	0.33	0.61	-0.90	Y
31	衡水市冀州区 Jizhou Qu, Hengshui Shi	344 658	804	603	72.51	0.75	0.75	1.43	Y
32	辛集市 Xinji Shi	635 039	1 363	827	82.32	0.15	0.61	-5.68	Y
33	太原市小店区 Xiaodian Qu, Taiyuan Shi	843 109	1 108	656	81.68	0.00	0.59	—	
34	太原市迎泽区 Yingze Qu, Taiyuan Shi	620 959	2 271	141	69.97	0.00	0.06	—	
35	太原市杏花岭区 Xinghualing Qu, Taiyuan Shi	668 948	2 165	1 203	55.84	2.68	0.56	17.73	Y
36	清徐县 Qingxu Xian	354 677	586	262	26.28	0.00	0.45	—	
37	阳泉市 Yangquan Shi	681 203	1 722	1 118	70.91	3.37	0.65	4.87	Y
38	平定县 Pingding Xian	317 523	699	463	58.51	0.00	0.66	-4.87	Y
39	盂县 Yu Xian	307 011	568	350	80.81	0.00	0.62	-5.33	Y
40	长治市 Changzhi Shi	483 628	933	442	59.38	0.00	0.47	—	
41	襄垣县 Xiangyuan Xian	276 897	702	400	68.66	0.43	0.57	—	Y
42	平顺县 Pingshun Xian	152 398	346	250	69.65	1.45	0.72	12.10	Y
43	沁源县 Qinyuan Xian	163 819	465	256	74.41	0.00	0.55	142.99	Y
44	阳城县 Yangcheng Xian	383 106	1 305	832	81.76	0.69	0.64	-11.75	Y
45	陵川县 Lingchuan Xian	250 943	214	154	54.21	0.00	0.72	—	
46	晋中市榆次区 Yuci Qu, Jizhong Shi	614 027	1 690	964	66.09	2.25	0.57	17.25	Y
47	晋中市太谷区 Taigu Qu, Jinzhong Shi	292 145	482	248	63.90	0.00	0.51	—	
48	昔阳县 Xiyang Xian	235 895	388	301	86.60	0.00	0.78	-16.43	
49	寿阳县 Shouyang Xian	214 640	663	438	58.07	4.68	0.66	7.76	Y
50	稷山县 Jishan Xian	360 943	583	403	59.01	0.17	0.69	-9.21	
51	新绛县 Xinjiang Xian	347 563	479	118	66.18	0.00	0.25	—	
52	绛县 Jiang Xian	285 752	555	359	36.22	12.25	0.65	82.87	
53	垣曲县 Yuanqu Xian	235 525	289	316	98.62	0.00	1.09	-41.52	
54	芮城县 Ruicheng Xian	410 707	173	338	91.91	0.00	1.95	-64.07	

序号 No.	肿瘤登记处 Cancer registries	人口数 Population	发病数 New cases	死亡数 Deaths	MV%	DCO%	M/I	发病率变化 Change for CR%	接受 Accepted
55	忻州市忻府区 Xinfu Qu, Xinzhou Shi	551 717	635	154	40.31	0.00	0.24	—	
56	定襄县 Dingxiang Xian	221 320	100	164	94.00	0.00	1.64	—	
57	原平市 Yuanping Shi	505 938	724	530	93.23	0.00	0.73	—	
58	临汾市尧都区 Yaodu Qu, Linfen Shi	817 493	1 048	228	33.40	0.00	0.22	—	
59	襄汾县 Xiangfen Xian	460 934	366	225	58.20	0.00	0.61	—	
60	洪洞县 Hongtong Xian	726 335	1 261	978	65.03	0.40	0.78	-24.49	
61	交城县 Jiaocheng Xian	239 093	390	103	34.62	0.00	0.26	—	
62	临县 Lin Xian	659 524	658	321	48.63	0.00	0.49	-4.66	
63	孝义市 Xiaoyi Shi	435 903	776	407	89.05	0.52	0.52	73.10	
64	汾阳市 Fenyang Shi	434 732	805	493	62.73	0.00	0.61	—	Y
65	托克托县 Togtoh Xian	211 701	227	29	56.83	8.37	0.13	—	
66	武川县 Wuchuan Xian	121 201	177	76	66.10	0.56	0.43	-5.16	
67	土默特右旗 Tumd Youqi	299 699	467	269	88.22	11.78	0.58	-20.42	
68	赤峰市红山区 Hongshan Qu, Chifeng Shi	462 000	1 042	539	72.55	0.00	0.52	-1.76	Y
69	赤峰市元宝山区 Yuanbaoshan Qu, Chifeng Shi	335 299	1 382	586	56.73	0.07	0.42	22.55	Y
70	赤峰市松山区 Songshan Qu, Chifeng Shi	601 399	1 535	859	65.60	0.26	0.56	-9.44	Y
71	敖汉旗 Aohan Qi	531 202	1 209	729	62.45	0.00	0.60	2.60	Y
72	通辽市科尔沁区 Horqin Qu, Tongliao Shi	824 968	1 797	949	71.06	0.00	0.53	-6.77	Y
73	科尔沁左翼中旗 Horqin Zuoyi Zhongqi	448 532	1 132	625	63.78	0.44	0.55	0.77	Y
74	科尔沁左翼后旗 Horqin Zuoyi Houqi	357 102	506	273	27.87	0.00	0.54		
75	开鲁县 Kailu Xian	398 300	1 095	675	65.84	0.46	0.62	-3.05	Y
76	库伦旗 Hure Qi	175 875	388	240	55.15	1.55	0.62	-10.37	Y
77	奈曼旗 Naiman Qi	423 299	1 097	703	72.47	0.00	0.64	10.68	Y
78	扎鲁特旗 Jarud Qi	303 000	666	386	75.83	0.00	0.58	-7.43	Y
79	霍林郭勒市 Holin Gol Shi	133 748	207	86	79.23	2.42	0.42	—	
80	呼伦贝尔市海拉尔区 Hailar Qu, Hulun Buir Shi	351 499	1 055	665	69.48	0.85	0.63	-19.96	Y

序号 No.	肿瘤登记处 Cancer registries	人口数 Population	发病数 New cases	死亡数 Deaths	MV%	DCO%	M/I	发病率变化 Change for CR%	接受 Accepted
81	呼伦贝尔市扎赉诺尔区 Dalai Nur Qu,Hulun Buir Shi	86 405	105	162	69.52	0.00	1.54	−36.26	
82	阿荣旗 Arun Qi	282 100	909	489	69.53	5.94	0.54	9.24	Y
83	莫力达瓦达斡尔族自治旗 Morin Dawa Daurzu Zizhiqi	280 800	546	324	46.70	9.34	0.59	53.80	Y
84	鄂温克族自治旗 Ewenkizu Zizhiqi	134 801	491	309	81.26	1.22	0.63	8.31	Y
85	陈巴尔虎旗 Chen Barag Qi	61 899	95	35	1.05	0.00	0.37	−22.95	
86	新巴尔虎左旗 Xin Barag Zuoqi	41 999	100	87	28.00	12.00	0.87	—	
87	新巴尔虎右旗 Xin Barag Youqi	34 298	24	35	0.00	0.00	1.46	—	
88	满洲里市 Manzhouli Shi	86 753	377	196	66.84	0.27	0.52	62.60	Y
89	牙克石市 Yakeshi Shi	331 000	1 017	874	57.92	12.09	0.86	−18.38	Y
90	扎兰屯市 Zalantun Shi	341 799	719	233	49.79	5.70	0.32	43.03	Y
91	根河市 Genhe Shi	137 301	554	343	47.29	20.22	0.62	30.67	Y
92	巴彦淖尔市临河区 Linhe Qu,Bayannur Shi	442 858	1 019	687	79.39	2.65	0.67	−12.04	Y
93	锡林浩特市 Xilin Hot Shi	251 759	783	381	73.31	0.13	0.49	−17.71	Y
94	西乌珠穆沁旗 Xi Ujimqin Qi	89 703	225	119	26.22	0.00	0.53	—	
95	沈阳市 Shenyang Shi	3 832 128	15 823	8 872	67.60	1.66	0.56	−1.07	Y
96	康平县 Kangping Xian	342 306	10 87	506	47.75	2.21	0.47	39.87	Y
97	法库县 Faku Xian	439 224	1 351	974	65.51	3.55	0.72	−5.35	Y
98	大连市 Dalian Shi	2 392 881	13 313	6 768	81.28	0.98	0.51	8.22	Y
99	庄河市 Zhuanghe Shi	889 345	3 924	2 276	80.30	0.74	0.58	3.94	Y
100	鞍山市 Anshan Shi	1 472 885	6 956	4 414	77.11	2.82	0.63	−0.48	Y
101	本溪市 Benxi Shi	894 691	3 295	1 971	60.12	0.24	0.60	12.64	Y
102	丹东市 Dandong Shi	775 607	2 994	1 873	75.45	5.21	0.63	13.37	Y
103	东港市 Donggang Shi	596 168	2 287	1 389	45.08	0.44	0.61	5.90	Y
104	营口市 Yingkou Shi	445 208	1 938	1 116	72.86	3.72	0.58	4.31	Y
105	阜新市 Fuxin Shi	612 249	2 374	1 777	58.34	5.56	0.75	2.20	Y
106	彰武县 Zhangwu Xian	399 455	1 103	761	51.41	1.36	0.69	3.98	Y
107	辽阳县 Liaoyang Xian	465 579	1 322	973	63.62	5.37	0.74	9.00	Y
108	盘锦市大洼区 Dawa Qu,Panjin Shi	329 890	1 040	585	44.81	0.38	0.56	−1.04	Y

序号 No.	肿瘤登记处 Cancer registries	人口数 Population	发病数 New cases	死亡数 Deaths	MV%	DCO%	M/I	发病率变化 Change for CR%	接受 Accepted
109	建平县 Jianping Xian	578 057	1 899	1 324	50. 34	4. 11	0. 70	11. 35	Y
110	长春市绿园区 Lüyuan Qu, Changchun Shi	601 792	540	21	94. 81	1. 30	0. 04	—	
111	德惠市 Dehui Shi	882 838	2 111	1 573	71. 10	1. 42	0. 75	−1. 52	Y
112	吉林市 Jilin Shi	1 983 170	5 989	3 174	55. 18	2. 40	0. 53	−18. 28	Y
113	永吉县 Yongji Xian	397 508	407	44	23. 10	2. 95	0. 11	−26. 67	
114	蛟河市 Jiaohe Shi	424 059	1 167	422	74. 64	0. 34	0. 36	−4. 00	
115	桦甸市 Huadian Shi	446 578	840	242	31. 19	1. 31	0. 29	−9. 75	
116	舒兰市 Shulan Shi	649 935	1 287	870	22. 92	0. 93	0. 68	—	
117	磐石市 Panshi Shi	510 232	892	122	85. 76	0. 34	0. 14	21. 66	
118	通化市 Tonghua Shi	241 138	99	9	81. 82	6. 06	0. 09	—	
119	梅河口市 Meihekou Shi	594 297	1 629	1 058	43. 28	2. 58	0. 65	0. 26	Y
120	集安市 Ji'an Shi	232 918	222	6	81. 98	0. 00	0. 03	—	
121	抚松县 Fusong Xian	280 263	376	191	58. 24	4. 52	0. 51	—	
122	松原市宁江区 Ningjiang Qu, Songyuan Shi	614 616	983	717	35. 50	0. 00	0. 73	—	
123	前郭尔罗斯蒙古族自治县 Qian Gorlos Mongolzu Zizhixian	573 101	1 754	329	21. 15	0. 06	0. 19	—	
124	乾安县 Qian'an Xian	301 438	339	119	74. 93	18. 58	0. 35	—	
125	通榆县 Tongyu Xian	353 492	245	74	60. 00	0. 00	0. 30	—	
126	大安市 Da'an Shi	409 011	374	250	40. 91	0. 00	0. 67	−71. 66	
127	延吉市 Yanji Shi	553 051	1 451	1 022	62. 85	0. 48	0. 70	−3. 83	Y
128	图们市 Tumen Shi	110 436	292	224	45. 89	0. 68	0. 77	−17. 40	Y
129	敦化市 Dunhua Shi	454 723	1 296	848	46. 14	0. 85	0. 65	3. 02	Y
130	珲春市 Hunchun Shi	227 871	550	389	15. 45	6. 18	0. 71	−21. 55	
131	龙井市 Longjing Shi	153 325	448	309	41. 74	0. 45	0. 69	0. 68	Y
132	和龙市 Helong Shi	188 088	422	346	29. 15	5. 45	0. 82	−13. 74	
133	汪清县 Wangqing Xian	218 922	792	540	33. 96	0. 00	0. 68	−1. 60	
134	安图县 Antu Xian	224 270	380	199	53. 95	0. 00	0. 52	2. 12	
135	哈尔滨市道里区 Daoli Qu, Harbin Shi	775 680	2 542	1 758	78. 91	1. 26	0. 69	−0. 43	Y
136	哈尔滨市南岗区 Nangang Qu, Harbin Shi	1 030 216	3 591	2 174	70. 09	1. 14	0. 61	5. 65	Y
137	哈尔滨市香坊区 Xiangfang Qu, Harbin Shi	790 737	2 877	1 666	77. 34	2. 88	0. 58	1. 56	Y

序号 No.	肿瘤登记处 Cancer registries	人口数 Population	发病数 New cases	死亡数 Deaths	MV%	DCO%	M/I	发病率变化 Change for CR%	接受 Accepted
138	尚志市 Shangzhi Shi	585 386	1 361	792	82. 51	0. 29	0. 58	0. 88	Y
139	五常市 Wuchang Shi	881 459	2 316	1 416	66. 71	0. 26	0. 61	11. 04	Y
140	勃利县 Boli Xian	288 677	755	570	80. 66	0. 53	0. 75	−0. 30	Y
141	牡丹江市东安区 Dong'an Qu,Mudanjiang Shi	190 797	624	386	78. 53	0. 64	0. 62	−0. 92	Y
142	牡丹江市阳明区 Yangming Qu,Mudanjiang Shi	232 530	546	356	77. 47	0. 37	0. 65	−0. 31	Y
143	牡丹江市爱民区 Aimin Qu,Mudanjiang Shi	266 482	961	669	81. 69	4. 06	0. 70	−1. 90	Y
144	牡丹江市西安区 Xi'an Qu,Mudanjiang Shi	246 453	714	465	75. 63	0. 56	0. 65	−2. 18	Y
145	海林市 Hailin Shi	377 859	1 023	731	69. 79	0. 49	0. 71	−0. 39	Y
146	上海市 Shanghai Shi	5 979 293	37 367	16 452	73. 18	0. 32	0. 44	8. 21	Y
147	上海市郊区 Rural Areas of Shanghai Shi	8 614 128	49 363	23 175	77. 17	0. 33	0. 47	—	Y
148	南京市溧水区 Lishui Qu,Nanjing Shi	441 061	1 399	978	71. 41	0. 00	0. 70	—	Y
149	南京市高淳区 Gaochun Qu,Nanjing Shi	447 689	1 460	888	74. 04	0. 27	0. 61	—	Y
150	无锡市 Wuxi Shi	2 614 225	10 832	5 944	74. 44	0. 26	0. 55	7. 75	Y
151	江阴市 Jiangyin Shi	1 257 612	5 053	2 856	79. 12	0. 10	0. 57	5. 91	Y
152	宜兴市 Yixing Shi	1 081 560	3 667	2 761	74. 31	0. 41	0. 75	4. 71	Y
153	徐州市 Xuzhou Shi	2 095 190	7 128	3 573	66. 53	2. 86	0. 50	7. 63	Y
154	邳州市 Pizhou Shi	1 945 275	5 019	2 891	66. 33	0. 44	0. 58	—	Y
155	常州市 Changzhou Shi	2 487 026	10 542	5 770	78. 99	0. 18	0. 55	3. 78	Y
156	溧阳市 Liyang Shi	790 545	2 853	1 700	77. 57	0. 07	0. 60	11. 49	Y
157	常州市金坛区 Jintan Qu,Changzhou Shi	548 678	2 436	1 468	73. 03	0. 08	0. 60	7. 14	Y
158	苏州市 Suzhou Shi	3 601 920	13 181	7 273	62. 51	3. 82	0. 55	−6. 47	Y
159	常熟市 Changshu Shi	1 068 524	4 102	2 554	63. 48	0. 49	0. 62	9. 42	Y
160	张家港市 Zhangjiagang Shi	929 223	4 508	2 415	71. 34	0. 80	0. 54	3. 19	Y
161	昆山市 Kunshan Shi	882 974	3 754	1 649	83. 80	0. 16	0. 44	3. 04	Y
162	太仓市 Taicang Shi	490 445	2 036	1 127	66. 70	0. 10	0. 55	5. 11	Y
163	南通市 Nantong Shi	1 951 790	8 044	5 445	65. 58	3. 58	0. 68	0. 90	Y
164	海安市 Hai'an Shi	926 661	3 761	2 646	67. 08	0. 19	0. 70	−3. 65	Y
165	如东县 Rudong Xian	1 023 787	4 336	2 829	71. 40	0. 05	0. 65	10. 73	Y

序号 No.	肿瘤登记处 Cancer registries	人口数 Population	发病数 New cases	死亡数 Deaths	MV%	DCO%	M/I	发病率变化 Change for CR%	接受 Accepted
166	启东市 Qidong Shi	1 113 112	5 773	3 418	62. 31	0. 02	0. 59	1. 45	Y
167	如皋市 Rugao Shi	1 422 236	5 604	3 871	65. 72	0. 11	0. 69	1. 67	Y
168	南通市海门区 Haimen Qu，Nantong Shi	997 130	4 441	2 845	67. 73	0. 05	0. 64	3. 39	Y
169	连云港市 Lianyungang Shi	1 040 878	2 832	1 768	68. 68	0. 71	0. 62	13. 85	Y
170	连云港市赣榆区 Ganyu Qu，Lianyungang Shi	1 201 480	2 892	1 835	60. 68	0. 76	0. 63	2. 28	Y
171	东海县 Donghai Xian	1 246 530	2 691	1 917	69. 97	1. 56	0. 71	0. 83	Y
172	灌云县 Guanyun Xian	1 037 435	2 385	1 778	66. 67	0. 21	0. 75	9. 08	Y
173	灌南县 Guannan Xian	820 441	1 962	1 206	62. 59	2. 24	0. 61	23. 19	Y
174	淮安市淮安区 Huai'an Qu，Huai'an Shi	1 151 449	3 702	2 637	67. 18	0. 08	0. 71	0. 97	Y
175	淮安市淮阴区 Huaiyin Qu，Huai'an Shi	917 956	2 392	1 754	68. 98	1. 17	0. 73	−1. 37	Y
176	淮安市清江浦区 Qingjiangpu Qu，Huai'an Shi	572 702	1 222	762	68. 99	3. 03	0. 62	−4. 01	Y
177	涟水县 Lianshui Xian	1 139 671	2 728	1 999	66. 75	0. 18	0. 73	2. 61	Y
178	淮安市洪泽区 Hongze Qu，Huai'an Shi	368 717	1 010	785	68. 32	0. 20	0. 78	−2. 44	Y
179	盱眙县 Xuyi Xian	798 211	2 034	1 254	81. 27	0. 29	0. 62	−0. 31	Y
180	金湖县 Jinhu Xian	344 378	1 049	725	75. 12	2. 48	0. 69	−4. 79	Y
181	盐城市亭湖区 Tinghu Qu，Yancheng Shi	695 150	2 328	1 517	65. 03	3. 87	0. 65	3. 96	Y
182	盐城市盐都区 Yandu Qu，Yancheng Shi	711 588	2 851	1 826	74. 96	0. 00	0. 64	1. 17	Y
183	响水县 Xiangshui Xian	623 260	1 669	1 181	75. 61	0. 18	0. 71	2. 39	Y
184	滨海县 Binhai Xian	1 225 771	3 027	2 094	66. 34	0. 03	0. 69	1. 55	Y
185	阜宁县 Funing Xian	1 122 771	3 399	2 627	69. 70	0. 12	0. 77	6. 88	Y
186	射阳县 Sheyang Xian	953 461	3 389	2 269	65. 80	0. 00	0. 67	6. 31	Y
187	建湖县 Jianhu Xian	783 485	2 612	1 814	58. 88	0. 00	0. 69	1. 31	Y
188	东台市 Dongtai Shi	1 097 723	4 146	2 841	73. 90	0. 07	0. 69	4. 75	Y
189	盐城市大丰区 Dafeng Qu，Yancheng Shi	710 929	3 262	2 037	65. 14	0. 18	0. 62	6. 64	Y
190	扬州市广陵区 Guangling Qu，Yangzhou Shi	493 513	1 858	1 276	51. 51	0. 27	0. 69	——	Y
191	宝应县 Baoying Xian	886 216	2 222	1 755	75. 61	2. 16	0. 79	−3. 83	Y

序号 No.	肿瘤登记处 Cancer registries	人口数 Population	发病数 New cases	死亡数 Deaths	MV%	DCO%	M/I	发病率变化 Change for CR%	接受 Accepted
192	仪征市 Yizheng Shi	559 804	2 064	1 612	43. 51	0. 15	0. 78	—	Y
193	丹阳市 Danyang Shi	804 788	3 647	2 569	71. 65	0. 44	0. 70	−1. 51	Y
194	扬中市 Yangzhong Shi	282 324	1 077	858	77. 07	0. 09	0. 80	1. 00	Y
195	泰兴市 Taixing Shi	1 177 976	3 898	2 924	78. 22	0. 00	0. 75	−8. 16	Y
196	宿迁市宿城区 Sucheng Qu,Suqian Shi	738 809	1 727	1 131	57. 56	1. 16	0. 65	12. 91	Y
197	泗阳县 Siyang Xian	1 054 649	3 152	2 205	73. 95	1. 40	0. 70	11. 09	Y
198	杭州市 Hangzhou Shi	7 613 736	33 440	13 282	86. 02	0. 68	0. 40	6. 78	Y
199	宁波市鄞州区 Yinzhou Qu, Ningbo Shi	789 069	3 961	1 404	83. 62	0. 08	0. 35	19. 31	Y
200	慈溪市 Cixi Shi	1 054 217	4 726	2 435	72. 26	0. 38	0. 52	13. 51	Y
201	温州市鹿城区 Lucheng Qu, Wenzhou Shi	774 071	3 282	1 367	86. 93	0. 24	0. 42	2. 67	Y
202	嘉兴市 Jiaxing Shi	562 884	2 728	1 107	76. 76	0. 00	0. 41	0. 37	Y
203	嘉善县 Jiashan Xian	396 157	2 240	1 001	79. 29	0. 00	0. 45	−0. 35	Y
204	海宁市 Haining Shi	694 108	2 748	1 239	79. 08	0. 00	0. 45	3. 05	Y
205	长兴县 Changxing Xian	634 486	2 947	1 297	80. 15	0. 00	0. 44	19. 40	Y
206	绍兴市上虞区 Shangyu Qu, Shaoxing Shi	722 235	3 910	1 652	89. 59	0. 00	0. 42	5. 52	Y
207	永康市 Yongkang Shi	621 111	2 584	1 178	79. 41	4. 68	0. 46	2. 67	Y
208	开化县 Kaihua Xian	361 213	1 146	567	74. 96	0. 00	0. 49	7. 19	Y
209	岱山县 Daishan Xian	180 388	1 256	559	77. 39	0. 08	0. 45	5. 35	Y
210	仙居县 Xianju Xian	517 744	2 327	984	65. 32	0. 00	0. 42	8. 15	Y
211	龙泉市 Longquan Shi	290 850	1 218	570	76. 85	2. 71	0. 47	13. 39	Y
212	合肥市 Hefei Shi	2 819 064	8 291	4 692	62. 75	0. 88	0. 57	−0. 99	Y
213	长丰县 Changfeng Xian	776 962	2 268	1 252	53. 92	0. 04	0. 55	3. 12	Y
214	肥东县 Feidong Xian	1 072 735	3 860	2 234	58. 89	0. 16	0. 58	7. 67	Y
215	肥西县 Feixi Xian	831 209	3 727	2 182	53. 98	0. 99	0. 59	−2. 32	Y
216	庐江县 Lujiang Xian	1 207 207	4 675	2 873	58. 63	0. 00	0. 61	−0. 71	Y
217	巢湖市 Chaohu Shi	858 597	2 542	1 677	48. 66	0. 00	0. 66	−8. 54	Y
218	芜湖市 Wuhu Shi	1 481 986	4 598	2 731	71. 73	0. 00	0. 59	0. 99	Y
219	芜湖市繁昌区 Fanchang Qu,Wuhu Shi	274 390	890	512	72. 25	0. 00	0. 58	—	Y
220	南陵县 Nanling Xian	548 153	1 761	805	75. 64	0. 00	0. 46	—	Y
221	蚌埠市 Bengbu Shi	1 164 366	2 441	1 237	74. 97	0. 04	0. 51	8. 49	Y

序号 No.	肿瘤登记处 Cancer registries	人口数 Population	发病数 New cases	死亡数 Deaths	MV%	DCO%	M/I	发病率变化 Change for CR%	接受 Accepted
222	五河县 Wuhe Xian	693 369	1 628	1 008	61. 18	0. 37	0. 62	−1. 49	Y
223	淮南市大通区 Datong Qu, Huainan Shi	184 996	416	101	79. 81	0. 00	0. 24	7. 83	
224	淮南市田家庵区 Tianjia'an Qu, Huainan Shi	525 299	1 752	460	69. 35	1. 66	0. 26	21. 75	
225	淮南市谢家集区 Xiejiaji Qu, Huainan Shi	308 277	901	315	95. 23	0. 00	0. 35	−7. 24	
226	淮南市八公山区 Bagongshan Qu, Huainan Shi	153 628	375	96	53. 33	4. 80	0. 26	14. 36	
227	淮南市潘集区 Panji Qu, Huainan Shi	456 348	1 106	498	41. 41	0. 36	0. 45	−10. 80	Y
228	凤台县 Fengtai Xian	598 000	1 364	562	60. 70	0. 00	0. 41	13. 69	
229	淮南市毛集区 Maoji Qu, Huainan Shi	134 679	360	89	96. 11	0. 56	0. 25	—	
230	淮南市高新区 Gaoxin Qu, Huainan Shi	48 701	117	36	89. 74	0. 00	0. 31	—	
231	马鞍山市 Ma'anshan Shi	636 763	2 133	1 301	80. 73	1. 83	0. 61	—	Y
232	当涂县 Dangtu Xian	477 996	1 614	933	70. 14	0. 81	0. 58	−0. 41	Y
233	铜陵市 Tongling Shi	442 960	1 381	944	69. 15	2. 46	0. 68	3. 47	Y
234	铜陵市义安区 Yi'an Qu, Tongling Shi	294 705	976	609	69. 47	0. 00	0. 62	5. 45	Y
235	安庆市迎江区 Yingjiang Qu, Anqing Shi	217 847	557	296	69. 30	7. 18	0. 53	—	Y
236	安庆市大观区 Daguan Qu, Anqing Shi	261 729	828	426	64. 25	1. 33	0. 51	—	Y
237	安庆市宜秀区 Yixiu Qu, Anqing Shi	170 828	520	267	54. 62	6. 15	0. 51	61. 18	Y
238	怀宁县 Huaining Xian	705 983	1 397	866	26. 06	7. 30	0. 62	—	
239	太湖县 Taihu Xian	580 978	1 464	775	45. 01	3. 96	0. 53	—	Y
240	望江县 Wangjiang Xian	631 136	1 399	503	58. 76	4. 50	0. 36	—	
241	岳西县 Yuexi Xian	413 408	1 355	467	38. 67	0. 00	0. 34	73. 47	
242	桐城市 Tongcheng Shi	681 535	1 979	685	43. 71	13. 34	0. 35	—	
243	潜山市 Qianshan Shi	576 454	1 274	686	67. 74	4. 47	0. 54	—	Y
244	天长市 Tianchang Shi	628 006	1 473	1 195	94. 30	0. 00	0. 81	0. 83	Y
245	阜阳市颍州区 Yingzhou Qu, Fuyang Shi	801 703	1 799	935	24. 07	0. 00	0. 52	−5. 85	

序号 No.	肿瘤登记处 Cancer registries	人口数 Population	发病数 New cases	死亡数 Deaths	MV%	DCO%	M/I	发病率变化 Change for CR%	接受 Accepted
246	阜阳市颍东区 Yingdong Qu, Fuyang Shi	667 120	1 475	999	46. 24	0. 14	0. 68	−2. 60	Y
247	太和县 Taihe Xian	1 773 939	5 137	3 157	70. 39	0. 25	0. 61	3. 50	Y
248	阜南县 Funan Xian	1 728 000	4 013	2 455	61. 28	1. 97	0. 61	7. 51	Y
249	颍上县 Yingshang Xian	1 763 793	3 433	1 752	70. 99	2. 27	0. 51	−9. 57	
250	宿州市埇桥区 Yongqiao Qu, Suzhou Shi	1 729 998	4 337	2 707	53. 82	1. 75	0. 62	1. 49	Y
251	灵璧县 Lingbi Xian	1 028 981	2 700	1 568	58. 33	0. 44	0. 58	−7. 85	Y
252	六安市金安区 Jin'an Qu, Lu'an Shi	845 041	1 889	1 026	82. 21	0. 00	0. 54	—	Y
253	六安市叶集区 Yeji Qu, Lu'an Shi	233 005	128	123	82. 03	0. 00	0. 96	—	
254	寿县 Shou Xian	1 220 244	3 184	1 954	81. 53	3. 14	0. 61	3. 60	Y
255	舒城县 Shucheng Xian	767 999	1 034	316	100. 00	0. 00	0. 31	—	
256	金寨县 Jinzhai Xian	683 502	1 462	895	50. 82	0. 34	0. 61	1. 38	Y
257	霍山县 Huoshan Xian	315 144	312	166	75. 96	6. 09	0. 53	—	
258	蒙城县 Mengcheng Xian	1 138 000	3 063	1 440	24. 03	0. 00	0. 47	30. 03	
259	东至县 Dongzhi Xian	480 977	1 787	1 233	64. 86	0. 00	0. 69	48. 08	Y
260	泾县 Jing Xian	304 998	792	477	81. 19	0. 51	0. 60	2. 22	Y
261	宁国市 Ningguo Shi	383 959	1 025	620	69. 27	5. 07	0. 60	572. 46	Y
262	福清市 Fuqing Shi	744 072	2 109	1 099	65. 34	0. 71	0. 52	9. 55	Y
263	福州市长乐区 Changle Qu, Fuzhou Shi	1 374 165	3 961	2 246	72. 25	7. 83	0. 57	7. 05	Y
264	厦门市 Xiamen Shi	1 700 118	5 078	2 743	85. 21	0. 00	0. 54	10. 96	Y
265	厦门市同安区 Tong'an Qu, Xiamen Shi	368 529	918	668	65. 90	0. 22	0. 73	−3. 77	Accepted
266	厦门市翔安区 Xiang'an Qu, Xiamen Shi	369 259	1 007	611	64. 05	0. 00	0. 61	−1. 28	Y
267	莆田市涵江区 Hanjiang Qu, Putian Shi	447 026	1 441	927	79. 25	2. 98	0. 64	1. 79	Y
268	永安市 Yong'an Shi	331 173	939	548	64. 64	0. 21	0. 58	5. 82	Y
269	惠安县 Hui'an Xian	809 561	2 169	1 707	70. 91	0. 18	0. 79	4. 16	
270	漳州市长泰区 Changtai Qu, Zhangzhou Shi	211 586	477	329	79. 04	0. 00	0. 69	9. 64	Y
271	建瓯市 Jian'ou Shi	551 946	1 345	995	60. 52	0. 07	0. 74	−4. 26	Y
272	龙岩市新罗区 Xinluo Qu, Longyan Shi	543 245	1 826	821	66. 16	0. 00	0. 45	12. 94	Y

序号 No.	肿瘤登记处 Cancer registries	人口数 Population	发病数 New cases	死亡数 Deaths	MV%	DCO%	M/I	发病率变化 Change for CR%	接受 Accepted
273	龙岩市永定区 Yongding Qu,Longyan Shi	505 447	1 175	817	77.45	0.26	0.70	−4.83	Y
274	南昌市青云谱区 Qingyunpu Qu,Nanchang Shi	265 946	601	379	66.72	3.83	0.63	10.54	Y
275	南昌市青山湖区 Qingshanhu Qu,Nanchang Shi	439 400	1 138	604	66.70	0.00	0.53	19.59	Y
276	南昌市新建区 Xinjian Qu,Nanchang Shi	658 700	1 356	972	68.95	1.55	0.72	4.74	Y
277	芦溪县 Luxi Xian	268 500	523	310	75.53	2.68	0.59	−2.79	Y
278	九江市浔阳区 Xunyang Qu,Jiujiang Shi	288 149	682	418	73.31	2.64	0.61	3.42	Y
279	武宁县 Wuning Xian	396 701	753	533	78.49	1.46	0.71	−11.84	Y
280	新余市渝水区 Yushui Qu,Xinyu Shi	868 136	1 902	922	63.41	2.16	0.48	16.21	Y
281	鹰潭市余江区 Yujiang Qu,Yingtan Shi	372 074	873	531	66.32	1.26	0.61	4.88	Y
282	赣州市章贡区 Zhanggong Qu,Ganzhou Shi	496 933	1 287	746	63.33	0.70	0.58	7.92	Y
283	赣州市南康区 Nankang Qu,Ganzhou Shi	807 347	1 871	842	55.64	0.00	0.45	—	Y
284	赣州市赣县区 Ganxian Qu,Ganzhou Shi	567 518	1 219	709	67.92	3.77	0.58	9.51	Y
285	信丰县 Xinfeng Xian	685 815	1 405	698	70.04	1.00	0.50	6.93	Y
286	大余县 Dayu Xian	298 600	571	378	61.47	3.68	0.66	−0.02	Y
287	上犹县 Shangyou Xian	267 227	557	349	68.04	4.31	0.63	8.19	Y
288	崇义县 Chongyi Xian	194 760	355	223	65.92	2.25	0.63	1.45	Y
289	龙南市 Longnan Shi	314 556	702	317	52.99	0.43	0.45	8.07	Y
290	宁都县 Ningdu Xian	830 462	1 409	1 001	54.65	1.99	0.71	—	
291	于都县 Yudu Xian	870 588	1 864	1 120	64.16	0.97	0.60	−4.35	Y
292	兴国县 Xingguo Xian	739 725	1 322	806	68.46	0.53	0.61	—	
293	吉安市吉州区 Jizhou Qu,Ji'anShi	345 084	722	380	61.91	0.00	0.53	−0.05	Y
294	峡江县 Xiajiang Xian	189 805	373	203	65.42	1.07	0.54	10.80	Y
295	安福县 Anfu Xian	398 151	808	560	68.32	0.62	0.69	−1.70	Y
296	万载县 Wanzai Xian	489 490	1 134	662	63.93	2.03	0.58	8.07	Y
297	上高县 Shanggao Xian	337 815	691	438	68.02	2.03	0.63	5.74	Y
298	靖安县 Jing'an Xian	152 617	296	219	65.20	2.03	0.74	0.97	Y

序号 No.	肿瘤登记处 Cancer registries	人口数 Population	发病数 New cases	死亡数 Deaths	MV%	DCO%	M/I	发病率变化 Change for CR%	接受 Accepted
299	樟树市 Zhangshu Shi	595 135	1 289	832	68.89	2.02	0.65	—	Y
300	乐安县 Le'an Xian	357 160	649	410	67.49	2.62	0.63	2.34	Y
301	宜黄县 Yihuang Xian	230 803	417	266	66.43	2.40	0.64	0.22	Y
302	抚州市东乡区 Dongxiang Qu,Fuzhou Shi	451 829	793	488	77.18	0.25	0.62	-0.60	
303	上饶市信州区 Xinzhou Qu,Shangrao Shi	428 196	1 174	724	66.18	2.73	0.62	5.18	Y
304	上饶市广丰区 Guangfeng Qu,Shangrao Shi	780 844	1 627	1 032	62.45	2.03	0.63	14.57	Y
305	上饶市广信区 Guangxin Qu,Shangrao Shi	716 585	1 292	948	61.53	3.56	0.73	—	Y
306	铅山县 Yanshan Xian	440 186	818	530	65.28	2.20	0.65	5.87	Y
307	横峰县 Hengfeng Xian	190 691	452	295	62.83	3.10	0.65	7.37	Y
308	弋阳县 Yiyang Xian	364 502	719	443	59.94	1.67	0.62	8.92	Y
309	余干县 Yugan Xian	928 021	1 674	1 051	61.17	1.08	0.63	-2.62	Y
310	鄱阳县 Poyang Xian	1 324 377	2 469	1 515	67.03	0.12	0.61	—	Y
311	万年县 Wannian Xian	370 246	728	468	63.05	1.65	0.64	2.50	Y
312	婺源县 Wuyuan Xian	345 636	731	472	63.34	4.51	0.65	3.50	Y
313	德兴市 Dexing Shi	303 386	558	339	65.41	1.79	0.61	2.61	Y
314	济南市 Jinan Shi	3 977 922	13 488	7 000	82.95	1.87	0.52	2.16	Y
315	济南市章丘区 Zhangqiu Qu,Jinan Shi	1 039 068	3 957	2 357	68.23	2.07	0.60	-0.90	Y
316	济南市莱芜区 Laiwu Qu, Jinan Shi	988 554	3 761	2 239	50.78	0.82	0.60	2.79	Y
317	青岛市 Qingdao Shi	1 880 695	5 437	3 076	80.03	7.96	0.57	1.16	Y
318	青岛市黄岛区 Huangdao Qu,Qingdao Shi	1 297 759	4 681	2 900	66.93	1.99	0.62	2.88	Y
319	淄博市临淄区 Linzi Qu, Zibo Shi	617 110	2 172	1 039	72.97	3.13	0.48	0.56	Y
320	沂源县 Yiyuan Xian	575 777	1 903	1 045	69.26	0.47	0.55	0.36	Y
321	滕州市 Tengzhou Shi	1 731 615	4 853	2 823	75.62	0.99	0.58	1.27	Y
322	广饶县 Guangrao Xian	532 794	1 836	1 061	79.58	0.16	0.58	9.66	Y
323	烟台市 Yantai Shi	2 212 772	8 756	3 986	69.27	1.86	0.46	3.58	Y
324	招远市 Zhaoyuan Shi	576 359	2 330	1 619	63.39	0.09	0.69	-5.12	Y
325	潍坊市潍城区 Weicheng Qu,Weifang Shi	372 859	1 316	620	85.41	0.08	0.47	—	Y

序号 No.	肿瘤登记处 Cancer registries	人口数 Population	发病数 New cases	死亡数 Deaths	MV%	DCO%	M/I	发病率变化 Change for CR%	接受 Accepted
326	临朐县 Linqu Xian	925 567	3 233	2 028	79.83	0.53	0.63	12.22	Y
327	青州市 Qingzhou Shi	969 747	3 771	2 001	68.89	0.11	0.53	—	Y
328	高密市 Gaomi Shi	904 235	3 111	1 915	70.85	0.61	0.62	8.92	Y
329	济宁市任城区 Rencheng Qu,Jining Shi	1 271 204	2 901	1 231	87.28	0.59	0.42	4.20	
330	汶上县 Wenshang Xian	823 177	2 308	1 394	86.53	1.13	0.60	−2.03	Y
331	梁山县 Liangshan Xian	820 826	2 432	1 220	70.44	0.00	0.50	2.10	Y
332	曲阜市 Qufu Shi	654 287	1 724	1 112	80.51	1.45	0.65	−10.37	Y
333	邹城市 Zoucheng Shi	1 157 634	3 316	2 129	77.41	0.48	0.64	−8.22	Y
334	宁阳县 Ningyang Xian	837 486	2 654	1 718	81.27	0.26	0.65	−1.21	Y
335	肥城市 Feicheng Shi	988 900	3 938	2 437	70.01	0.66	0.62	3.14	Y
336	乳山市 Rushan Shi	547 486	2 762	1 390	63.07	7.71	0.50	22.41	Y
337	日照市东港区 Donggang Qu,Rizhao Shi	928 955	2 762	1 651	84.50	3.04	0.60	7.59	Y
338	莒县 Ju Xian	1 160 585	3 406	1 527	66.79	0.06	0.45	—	Y
339	沂南县 Yinan Xian	976 473	3 229	1 652	73.68	0.09	0.51	23.59	Y
340	沂水县 Yishui Xian	1 184 445	3 094	1 947	67.84	2.04	0.63	−2.38	Y
341	莒南县 Junan Xian	861 342	2 416	1 512	56.46	0.33	0.63	−11.96	Y
342	德州市德城区 Decheng Qu,Dezhou Shi	401 382	1 415	531	48.20	0.00	0.38	85.78	
343	聊城市东昌府区 Dongchang-fu Qu,Liaocheng Shi	1 282 297	3 709	1 563	78.40	3.18	0.42	—	Y
344	高唐县 Gaotang Xian	512 634	1 573	868	69.55	0.00	0.55	4.17	Y
345	滨州市滨城区 Bincheng Qu,Binzhou Shi	695 653	2 290	1 188	77.77	0.00	0.52	8.69	Y
346	菏泽市牡丹区 Mudan Qu,Heze Shi	1 388 495	4 079	2 891	32.02	1.40	0.71	25.17	Y
347	单县 Shan Xian	1 275 499	3 433	1 666	80.37	0.17	0.49	−3.68	Y
348	巨野县 Juye Xian	1 098 154	3 037	1 919	37.93	0.92	0.63	2.57	Y
349	郑州市 Zhengzhou Shi	2 988 991	8 178	1 817	75.02	1.01	0.22	6.64	
350	巩义市 Gongyi Shi	847 567	1 982	1 031	50.25	4.09	0.52	1.61	Y
351	开封市祥符区 Xiangfu Qu,Kaifeng Shi	667 086	1 738	854	71.98	0.58	0.49	10.59	Y
352	洛阳市 Luoyang Shi	1 613 610	5 189	2 728	76.82	2.00	0.53	10.68	Y
353	洛阳市孟津区 Mengjin Qu,Luoyang Shi	468 250	1 404	796	74.79	1.50	0.57	2.66	Y

序号 No.	肿瘤登记处 Cancer registries	人口数 Population	发病数 New cases	死亡数 Deaths	MV%	DCO%	M/I	发病率变化 Change for CR%	接受 Accepted
354	新安县 Xin'an Xian	539 740	1 542	949	67.06	0.84	0.62	11.41	Y
355	栾川县 Luanchuan Xian	355 734	979	628	76.51	0.31	0.64	10.73	Y
356	嵩县 Song Xian	638 907	1 724	1 176	73.14	1.51	0.68	6.54	Y
357	汝阳县 Ruyang Xian	526 693	1 249	701	73.74	3.12	0.56	−2.23	Y
358	宜阳县 Yiyang Xian	711 526	1 988	1 261	71.03	0.86	0.63	3.31	Y
359	洛宁县 Luoning Xian	509 488	1 371	853	72.72	0.22	0.62	5.63	Y
360	伊川县 Yichuan Xian	924 743	2 063	1 436	83.42	1.02	0.70	−1.86	Y
361	洛阳市偃师区 Yanshi Qu, Luoyang Shi	632 704	1 900	1 049	73.37	1.58	0.55	4.16	Y
362	平顶山市 Pingdingshan Shi	898 044	2 666	1 295	75.96	0.15	0.49	27.97	Y
363	鲁山县 Lushan Xian	950 786	2 365	1 794	84.40	0.42	0.76	−1.03	Y
364	郏县 Jia Xian	644 259	1 776	1 033	62.05	0.28	0.58	15.16	Y
365	安阳市 Anyang Shi	1 179 532	3 308	1 241	85.55	0.00	0.38	6.37	
366	林州市 Linzhou Shi	1 129 335	3 754	2 266	82.07	0.77	0.60	7.22	Y
367	鹤壁市 Hebi Shi	650 048	1 839	1 138	69.98	2.07	0.62	1.93	Y
368	新乡市 Xinxiang Shi	958 783	2 415	611	86.63	0.04	0.25	−3.47	
369	辉县市 Huixian Shi	898 852	2 360	1 445	79.49	0.59	0.61	−4.04	Y
370	焦作市 Jiaozuo Shi	803 162	2 296	693	89.29	1.44	0.30	−0.19	
371	濮阳市华龙区 Hualong Qu, Puyang Shi	436 597	1 641	763	79.52	4.45	0.46	21.58	Y
372	濮阳县 Puyang Xian	1 130 427	3 370	1 727	67.45	0.18	0.51	8.11	Y
373	禹州市 Yuzhou Shi	1 315 977	3 520	2 842	82.56	1.16	0.81	6.40	Y
374	漯河市 Luohe Shi	832 256	2 125	1 371	72.75	1.46	0.65	−4.78	Y
375	漯河市郾城区 Yancheng Qu, Luohe Shi	500 538	1 309	865	66.31	2.98	0.66	0.32	Accepted
376	舞阳县 Wuyang Xian	545 479	1 435	929	59.86	7.04	0.65	−0.22	Y
377	临颍县 Linying Xian	732 269	1 484	645	73.65	0.88	0.43	3.08	
378	三门峡市湖滨区 Hubin Qu, Sanmenxia Shi	290 026	987	520	87.94	0.51	0.53	10.66	Y
379	南阳市卧龙区 Wolong Qu, Nanyang Shi	933 468	2 506	1 500	67.28	3.87	0.60	4.25	Y
380	南召县 Nanzhao Xian	553 949	1 739	886	75.16	0.63	0.51	18.10	Y
381	方城县 Fangcheng Xian	1 158 481	2 915	1 777	77.08	0.51	0.61	1.41	Y
382	内乡县 Neixiang Xian	735 699	2 027	1 321	71.48	1.09	0.65	2.19	Y
383	睢县 Sui Xian	859 688	2 134	780	50.98	0.00	0.37	1.40	

序号 No.	肿瘤登记处 Cancer registries	人口数 Population	发病数 New cases	死亡数 Deaths	MV%	DCO%	M/I	发病率变化 Change for CR%	接受 Accepted
384	虞城县 Yucheng Xian	1 136 037	3 185	1 915	67. 91	0. 00	0. 60	15. 35	Y
385	信阳市浉河区 Shihe Qu, Xinyang Shi	640 884	1 635	832	82. 20	3. 00	0. 51	12. 68	Y
386	罗山县 Luoshan Xian	761 677	1 899	973	77. 51	0. 21	0. 51	−10. 29	Y
387	固始县 Gushi Xian	1 846 659	5 483	1 552	81. 52	3. 43	0. 28	−16. 46	
388	沈丘县 Shenqiu Xian	1 192 576	3 272	2 173	63. 97	2. 20	0. 66	−2. 08	Y
389	郸城县 Dancheng Xian	1 395 356	3 774	2 428	66. 53	2. 38	0. 64	3. 35	Y
390	太康县 Taikang Xian	1 615 914	5 899	2 089	63. 69	0. 00	0. 35	17. 84	
391	西平县 Xiping Xian	8872 68	2 404	1 546	72. 96	2. 75	0. 64	4. 35	Y
392	济源市 Jiyuan Shi	725 524	2 074	1 277	71. 84	0. 96	0. 62	6. 02	Y
393	武汉市 Wuhan Shi	5 024 001	19 284	10 228	83. 30	5. 17	0. 53	−0. 48	Y
394	大冶市 Daye Shi	885 702	2 329	1 400	73. 51	5. 24	0. 60	1. 75	Y
395	十堰市郧阳区 Yunyang Qu, Shiyan Shi	567 928	1 263	957	68. 17	0. 63	0. 76	0. 51	Y
396	丹江口市 Danjiangkou Shi	449 200	1 154	777	50. 61	0. 00	0. 67	—	Y
397	宜昌市 Yichang Shi	1 312 927	4 290	2 303	67. 97	3. 89	0. 54	10. 72	Y
398	秭归县 Zigui Xian	370 788	1 128	687	44. 33	25. 53	0. 61		Y
399	五峰土家族自治县 Wufeng Tujiazu Zizhixian	197 832	509	369	69. 74	1. 38	0. 72	3. 71	Y
400	宜都市 Yidu Shi	388 332	1 239	803	58. 27	0. 32	0. 65	—	Y
401	襄阳市 Xiangyang Shi	1 413 726	4 680	2 521	66. 69	6. 09	0. 54	40. 72	Y
402	枣阳市 Zaoyang Shi	1 002 000	2 770	1 644	44. 08	0. 65	0. 59	—	Y
403	宜城市 Yicheng Shi	525 401	1 228	816	50. 49	1. 47	0. 66	−2. 00	Y
404	京山市 Jingshan Shi	629 879	1 425	859	64. 70	0. 07	0. 60	−1. 01	
405	钟祥市 Zhongxiang Shi	1 013 800	2 345	1 485	82. 43	0. 21	0. 63	2. 85	Y
406	云梦县 Yunmeng Xian	541 159	1 358	783	61. 05	0. 59	0. 58	−12. 08	Y
407	荆州市 Jingzhou Shi	1 251 797	3 447	1 777	67. 22	8. 73	0. 52	23. 32	Y
408	公安县 Gong'an Xian	862 802	2 641	1 719	82. 36	0. 19	0. 65	0. 98	Y
409	洪湖市 Honghu Shi	813 201	2 174	1 330	72. 22	0. 23	0. 61	18. 85	Y
410	麻城市 Macheng Shi	1 159 377	3 085	2 033	74. 98	0. 45	0. 66	1. 83	Y
411	嘉鱼县 Jiayu Xian	371 968	818	491	62. 71	3. 42	0. 60	3. 74	Y
412	通城县 Tongcheng Xian	415 396	1 028	594	62. 74	1. 07	0. 58	9. 56	Y
413	恩施市 Enshi Shi	809 188	1 938	1 110	63. 21	1. 19	0. 57	−5. 64	Y
414	天门市 Tianmen Shi	1 272 303	3 376	2 255	66. 82	0. 09	0. 67	2. 37	Y

序号 No.	肿瘤登记处 Cancer registries	人口数 Population	发病数 New cases	死亡数 Deaths	MV%	DCO%	M/I	发病率变化 Change for CR%	接受 Accepted
415	长沙市芙蓉区 Furong Qu， Changsha Shi	414 322	1 471	881	77.77	3.40	0.60	−7.83	Y
416	长沙市天心区 Tianxin Qu， Changsha Shi	485 699	1 927	1 046	78.31	0.05	0.54	8.72	Y
417	长沙市岳麓区 Yuelu Qu， Changsha Shi	751 869	1 494	911	73.03	4.28	0.61	2.24	Y
418	长沙市开福区 Kaifu Qu， Changsha Shi	496 543	1 852	1 185	79.97	0.59	0.64	−0.37	Y
419	长沙市雨花区 Yuhua Qu， Changsha Shi	705 419	1 830	1 044	78.09	0.27	0.57	2.63	Y
420	长沙市望城区 Wangcheng Qu，Changsha Shi	623 785	1 665	1 054	77.54	1.02	0.63	12.89	Y
421	长沙县 Changsha Xian	795 988	2 547	1 495	79.58	0.94	0.59	9.90	Y
422	浏阳市 Liuyang Shi	1 488 741	3 205	2 151	73.79	0.37	0.67	—	Y
423	株洲市芦淞区 Lusong Qu， Zhuzhou Shi	236 818	726	423	77.13	2.48	0.58	8.18	Y
424	株洲市石峰区 Shifeng Qu， Zhuzhou Shi	244 177	626	429	73.16	6.55	0.69	4.25	Y
425	攸县 You Xian	810 098	1 801	1 376	71.74	0.11	0.76	11.03	Y
426	湘潭市雨湖区 Yuhu Qu， Xiangtan Shi	513 375	1 660	744	73.37	0.96	0.45	8.30	Y
427	衡东县 Hengdong Xian	757 903	1 545	1 083	71.78	0.91	0.70	4.76	Y
428	常宁市 Changning Shi	961 700	2 110	1 396	78.63	0.19	0.66	21.91	Y
429	邵东市 Shaodong Shi	1 341 199	3 460	2 110	76.33	4.54	0.61	9.46	Y
430	新宁县 Xinning Xian	651 500	1 178	824	71.99	2.12	0.70	3.93	Y
431	岳阳市岳阳楼区 Yueyang- glou Qu，Yueyang Shi	518 550	1 465	785	77.41	0.82	0.54	9.61	Y
432	常德市武陵区 Wuling Qu， Changde Shi	430 415	1 202	804	74.04	6.16	0.67	3.57	Y
433	津市市 Jinshi Shi	234 310	783	422	74.20	5.49	0.54	—	Y
434	慈利县 Cili Xian	699 525	1 849	1 047	75.01	0.97	0.57	19.13	Y
435	益阳市资阳区 Ziyang Qu， Yiyang Shi	434 892	1 033	730	75.22	3.00	0.71	2.10	Y
436	桃江县 Taojiang Xian	887 149	2 034	1 204	77.58	4.62	0.59	3.29	Y
437	临武县 Linwu Xian	393 401	819	528	81.32	1.83	0.64	−3.76	Y
438	资兴市 Zixing Shi	377 902	897	603	75.36	3.12	0.67	6.88	Y

序号 No.	肿瘤登记处 Cancer registries	人口数 Population	发病数 New cases	死亡数 Deaths	MV%	DCO%	M/I	发病率变化 Change for CR%	接受 Accepted
439	道县 Dao Xian	802 150	1 771	1 130	73. 91	7. 62	0. 64	0. 82	Y
440	宁远县 Ningyuan Xian	893 900	1 948	1 153	77. 36	0. 62	0. 59	3. 86	Y
441	新田县 Xintian Xian	448 250	1 208	667	74. 01	0. 33	0. 55	53. 98	Y
442	麻阳苗族自治县 Mayang Miaozu Zizhixian	398 250	784	503	66. 71	3. 70	0. 64	3. 44	Y
443	洪江市 Hongjiang Shi	428 696	847	636	69. 89	1. 53	0. 75	11. 73	Y
444	娄底市娄星区 Louxing Qu, Loudi Shi	613 553	1 520	983	79. 54	2. 89	0. 65	—	Y
445	冷水江市 Lengshuijiang Shi	369 550	974	597	75. 26	3. 08	0. 61	5. 17	Y
446	涟源市 Lianyuan Shi	1 145 000	2 299	1 501	77. 69	0. 00	0. 65	−3. 24	Y
447	广州市 Guangzhou Shi	4 486 633	17 734	8 493	78. 44	0. 24	0. 48	2. 20	Y
448	广州市郊区 Rural Areas of Guangzhou Shi	4 641 183	13 311	6 102	77. 82	0. 17	0. 46	7. 29	Y
449	韶关市曲江区 Qujiang Qu, Shaoguan Shi	265 926	1 062	590	53. 58	0. 00	0. 56	—	Y
450	翁源县 Wengyuan Xian	397 284	1 174	649	52. 73	0. 00	0. 55	—	Y
451	南雄市 Nanxiong Shi	507 074	1 205	815	57. 51	4. 40	0. 68	6. 41	Y
452	深圳市 Shenzhen Shi	4 378 296	8 946	2 176	78. 27	2. 11	0. 24	−11. 02	Y
453	珠海市 Zhuhai Shi	1 238 717	3 610	1 641	73. 30	0. 72	0. 45	0. 86	Y
454	佛山市禅城区 Chancheng Qu, Foshan Shi	687 711	2 657	1 173	57. 62	0. 00	0. 44	—	Y
455	佛山市南海区 Nanhai Qu, Foshan Shi	1 497 607	4 478	2 271	68. 71	0. 00	0. 51	3. 55	Y
456	佛山市顺德区 Shunde Qu, Foshan Shi	1 475 826	5 109	2 604	62. 97	0. 00	0. 51	2. 82	Y
457	佛山市三水区 Sanshui Qu, Foshan Shi	438 336	969	742	66. 56	0. 83	0. 77	—	Y
458	佛山市高明区 Gaoming Qu, Foshan Shi	322 448	1 397	472	56. 98	0. 00	0. 34	—	
459	江门市 Jiangmen Shi	687 335	2 441	1 281	76. 65	0. 16	0. 52	8. 11	Y
460	湛江市赤坎区 Chikan Qu, Zhanjiang Shi	261 444	1 315	138	73. 00	0. 00	0. 10	—	
461	湛江市霞山区 Xiashan Qu, Zhanjiang Shi	376 922	2 577	370	80. 79	0. 00	0. 14	—	
462	徐闻县 Xuwen Xian	727 268	31	414	12. 90	0. 00	13. 35	—	
463	肇庆市端州区 Duanzhou Qu, Zhaoqing Shi	417 377	1 473	692	69. 31	0. 00	0. 47	18. 01	Y

序号 No.	肿瘤登记处 Cancer registries	人口数 Population	发病数 New cases	死亡数 Deaths	MV%	DCO%	M/I	发病率变化 Change for CR%	接受 Accepted
464	四会市 Sihui Shi	429 374	788	706	31.35	0.76	0.90	−17.50	Y
465	惠州市惠阳区 Huiyang Qu, Huizhou Shi	401 139	1 025	619	74.05	7.22	0.60	−13.75	Y
466	梅州市梅江区 Meijiang Qu, Meizhou Shi	356 527	1 170	512	82.22	1.54	0.44	10.82	Y
467	梅州市梅县区 Meixian Qu, Meizhou Shi	612 499	1 861	1 034	53.95	2.53	0.56	8.96	Y
468	河源市源城区 Yuancheng Qu, Heyuan Shi	350 815	1 396	253	35.96	0.29	0.18	—	
469	阳江市阳东区 Yangdong Qu, Yangjiang Shi	518 233	1 098	635	69.22	0.00	0.58	0.30	Y
470	清远市清城区 Qingcheng Qu, Qingyuan Shi	763 192	666	974	63.96	0.00	1.46	—	
471	阳山县 Yangshan Xian	575 637	1 397	868	51.83	7.30	0.62	15.26	Y
472	东莞市 Dongguan Shi	2 217 578	6 253	2 987	71.10	0.03	0.48	1.21	Y
473	中山市 Zhongshan Shi	1 760 787	5 691	2 836	77.79	0.00	0.50	1.04	Y
474	潮州市潮安区 Chaoan Qu, Chaozhou Shi	1 143 775	153	1 574	35.29	0.00	10.29	—	
475	揭西县 Jiexi Xian	1 006 515	2 282	1 106	55.13	0.00	0.48	−23.21	Y
476	普宁市 Puning Shi	2 462 731	4 815	2 507	70.63	7.17	0.52	—	Y
477	罗定市 Luoding Shi	1 292 822	2 497	1 666	55.63	2.88	0.67	6.12	Y
478	南宁市兴宁区 Xingning Qu, Nanning Shi	349 414	916	535	61.68	1.75	0.58	−1.80	Y
479	南宁市青秀区 Qingxiu Qu, Nanning Shi	766 901	1 791	1 025	82.30	1.45	0.57	12.85	Y
480	南宁市江南区 Jiangnan Qu, Nanning Shi	373 600	796	582	54.40	3.27	0.73	6.64	Y
481	南宁经济技术开发区 Nanning Economic & Technological Development Zone	161 985	314	186	60.83	0.32	0.59	16.09	Y
482	南宁市西乡塘区 Xixiangtang Qu, Nanning Shi	815 000	2 176	1 307	74.82	0.14	0.60	−1.10	Y
483	南宁市良庆区 Liangqing Qu, Nanning Shi	305 167	636	376	67.92	0.31	0.59	−14.60	Y
484	南宁市邕宁区 Yongning Qu, Nanning Shi	274 498	641	413	55.38	1.09	0.64	—	Y
485	南宁东盟经济开发区 National Nanning-ASEAN Economic Development Zone	39 219	92	68	63.04	1.09	0.74	0.33	Y

序号 No.	肿瘤登记处 Cancer registries	人口数 Population	发病数 New cases	死亡数 Deaths	MV%	DCO%	M/I	发病率变化 Change for CR%	接受 Accepted
486	南宁市武鸣区 Wuming Qu, Nanning Shi	683 867	1 394	811	65.35	0.22	0.58	—	Y
487	隆安县 Long'an Xian	422 396	946	547	60.99	0.21	0.58	6.29	Y
488	马山县 Mashan Xian	575 174	1 077	647	42.99	1.39	0.60	—	Y
489	上林县 Shanglin Xian	506 942	962	633	30.15	0.00	0.66	—	
490	宾阳县 Binyang Xian	1 055 912	2 480	1 577	50.08	0.40	0.64	−8.62	Y
491	横州市 Hengzhou Shi	1 265 620	2 485	1 650	40.93	5.59	0.66	—	Y
492	柳州市 Liuzhou Shi	1 827 300	4 773	3 033	73.45	0.04	0.64	2.12	Y
493	鹿寨县 Luzhai Xian	352 001	722	455	82.83	6.65	0.63	—	Y
494	桂林市 Guilin Shi	802 204	2 298	1 366	62.49	0.83	0.59	−2.46	Y
495	梧州市 Wuzhou Shi	801 233	1 951	1 262	68.48	0.31	0.65	0.15	Y
496	苍梧县 Cangwu Xian	410 733	892	606	56.73	1.35	0.68	−5.52	Y
497	岑溪市 Cenxi Shi	777 875	1 578	805	57.35	0.44	0.51	—	Y
498	北海市 Beihai Shi	727 602	2 204	1 190	66.70	0.45	0.54	3.21	Y
499	合浦县 Hepu Xian	935 702	2 418	1 786	53.06	2.23	0.74	0.12	Y
500	钦州市钦南区 Qinnan Qu, Qinzhou Shi	627 428	1 208	723	62.33	0.75	0.60	−6.19	Y
501	贵港市港北区 Gangbei Qu, Guigang Shi	724 602	1 440	962	75.14	2.99	0.67	4.42	Y
502	贵港市港南区 Gangnan Qu, Guigang Shi	704 497	1 346	838	67.16	0.07	0.62	−2.04	Y
503	贵港市覃塘区 Qintang Qu, Guigang Shi	607 113	1 146	975	43.46	1.13	0.85	4.01	Y
504	平南县 Pingnan Xian	1 538 894	4 148	2 263	69.77	0.96	0.55	2.51	Y
505	桂平市 Guiping Shi	2 034 209	3 820	2 529	44.27	0.68	0.66	—	Y
506	陆川县 Luchuan Xian	800 186	1 430	1 077	68.53	0.00	0.75	−2.98	
507	北流市 Beiliu Shi	1 536 902	2 825	1 785	57.66	0.00	0.63	35.51	Y
508	百色市右江区 Youjiang Qu, Bose Shi	353 661	672	398	73.96	6.70	0.59	−3.72	Y
509	百色市田阳区 Tianyang Qu, Bose Shi	342 938	642	480	71.03	0.00	0.75	−1.53	Y
510	田东县 Tiandong Xian	434 084	769	480	66.19	0.00	0.62	—	
511	凌云县 Lingyun Xian	195 300	337	191	79.82	0.00	0.57	—	
512	贺州市平桂区 Pinggui Qu, Hezhou Shi	412 299	991	475	41.98	2.02	0.48	—	Y

序号 No.	肿瘤登记处 Cancer registries	人口数 Population	发病数 New cases	死亡数 Deaths	MV%	DCO%	M/I	发病率变化 Change for CR%	接受 Accepted
513	罗城仫佬族自治县 Luocheng Mulaozu Zizhixian	389 439	736	494	74.73	0.41	0.67	−1.98	Y
514	来宾市兴宾区 Xingbin Qu, Laibin Shi	969 700	1 755	1 172	41.48	0.17	0.67	—	Y
515	合山市 Heshan Shi	118 196	355	281	68.45	0.00	0.79	4.30	Y
516	崇左市江州区 Jiangzhou Qu, Chongzuo Shi	377 256	666	386	87.99	0.45	0.58	—	
517	扶绥县 Fusui Xian	461 786	1 147	855	38.71	1.39	0.75	−3.66	Y
518	大新县 Daxin Xian	385 013	742	544	69.54	0.00	0.73	—	Y
519	三亚市 Sanya Shi	592 206	1 695	765	31.27	1.42	0.45	6.83	Y
520	五指山市 Wuzhishan Shi	104 457	246	101	34.96	0.00	0.41	−5.08	Y
521	琼海市 Qionghai Shi	499 312	1 200	752	76.83	0.08	0.63	−0.17	Y
522	定安县 Ding'an Xian	294 800	985	363	26.60	1.73	0.37	36.03	
523	昌江黎族自治县 Changjiang Lizu Zizhixian	233 500	713	340	33.80	0.00	0.48	24.94	Y
524	陵水黎族自治县 Lingshui Lizu Zizhixian	373 535	901	329	32.08	0.00	0.37	−13.49	
525	重庆市万州区 Wanzhou Qu, Chongqing Shi	1 635 799	4 952	3 298	76.51	0.00	0.67	0.36	Y
526	重庆市涪陵区 Fuling Qu, Chongqing Shi	1 160 201	3 131	1 933	60.43	2.17	0.62	2.75	Y
527	重庆市渝中区 Yuzhong Qu, Chongqing Shi	659 001	2 207	1 123	65.47	3.94	0.51	4.67	Y
528	重庆市大渡口区 Dadukou Qu, Chongqing Shi	355 000	822	377	73.11	0.85	0.46	−29.58	Y
529	重庆市江北区 Jiangbei Qu, Chongqing Shi	874 400	2 420	1 554	70.45	0.25	0.64	41.26	Y
530	重庆市沙坪坝区 Shapingba Qu, Chongqing Shi	1 120 013	3 465	2 132	68.51	0.43	0.62	21.75	Y
531	重庆市九龙坡区 Jiulongpo Qu, Chongqing Shi	951 816	2 283	1 421	79.68	0.88	0.62	−15.98	Y
532	重庆市南岸区 Nan'an Qu, Chongqing Shi	891 001	2 806	1 401	45.87	0.00	0.50	−21.72	Y
533	重庆市北碚区 Beibei Qu, Chongqing Shi	805 801	2 663	1 412	72.81	0.56	0.53	−0.69	Y
534	重庆市綦江区 Qijiang Qu, Chongqing Shi	820 003	2 224	1 152	74.37	0.63	0.52	13.28	Y

序号 No.	肿瘤登记处 Cancer registries	人口数 Population	发病数 New cases	死亡数 Deaths	MV%	DCO%	M/I	发病率变化 Change for CR%	接受 Accepted
535	重庆市大足区 Dazu Qu, Chongqing Shi	787 399	2 484	1 599	70.21	0.04	0.64	−7.60	Y
536	重庆市渝北区 Yubei Qu, Chongqing Shi	1 486 446	4 726	2 981	60.92	3.96	0.63	−3.28	Y
537	重庆市巴南区 Banan Qu, Chongqing Shi	1 016 429	3 252	1 832	71.19	2.03	0.56	19.81	Y
538	重庆市黔江区 Qianjiang Qu, Chongqing Shi	466 882	922	766	78.63	0.11	0.83	−26.48	Y
539	重庆市长寿区 Changshou Qu, Chongqing Shi	837 501	2 962	1 932	71.47	0.14	0.65	27.10	Y
540	重庆市江津区 Jiangjin Qu, Chongqing Shi	1 368 762	3 785	2 342	45.13	4.97	0.62	−1.05	Y
541	重庆市合川区 Hechuan Qu, Chongqing Shi	1 390 098	3 332	2 225	86.16	0.27	0.67	−6.61	Y
542	重庆市永川区 Yongchuan Qu, Chongqing Shi	1 120 007	3 313	2 625	64.17	3.23	0.79	−9.61	Y
543	重庆市南川区 Nanchuan Qu, Chongqing Shi	582 098	969	759	71.72	2.17	0.78	240.35	
544	重庆市璧山区 Bishan Qu, Chongqing Shi	272 451	698	397	71.20	0.00	0.57	10.62	Y
545	重庆市潼南区 Tongnan Qu, Chongqing Shi	715 701	2 399	1 053	67.40	1.17	0.44	18.13	Y
546	重庆市铜梁区 Tongliang Qu, Chongqing Shi	848 316	2 312	1 524	65.96	4.89	0.66	−14.48	Y
547	重庆市荣昌区 Rongchang Qu, Chongqing Shi	667 478	1 052	765	67.49	1.33	0.73	30.59	Y
548	重庆市万盛经济开发区 Wansheng Economic Development Zone, Chongqing Shi	702 547	2 047	1 249	76.94	0.00	0.61	21.08	Y
549	重庆市梁平区 Liangping Qu, Chongqing Shi	681 124	1 259	802	26.69	0.71	0.64	31.14	
550	城口县 Chengkou Xian	188 270	425	255	74.12	1.65	0.60	—	Y
551	丰都县 Fengdu Xian	632 212	1 397	858	61.06	0.00	0.61	−6.72	Y
552	垫江县 Dianjiang Xian	692 285	1 615	1 182	73.07	0.68	0.73	10.43	Y
553	重庆市武隆区 Wulong Qu, Chongqing Shi	350 366	1 369	670	19.36	3.58	0.49	51.87	
554	忠县 Zhong Xian	788 834	2 400	1 448	70.42	0.21	0.60	3.72	Y

序号 No.	肿瘤登记处 Cancer registries	人口数 Population	发病数 New cases	死亡数 Deaths	MV%	DCO%	M/I	发病率变化 Change for CR%	接受 Accepted
555	重庆市开州区 Kaizhou Qu, Chongqing Shi	1 180 500	4 242	2 807	67.73	0.26	0.66	4.68	Y
556	云阳县 Yunyang Xian	926 700	2 855	2 275	55.62	0.04	0.80	16.95	Y
557	奉节县 Fengjie Xian	727 899	2 574	1 496	70.28	4.47	0.58	21.71	Y
558	巫山县 Wushan Xian	467 185	1 413	909	70.77	0.00	0.64	42.10	Y
559	巫溪县 Wuxi Xian	395 133	905	619	71.27	0.11	0.68	-6.63	Y
560	石柱土家族自治县 Shizhu Tujiazu Zizhixian	390 586	960	631	80.00	0.00	0.66	0.63	Y
561	秀山土家族苗族自治县 Xiushan Tujiazu Miaozu Zizhixian	496 493	767	703	56.32	0.00	0.92	50.89	
562	酉阳土家族苗族自治县 Youyang Tujiazu Miaozu Zizhixian	549 102	1 042	599	63.05	4.70	0.57	43.09	Y
563	彭水苗族土家族自治县 Pengshui Miaozu Tujiazu Zizhixian	490 800	1 471	890	46.43	0.14	0.61	49.97	Y
564	成都市锦江区 Jinjiang Qu, Chengdu Shi	581 793	1 223	912	75.55	3.03	0.75	—	Y
565	成都市青羊区 Qingyang Qu, Chengdu Shi	681 411	2 440	1 554	83.61	1.64	0.64	-2.28	Y
566	成都市金牛区 Jinniu Qu, Chengdu Shi	763 608	2 521	1 527	53.35	7.62	0.61	—	Y
567	成都市武侯区 Wuhou Qu, Chengdu Shi	650 954	1 650	991	80.85	4.79	0.60	—	Y
568	成都市成华区 Chenghua Qu, Chengdu Shi	749 335	2 299	1 431	67.25	3.35	0.62	-9.01	Y
569	成都市高新区 Gaoxin Qu, Chengdu Shi	522 567	1 740	606	89.71	2.30	0.35	—	Y
570	成都市龙泉驿区 Longquanyi Qu, Chengdu Shi	699 605	2 053	1 381	67.17	0.83	0.67	2.65	Y
571	成都市青白江区 Qingbaijiang Qu, Chengdu Shi	420 296	1 740	1 087	67.76	0.06	0.62	—	Y
572	成都市新都区 Xindu Qu, Chengdu Shi	799 448	2 307	1 528	78.50	0.00	0.66	18.97	Y
573	成都市温江区 Wenjiang Qu, Chengdu Shi	453 584	1 585	684	66.25	25.17	0.43	—	Y

序号 No.	肿瘤登记处 Cancer registries	人口数 Population	发病数 New cases	死亡数 Deaths	MV%	DCO%	M/I	发病率变化 Change for CR%	接受 Accepted
574	金堂县 Jintang Xian	902 853	2 947	1 478	81.61	0.03	0.50	-0.80	Y
575	成都市双流区 Shuangliu Qu,Chengdu Shi	582 093	1 675	1 149	54.39	1.31	0.69	-0.89	Y
576	成都市天府新区 Tianfu Xinqu,Chengdu Shi	589 218	1 165	710	82.66	3.69	0.61	-24.10	Y
577	成都市郫都区 Pidu Qu, Chengdu Shi	616 884	1 467	1 022	70.69	2.59	0.70	-2.96	Y
578	大邑县 Dayi Xian	509 495	1 055	859	34.98	7.01	0.81	—	
579	蒲江县 Pujiang Xian	267 781	629	379	66.93	0.32	0.60		Y
580	成都市新津区 Xinjin Qu, Chengdu Shi	318 898	1 129	677	72.72	2.92	0.60	-7.89	Y
581	简阳市 Jianyang Shi	1 175 921	2 582	1 657	75.06	3.06	0.64	—	Y
582	都江堰市 Dujiangyan Shi	622 431	1 513	1 373	65.17	0.00	0.91	—	Y
583	彭州市 Pengzhou Shi	802 730	2 834	1 742	70.36	1.45	0.61	-1.82	Y
584	邛崃市 Qionglai Shi	655 023	2 605	1 566	58.04	3.88	0.60	—	Y
585	崇州市 Chongzhou Shi	663 214	2 060	1 262	72.04	11.60	0.61	—	Y
586	自贡市自流井区 Ziliujing Qu,Zigong Shi	404 417	1 761	865	84.89	0.17	0.49	25.96	Y
587	自贡市贡井区 Gongjing Qu, Zigong Shi	285 672	1 285	737	56.34	1.01	0.57	49.18	Y
588	自贡市大安区 Da'an Qu, Zigong Shi	439 944	1 103	858	53.85	0.00	0.78	-3.04	Y
589	自贡市沿滩区 Yantan Qu, Zigong Shi	357 096	792	539	51.89	0.38	0.68	4.35	Y
590	荣县 Rong Xian	679 574	1 719	1 308	36.59	1.80	0.76	31.57	
591	富顺县 Fushun Xian	1 074 971	2 648	1 966	65.22	0.00	0.74	1.67	Y
592	攀枝花市东区 Dong Qu, Panzhihua Shi	292 667	886	643	77.88	3.95	0.73	5.35	Y
593	攀枝花市西区 Xi Qu,Pan-zhihua Shi	131 270	477	351	80.29	0.00	0.74	-6.99	Y
594	攀枝花市仁和区 Renhe Qu,Panzhihua Shi	233 813	530	307	69.06	2.45	0.58	0.59	Y
595	米易县 Miyi Xian	222 063	458	284	76.20	0.66	0.62	0.29	Y
596	盐边县 Yanbian Xian	211 472	263	191	58.94	4.18	0.73	1.47	Y
597	泸州市江阳区 Jiangyang Qu,Luzhou Shi	682 192	1 944	1 247	52.88	0.10	0.64	-3.68	Y

序号 No.	肿瘤登记处 Cancer registries	人口数 Population	发病数 New cases	死亡数 Deaths	MV%	DCO%	M/I	发病率变化 Change for CR%	接受 Accepted
598	泸州市纳溪区 Naxi Qu，Luzhou Shi	466 170	1 004	586	58.76	3.69	0.58	13.85	Y
599	泸州市龙马潭区 Longma-tan Qu，Luzhou Shi	372 745	1 388	924	78.24	0.22	0.67	20.47	Y
600	泸县 Lu Xian	1 073 739	3 596	2 255	41.10	1.03	0.63	12.62	Y
601	合江县 Hejiang Xian	898 339	2 864	1 801	60.82	0.94	0.63	30.25	Y
602	叙永县 Xuyong Xian	725 489	1 297	815	53.74	2.24	0.63	-2.90	
603	古蔺县 Gulin Xian	876 241	1 714	963	52.04	0.47	0.56	12.25	Y
604	德阳市旌阳区 Jingyang Qu，Deyang Shi	698 366	2 475	1 631	69.86	0.32	0.66	14.10	Y
605	中江县 Zhongjiang Xian	245 805	817	532	71.48	0.86	0.65	29.36	Y
606	德阳市罗江区 Luojiang Qu，Deyang Shi	1 394 765	3 247	2 008	55.44	1.32	0.62	22.64	Y
607	广汉市 Guanghan Shi	590 630	1 996	1 436	80.66	0.35	0.72	16.78	Y
608	什邡市 Shifang Shi	428 932	1 348	941	69.36	0.15	0.70	3.00	Y
609	绵竹市 Mianzhu Shi	500 318	1 829	1 260	65.77	0.66	0.69	14.85	Y
610	绵阳市涪城区 Fucheng Qu，Mianyang Shi	741 844	1 849	1 188	70.52	7.63	0.64	-26.14	Y
611	绵阳市游仙区 Youxian Qu，Mianyang Shi	489 661	1 296	910	71.91	0.08	0.70	-8.42	Y
612	绵阳市安州区 Anzhou Qu，Mianyang Shi	444 236	1 024	757	59.77	0.68	0.74	7.52	Y
613	三台县 Santai Xian	1 414 061	3 114	2 022	61.37	0.61	0.65	-19.62	Y
614	盐亭县 Yanting Xian	594 918	2 295	1 725	69.15	0.17	0.75	1.02	Y
615	梓潼县 Zitong Xian	377 136	911	824	73.11	6.59	0.90	20.15	Accepted
616	北川羌族自治县 Beichuan Qiangzu Zizhixian	234 455	503	337	43.74	1.19	0.67	1.54	Y
617	平武县 Pingwu Xian	177 413	180	125	55.00	20.56	0.69	57.78	
618	江油市 Jiangyou Shi	864 903	2 491	1 680	75.27	0.56	0.67	5.21	Y
619	广元市利州区 Lizhou Qu，Guangyuan Shi	491 251	1 277	935	74.71	0.47	0.73	-4.11	Y
620	广元市昭化区 Zhaohua Qu，Guangyuan Shi	231 716	600	352	51.83	0.17	0.59	-5.61	Y
621	广元市朝天区 Chaotian Qu，Guangyuan Shi	201 901	424	335	80.66	0.00	0.79	-35.04	Y
622	旺苍县 Wangcang Xian	445 912	932	631	72.32	1.29	0.68	-5.56	Y

序号 No.	肿瘤登记处 Cancer registries	人口数 Population	发病数 New cases	死亡数 Deaths	MV%	DCO%	M/I	发病率变化 Change for CR%	接受 Accepted
623	青川县 Qingchuan Xian	227 480	520	356	68. 46	0. 00	0. 68	1. 88	Y
624	剑阁县 Jiange Xian	653 453	2 099	1 402	68. 94	0. 14	0. 67	18. 02	Y
625	苍溪县 Cangxi Xian	764 388	1 631	1 142	72. 29	0. 18	0. 70	−4. 06	Y
626	遂宁市船山区 Chuanshan Qu,Suining Shi	653 496	2 031	1 302	73. 90	0. 49	0. 64	31. 76	Y
627	遂宁市安居区 Anju Qu, Suining Shi	779 325	1 827	1 356	69. 35	0. 38	0. 74	10. 01	Y
628	蓬溪县 Pengxi Xian	700 563	2 034	1 305	76. 50	0. 00	0. 64	26. 84	Y
629	射洪市 Shehong Shi	958 343	2 696	1 800	80. 04	0. 45	0. 67	25. 54	Y
630	大英县 Daying Xian	552 215	1 289	841	77. 66	0. 23	0. 65	9. 29	Y
631	内江市市中区 Shizhong Qu,Neijiang Shi	517 355	1 759	904	75. 04	5. 34	0. 51	79. 51	Y
632	内江市东兴区 Dongxing Qu,Neijiang Shi	882 512	2 138	1 508	61. 37	5. 19	0. 71	32. 46	Y
633	威远县 Weiyuan Xian	692 931	1 424	928	21. 77	2. 88	0. 65	31. 39	
634	资中县 Zizhong Xian	1 250 820	3 842	2 207	64. 00	0. 57	0. 57	34. 22	Y
635	隆昌市 Longchang Shi	770 024	1 930	1 347	64. 20	0. 21	0. 70	17. 86	Y
636	乐山市市中区 Shizhong Qu, Leshan Shi	637 204	1 252	1 105	55. 83	1. 36	0. 88	−35. 05	Y
637	乐山市沙湾区 Shawan Qu, Leshan Shi	175 073	506	308	70. 75	3. 56	0. 61	58. 12	Y
638	乐山市五通桥区 Wutongqiao Qu,Leshan Shi	301 658	784	554	88. 65	1. 79	0. 71	25. 04	Y
639	乐山市金口河区 Jinkouhe Qu,Leshan Shi	48 513	39	13	76. 92	2. 56	0. 33	−9. 98	
640	犍为县 Qianwei Xian	556 473	1 136	680	46. 13	0. 35	0. 60	3. 84	Y
641	井研县 Jingyan Xian	396 549	971	740	41. 30	0. 00	0. 76	26. 59	Y
642	夹江县 Jiajiang Xian	345 058	783	482	89. 66	0. 00	0. 62	41. 64	Y
643	沐川县 Muchuan Xian	251 254	357	125	67. 51	1. 12	0. 35	201. 76	
644	峨边彝族自治县 Ebian Yi-zu Zizhixian	146 486	87	18	54. 02	3. 45	0. 21	−7. 58	
645	马边彝族自治县 Mabian Yizu Zizhixian	221 209	183	16	49. 73	7. 10	0. 09	61. 34	
646	峨眉山市 Emeishan Shi	429 044	1 036	784	70. 27	0. 77	0. 76	4. 52	Y
647	南充市顺庆区 Shunqing Qu,Nanchong Shi	660 780	2 560	1 011	52. 46	23. 20	0. 39	−24. 83	

序号 No.	肿瘤登记处 Cancer registries	人口数 Population	发病数 New cases	死亡数 Deaths	MV%	DCO%	M/I	发病率变化 Change for CR%	接受 Accepted
648	南充市高坪区 Gaoping Qu, Nanchong Shi	597 172	1 276	1 094	86.21	0.31	0.86	−16.32	Y
649	南充市嘉陵区 Jialing Qu, Nanchong Shi	683 658	1 615	1 111	28.30	1.30	0.69	−9.76	
650	南部县 Nanbu Xian	1 247 996	1 910	933	83.87	0.58	0.49	−26.39	
651	营山县 Yingshan Xian	906 662	1 644	997	34.85	0.36	0.61	−27.24	
652	蓬安县 Peng'an Xian	677 586	1 407	1 035	54.94	0.85	0.74	−13.09	Y
653	仪陇县 Yilong Xian	1 075 855	2 650	1 951	68.91	1.32	0.74	13.17	Y
654	西充县 Xichong Xian	598 133	1 218	709	45.89	0.00	0.58	−25.22	Y
655	阆中市 Langzhong Shi	839 173	2 722	1 799	67.34	0.70	0.66	−7.37	Y
656	眉山市东坡区 Dongpo Qu, Meishan Shi	876 254	2 198	1 461	81.39	0.27	0.66	4.80	Y
657	眉山市彭山区 Pengshan Qu, Meishan Shi	327 809	908	390	67.62	0.33	0.43	28.43	Y
658	仁寿县 Renshou Xian	1 540 446	4 226	2 521	41.24	0.17	0.60	19.12	Y
659	洪雅县 Hongya Xian	345 753	477	356	74.42	0.42	0.75	125.10	
660	丹棱县 Danling Xian	144 679	380	194	53.16	7.89	0.51	30.39	Y
661	青神县 Qingshen Xian	193 741	432	331	80.09	0.23	0.77	7.12	Y
662	宜宾市翠屏区 Cuiping Qu, Yibin Shi	843 383	2 323	1 509	47.01	0.39	0.65	7.86	Y
663	宜宾市南溪区 Nanxi Qu, Yibin Shi	432 688	894	664	54.36	0.45	0.74	—	Y
664	宜宾市叙州区 Xuzhou Qu, Yibing Shi	1 022 307	2 024	1 086	55.88	0.54	0.54	1.72	Y
665	江安县 Jiang'an Xian	564 056	1 158	745	50.35	0.60	0.64	30.26	Y
666	长宁县 Changning Xian	462 854	1 113	757	72.78	0.18	0.68	7.05	Y
667	高县 Gao Xian	412 420	722	367	50.69	0.14	0.51	30.06	
668	珙县 Gong Xian	430 919	571	308	79.16	4.90	0.54	—	
669	筠连县 Junlian Xian	450 986	658	320	76.75	0.61	0.49	9.52	
670	兴文县 Xingwen Xian	482 324	769	529	72.82	0.26	0.69		
671	屏山县 Pingshan Xian	311 986	425	277	45.65	5.88	0.65	46.42	
672	广安市广安区 Guang'an Qu, Guang'an Shi	897 164	2 590	1 878	72.32	2.08	0.73	2.82	Y
673	广安市前锋区 Qianfeng Qu, Guang'an Shi	368 974	864	620	60.30	0.12	0.72	−6.69	Y
674	岳池县 Yuechi Xian	1 163 510	2 484	1 893	69.12	0.72	0.76	15.88	Y

序号 No.	肿瘤登记处 Cancer registries	人口数 Population	发病数 New cases	死亡数 Deaths	MV%	DCO%	M/I	发病率变化 Change for CR%	接受 Accepted
675	武胜县 Wusheng Xian	826 659	1 709	1 274	32.42	2.28	0.75	−1.09	
676	邻水县 Linshui Xian	1 019 829	2 267	1 538	34.01	2.29	0.68	65.53	
677	华蓥市 Huaying Shi	358 372	808	617	60.15	10.02	0.76	65.78	Y
678	达州市通川区 Tongchuan Qu, Dazhou Shi	594 093	910	710	52.20	3.85	0.78	—	
679	达州市达川区 Dachuan Qu, Dazhou Shi	1 185 241	2 062	1 130	55.33	2.04	0.55	−8.07	
680	宣汉县 Xuanhan Xian	1 299 559	3 119	2 013	75.79	0.42	0.65	33.85	Y
681	开江县 Kaijiang Xian	586 306	637	691	54.95	8.95	1.08	−31.12	
682	大竹县 Dazhu Xian	1 092 694	2 510	1 539	68.37	1.00	0.61	−1.53	Y
683	渠县 Qu Xian	1 343 760	2 676	2 136	49.10	0.75	0.80	6.01	Y
684	万源市 Wanyuan Shi	578 072	581	463	64.72	0.52	0.80	−14.94	
685	雅安市雨城区 Yucheng Qu, Ya'an Shi	342 117	922	601	67.68	3.80	0.65	6.72	Y
686	雅安市名山区 Mingshan Qu, Ya'an Shi	278 876	669	401	68.61	0.90	0.60	6.22	Y
687	荥经县 Yingjing Xian	146 554	394	250	77.66	1.02	0.63	−0.19	Y
688	汉源县 Hanyuan Xian	319 070	773	485	59.51	0.78	0.63	6.67	Y
689	石棉县 Shimian Xian	121 442	315	209	66.35	3.49	0.66	1.47	Y
690	天全县 Tianquan Xian	150 804	422	271	61.85	0.24	0.64	0.70	Y
691	芦山县 Lushan Xian	119 404	352	207	75.28	0.57	0.59	9.76	Y
692	宝兴 Baoxing Xian	58 335	146	83	66.44	1.37	0.57	2.31	Y
693	巴中市巴州区 Bazhou Qu, Bazhong Shi	711 390	1 837	688	32.83	1.96	0.37	61.02	
694	巴中市恩阳区 Enyang Qu, Bazhong Shi	571 167	779	716	55.84	0.77	0.92	16.42	
695	通江县 Tongjiang Xian	735 908	1 374	829	63.76	0.00	0.60	22.74	Y
696	南江县 Nanjiang Xian	660 096	1 297	799	69.47	0.62	0.62	18.98	Y
697	平昌县 Pingchang Xian	943 088	1 311	1 040	58.43	1.37	0.79	−9.08	
698	资阳市雁江区 Yanjiang Qu, Ziyang Shi	1 080 782	3 228	2 184	49.88	0.09	0.68	13.42	Y
699	安岳县 Anyue Xian	1 580 035	2 395	1 157	61.46	0.79	0.48	13.41	
700	乐至县 Lezhi Xian	814 674	2 383	1 394	53.97	0.63	0.58	16.65	Y
701	马尔康市 Barkam Shi	54 162	59	44	100.00	0.00	0.75	37.81	
702	汶川县 Wenchuan Xian	94 114	117	108	83.76	0.85	0.92	−16.04	

序号 No.	肿瘤登记处 Cancer registries	人口数 Population	发病数 New cases	死亡数 Deaths	MV%	DCO%	M/I	发病率变化 Change for CR%	接受 Accepted
703	理县 Li Xian	44 459	40	42	82.50	2.50	1.05	−58.53	
704	茂县 Mao Xian	111 029	116	92	48.28	31.90	0.79	−31.27	
705	松潘县 Songpan Xian	74 066	47	31	95.74	0.00	0.66	−32.86	
706	九寨沟县 Jiuzhaigou Xian	67 511	87	54	21.84	0.00	0.62	—	
707	金川县 Jinchuan Xian	74 000	24	31	8.33	0.00	1.29	−47.80	
708	小金县 Xiaojin Xian	80 402	57	44	15.79	38.60	0.77	−7.85	
709	阿坝县 Aba Xian	81 669	25	19	4.00	96.00	0.76		
710	红原县 Hongyuan Xian	48 200	25	26	32.00	52.00	1.04	−38.17	
711	泸定县 Luding Xian	86 820	22	0	31.82	0.00	0.00	—	
712	白玉县 Baiyu Xian	56 922	18	0	100.00	0.00	0.00	—	
713	理塘县 Litang Xian	68 220	18	5	33.33	33.33	0.28	—	
714	贵阳市花溪区 Huaxi Qu, Guiyang Shi	617 006	1 042	642	56.43	0.58	0.62	38.67	
715	开阳县 Kaiyang Xian	373 634	858	704	69.93	1.63	0.82	−9.25	Y
716	息烽县 Xifeng Xian	229 798	525	241	35.24	5.52	0.46	92.96	Y
717	修文县 Xiuwen Xian	289 036	542	280	86.90	0.18	0.52	—	Y
718	清镇市 Qingzhen Shi	492 792	935	459	87.59	1.07	0.49	−11.05	Y
719	六盘水市钟山区 Zhongshan Qu, Liupanshui Shi	546 271	1 327	477	33.76	1.66	0.36	46.03	Y
720	六盘水市六枝特区 Luzhi Tequ, Lupanshui Shi	503 999	1 337	827	40.91	0.00	0.62	1.88	Y
721	六盘水市水城区 Shuicheng Qu, Liupanshui Shi	682 074	1 044	486	26.82	3.07	0.47	82.14	
722	盘州市 Panzhou Shi	1 051 863	2 957	1 890	96.65	0.17	0.64	24.35	Y
723	遵义市红花岗区 Honghuagang Qu, Zunyi Shi	856 701	600	131	75.00	13.17	0.22	93.63	
724	遵义市汇川区 Huichuan Qu, Zunyi Shi	572 499	1 471	523	76.00	1.22	0.36	98.08	
725	习水县 Xishui Xian	521 230	712	578	36.52	14.04	0.81	5.00	
726	赤水市 Chishui Shi	244 803	846	449	58.75	0.59	0.53	71.31	Y
727	安顺市西秀区 Xixiu Qu, Anshun Shi	612 803	1 458	952	84.71	0.27	0.65	−11.83	Y
728	普定县 Puding Xian	392 802	635	339	22.20	1.89	0.53	—	

序号 No.	肿瘤登记处 Cancer registries	人口数 Population	发病数 New cases	死亡数 Deaths	MV%	DCO%	M/I	发病率变化 Change for CR%	接受 Accepted
729	镇宁布依族苗族自治县 Zhenning Buyeizu Miaozu ZizhiXian	272 094	718	447	52. 23	0. 00	0. 62	−17. 17	Y
730	毕节市七星关区 Qixing-guan Qu,Bijie Shi	1 158 505	1 832	757	37. 55	0. 05	0. 41	4. 82	
731	黔西市 Qianxi Shi	672 293	426	145	49. 06	0. 23	0. 34	—	
732	铜仁市碧江区 Bijiang Qu, Tongren Shi	305 448	746	543	88. 07	2. 68	0. 73	−1. 34	Y
733	玉屏侗族自治县 Yuping Dongzu Zizhixian	127 703	393	263	42. 75	3. 82	0. 67	44. 47	Y
734	沿河土家族自治县 Yanhe Tujiazu Zizhixian	453 402	396	137	44. 19	8. 59	0. 35	—	
735	铜仁市万山区 Wanshan Qu,Tongren Shi	117 012	171	48	59. 06	0. 58	0. 28	—	
736	兴义市 Xingyi Shi	707 295	1 464	414	94. 60	0. 96	0. 28	—	
737	册亨县 Ceheng Xian	254 147	524	298	67. 56	0. 00	0. 57	−18. 52	Y
738	安龙县 Anlong Xian	228 460	376	28	56. 12	0. 00	0. 07	—	
739	黄平县 Huangping Xian	265 657	531	220	34. 09	0. 38	0. 41	26. 82	
740	剑河县 Jianhe Xian	182 640	91	58	10. 99	1. 10	0. 64	—	
741	榕江县 Rongjiang Xian	289 199	333	173	30. 93	3. 60	0. 52	−10. 10	
742	雷山县 Leishan Xian	116 800	188	83	63. 30	0. 00	0. 44	−9. 91	
743	麻江县 Majiang Xian	123 633	173	126	21. 97	4. 62	0. 73	−12. 00	
744	丹寨县 Danzhai Xian	123 886	315	93	18. 41	0. 63	0. 30	—	
745	都匀市 Duyun Shi	467 452	1 127	405	67. 88	1. 33	0. 36	−25. 34	
746	福泉市 Fuquan Shi	296 003	581	321	48. 36	0. 69	0. 55	18. 48	Y
747	荔波县 Libo Xian	133 708	180	139	34. 44	6. 67	0. 77	−9. 44	
748	瓮安县 Weng'an Xian	394 300	312	156	34. 94	12. 82	0. 50	—	
749	龙里县 Longli Xian	161 602	467	238	47. 54	5. 14	0. 51	2. 20	Y
750	昆明市五华区 Wuhua Qu, Kunming Shi	589 019	1 605	915	58. 63	0. 06	0. 57	−13. 74	Y
751	昆明市盘龙区 Panlong Qu, Kunming Shi	571 078	1 572	986	56. 55	13. 30	0. 63	0. 54	Y
752	昆明市官渡区 Guandu Qu, Kunming Shi	535 331	1 244	742	62. 46	0. 00	0. 60	1. 12	Y

序号 No.	肿瘤登记处 Cancer registries	人口数 Population	发病数 New cases	死亡数 Deaths	MV%	DCO%	M/I	发病率变化 Change for CR%	接受 Accepted
753	昆明市西山区 Xishan Qu, Kunming Shi	559 574	1 483	1 004	71. 54	0. 20	0. 68	−0. 88	Y
754	昆明市呈贡区 Chenggong Qu, Kunming Shi	126 198	265	100	88. 30	0. 00	0. 38	—	
755	昆明市晋宁区 Jinning Qu, Kunming Shi	286 224	630	373	63. 81	0. 00	0. 59	—	Y
756	富民县 Fumin Xian	153 202	272	153	1. 84	0. 00	0. 56	2. 56	
757	宜良县 Yiliang Xian	435 471	1 642	417	19. 06	0. 00	0. 25	—	
758	石林彝族自治县 Shilin Yi- zu Zizhixian	254 245	323	252	37. 46	0. 00	0. 78	—	
759	嵩明县 Songming Xian	310 010	549	313	62. 48	0. 55	0. 57	−4. 13	
760	禄劝彝族苗族自治县 Lu- chuan Yizu Miaozu Zizhix- ian	488 731	849	498	47. 70	0. 12	0. 59	1. 71	Y
761	安宁市 Anning Shi	279 729	707	367	98. 59	0. 00	0. 52	−10. 01	
762	曲靖市麒麟区 Qilin Qu, Qujing Shi	731 260	1 513	847	52. 35	3. 44	0. 56	2. 44	Y
763	曲靖市沾益区 Zhanyi Qu, Qujing Shi	453 099	843	575	53. 26	0. 00	0. 68	1. 30	Y
764	曲靖市马龙区 Malong Qu, Qujing Shi	208 255	373	220	52. 55	5. 09	0. 59	9. 43	
765	陆良县 Luliang Xian	644 099	1 211	592	15. 94	12. 55	0. 49	−45. 35	
766	师宗县 Shizong Xian	545 000	1 144	831	39. 34	7. 60	0. 73	—	Y
767	罗平县 Luoping Xian	1 306 030	1 130	533	27. 52	8. 23	0. 47	—	
768	富源县 Fuyuan Xian	745 797	1 989	1 008	71. 34	5. 73	0. 51	16. 37	Y
769	宣威市 Xuanwei Shi	1 548 585	3 546	2 100	56. 06	0. 00	0. 59	7. 93	Y
770	玉溪市红塔区 Hongta Qu, Yuxi Shi	455 243	972	590	76. 65	4. 12	0. 61	−6. 74	Y
771	玉溪市江川区 Jiangchuan Qu, Yuxi Shi	284 809	570	332	75. 26	0. 00	0. 58	8. 47	Y
772	澄江市 Chengjiang Shi	147 077	322	172	76. 09	0. 00	0. 53	−3. 56	Y
773	通海县 Tonghai Xian	290 700	641	363	79. 41	0. 00	0. 57	11. 79	Y
774	华宁县 Huaning Xian	213 215	387	204	57. 88	0. 00	0. 53	7. 31	Y
775	易门县 Yimen Xian	165 654	431	267	68. 45	0. 00	0. 62	9. 44	Y

序号 No.	肿瘤登记处 Cancer registries	人口数 Population	发病数 New cases	死亡数 Deaths	MV%	DCO%	M/I	发病率变化 Change for CR%	接受 Accepted
776	峨山彝族自治县 Eshan Yi-zu Zizhixian	155 828	443	251	61.17	1.81	0.57	13.14	Y
777	新平彝族傣族自治县 Xin-ping Yizu Daizu Zizhixian	279 829	517	333	69.44	0.39	0.64	0.09	Y
778	元江哈尼族彝族傣族自治县 Yuanjiang Hanizu Yizu Daizu Zizhixian	211 319	470	262	71.06	0.00	0.56	-3.10	Y
779	保山市隆阳区 Longyang Qu,Baoshan Shi	944 600	1 703	1 105	71.52	0.00	0.65	-8.11	Y
780	施甸县 Shidian Xian	347 941	611	363	62.19	0.82	0.59	-2.46	Y
781	龙陵县 Longling Xian	292 001	519	274	51.45	0.00	0.53	27.13	
782	昌宁县 Changning Xian	354 909	641	382	73.48	0.00	0.60	1.14	Y
783	腾冲市 Tengchong Shi	670 000	1 346	801	75.41	0.00	0.60	—	Y
784	巧家县 Qiaojia Xian	541 887	737	456	85.07	0.00	0.62	-10.94	
785	绥江县 Suijiang Xian	170 766	331	221	29.91	0.00	0.67	8.32	
786	水富市 Shuifu Shi	109 097	206	160	14.56	0.49	0.78	0.33	
787	丽江市古城区 Gucheng Qu,Lijiang Shi	159 126	349	225	69.05	0.86	0.64	-11.26	Y
788	玉龙纳西族自治县 Yulong Naxizu Zizhixian	223 000	410	252	79.27	1.95	0.61	-2.71	Y
789	华坪县 Huaping Xian	161 816	294	181	75.17	3.74	0.62	8.49	Y
790	宁蒗彝族自治县 Ninglang Yizu Zizhixian	270 627	501	305	73.25	6.59	0.61	—	Y
791	景东彝族自治县 Jingdong Yizu Zizhixian	366 226	913	521	69.00	14.13	0.57	69.75	Y
792	景谷傣族彝族自治县 Jing-gu Daizu Yizu Zizhixian	299 799	522	364	82.57	0.00	0.70	-2.15	Y
793	江城哈尼族彝族自治县 Jiangcheng Hanizu Yizu Zizhixian	117 996	216	128	75.00	0.00	0.59	-23.04	Y
794	临沧市临翔区 Linxiang Qu,Lincang Shi	326 871	630	346	83.81	0.00	0.55	5.22	Y
795	凤庆县 Fengqing Xian	444 133	905	494	67.18	2.43	0.55	—	Y
796	镇康县 Zhenkang Xian	184 343	340	198	63.24	0.88	0.58	34.95	Y
797	沧源佤族自治县 Cangyuan Vazu Zizhixian	171 115	300	186	81.33	4.67	0.62	8.56	

序号 No.	肿瘤登记处 Cancer registries	人口数 Population	发病数 New cases	死亡数 Deaths	MV%	DCO%	M/I	发病率变化 Change for CR%	接受 Accepted
798	楚雄市 Chuxiong Shi	535 986	1 034	674	65.96	0.00	0.65	−13.34	Y
799	双柏县 Shuangbai Xian	160 800	277	164	65.70	0.00	0.59	−7.77	
800	牟定县 Mouding Xian	212 500	423	216	76.60	0.00	0.51	−4.39	Y
801	姚安县 Yao'an Xian	203 652	391	210	66.24	0.00	0.54	9.83	Y
802	大姚县 Dayao Xian	279 706	555	313	58.20	0.00	0.56	13.39	Y
803	永仁县 Yongren Xian	111 401	236	97	83.90	0.00	0.41	23.43	
804	元谋县 Yuanmou Xian	221 101	389	231	73.26	0.00	0.59	−1.13	Y
805	武定县 Wuding Xian	279 798	414	220	23.19	0.00	0.53	1.13	
806	禄丰市 Lufeng Shi	431 699	825	485	66.18	0.00	0.59	−19.14	Y
807	个旧市 Gejiu Shi	378 892	926	627	66.74	0.00	0.68	−5.11	Y
808	开远市 Kaiyuan Shi	283 162	654	310	41.13	0.00	0.47	9.10	Y
809	蒙自市 Mengzi Shi	425 429	843	493	81.26	0.00	0.58	—	Y
810	屏边苗族自治县 Pingbian Miaozu Zizhixian	160 889	342	214	67.54	0.00	0.63	−3.90	Y
811	建水县 Jianshui Xian	546 580	928	685	71.12	0.65	0.74	−3.18	
812	石屏县 Shiping Xian	317 867	719	438	70.65	0.00	0.61	20.84	Y
813	弥勒市 Mile Shi	544 787	976	535	74.28	0.00	0.55	—	
814	泸西县 Luxi Xian	448 960	884	564	67.53	0.00	0.64	6.04	Y
815	文山市 Wenshan Shi	500 992	820	508	90.61	0.00	0.62	—	
816	砚山县 Yanshan Xian	500 992	602	551	100.00	0.00	0.92	−27.11	
817	西畴县 Xichou Xian	262 996	461	291	64.21	3.90	0.63	5.81	
818	丘北县 Qiubei Xian	493 471	864	594	62.04	0.00	0.69	−2.92	
819	富宁县 Funing Xian	421 829	629	396	56.92	0.00	0.63	41.52	
820	景洪市 Jinghong Shi	532 475	1 278	748	86.23	0.00	0.59	−2.85	Y
821	大理市 Dali Shi	638 053	761	138	52.56	0.00	0.18	−26.28	
822	祥云县 Xiangyun Xian	475 129	1 101	449	59.22	0.00	0.41	58.00	
823	宾川县 Binchuan Xian	361 129	383	254	23.24	0.00	0.66	—	
824	弥渡县 Midu Xian	322 577	522	282	7.09	0.00	0.54	10.31	
825	南涧彝族自治县 Nanjian Yizu Zizhixian	220 287	308	180	28.90	0.00	0.58	—	
826	兰坪白族普米族自治县 Lanping Baizu Pumizu Zizhi Xian	218 001	306	205	73.86	0.00	0.67	8.03	

序号 No.	肿瘤登记处 Cancer registries	人口数 Population	发病数 New cases	死亡数 Deaths	MV%	DCO%	M/I	发病率变化 Change for CR%	接受 Accepted
827	香格里拉市 Shangêlila Shi	151 125	270	148	32. 96	0. 00	0. 55	—	
828	德钦县 Dêqên Xian	61 044	75	51	6. 67	1. 33	0. 68	—	
829	维西傈僳族自治县 Weixi Lisuzu Zizhixian	157 184	219	130	67. 58	19. 63	0. 59	—	
830	拉萨市城关区 Chengguan Qu,Lhasa Shi	340 042	183	3	48. 63	0. 00	0. 02	−7. 94	
831	林芝市巴宜区 Bayi Qu, Linzhi Shi	48 575	144	66	30. 56	39. 58	0. 46	—	Y
832	昌都市卡若区 Karuo Qu, Qamdo Shi	119 772	48	5	37. 50	0. 00	0. 10	—	
833	日喀则市 Xigazê Shi	798 015	18	0	61. 11	0. 00	0. 00	—	
834	西安市碑林区 Beilin Qu, Xi'an Shi	717 497	1 519	1 082	83. 67	5. 46	0. 71	−14. 10	Y
835	西安市莲湖区 Lianhu Qu, Xi'an Shi	737 800	2 059	1 425	71. 25	0. 39	0. 69	−52. 90	Y
836	西安市未央区 Weiyang Qu,Xi'an Shi	653 100	2 235	1 253	82. 64	2. 19	0. 56	9. 00	Y
837	西安市雁塔区 Yanta Qu, Xi'an Shi	948 968	1 928	1 465	87. 71	0. 26	0. 76	−7. 50	Y
838	西安市高陵区 Gaoling Qu, Xi'an Shi	356 999	770	558	59. 74	0. 78	0. 72	−8. 93	Y
839	西安市鄠邑区 Huyi Qu, Xi'an Shi	543 471	1 038	820	75. 43	6. 74	0. 79	−1. 33	Y
840	铜川市耀州区 Yaozhou Qu,Tongchuan Shi	336 403	490	271	86. 94	0. 82	0. 55	−27. 07	
841	宝鸡市渭滨区 Weibin Qu, Baoji Shi	350 652	478	473	67. 36	0. 00	0. 99	—	
842	宝鸡市金台区 Jintai Qu, Baoji Shi	380 101	638	385	58. 62	0. 00	0. 60	−9. 11	
843	宝鸡市陈仓区 Chencang Qu,Baoji Shi	439 958	820	551	76. 59	1. 59	0. 67	3. 64	Y
844	宝鸡市凤翔区 Fengxiang Qu,Baoji Shi	491 400	999	757	69. 67	0. 70	0. 76	7. 42	Y
845	岐山县 Qishan Xian	466 500	831	615	73. 29	0. 60	0. 74	−1. 45	Y
846	扶风县 Fufeng Xian	423 100	471	139	66. 88	0. 00	0. 30		
847	眉县 Mei Xian	305 000	547	375	98. 54	0. 73	0. 69	−3. 11	

序号 No.	肿瘤登记处 Cancer registries	人口数 Population	发病数 New cases	死亡数 Deaths	MV%	DCO%	M/I	发病率变化 Change for CR%	接受 Accepted
848	陇县 Long Xian	272 437	572	371	82.87	4.20	0.65	13.40	Y
849	千阳县 Qianyang Xian	125 200	269	177	82.53	0.37	0.66	6.87	Y
850	麟游县 Linyou Xian	91 621	190	128	61.58	3.16	0.67	0.07	Y
851	凤县 Feng Xian	94 825	100	99	14.00	0.00	0.99	—	
852	太白县 Taibai Xian	51 999	101	51	8.91	1.98	0.50	—	
853	三原县 Sanyuan Xian	414 461	691	592	35.60	0.00	0.86	—	
854	泾阳县 Jingyang Xian	316 600	725	574	63.31	0.14	0.79	9.94	Y
855	武功县 Wugong Xian	457 158	926	575	63.28	1.08	0.62	—	Y
856	渭南市临渭区 Linwei Qu, Weinan Shi	753 899	1 708	997	80.97	1.00	0.58	6.34	Y
857	渭南市华州区 Huazhou Qu, Weinan Shi	327 904	673	493	60.62	0.45	0.73	−1.75	Y
858	潼关县 Tongguan Xian	160 037	211	170	78.20	4.27	0.81	−25.41	
859	大荔县 Dali Xian	704 400	1 581	1 114	68.18	0.19	0.70	0.94	Y
860	合阳县 Heyang Xian	442 963	761	458	97.77	2.10	0.60	3.55	
861	澄城县 Chengcheng Xian	393 096	570	428	94.91	0.18	0.75	−13.98	
862	蒲城县 Pucheng Xian	752 000	1 491	1 158	74.04	0.80	0.78	4.89	Y
863	富平县 Fuping Xian	753 701	1 522	1 125	72.40	0.85	0.74	5.61	Y
864	韩城市 Hancheng Shi	400 600	253	222	66.80	8.70	0.88	—	
865	华阴市 Huayin Shi	263 400	505	304	79.41	0.20	0.60	11.11	Y
866	延安市宝塔区 Baota Qu, Yan'an Shi	471 879	892	514	79.04	1.68	0.58	12.49	Y
867	延安市安塞区 Ansai Qu, Yan'an Shi	175 400	204	64	79.90	0.49	0.31	—	
868	延川县 Yanchuan Xian	171 939	145	56	75.86	7.59	0.39	—	
869	富县 Fu Xian	157 484	387	174	68.73	0.00	0.45	22.33	Y
870	黄龙县 Huanglong Xian	49 592	72	52	100.00	0.00	0.72	—	
871	黄陵县 Huangling Xian	125 579	254	139	87.01	0.79	0.55	93.96	Y
872	汉中市汉台区 Hantai Qu, Hanzhong Shi	540 801	1 188	803	67.93	4.29	0.68	−10.24	Y
873	城固县 Chenggu Xian	559 434	1 080	724	83.52	0.09	0.67	3.61	Y
874	宁强县 Ningqiang Xian	308 809	727	281	95.60	0.28	0.39	−20.73	
875	绥德县 Suide Xian	359 281	460	498	85.43	0.87	1.08	−9.09	

序号 No.	肿瘤登记处 Cancer registries	人口数 Population	发病数 New cases	死亡数 Deaths	MV%	DCO%	M/I	发病率变化 Change for CR%	接受 Accepted
876	安康市汉滨区 Hanbin Qu, Ankang Shi	960 587	1 765	1 247	65.78	1.87	0.71	−2.56	Y
877	汉阴县 Hanyin Xian	249 000	461	292	93.93	0.00	0.63	34.61	Y
878	石泉县 Shiquan Xian	182 437	376	177	95.48	2.13	0.47	26.83	
879	宁陕县 Ningshan Xian	71 303	155	98	89.03	3.23	0.63	−10.61	Y
880	紫阳县 Ziyang Xian	287 201	770	517	84.03	0.26	0.67	4.43	Y
881	岚皋县 Langao Xian	151 220	375	125	99.73	0.00	0.33	—	
882	平利县 Pingli Xian	431 702	136	34	86.03	0.74	0.25	—	
883	镇坪县 Zhenping Xian	51 386	164	46	86.59	0.00	0.28	7.19	
884	旬阳市 Xunyang Shi	431 702	1 013	668	78.97	0.10	0.66	29.33	Y
885	商洛市商州区 Shangzhou Qu, Shangluo Shi	560 374	1 420	981	96.55	0.00	0.69	−12.90	Y
886	洛南县 Luonan Xian	462 192	502	410	95.22	0.00	0.82	—	
887	镇安县 Zhen'an Xian	280 108	618	473	85.60	0.16	0.77	8.67	Y
888	兰州市城关区 Chengguan Qu, Lanzhou Shi	955 845	3 868	925	49.22	0.00	0.24	21.56	
889	兰州市七里河区 Qilihe Qu, Lanzhou Shi	574 576	1 067	797	46.02	15.56	0.75	−28.22	
890	兰州市西固区 Xigu Qu, Lanzhou Shi	325 217	593	404	42.83	5.23	0.68	−47.07	
891	兰州市安宁区 Anning Qu, Lanzhou Shi	208 886	152	71	7.89	0.00	0.47	−71.45	
892	兰州市红古区 Honggu Qu, Lanzhou Shi	144 112	155	125	0.65	4.52	0.81	−48.78	
893	白银市白银区 Baiyin Qu, Baiyin Shi	316 205	754	329	42.84	0.27	0.44	−15.20	Y
894	白银市平川区 Pingchuan Qu, Baiyin Shi	211 078	629	292	30.84	13.20	0.46	107.70	Y
895	靖远县 Jingyuan Xian	460 813	939	514	34.93	0.00	0.55	0.54	Y
896	会宁县 Huining Xian	550 807	1 237	703	45.92	3.56	0.57	—	Y
897	景泰县 Jingtai Xian	239 617	605	379	68.26	1.82	0.63	−2.75	Y
898	天水市秦州区 Qinzhou Qu, Tianshui Shi	663 300	212	50	57.55	0.00	0.24	−80.32	
899	天水市麦积区 Maiji Qu, Tianshui Shi	1 113 692	172	65	30.81	8.72	0.38	−92.19	

序号 No.	肿瘤登记处 Cancer registries	人口数 Population	发病数 New cases	死亡数 Deaths	MV%	DCO%	M/I	发病率变化 Change for CR%	接受 Accepted
900	武威市凉州区 Liangzhou Qu,Wuwei Shi	1 081 317	3 034	1 606	75.97	0.07	0.53	-9.66	Y
901	民勤县 Minqin Xian	242 894	730	343	76.44	2.74	0.47	2.94	Y
902	古浪县 Gulang Xian	388 877	895	602	59.33	2.46	0.67	-12.61	Y
903	天祝藏族自治县 Tianzhu Zangzu Zizhixian	179 100	410	271	47.32	0.00	0.66	-23.79	Y
904	张掖市甘州区 Ganzhou Qu,Zhangye Shi	519 840	1 249	841	65.09	0.48	0.67	-16.75	Y
905	高台县 Gaotai Xian	147 100	403	197	57.57	0.00	0.49	-27.62	Y
906	静宁县 Jingning Xian	484 086	1 477	817	69.33	5.62	0.55	-1.04	Y
907	敦煌市 Dunhuang Shi	144 719	348	196	59.20	0.86	0.56	3.08	Y
908	庆城县 Qingcheng Xian	265 924	609	267	49.26	0.99	0.44	13.38	Y
909	临洮县 Lintao Xian	545 255	881	242	48.13	8.17	0.27	81.72	
910	临潭县 Lintan Xian	140 473	315	212	77.14	2.54	0.67	45.19	Y
911	西宁市 Xining Shi	994 980	3 127	1 473	71.63	0.58	0.47	10.51	Y
912	大通回族土族自治县 Datong Huizu Tuzu ZizhiXian	467 429	865	595	44.62	0.00	0.69	24.99	Y
913	西宁市湟中区 Huangzhong Qu,Xining Shi	481 735	1 307	677	73.91	0.23	0.52	41.78	Y
914	海东市乐都区 Ledu Qu,Haidong Shi	288 040	562	397	61.03	0.00	0.71	-3.80	Y
915	民和回族土族自治县 Minhe Huizu Tuzu ZizhiXian	438 517	696	481	67.82	0.29	0.69	-1.25	
916	互助土族自治县 Huzhu Tuzu Zizhixian	401 659	666	513	68.77	0.00	0.77	-7.66	Y
917	循化撒拉族自治县 Xunhua Salarzu Zizhixian	163 653	300	223	87.33	0.33	0.74	-1.90	Y
918	海南藏族自治州 Hainan Zangzu Zizhizhou	470 309	1 033	683	42.11	0.58	0.66	-3.48	Y
919	银川市兴庆区 Xingqing Qu,Yinchuan Shi	585 138	1 091	770	93.77	0.00	0.71	-29.07	Y
920	银川市西夏区 Xixia Qu,Yinchuan Shi	244 850	926	428	66.09	2.70	0.46	60.47	Y
921	银川市金凤区 Jinfeng Qu,Yinchuan Shi	315 481	906	402	68.10	0.77	0.44	12.92	Y
922	贺兰县 Helan Xian	241 245	591	388	68.70	1.02	0.66	-9.90	Y

序号 No.	肿瘤登记处 Cancer registries	人口数 Population	发病数 New cases	死亡数 Deaths	MV%	DCO%	M/I	发病率变化 Change for CR%	接受 Accepted
923	石嘴山市大武口区 Dawukou Qu, Shizuishan Shi	255 934	863	476	80.19	0.12	0.55	8.54	Y
924	石嘴山市惠农区 Huinong Qu, Shizuishan Shi	170 997	545	362	67.52	0.37	0.66	−6.01	Y
925	平罗县 Pingluo Xian	312 087	684	448	72.37	0.73	0.65	17.32	Y
926	青铜峡市 Qingtongxia Shi	291 649	747	475	72.96	0.54	0.64	21.74	Y
927	固原市原州区 Yuanzhou Qu, Guyuan Shi	431 133	884	502	74.77	5.09	0.57	−7.59	Y
928	中卫市沙坡头区 Shapotou Qu, Zhongwei Shi	406 181	1 113	650	72.96	2.07	0.58	1.16	Y
929	中宁县 Zhongning Xian	333 029	605	391	67.11	4.13	0.65	24.60	Y
930	乌鲁木齐市天山区 Tianshan Qu, Ürümqi Shi	421 545	1 363	746	52.38	13.65	0.55	0.11	Y
931	乌鲁木齐市沙依巴克区 Saybag Qu, Ürümqi Shi	793 656	1 228	36	88.11	0.33	0.03	—	
932	乌鲁木齐市新市区 Xinshi Qu, Ürümqi Shi	866 126	2 651	20	88.23	0.04	0.01	—	
933	乌鲁木齐市水磨沟区 Shuimogou Qu, Ürümqi Shi	463 237	332	10	86.75	0.90	0.03	—	
934	乌鲁木齐市头屯河区 Toutunhe Qu, Ürümqi Shi	206 558	160	36	77.50	6.88	0.23	—	
935	乌鲁木齐市米东区 Midong Qu, Ürümqi Shi	276 464	467	328	81.37	1.50	0.70	−15.56	
936	克拉玛依市 Karamay Shi	431 663	1 988	1 077	70.72	1.61	0.54	31.13	Y
937	阜康市 Fukang Shi	186 613	119	17	35.29	1.68	0.14	—	
938	库尔勒市 Korla Shi	566 610	383	1	84.60	0.00	0.00	35.80	
939	阿克苏市 Aksu Shi	577 339	135	5	36.30	15.56	0.04	—	
940	拜城县 Baicheng Xian	248 144	32	2	46.88	0.00	0.06	—	
941	和田市 Hotan Shi	349 022	258	84	98.45	0.00	0.33	47.70	
942	和田县 Hotan Xian	292 430	109	26	96.33	0.00	0.24	26.12	
943	霍城县 Huocheng Xian	315 231	15	6	53.33	6.67	0.40	—	
944	新源县 Xinyuan Xian	294 318	574	369	64.29	1.92	0.64	49.53	Y
945	第二师 Di'ershi	211 914	316	99	63.92	0.95	0.31	11.45	
946	第七师 Diqishi	125 854	366	213	80.33	0.00	0.58	2.92	Y
947	第八师 Dibashi	591 637	1 806	1 093	60.69	3.65	0.61	−0.18	Y

4 本年报收录登记地区的选取与数据质量评价

4.1 年报收录登记地区的选取

国家癌症中心审核了 947 个登记地区提交的 2018 年登记资料,经质量控制,700 个肿瘤登记地区的数据被本年报收录,覆盖了全国 31 个省(自治区、直辖市)及新疆生产建设兵团(未包括香港特别行政区、澳门特别行政区和台湾省)。该数据作为全国肿瘤登记地区样本数据,用于分析中国癌症的发病与死亡。

4.2 全国登记地区数据质量评价指标

700 个肿瘤登记地区合计形态学诊断比例为 69.94%,仅有死亡证明书比例为 1.34%,死亡发病比为 0.58;全国城市登记地区合计形态学诊断比例为 71.50%,仅有死亡证明书比例为 1.58%,死亡发病比为 0.55;全国农村登记地区合计形态学诊断比例为 68.48%,仅有死亡证明书比例为 1.11%,死亡发病比为 0.61(表 3-3)。

4 Coverage and data quality of cancer registries in this annual report

4.1 Coverage of cancer registries in this annual report

Among 947 cancer registries which provided cancer data to NCC, 700 cancer registries' data were included in this annual report, covering all 31 provinces (autonomous regions and municipalities) and Xinjiang Production and Construction Corps in China (not including Hongkong Tebiexingzhengqu, Macau Tebiexingzhengqu and Taiwan Sheng). The qualified data were included in the final database for further analysis.

4.2 Evaluation of data quality

Among the 700 cancer registries, the MV%, DCO%, M/I was 69.94%, 1.34% and 0.58, respectively. In urban cancer registries, the MV%, DCO% and M/I was 71.50%, 1.58% and 0.55, respectively. In rural cancer registries, the MV%, DCO% and M/I was 68.48%, 1.11% and 0.61, respectively (Table 3-3).

表 3-3 中国肿瘤登记地区合计数据质量评价
Table 3-3 Quality indicators of the qualified national cancer registries

部位 Site	ICD-10 编码范围	全国合计 All			城市 Urban			农村 Rural		
		MV%	DCO%	M/I	MV%	DCO%	M/I	MV%	DCO%	M/I
口腔和咽喉（除外鼻咽癌）Oral cavity & pharynx but nasopharynx	C00-C10，C12-C14	76.85	1.01	0.49	79.85	1.28	0.51	73.84	0.74	0.48
鼻咽癌 Nasopharynx	C11	75.11	1.01	0.52	74.76	1.11	0.52	75.42	0.92	0.51
食管 Esophagus	C15	74.61	1.36	0.80	72.79	1.91	0.81	75.62	1.05	0.79
胃 Stomach	C16	75.51	1.51	0.73	74.36	1.87	0.71	76.35	1.24	0.74
结直肠肛门 Colon, rectum & anus	C18-C21	79.28	0.96	0.48	79.44	1.12	0.47	79.09	0.79	0.48
肝脏 Liver	C22	40.77	2.50	0.88	40.27	2.92	0.87	41.16	2.17	0.89
胆囊及其他 Gallbladder etc.	C23-C24	50.24	1.79	0.76	49.38	2.33	0.79	51.05	1.28	0.73
胰腺 Pancreas	C25	43.37	2.11	0.89	43.54	2.62	0.91	43.20	1.59	0.87
喉 Larynx	C32	75.22	1.26	0.57	76.31	1.47	0.55	74.04	1.05	0.59
气管,支气管,肺 Trachea, bronchus & lung	C33-C34	61.63	1.86	0.75	63.84	2.26	0.73	59.63	1.50	0.76
其他胸腔器官 Other thoracic organs	C37-C38	59.24	1.39	0.50	63.29	1.96	0.53	54.99	0.79	0.47
骨 Bone	C40-C41	45.19	2.44	0.72	47.28	3.22	0.75	43.85	1.94	0.69
皮肤黑色素瘤 Melanoma of skin	C43	93.95	0.59	0.51	93.08	0.75	0.48	94.86	0.43	0.54
乳房 Breast	C50	86.62	0.40	0.23	87.89	0.52	0.22	85.12	0.26	0.24
子宫颈 Cervix uteri	C53	84.79	0.55	0.32	84.89	0.83	0.31	84.72	0.35	0.32
子宫体及子宫部位不明 Uterus & unspecified	C54-C55	83.04	0.45	0.25	85.43	0.49	0.23	80.74	0.41	0.27
卵巢 Ovary	C56	76.05	0.78	0.47	77.15	1.07	0.49	74.88	0.48	0.44
前列腺 Prostate	C61	74.35	0.78	0.40	75.81	0.91	0.38	72.38	0.61	0.42
睾丸 Testis	C62	76.99	0.08	0.23	79.81	0.16	0.18	74.12	0.00	0.27
肾及泌尿系统不明 Kidney & unspecified urinary organs	C64-C66，C68	74.30	0.60	0.36	76.56	0.74	0.36	71.24	0.42	0.36
膀胱 Bladder	C67	76.15	1.05	0.44	78.02	1.28	0.43	74.09	0.80	0.44
脑,神经系统 Brain & central nervous system	C70-C72，D32-D33，D42-D43	49.86	1.65	0.55	52.17	1.97	0.52	47.91	1.38	0.58
甲状腺 Thyroid gland	C73	91.87	0.06	0.04	93.29	0.06	0.03	89.78	0.07	0.05
淋巴瘤 Lymphoma	C81-C86，C88,C90,C96	93.59	0.69	0.56	93.31	0.91	0.54	93.91	0.44	0.59
白血病 Leukemia	C91-C95，D45-D47	92.23	0.84	0.63	92.22	1.17	0.62	92.24	0.54	0.64
不明及其他癌症 Other and unspecified	O&U	63.27	1.64	0.50	63.90	2.01	0.51	62.63	1.26	0.49
所有部位合计 All sites	C00-C97，D32-D33，D42-D43，D45-D47	69.94	1.34	0.58	71.50	1.58	0.55	68.48	1.11	0.61

第四章 2018年中国肿瘤登记地区癌症发病与死亡

本年报收录的肿瘤登记处覆盖人口 523 160 249 人,占 2018 年中国总人口(1 405 410 000)的 37.22%。本年报收录的数据反映了目前我国癌症的发病与死亡情况,为我国的癌症防治与研究提供了基础数据。

1 中国肿瘤登记地区覆盖人口

2018 年纳入年报的中国肿瘤登记地区覆盖人口 523 160 249 人(男性 265 488 549 人,女性 257 671 700 人),占全国 2018 年末人口数的 37.22%。其中城市人口 236 047 481 人(男性 118 492 370 人,女性 117 555 111 人),占全国登记地区人口的 45.12%;农村人口 287 112 768 人(男性 146 996 179 人,女性 140 116 589 人),占全国登记地区人口的 54.88%(表 4-1a,图 4-1)。

东部登记地区覆盖人口 217 144 390 人(男性 109 052 317 人,女性 108 092 073 人),占全国登记地区人口的 41.51%;中部登记地区覆盖人口 129 694 438 人(男性 66 273 553 人,女性 63 420 885 人),占全国登记地区人口的 24.79%;西部登记地区覆盖人口 176 321 421 人(男性 90 162 679 人,女性 86 158 742 人),占全国登记地区人口的 33.70%(表 4-1b,图 4-1)。

Chapter 4 Cancer incidence and mortality in the registration areas of China,2018

In this annual report, a total of 523 160 249 people were covered in the registration system in China, accounting for 37.22% of the total population (1 405 410 000) in China in 2018. This annual report represented the current status of cancer incidence and mortality rates in China and provided the basic data for cancer prevention and control.

1 Population coverage in cancer registration areas of China

The population covered by cancer registration areas included in the annual report in 2018 was 523 160 249 (265 488 549 males and 257 671 700females), which accounted for 37.22% of the total population at the end of 2018. There were 236 047 481 people in urban areas(118 492 370males and 117 555 111 females)and 287 112 768 people in the rural areas(146 996 179 males and 140 116 589 females), accounting for 45.12% and 54.88% of the covered population in all cancer registration areas,respectively(Table 4-1a, Figure 4-1).

The population covered by cancer registration in eastern areas was 217 144 390(109 052 317 males and 108 092 073 females), which accounted for 41.51% of the covered population in all cancer registration areas. The population covered by the cancer registration in the central areas was 129 694 438 (66 273 553males and 63 420 885 females), which accounted for 24.79% of the population in all cancer registration areas. The population covered by the cancer registration in western areas was 176 321 421 (90 162 679 males and 86 158 742 females), which accounted for 33.70% of the population in all cancer registration areas(Table 4-1b, Figure 4-1).

表 4-1a 2018 年中国肿瘤登记地区覆盖人口

Table 4-1a Population in all cancer registration areas of China, 2018

年龄组/岁 Age group/years	全国 All areas			城市地区 Urban areas			农村地区 Rural areas		
	合计 All	男性 Male	女性 Female	合计 All	男性 Male	女性 Female	合计 All	男性 Male	女性 Female
合计	523 160 249	265 488 549	257 671 700	236 047 481	118 492 370	117 555 111	287 112 768	146 996 179	140 116 589
0~	5 351 889	2 831 943	2 519 946	2 408 681	1 266 213	1 142 468	2 943 208	1 565 730	1 377 478
1~	23 931 238	12 729 464	11 201 774	10 546 850	5 551 171	4 995 679	13 384 388	7 178 293	6 206 095
5~	28 842 375	15 279 403	13 562 972	12 070 648	6 372 389	5 698 259	16 771 727	8 907 014	7 864 713
10~	26 591 483	14 201 472	12 390 011	10 897 060	5 765 779	5 131 281	15 694 423	8 435 693	7 258 730
15~	27 727 794	14 585 468	13 142 326	11 359 200	5 929 630	5 429 570	16 368 594	8 655 838	7 712 756
20~	34 515 110	17 702 871	16 812 239	14 658 239	7 503 030	7 155 209	19 856 871	10 199 841	9 657 030
25~	38 605 303	19 615 180	18 990 123	17 177 709	8 564 297	8 613 412	21 427 594	11 050 883	10 376 711
30~	38 663 141	19 464 756	19 198 385	18 467 999	9 102 943	9 365 056	20 195 142	10 361 813	9 833 329
35~	39 956 042	20 154 570	19 801 472	19 162 520	9 494 576	9 667 944	20 793 522	10 659 994	10 133 528
40~	41 246 056	20 862 589	20 383 467	18 676 972	9 322 529	9 354 443	22 569 084	11 540 060	11 029 024
45~	46 480 021	23 439 973	23 040 048	21 022 330	10 548 766	10 473 564	25 457 691	12 891 207	12 566 484
50~	39 175 921	19 869 722	19 306 199	17 586 441	8 888 089	8 698 352	21 589 480	10 981 633	10 607 847
55~	33 671 990	16 963 128	16 708 862	15 765 361	7 912 339	7 853 022	17 906 629	9 050 789	8 855 840
60~	31 384 128	15 772 987	15 611 141	14 871 872	7 398 653	7 473 219	16 512 256	8 374 334	8 137 922
65~	24 472 174	12 153 174	12 319 000	11 388 103	5 590 416	5 797 687	13 084 071	6 562 758	6 521 313
70~	16 823 799	8 276 466	8 547 333	7 730 530	3 761 272	3 969 258	9 093 269	4 515 194	4 578 075
75~	11 984 179	5 682 100	6 302 079	5 542 420	2 601 765	2 940 655	6 441 759	3 080 335	3 361 424
80~	8 101 104	3 644 185	4 456 919	3 904 609	1 759 667	2 144 942	4 196 495	1 884 518	2 311 977
85+	5 636 502	2 259 098	3 377 404	2 809 937	1 158 846	1 651 091	2 826 565	1 100 252	1 726 313

表 4-1b　2018 年中国肿瘤登记地区东、中、西部地区覆盖人口

Table4-1b　Population in eastern, central and western areas in cancer registration areas of China, 2018

年龄组/岁 Age group/ years	东部地区 Eastern areas			中部地区 Central areas			西部地区 Western areas		
	合计 All	男性 Male	女性 Female	合计 All	男性 Male	女性 Female	合计 All	男性 Male	女性 Female
合计	217 144 390	109 052 317	108 092 073	129 694 438	66 273 553	63 420 885	176 321 421	90 162 679	86 158 742
0~	2 230 676	1 173 760	1 056 916	1 350 104	719 993	630 111	1 771 109	938 190	832 919
1~	10 170 421	5 387 349	4 783 072	6 260 676	3 376 756	2 883 920	7 500 141	3 965 359	3 534 782
5~	11 394 983	6 060 802	5 334 181	7 829 534	4 182 703	3 646 831	9 617 858	5 035 898	4 581 960
10~	9 777 558	5 214 587	4 562 971	7 061 465	3 829 356	3 232 109	9 752 460	5 157 529	4 594 931
15~	9 175 409	4 845 074	4 330 335	7 308 273	3 882 564	3 425 709	11 244 112	5 857 830	5 386 282
20~	11 863 454	6 136 149	5 727 305	9 136 981	4 678 354	4 458 627	13 514 675	6 888 368	6 626 307
25~	15 977 454	8 104 296	7 873 158	10 229 996	5 168 443	5 061 553	12 397 853	6 342 441	6 055 412
30~	17 381 304	8 622 478	8 758 826	9 748 435	4 920 603	4 827 832	11 533 402	5 921 675	5 611 727
35~	16 444 057	8 160 167	8 283 890	9 884 084	5 015 507	4 868 577	13 627 901	6 978 896	6 649 005
40~	15 284 683	7 602 130	7 682 553	10 657 711	5 416 967	5 240 744	15 303 662	7 843 492	7 460 170
45~	18 150 199	9 052 329	9 097 870	11 470 188	5 800 251	5 669 937	16 859 634	8 587 393	8 272 241
50~	17 717 884	8 890 178	8 827 706	9 263 444	4 703 317	4 560 127	12 194 593	6 276 227	5 918 366
55~	15 187 677	7 618 293	7 569 384	7 862 477	3 981 741	3 880 736	10 621 836	5 363 094	5 258 742
60~	15 267 128	7 591 816	7 675 312	6 812 571	3 443 152	3 369 419	9 304 429	4 738 019	4 566 410
65~	11 500 752	5 647 212	5 853 540	5 281 774	2 647 987	2 633 787	7 689 648	3 857 975	3 831 673
70~	7 504 424	3 637 584	3 866 840	3 790 084	1 880 849	1 909 235	5 529 291	258 033	2 771 258
75~	5 220 690	2 438 548	2 782 142	2 839 223	1 348 393	1 490 830	3 924 266	1 895 159	2 029 107
80~	3 953 368	1 735 135	2 218 233	1 756 283	802 371	953 912	2 391 453	1 106 679	1 284 774
85+	2 942 269	1 134 430	1 807 839	1 151 135	474 246	676 889	1 543 098	650 422	892 676

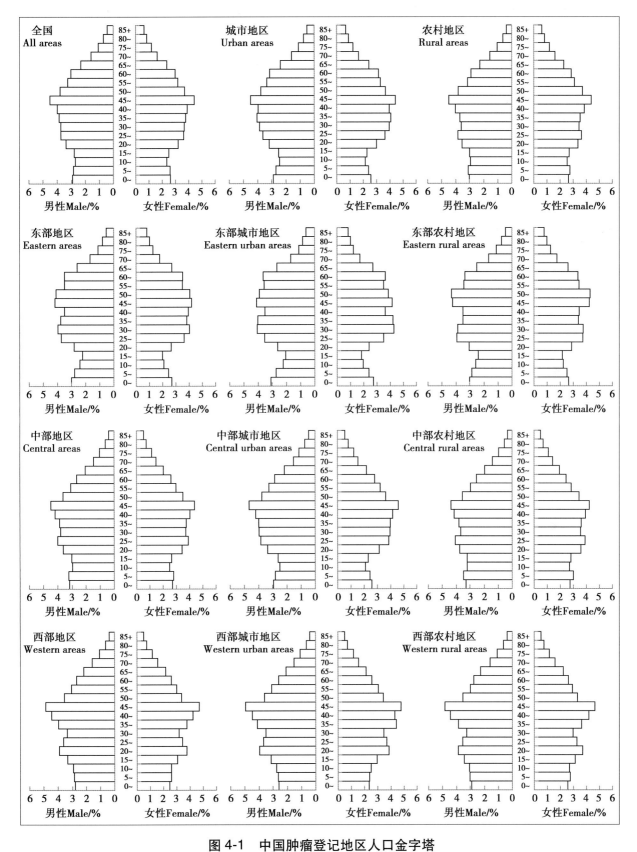

图 4-1 中国肿瘤登记地区人口金字塔

Figure 4-1 Population pyramid in cancer registration areas of China

2 中国肿瘤登记地区全部癌症发病与死亡

2.1 中国肿瘤登记地区全部癌症发病情况

2018 年中国肿瘤登记地区新发病例数 1 563 923 例（男性 860 417 例，女性 703 506 例），其中城市地区的新发病例数 757 307 例，占 48.42%，农村地区 806 616 例，占 51.58%。东部地区 767 093 例，占新发病例数的 49.05%；中部地区 349 489 例，占新发病例数的 22.35%；西部地区 447 341 例，占新发病例数的 28.60%（表 4-2）。

中国肿瘤登记地区发病率为 298.94/10 万（男性 324.09/10 万，女性 273.02/10 万），中标率 190.16/10 万，世标率 185.49/10 万，累积率（0~74 岁）为 21.34%。城市地区发病率为 320.83/10 万（男性 343.02/10 万，女性 298.46/10 万），中标率 198.15/10 万，世标率 192.91/10 万，累积率（0~74 岁）为 21.98%。农村地区发病率为 280.94/10 万（男性 308.83/10 万，女性 251.68/10 万），中标率 183.13/10 万，世标率 178.95/10 万，累积率（0~74 岁）为 20.79%。城市与农村相比，城市男女的发病率、中标率、世标率、累积率均高于农村地区男女相应的指标（表 4-2）。

东部地区发病率为 353.26/10 万（男性 375.12/10 万，女性 331.22/10 万），中标率 208.16/10 万，世标率 201.84/10 万，累积率（0~74 岁）为 23.04%。中部地区发病率为 269.47/10 万（男性 288.64/10 万，女性 249.44/10 万），中标率 185.23/10 万，世标率 181.66/10 万，累积率（0~74 岁）为 21.14%。西部地区发病率为 253.71/10 万（男性 288.43/10 万，女性 217.38/10 万），中标率 170.24/10 万，世标率 166.68/10 万，累积率（0~74 岁）为 19.24%。东中西部地区相比，东部地区的男性和女性发病率、中标率、世标率和累积率均高于中部和西部地区。西部地区的女性发病率、中标率、世标率和累积率均低于东部和中部地区（表 4-2）。

2 Incidence and mortality for all cancer sites in the registration areas of China

2.1 Incidence for all cancer sites in the registration areas of China

In 2018, there were 1 563 923 new cases (860 417 males and 703 506 females) in cancer registration areas of China. Among all the new cases, 757 307 (48.42%) came from urban areas, and 806 616 (51.58%) were from rural areas. There were 767 093 (49.05%) cases in eastern areas, 349 489 (22.35%) cases in the central areas, and 447 341 (28.60%) cases in western areas (Table 4-2).

The incidence rate for all cancer sites was 298.94 per 100 000 in 2018 (324.09 per 100 000 in males, and 273.02 per 100 000 in females). The ASR China was 190.16 per 100 000, and the ASR World was 185.49 per 100 000. The cumulative rate (0-74 years old) was 21.34%. The incidence rate in the urban areas was 320.83 per 100 000 in 2018 (343.02 per 100 000 in males and 298.46 per 100 000 in females). The ASR China was 198.15 per 100 000, and the ASR world was 192.91 per 100 000. The cumulative rate (0-74 years old) was 21.98%. The incidence rate in the rural areas was 280.94 per 100 000 (308.83 per 100 000 in males and 251.68 per 100 000 in females). The ASR China was 183.13 per 100 000, and the ASR world was 178.95 per 100 000. The cumulative rate (0-74 years old) was 20.79%. The incidence rate, ASR China, ASR World, and the cumulative rate of all cancer sites were higher in the urban areas than those in the rural areas for both sexes (Table 4-2).

The incidence rate in eastern areas was 353.26 per 100 000 (375.12 per 100 000 in males and 331.22 per 100 000 in females). The ASR China was 208.16 per 100 000, and the ASR world was 201.84 per 100 000. The cumulative rate (0-74 years old) was 23.04%. The incidence rate in the central areas was 269.47 per 100 000 in 2018 (288.64 per 100 000 in males and 249.44 per 100 000 in females). The ASR China was 185.23 per 100 000, and the ASR World was 181.66 per 100 000. The cumulative rate (0-74 years old) was 21.14%. The incidence rate in western areas was 253.71 per 100 000 (288.43 per 100 000 in males and 217.38 per 100 000 in females). The ASR China was 170.24 per 100 000, and the ASR World was 166.68 per 100 000. The cumulative rate (0-74 years old) was 19.24%. The incidence rate, ASR China, ASR World, and the cumulative rate of both males and females in eastern areas were higher than those in central and western areas. The incidence rate, ASR China, ASR World, and cumulative rate for females in western areas were lower than those in eastern and central areas (Table 4-2).

表 4-2　2018 年中国肿瘤登记地区全部癌症发病情况

Table 4-2　Incidence rate for all cancer sites in the registration areas of China,2018

地区 Area	性别 Sex	病例数 No. cases	发病率 Incidence rate/ 100 000^{-1}	中标率 ASR China/ 100 000^{-1}	世标率 ASR World/ 100 000^{-1}	累积率 Cum. rate 0~74/%
全国 All areas	合计 Both	1 563 923	298. 94	190. 16	185. 49	21. 34
	男性 Male	860 417	324. 09	205. 39	203. 62	24. 08
	女性 Female	703 506	273. 02	176. 98	169. 40	18. 68
城市地区 Urban areas	合计 Both	757 307	320. 83	198. 15	192. 91	21. 98
	男性 Male	406 447	343. 02	209. 37	207. 52	24. 35
	女性 Female	350 860	298. 46	189. 02	180. 46	19. 74
农村地区 Rural areas	合计 Both	806 616	280. 94	183. 13	178. 95	20. 79
	男性 Male	453 970	308. 83	201. 84	200. 10	23. 85
	女性 Female	352 646	251. 68	166. 28	159. 60	17. 75
东部地区 Eastern areas	合计 Both	767 093	353. 26	208. 16	201. 84	23. 04
	男性 Male	409 072	375. 12	217. 56	214. 86	25. 27
	女性 Female	358 021	331. 22	201. 39	191. 52	20. 94
中部地区 Central areas	合计 Both	349 489	269. 47	185. 23	181. 66	21. 14
	男性 Male	191 292	288. 64	199. 39	198. 53	23. 82
	女性 Female	158 197	249. 44	172. 65	166. 30	18. 48
西部地区 Western areas	合计 Both	447 341	253. 71	170. 24	166. 68	19. 24
	男性 Male	260 053	288. 43	193. 66	192. 26	22. 70
	女性 Female	187 288	217. 38	147. 87	142. 11	15. 75

2.2　中国肿瘤登记地区全部癌症年龄别发病率

2018 年中国肿瘤登记地区全部癌症的年龄别发病率在 0~34 岁时处于较低水平,35~39 岁年龄组发病率快速上升,为 95. 49/10 万,80~84 岁年龄组发病率处于最高水平,为 1 422. 68/10 万,85 岁及以上年龄组的发病率有所下降,为 1 318. 34/10 万。城市和农村地区的癌症年龄别发病率变化模式基本相同。除 5~19 岁年龄组农村发病率略高于城市以外,城市发病率均高于农村。城市男性癌症发病率在 5~19 岁、45~54 岁和 70~74 岁年龄组低于农村,其他年龄组高于农村;城市女性癌症发病率在 5~19 岁年龄组低于农村,其他年龄组高于农村(表 4-3a,图 4-2)。

东部、中部和西部地区的年龄别发病率均在 80~84 岁年龄组达到最高,85 岁及以上年龄组时有所下降。除少数几个年龄组外,东部地区男女性年龄组发病率均高于中部和西部地区。三个区域的城市癌症发病率均高于农村,分城乡、分性别的年龄别发病率曲线基本类似(表 4-3b,图 4-2)。

2.2　Age-specific incidence rates for all cancer sites in the registration areas of China

In 2018,incidence rate for all cancer sites was relatively low in the age group of 0-34 years,and dramatically increased from age group 35-39 years old(95. 49 per 100 100),and reached the peak at the age of 80-84 years old(1 422. 68 per 100 000)and then decreased slightly after 85 years old(1 318. 34 per 100 000). The overall trends of the age-specific incidence in urban areas were similar as that in rural areas. The incidence rate in urban areas was higher than that in rural areas except the age group of 5-19. The incidence rates for males in urban areas were lower than those in rural areas in the age group of 5-19、45-54 and 70-74,and higher in other age groups. The incidence rate of cancer among urban women in the 5-19 age group is lower than that in rural areas,and other age groups are higher than that in rural areas(Table 4-3a,Figure 4-2).

The age-specific incidence rates in eastern,central and western areas reached peak at the age group of 80-84 years old,and declined after 85-year-old. Overall,the incidence rates in eastern areas were higher than those in central and western areas for both sexes. The incidence rates in urban areas were higher than those in rural areas in the all three geographic areas and the age-specific incidence curves by urban and rural areas and by sex are basically similar(Table 4-3b,Figure 4-2).

表 4-3a　2018 年中国肿瘤登记地区癌症年龄别发病率

Table 4-3a　Age-specific incidence rates for all cancer sites in
the registration areas of China, 2018

单位:100 000^{-1}

年龄组/ 岁 Age group/ years	全国 All areas			城市地区 Urban areas			农村地区 Rural areas		
	合计 All	男性 Male	女性 Female	合计 All	男性 Male	女性 Female	合计 All	男性 Male	女性 Female
合计	298.94	324.09	273.02	320.83	343.02	298.46	280.94	308.83	251.68
0~	12.63	13.07	12.14	13.29	13.35	13.22	12.10	12.84	11.25
1~	11.51	12.41	10.48	12.24	13.51	10.83	10.93	11.56	10.20
5~	8.02	8.63	7.33	7.80	8.32	7.21	8.18	8.86	7.41
10~	9.22	9.67	8.70	8.53	9.02	7.97	9.70	10.11	9.22
15~	11.48	11.45	11.51	11.12	11.35	10.87	11.73	11.52	11.97
20~	17.71	14.21	21.40	19.04	14.89	23.40	16.73	13.72	19.91
25~	40.30	29.77	51.17	46.01	33.79	58.17	35.72	26.66	45.37
30~	68.10	48.25	88.22	75.97	52.24	99.04	60.90	44.75	77.92
35~	95.49	66.65	124.85	106.01	71.39	140.01	85.81	62.44	110.39
40~	149.08	107.27	191.87	161.05	109.87	212.06	139.17	105.17	174.74
45~	244.07	193.49	295.54	252.38	191.92	313.28	237.21	194.77	280.75
50~	394.65	366.82	423.30	402.22	365.24	440.01	388.49	368.10	409.59
55~	448.56	478.73	417.92	484.11	504.83	463.22	417.26	455.92	377.75
60~	722.19	859.61	583.35	748.53	878.63	619.72	698.47	842.80	549.94
65~	930.79	1 167.76	697.00	938.93	1 170.13	715.99	923.70	1 165.74	680.12
70~	1 117.21	1 441.38	803.31	1 121.71	1 434.17	825.62	1 113.38	1 447.38	783.98
75~	1 283.80	1 681.77	924.98	1 326.21	1 708.61	987.88	1 247.31	1 659.11	869.96
80~	1 422.68	1 868.79	1 057.93	1 504.91	1 950.71	1 139.19	1 346.17	1 792.29	982.54
85+	1 318.34	1 798.64	997.07	1 427.22	1 917.51	1 083.10	1 210.09	1 673.43	914.78

表 4-3b 2018 年中国不同肿瘤登记地区癌症年龄别发病率
Table 4-3b Age-specific incidence rates for all cancer sites in different registration areas of China,2018

单位:100 000^{-1}

年龄组/岁 Age group/ years	东部地区 Eastern areas			中部地区 Central areas			西部地区 Western areas		
	合计 All	男性 Male	女性 Female	合计 All	男性 Male	女性 Female	合计 All	男性 Male	女性 Female
合计	353.26	375.12	331.22	269.47	288.64	249.44	253.71	288.43	217.38
0~	15.96	16.02	15.90	12.52	12.50	12.54	8.53	9.81	7.08
1~	13.03	14.46	11.42	11.72	12.17	11.20	9.27	9.84	8.63
5~	8.13	8.60	7.59	9.09	10.14	7.90	7.02	7.43	6.57
10~	9.29	9.53	9.01	10.78	11.41	10.02	8.02	8.51	7.46
15~	13.21	13.00	13.44	11.78	11.59	12.00	9.87	10.07	9.65
20~	22.49	17.34	28.01	15.91	12.95	19.02	14.73	12.28	17.28
25~	49.48	35.59	63.77	37.61	27.63	47.81	30.69	24.09	37.60
30~	80.65	54.45	106.44	57.88	40.69	75.40	57.82	45.51	70.82
35~	122.61	80.79	163.80	83.30	56.03	111.39	71.63	57.76	86.18
40~	178.36	117.72	238.37	134.28	92.52	177.44	130.14	107.34	154.11
45~	272.86	199.58	345.76	239.99	186.08	295.14	215.87	192.06	240.59
50~	384.57	337.88	431.58	403.46	366.70	441.37	402.62	407.90	397.02
55~	518.44	535.21	501.56	427.78	448.25	406.78	364.01	421.14	305.76
60~	753.49	872.90	635.37	713.55	847.42	576.75	677.16	847.17	500.77
65~	967.74	1 196.56	746.98	971.57	1 219.00	722.80	847.52	1 090.44	602.92
70~	1 212.36	1 560.65	884.73	1 098.50	1 421.54	780.26	1 000.89	1 297.59	705.60
75~	1 416.92	1 854.38	1 033.48	1 198.60	1 571.57	861.27	1 168.35	1 538.08	823.02
80~	1 547.72	2 048.83	1 155.74	1 378.37	1 799.42	1 024.20	1 248.53	1 636.79	914.09
85+	1 409.69	1 940.36	1 076.70	1 253.46	1 668.12	962.93	1 192.54	1 646.62	861.68

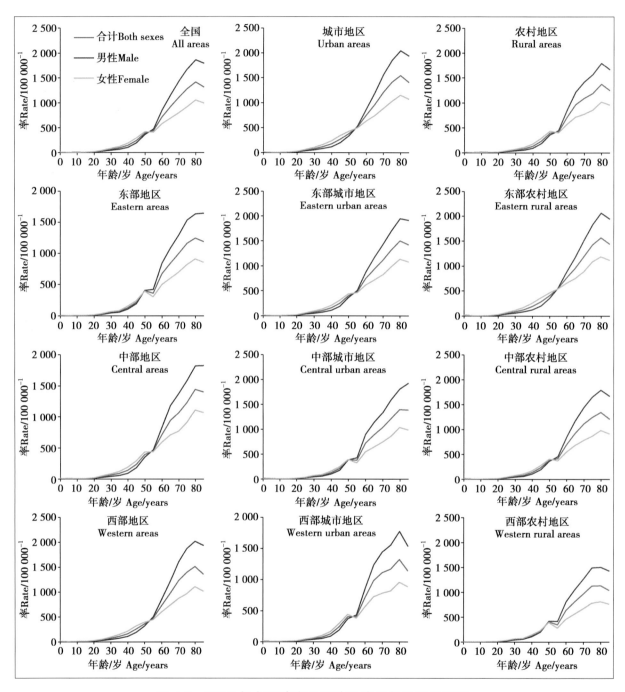

图 4-2 2018 年中国肿瘤登记地区癌症年龄别发病率

Figure 4-2 Age-specific incidence rates for all cancer sites in
the registration areas of China,2018

2.3 中国肿瘤登记地区全部癌症死亡情况

2018 年中国肿瘤登记地区报告癌症死亡 912 425 例（男性 584 397 例，女性 328 028 例），其中城市地区 420 199 例，占全国癌症死亡的 46.05%，农村地区 492 226 例，占全国癌症死亡的 53.95%。东部地区 418 659 例，占全国癌症死亡的 45.88%；中部地区 210 484 例，占全国癌症死亡的 23.07%；西部地区 283 282 例，占全国癌症死亡的 31.05%（表 4-4）。

中国肿瘤登记地区 2018 年癌症死亡率为 174.41/10 万（男性 220.12/10 万，女性 127.30/10 万），中标率 100.82/10 万，世标率 100.15/10 万，累积率（0~74 岁）为 11.31%。城市地区死亡率为 178.01/10 万（男性 224.91/10 万，女性 130.75/10 万），中标率 98.01/10 万，世标率 97.55/10 万，累积率（0~74 岁）为 10.80%。农村地区死亡率为 171.44/10 万（男性 216.26/10 万，女性 124.42/10 万），中标率 103.14/10 万，世标率 102.27/10 万，累积率（0~74 岁）为 11.75%。城市与农村相比，城市地区男性和女性死亡率均高于农村，而城市男性和女性的中标率、世标率和累积率均低于农村（表 4-4）。

东部、中部和西部地区死亡率分别为 192.80/10 万（男性 241.83/10 万，女性 143.34/10 万）、162.29 万（男性 202.53/10 万，女性 120.24/10 万）和 160.66/10 万（男性 206.79/10 万，女性 112.39/10 万）。东部地区的中标率为 98.43/10 万、中部地区 103.81/10 万、西部地区 101.74/10 万。东部地区的世标率为 97.74/10 万、中部地区 103.22/10 万、西部地区 101.03/10 万。东部、中部和西部地区累积率（0~74 岁）分别为 10.84%、11.96% 和 11.56%。东部地区男女性的死亡率均高于中部和西部，男女合计的中标率、世标率和累积率均低于中部和西部地区（表 4-4）。

2.3 Mortality for all cancer sites in the registration areas of China

In 2018, there were 912 425 cancer deaths (584 397 males and 328 028 females) in the registration areas of China. Among those, 420 199 (46.05%) came from urban areas, and 492 226 (53.95%) came from rural areas. There were 418 659 (45.88%) death cases in eastern areas, 210 484 (23.07%) in central areas and 283 282 (31.05%) in western areas (Table 4-4).

The mortality rate of all cancer sites was 174.41 per 100 000 in 2018 (220.12 per 100 000 in males and 127.30 per 100 000 in females). The ASR China was 100.82 per 100 000, and the ASR World was 100.15 per 100 000. The cumulative rate (0-74 years old) was 11.31%. The mortality for all cancer sites in urban areas was 178.01 per 100 000 (224.91 per 100 000 in males and 130.75 per 100 000 in females). The ASR China was 98.01 per 100 000, and the ASR World was 97.55 per 100 000. The cumulative rate (0-74 years old) was 10.80%. The mortality for all cancer sites in rural areas was 171.44 per 100 000 in 2018 (216.26 per 100 000 in males and 124.42 per 100 000 in females). The ASR China was 103.14 per 100 000, and the ASR World was 102.27 per 100 000. The cumulative rate (0-74 years old) was 11.75%. The mortality rates for all cancer sites in urban areas were higher than those in rural areas for both sexes. The ASR China, ASR World and cumulative rates of all cancer sites were lower in urban areas than those in rural areas for both sexes (Table 4-4).

The mortality rates for all cancer sites in eastern, central and western areas were 192.80 per 100 000 (241.83 per 100 000 in males and 143.34 per 100 000 in females), 162.29 per 100 000 (202.53 per 100 000 in males and 120.24 per 100 000 in females), and 160.66 per 100 000 (206.79 per 100 000 in males and 112.39 per 100 000 in females), respectively. The ASR China were 98.43 per 100 000 in eastern areas, 103.81 per 100 000 in central areas, and 101.74 per 100 000 in western areas, respectively. The ASR World were 97.74 per 100 000 in eastern areas, 103.22 per 100 000 in central areas, and 101.03 per 100 000 in western areas. The cumulative rates (0-74 years old) in the eastern, central and western areas were 10.84%, 11.96% and 11.56%, respectively. The mortality rate for all cancer sites in eastern areas was higher than that in central and western areas for both sexes. The ASR China, ASR World and cumulative rates were the lowest in eastern areas for both sexes combined (Table 4-4).

表 4-4　2018 年中国肿瘤登记地区全部癌症死亡情况

Table 4-4　Mortality for all cancer sites in the registration areas of China,2018

地区 Area	性别 Sex	死亡数 No. deaths	粗率 Crude rate/ 100 000^{-1}	中标率 ASR China/ 100 000^{-1}	世标率 ASR World/ 100 000^{-1}	累积率 Cum. rate 0~74/%
全国 All areas	合计 Both	912 425	174. 41	100. 82	100. 15	11. 31
	男性 Male	584 397	220. 12	133. 06	132. 70	15. 14
	女性 Female	328 028	127. 30	70. 17	69. 29	7. 53
城市地区 Urban areas	合计 Both	420 199	178. 01	98. 01	97. 55	10. 80
	男性 Male	266 498	224. 91	129. 19	129. 26	14. 55
	女性 Female	153 701	130. 75	68. 81	67. 93	7. 17
农村地区 Rural areas	合计 Both	492 226	171. 44	103. 14	102. 27	11. 75
	男性 Male	317 899	216. 26	136. 18	135. 41	15. 64
	女性 Female	174 327	124. 42	71. 30	70. 43	7. 84
东部地区 Eastern areas	合计 Both	418 659	192. 80	98. 43	97. 74	10. 84
	男性 Male	263 723	241. 83	130. 20	129. 89	14. 56
	女性 Female	154 936	143. 34	69. 29	68. 37	7. 25
中部地区 Central areas	合计 Both	210 484	162. 29	103. 81	103. 22	11. 96
	男性 Male	134 227	202. 53	135. 05	134. 67	15. 73
	女性 Female	76 257	120. 24	73. 66	72. 90	8. 17
西部地区 Western areas	合计 Both	283 282	160. 66	101. 74	101. 03	11. 56
	男性 Male	186 447	206. 79	135. 16	134. 74	15. 57
	女性 Female	96 835	112. 39	68. 71	67. 78	7. 49

2.4　中国肿瘤登记地区全部癌症年龄别死亡率

中国肿瘤登记地区癌症年龄别死亡率在 25~29 岁组为 7.84/10 万(男性 8.93/10 万,女性 6.71/10 万),在 40~44 岁年龄组时达到 43.50/10 万,在这以后死亡率随年龄增长而明显升高,在 85 岁以上年龄组达最高,死亡率为 1 479.18/10 万。城乡年龄别死亡率的变化模式基本相似,城市地区和农村地区的癌症死亡率均在 85 岁及以上年龄组达到最高,死亡率分别为 1 596.98/10 万和 1 362.08/10 万。城市多数年龄组的死亡率低于农村(表 4-5a,图 4-3)。

东部、中部和西部地区的年龄别癌症死亡率曲线与全国的基本一致。东部、中部和西部地区男女年龄别死亡率均在 85 岁以后达到高峰,死亡率分别为 1 628.61/10 万、1 369.26/10 万和 1 276.26/10 万。在 0~64 岁的各个组别中,西部多数年龄组的死亡率高于东部和中部,65~69 岁年龄组以中部最高,而 75 岁以上的年龄组以东部地区最高。三个区域的城市癌症死亡率均高于农村,城市与农村的年龄别死亡率曲线基本相似(表 4-5b,图 4-3)。

2.4　Age-specific mortality rates for all cancer sites in the registration areas of China

The age-specific mortality rate for all cancer sites was 7. 84 per 100 000(8. 93 per 100 000 in males and 6. 71 per 100 000 in females) in the 25-29 age group and 43. 50 per 100 000 in the 40-44 age group. The mortality rate increased significantly after the age group of 40-44 years old and reached the peak in the over 85 age group,with a mortality rate of 1 479. 18/100 000. The trends of age-specific mortality in urban and rural areas were similar,the mortality rate in urban areas and rural areas reaches the highest in the age group of 85 years and above,with a mortality rate of 1 596. 98 per 100 000 and 1 362. 08 per 100 000,respectively. Most age groups had lower mortality rates in urban areas than in rural areas(Table 4-5a,Figure 4-3).

The trends of age-specific mortality rates in different areas(eastern areas,central areas,and western areas) were similar to those of the overall country. The age-specific mortality rates for both sexes in eastern,central and western areas reached peak after 85 years old,with mortality rates of 1 628. 61 per 100 000,1 369. 26 per 100 000 and 1 276. 26 per 100 000,respectively. Most age groups in the age range of 0-64 had the highest mortality rate in western areas. The mortality rate was the highest in the central areas in the 65-69 age group,and it was the highest in eastern areas in above 75 years old age groups. The trends of the age-specific mortality rates were similar in urban and rural areas,although the rates in urban areas were generally higher than those in rural areas in all three geographic areas(Table 4-5b,Figure 4-3).

表 4-5a 2018 年中国肿瘤登记地区癌症年龄别死亡率

Table 4-5a Age-specific mortality rates for all cancer sites in the registration areas of China, 2018

单位:100 000⁻¹

年龄组/岁 Age group/years	全国 All areas			城市地区 Urban areas			农村地区 Rural areas		
	合计 All	男性 Male	女性 Female	合计 All	男性 Male	女性 Female	合计 All	男性 Male	女性 Female
合计	174.41	220.12	127.30	178.01	224.91	130.75	171.44	216.26	124.42
0~	4.75	4.06	5.52	4.36	4.03	4.73	5.06	4.09	6.17
1~	3.38	3.61	3.12	3.33	3.58	3.04	3.43	3.64	3.19
5~	3.15	3.49	2.76	3.01	3.28	2.70	3.26	3.65	2.81
10~	3.29	3.78	2.73	3.07	3.50	2.59	3.44	3.97	2.82
15~	4.01	4.60	3.35	3.76	4.28	3.19	4.18	4.82	3.46
20~	4.33	5.09	3.53	3.97	4.68	3.23	4.59	5.39	3.75
25~	7.84	8.93	6.71	7.11	7.89	6.34	8.42	9.74	7.02
30~	14.16	15.68	12.62	12.97	13.96	12.01	15.25	17.20	13.19
35~	22.15	25.19	19.06	20.38	22.53	18.28	23.78	27.55	19.81
40~	43.50	50.31	36.53	40.82	46.36	35.30	45.72	53.51	37.57
45~	83.35	99.59	66.83	78.29	91.84	64.64	87.53	105.94	68.65
50~	160.08	199.89	119.11	152.28	189.78	113.95	166.44	208.07	123.34
55~	204.86	272.03	136.67	207.19	275.78	138.09	202.81	268.75	135.41
60~	377.41	518.23	235.14	364.39	505.02	225.16	389.14	529.89	244.30
65~	560.11	770.77	352.28	529.55	738.67	327.91	586.70	798.11	373.94
70~	770.99	1 046.52	504.18	730.13	997.96	476.34	805.72	1 086.97	528.32
75~	1 037.95	1 396.54	714.64	1 030.83	1 368.92	731.71	1 044.08	1 419.88	699.70
80~	1 336.25	1 772.99	979.15	1 383.93	1 799.43	1 043.06	1 291.89	1 748.30	919.86
85+	1 479.18	2 018.59	1 118.37	1 596.98	2 154.82	1 205.45	1 362.08	1 875.12	1 035.10

表 4-5b 2018 年中国不同肿瘤登记地区癌症年龄别死亡率
Table 4-5b Age-specific mortality rates for all cancer sites in different registration areas of China, 2018

单位:100 000^{-1}

年龄组/ 岁 Age group/ years	东部地区 Eastern areas			中部地区 Central areas			西部地区 Western areas		
	合计 All	男性 Male	女性 Female	合计 All	男性 Male	女性 Female	合计 All	男性 Male	女性 Female
合计	192.80	241.83	143.34	162.29	202.53	120.24	160.66	206.79	112.39
0~	5.16	3.49	7.00	4.52	4.17	4.92	4.40	4.69	4.08
1~	3.21	3.29	3.12	2.94	3.20	2.64	4.00	4.41	3.54
5~	2.88	3.10	2.62	3.41	3.87	2.88	3.26	3.65	2.84
10~	2.94	3.05	2.81	3.55	4.26	2.72	3.46	4.17	2.66
15~	4.12	4.77	3.39	4.08	4.61	3.47	3.87	4.46	3.23
20~	3.83	4.47	3.14	4.48	5.30	3.61	4.67	5.50	3.80
25~	6.25	7.06	5.41	8.54	9.73	7.33	9.31	10.67	7.88
30~	10.97	11.27	10.66	14.18	15.40	12.93	18.96	22.34	15.40
35~	20.31	21.26	19.37	21.54	23.85	19.16	24.81	30.74	18.59
40~	38.51	41.73	35.33	40.78	46.69	34.67	50.39	61.15	39.07
45~	75.13	87.68	62.65	84.37	98.41	70.00	91.51	112.96	69.24
50~	133.03	164.66	101.17	164.98	198.16	130.76	195.66	251.07	136.90
55~	207.15	273.72	140.14	206.27	264.06	146.98	200.55	275.55	124.06
60~	349.24	480.90	219.01	397.87	537.21	255.47	408.67	564.24	247.24
65~	527.77	731.92	330.81	626.27	842.04	409.33	563.03	778.72	345.85
70~	782.71	1 072.50	510.11	808.21	1 088.82	531.78	729.55	983.42	476.90
75~	1 108.15	1 499.13	765.45	1 014.33	1 373.78	689.21	961.66	1 280.74	663.64
80~	1 453.14	1 941.98	1 070.76	1 351.09	1 788.08	983.53	1 132.12	1 497.09	817.73
85+	1 628.61	2 262.37	1 230.92	1 369.26	1 827.11	1 048.47	1 276.26	1 733.03	943.46

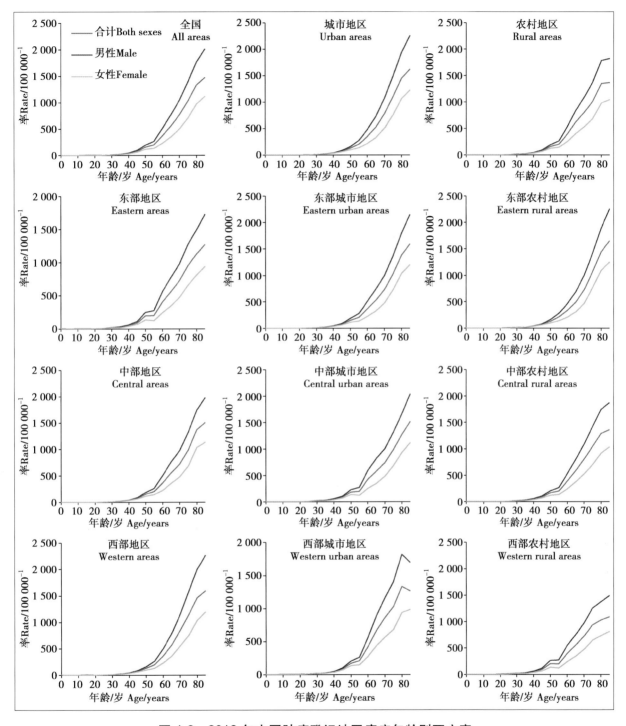

图 4-3 2018 年中国肿瘤登记地区癌症年龄别死亡率

Figure 4-3 Age-specific mortality rates for all cancer sites in the registration areas of China, 2018

2.5 中国不同肿瘤登记地区全部癌症发病与死亡情况

总体而言,七大区发病率与死亡率相差不大。华南地区男性发病率和死亡率均最高,华北地区男性发病率和死亡率最低;东北地区女性发病率最高,西南地区女性发病率最低;东北地区女性死亡率最高,西南地区女性死亡率最低。城市地区男女合计的发病率与死亡率相差不大。华南城市地区男性癌症发病率最高,华北城市男性发病率最低;华东城市地区女性发病率最高,西南城市地区女性发病率最低。华南城市地区男性死亡率最高,华北城市地区男性死亡率最低;华东城市地区女性死亡率最高。华东农村地区男性发病率最高,东北农村地区男性死亡率最高,华北农村地区男性发病率和死亡率最低;华东地区农村女性发病率最高,西南地区农村女性发病率最低;东北地区农村女性死亡率最高,西南地区农村女性死亡率最低(图4-4)。

2.5 Incidence and mortality for all cancer sites in different registration areas of China

In general, there was little difference among the seven administrative districts for the incidence and mortality rates. The incidence and mortality rates were highest in South China and lowest in North China for males. For females, the incidence rate was highest in Northeast China and lowest in Southwest China, and the mortality was highest in Northeast China and lowest in Southwest China. There was little difference of the incidence and mortality rates in the urban areas for both sexes. The incidence rate in the urban areas was highest in South China and lowest in North China for males, and highest in East China and lowest in Southwest for females. The mortality rate in the urban areas was highest in South China and lowest in North China for males, and highest in East China for females. In the rural areas, the incidence rate of males were highest in East China and lowest in North China, the mortality rate were highest in Northeast China and lowest in North China. For females, the incidence rate was highest in East China and lowest in Southwest China, and the mortality rate was highest in Northeast China and lowest in Southwest China(Figure 4-4).

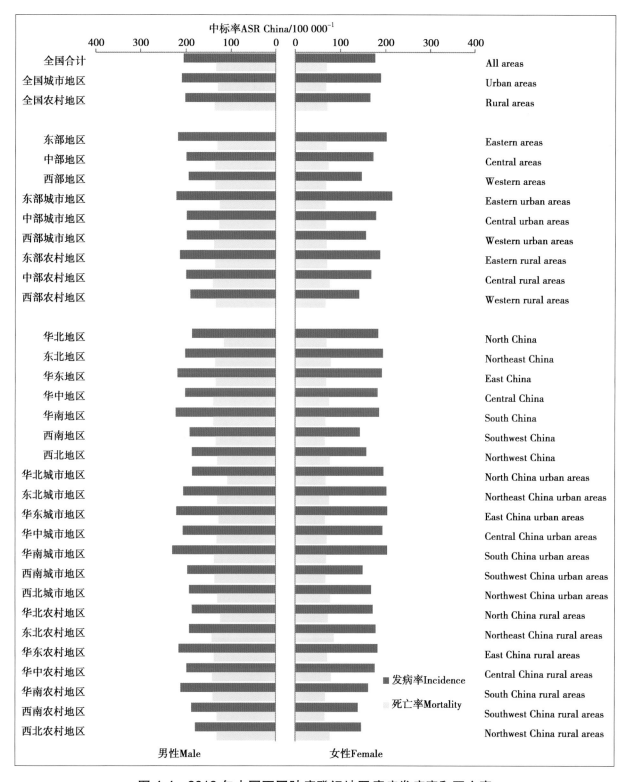

中标率ASR China/100 000⁻¹

全国合计	All areas
全国城市地区	Urban areas
全国农村地区	Rural areas
东部地区	Eastern areas
中部地区	Central areas
西部地区	Western areas
东部城市地区	Eastern urban areas
中部城市地区	Central urban areas
西部城市地区	Western urban areas
东部农村地区	Eastern rural areas
中部农村地区	Central rural areas
西部农村地区	Western rural areas
华北地区	North China
东北地区	Northeast China
华东地区	East China
华中地区	Central China
华南地区	South China
西南地区	Southwest China
西北地区	Northwest China
华北城市地区	North China urban areas
东北城市地区	Northeast China urban areas
华东城市地区	East China urban areas
华中城市地区	Central China urban areas
华南城市地区	South China urban areas
西南城市地区	Southwest China urban areas
西北城市地区	Northwest China urban areas
华北农村地区	North China rural areas
东北农村地区	Northeast China rural areas
华东农村地区	East China rural areas
华中农村地区	Central China rural areas
华南农村地区	South China rural areas
西南农村地区	Southwest China rural areas
西北农村地区	Northwest China rural areas

■ 发病率Incidence
　 死亡率Mortality

男性Male　　女性Female

图 4-4　2018 年中国不同肿瘤登记地区癌症发病率和死亡率
Figure 4-4　Incidence and mortality for all cancer sites in different
registration areas of China,2018

3 中国肿瘤登记地区前 10 位癌症发病与死亡

3 Top ten leading causes of new cancer cases and deaths in the registration areas of China

3.1 中国肿瘤登记地区前 10 位癌症发病情况

中国肿瘤登记地区癌症发病第 1 位的是肺癌,其次为女性乳腺癌、结直肠癌、肝癌和胃癌。男性发病第 1 位癌症为肺癌,其次为肝癌、胃癌、结直肠癌和食管癌;女性发病第 1 位癌症为肺癌,其次为乳腺癌、结直肠癌、甲状腺癌和子宫颈癌(表 4-6,图 4-5a,图 4-5b)。

3.1 Top ten leading causes of new cancer cases in the registration areas of China

Lung cancer was the most common cancer in cancer registration areas of China, followed by female breast cancer, colorectal cancer, liver cancer and stomach cancer. The top five cancers in males were lung cancer, liver cancer, stomach cancer, colorectal cancer, and esophageal cancer. The most common cancer in females was lung cancer, followed by breast cancer, colorectal cancer, thyroid cancer and cervix cancer (Table 4-6, Figure 4-5a, Figure 4-5b).

表 4-6　2018 年中国肿瘤登记地区前 10 位癌症发病率

Table 4-6　Incidence rates of top ten leading cancer sites in the registration areas of China, 2018

单位:100 000^{-1}

顺位 Rank	合计 All				男性 Male				女性 Female			
	部位 Site	粗率 Crude rate	世标率 ASR World	中标率 ASR China	部位 Site	粗率 Crude rate	世标率 ASR World	中标率 ASR China	部位 Site	粗率 Crude rate	世标率 ASR World	中标率 ASR China
1	肺 Lung	65.05	38.20	38.23	肺 Lung	83.45	50.72	50.48	肺 Lung	46.10	26.25	26.54
2	乳腺 Breast	43.02	28.39	30.35	肝 Liver	40.02	25.68	26.22	乳腺 Breast	43.02	28.39	30.35
3	结直肠 Colon-rectum	30.51	18.05	18.23	胃 Stomach	37.12	22.60	22.55	结直肠 Colon-rectum	25.56	14.49	14.75
4	肝 Liver	27.42	16.90	17.21	结直肠 Colon-rectum	35.32	21.74	21.84	甲状腺 Thyroid	24.60	18.09	20.95
5	胃 Stomach	27.03	15.84	15.92	食管 Esophagus	26.30	15.90	15.67	子宫颈 Cervix	18.10	12.00	12.95
6	子宫颈 Cervix	18.10	12.00	12.95	前列腺 Prostate	12.75	7.14	7.24	胃 Stomach	16.64	9.32	9.54
7	食管 Esophagus	17.96	10.29	10.20	膀胱 Bladder	9.09	5.40	5.43	肝 Liver	14.43	8.17	8.25
8	甲状腺 Thyroid	16.17	12.01	13.99	胰腺 Pancreas	8.12	4.92	4.91	子宫体 Uterus	10.56	6.85	7.08
9	前列腺 Prostate	12.75	7.14	7.24	甲状腺 Thyroid	7.98	6.04	7.16	食管 Esophagus	9.36	4.86	4.89
10	子宫体 Uterus	10.56	6.85	7.08	淋巴瘤 Lymphoma	7.44	4.98	5.07	脑 Brain	8.35	5.62	5.71

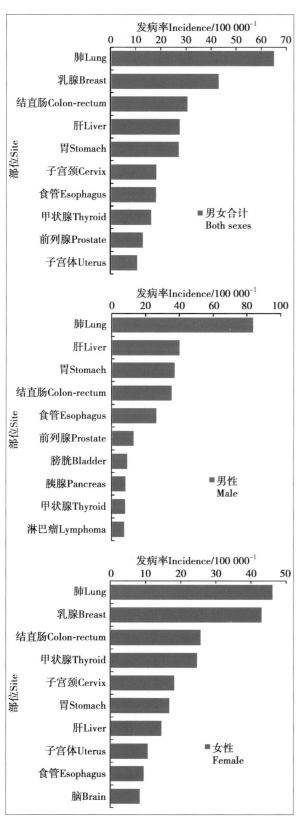

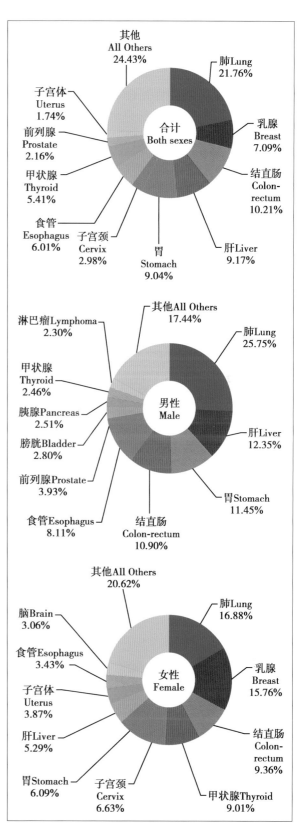

图 4-5a 2018 年中国肿瘤登记地区
前 10 位癌症发病率
Figure 4-5a Incidence rates of top ten
leading cancer sites in the registration
areas of China, 2018

图 4-5b 2018 年中国肿瘤登记地区
前 10 位癌症发病构成
Figure 4-5b Distribution of top ten leading
causes of new cancer cases in the
registration areas of China, 2018

3.2 中国肿瘤登记地区前 10 位癌症死亡情况

中国肿瘤登记地区男女合计癌症死亡第 1 位的为肺癌,其次为肝癌、胃癌、结直肠癌和食管癌;男性死亡第 1 位癌症为肺癌,其次为肝癌、胃癌、食管癌和结直肠癌;女性死亡第 1 位癌症为肺癌,其次为肝癌、胃癌、结直肠癌和乳腺癌(表 4-7,图 4-6a,图 4-6b)。

3.2 Top ten leading causes of cancer deaths in the registration areas of China

For both sexes combined, lung cancer was the leading cause of cancer deaths, followed by liver cancer, stomach cancer, colorectal cancer and esophageal cancer. For males, the top five leading causes of cancer death were lung cancer, liver cancer, stomach cancer, esophageal cancer and colorectal cancer. For females, the top five leading causes of cancer death were lung cancer, liver cancer, stomach cancer, colorectal cancer and breast cancer (Table 4-7, Figure 4-6a, Figure 4-6b).

表 4-7 2018 年中国肿瘤登记地区前 10 位癌症死亡率

Table 4-7 Mortality rates of top ten leading cancer sites in the registration areas of China, 2018

单位:100 000^{-1}

顺位 Rank	合计 All				男性 Male				女性 Female			
	部位 Site	粗率 Crude rate	世标率 ASR World	中标率 ASR China	部位 Site	粗率 Crude rate	世标率 ASR World	中标率 ASR China	部位 Site	粗率 Crude rate	世标率 ASR World	中标率 ASR China
1	肺 Lung	48.49	27.16	27.18	肺 Lung	67.06	39.69	39.61	肺 Lung	29.36	15.24	15.35
2	肝 Liver	24.11	14.54	14.77	肝 Liver	34.99	22.15	22.54	肝 Liver	12.89	7.01	7.08
3	胃 Stomach	19.76	10.98	11.09	胃 Stomach	27.18	15.95	16.05	胃 Stomach	12.12	6.28	6.40
4	结直肠 Colon-rectum	14.52	7.94	8.00	食管 Esophagus	20.96	12.36	12.27	结直肠 Colon-rectum	12.02	6.12	6.19
5	食管 Esophagus	14.32	7.89	7.87	结直肠 Colon-rectum	16.95	9.90	9.93	乳腺 Breast	9.66	5.81	5.98
6	乳腺 Breast	9.66	5.81	5.98	胰腺 Pancreas	7.31	4.36	4.35	食管 Esophagus	7.47	3.60	3.65
7	胰腺 Pancreas	6.39	3.58	3.59	前列腺 Prostate	5.07	2.68	2.64	子宫颈 Cervix	5.72	3.49	3.62
8	子宫颈 Cervix	5.72	3.49	3.62	脑 Brain	4.60	3.19	3.22	胰腺 Pancreas	5.45	2.83	2.85
9	前列腺 Prostate	5.07	2.68	2.64	淋巴瘤 Lymphoma	4.43	2.77	2.81	脑 Brain	3.84	2.45	2.44
10	脑 Brain	4.23	2.82	2.83	白血病 Leukemia	4.42	3.15	3.17	卵巢 Ovary	3.65	2.21	2.24

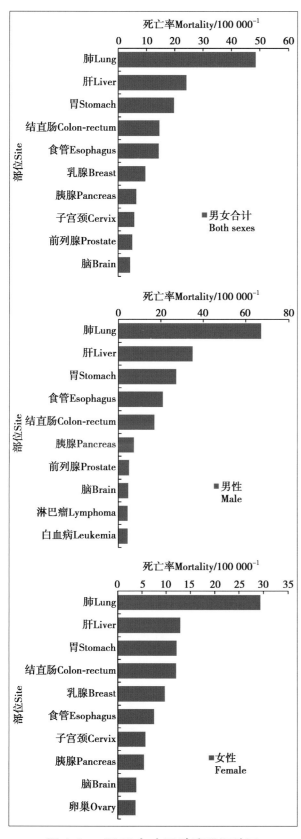

图 4-6a　2018 年中国肿瘤登记地区
前 10 位癌症死亡率
Figure 4-6a　Mortality rates of top ten
leading cancer sites in the registration
areas of China,2018

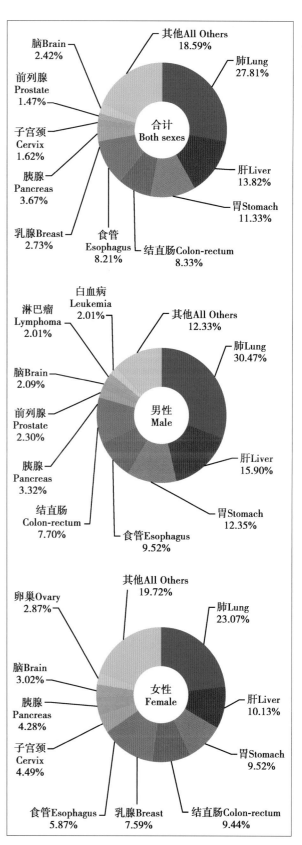

图 4-6b　2018 年中国肿瘤登记地区
前 10 位癌症死亡构成
Figure 4-6b　Distribution of top ten leading
causes of cancer deaths in the
registration areas of China,2018

3.3 中国城市肿瘤登记地区前10位癌症发病情况

中国城市肿瘤登记地区癌症发病第1位的是肺癌,其次为女性乳腺癌、结直肠癌、肝癌和胃癌。男性癌症发病第1位的是肺癌,其次为结直肠癌、肝癌、胃癌和食管癌;女性癌症发病第1位的是乳腺癌,其次为肺癌、甲状腺癌、结直肠癌和子宫颈癌(表4-8,图4-7a,图4-7b)。

3.3 Top ten leading causes of new cancer cases in urban registration areas of China

Lung cancer was the most common cancer in urban areas of China, followed by female breast cancer, colorectal cancer, liver cancer and stomach cancer. In males, lung cancer was the most common cancer, followed by colorectal cancer, liver cancer, stomach cancer and esophageal cancer. In females, breast cancer was the most common cancer, followed by lung cancer, thyroid cancer, colorectal cancer and cervix cancer(Table 4-8, Figure 4-7a, Figure 4-7b).

表 4-8 2018 年中国城市肿瘤登记地区前 10 位癌症发病率

Table 4-8 Incidence rates of top ten leading cancer sites in urban registration areas of China, 2018

单位:100 000^{-1}

顺位 Rank	合计 All				男性 Male				女性 Female			
	部位 Site	粗率 Crude rate	世标率 ASR World	中标率 ASR China	部位 Site	粗率 Crude rate	世标率 ASR World	中标率 ASR China	部位 Site	粗率 Crude rate	世标率 ASR World	中标率 ASR China
1	肺 Lung	68.62	38.84	38.83	肺 Lung	87.23	50.89	50.53	乳腺 Breast	51.38	32.87	34.95
2	乳腺 Breast	51.38	32.87	34.95	结直肠 Colon-rectum	42.10	24.82	24.85	肺 Lung	49.86	27.53	27.86
3	结直肠 Colon-rectum	36.00	20.42	20.57	肝 Liver	38.68	23.95	24.33	甲状腺 Thyroid	31.60	22.86	26.60
4	肝 Liver	26.27	15.61	15.84	胃 Stomach	34.72	20.28	20.23	结直肠 Colon-rectum	29.84	16.23	16.51
5	胃 Stomach	25.41	14.33	14.42	食管 Esophagus	21.78	12.72	12.50	子宫颈 Cervix	17.11	11.15	12.02
6	甲状腺 Thyroid	21.32	15.58	18.26	前列腺 Prostate	16.41	8.74	8.87	胃 Stomach	16.02	8.70	8.92
7	子宫颈 Cervix	17.11	11.15	12.02	甲状腺 Thyroid	11.13	8.29	9.89	肝 Liver	13.76	7.44	7.53
8	前列腺 Prostate	16.41	8.74	8.87	膀胱 Bladder	10.54	5.97	6.00	子宫体 Uterus	11.37	7.21	7.42
9	食管 Esophagus	14.23	7.91	7.81	胰腺 Pancreas	9.04	5.24	5.22	卵巢 Ovary	8.83	5.80	6.09
10	子宫体 Uterus	11.37	7.21	7.42	淋巴瘤 Lymphoma	8.68	5.58	5.70	脑 Brain	8.53	5.53	5.61

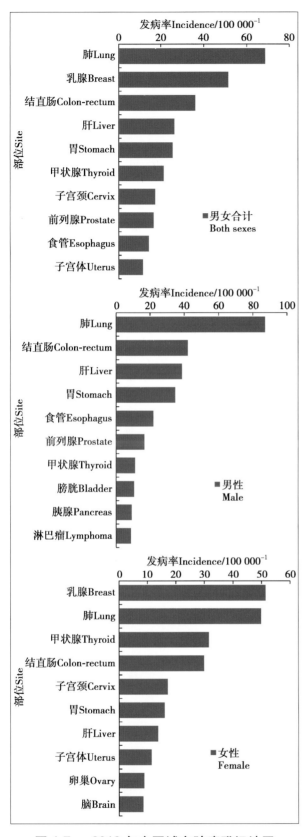

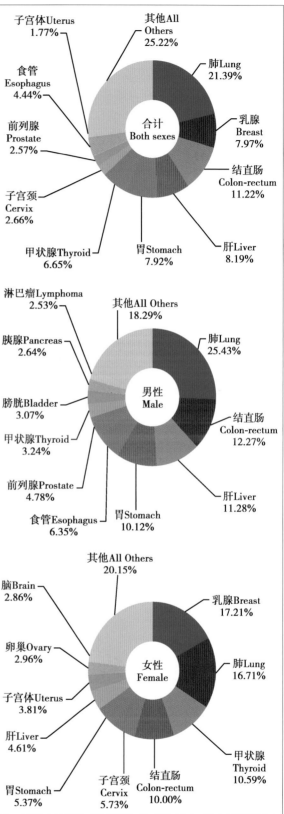

图 4-7a　2018 年中国城市肿瘤登记地区
前 10 位癌症发病率
Figure 4-7a　Incidence rates of top ten
leading cancer sites in urban registration
areas of China, 2018

图 4-7b　2018 年中国城市肿瘤登记地区
前 10 位癌症发病构成
Figure 4-7b　Distribution of top ten leading
causes of new cancer cases in urban
registration areas of China, 2018

3.4 中国城市肿瘤登记地区前 10 位癌症死亡情况

中国城市肿瘤登记地区合计癌症死亡第 1 位的为肺癌,其次为肝癌、胃癌、结直肠癌和食管癌。男性癌症死亡第 1 位的为肺癌,其次为肝癌、胃癌、结直肠癌和食管癌;女性癌症死亡率第 1 位的为肺癌,其次为结直肠癌、肝癌、胃癌和乳腺癌(表 4-9,图 4-8a,图 4-8b)。

3.4 Top ten leading causes of cancer deaths in urban registration areas of China

Lung cancer was the leading cause of cancer deaths in urban areas of China, followed by cancers of liver, stomach, colon-rectum and esophagus. In males, lung cancer was the leading cause of cancer deaths, followed by liver cancer, stomach cancer, colorectal cancer and esophageal cancer. In females, lung cancer ranked as the leading cancer cause of cancer death, followed by colorectal cancer, liver cancer, stomach cancer and breast cancer (Table 4-9, Figure 4-8a, Figure 4-8b).

表 4-9 2018 年中国城市肿瘤登记地区前 10 位癌症死亡率

Table 4-9 Mortality rates of top ten leading cancer sites in urban registration areas of China, 2018

单位:100 000^{-1}

顺位 Rank	合计 All				男性 Male				女性 Female			
	部位 Site	粗率 Crude rate	世标率 ASR World	中标率 ASR China	部位 Site	粗率 Crude rate	世标率 ASR World	中标率 ASR China	部位 Site	粗率 Crude rate	世标率 ASR World	中标率 ASR China
1	肺 Lung	49.77	26.56	26.54	肺 Lung	69.36	39.15	38.97	肺 Lung	30.03	14.75	14.89
2	肝 Liver	22.79	13.19	13.35	肝 Liver	33.30	20.29	20.54	结直肠 Colon-rectum	13.88	6.68	6.76
3	胃 Stomach	18.09	9.61	9.72	胃 Stomach	24.90	13.93	14.02	肝 Liver	12.20	6.28	6.34
4	结直肠 Colon-rectum	17.03	8.82	8.86	结直肠 Colon-rectum	20.15	11.15	11.13	胃 Stomach	11.23	5.60	5.72
5	食管 Esophagus	11.47	6.12	6.08	食管 Esophagus	17.63	10.05	9.93	乳腺 Breast	11.11	6.39	6.56
6	乳腺 Breast	11.11	6.39	6.56	胰腺 Pancreas	8.28	4.71	4.70	胰腺 Pancreas	6.25	3.09	3.12
7	胰腺 Pancreas	7.27	3.89	3.89	前列腺 Prostate	6.30	3.09	3.04	子宫颈 Cervix	5.37	3.22	3.36
8	前列腺 Prostate	6.30	3.09	3.04	淋巴瘤 Lymphoma	5.04	2.99	3.03	食管 Esophagus	5.25	2.39	2.42
9	子宫颈 Cervix	5.37	3.22	3.36	白血病 Leukemia	4.64	3.11	3.10	卵巢 Ovary	4.34	2.53	2.56
10	卵巢 Ovary	4.34	2.53	2.56	膀胱 Bladder	4.51	2.31	2.26	脑 Brain	3.63	2.24	2.22

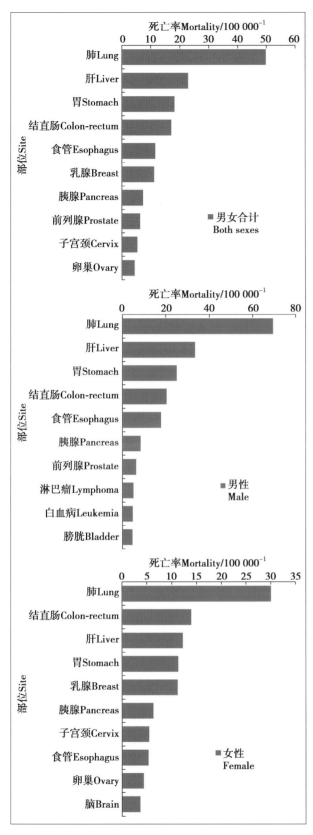

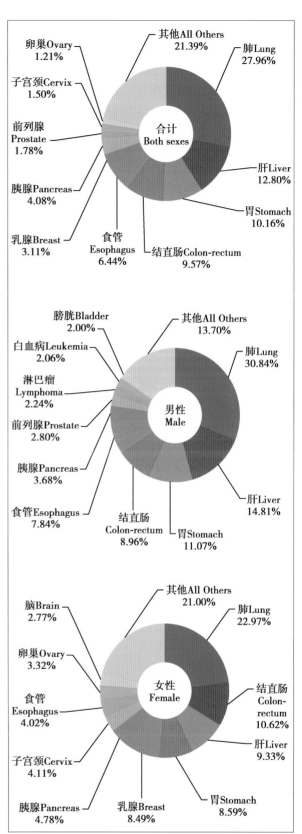

图 4-8a　2018 年中国城市肿瘤登记地区
前 10 位癌症死亡率
Figure 4-8a　Mortality rates of top ten
leading cancer sites in urban registration
areas of China,2018

图 4-8b　2018 年中国城市肿瘤登记地区
前 10 位癌症死亡构成
Figure 4-8b　Distribution of top ten leading
causes of cancer deaths in urban
registration areas of China,2018

3.5 中国农村肿瘤登记地区前 10 位癌症发病情况

中国农村肿瘤登记地区合计发病第 1 位癌症为肺癌,其次为女性乳腺癌、肝癌、胃癌和结直肠癌。男性发病第 1 位癌症为肺癌,其次为肝癌、胃癌、食管癌和结直肠癌;女性发病第 1 位癌症为肺癌,其次为乳腺癌、结直肠癌、子宫颈癌和甲状腺癌(表 4-10,图 4-9a,图 4-9b)。

3.5 Top ten leading causes of new cancer cases in rural registration areas of China

Lung cancer was the most common cancer in rural areas of China, followed by cancers of female breast, liver, stomach and colon-rectum. In males, lung cancer was the most common cancer, followed by liver cancer, stomach cancer, esophageal cancer and colorectal cancer. In females, lung cancer was the most common cancer, followed by breast cancer, colorectal cancer, cervical cancer and thyroid cancer (Table 4-10, Figure 4-9a, Figure 4-9b).

表 4-10　2018 年中国农村肿瘤登记地区前 10 位癌症发病率

Table 4-10　Incidence rates of top ten leading cancer sites in rural registration areas of China, 2018

单位:100 000^{-1}

顺位 Rank	合计 All				男性 Male				女性 Female			
	部位 Site	粗率 Crude rate	世标率 ASR World	中标率 ASR China	部位 Site	粗率 Crude rate	世标率 ASR World	中标率 ASR China	部位 Site	粗率 Crude rate	世标率 ASR World	中标率 ASR China
1	肺 Lung	62.12	37.62	37.68	肺 Lung	80.41	50.53	50.40	肺 Lung	42.94	25.11	25.36
2	乳腺 Breast	36.02	24.44	26.30	肝 Liver	41.10	27.14	27.80	乳腺 Breast	36.02	24.44	26.30
3	肝 Liver	28.36	18.00	18.39	胃 Stomach	39.05	24.57	24.53	结直肠 Colon-rectum	21.98	12.94	13.18
4	胃 Stomach	28.36	17.14	17.22	食管 Esophagus	29.94	18.65	18.41	子宫颈 Cervix	18.92	12.75	13.76
5	结直肠 Colon-rectum	26.01	15.95	16.18	结直肠 Colon-rectum	29.85	19.05	19.24	甲状腺 Thyroid	18.73	13.92	15.97
6	食管 Esophagus	21.02	12.39	12.28	前列腺 Prostate	9.80	5.73	5.81	胃 Stomach	17.15	9.87	10.08
7	子宫颈 Cervix	18.92	12.75	13.76	膀胱 Bladder	7.92	4.89	4.94	肝 Liver	15.00	8.80	8.89
8	甲状腺 Thyroid	11.93	8.95	10.31	胰腺 Pancreas	7.38	4.63	4.64	食管 Esophagus	11.66	6.26	6.29
9	子宫体 Uterus	9.88	6.53	6.78	脑 Brain	7.01	5.21	5.31	子宫体 Uterus	9.88	6.53	6.78
10	前列腺 Prostate	9.80	5.73	5.81	淋巴瘤 Lymphoma	6.44	4.46	4.53	脑 Brain	8.20	5.69	5.79

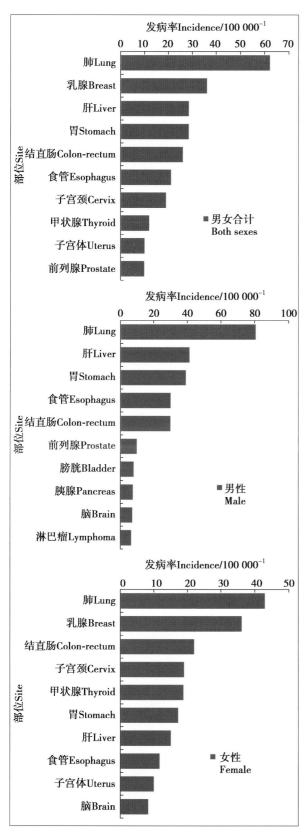

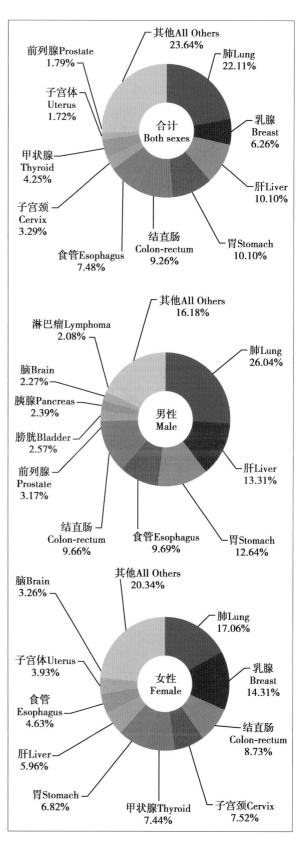

图 4-9a 2018 年中国农村肿瘤登记地区
前 10 位癌症发病率
Figure 4-9a Incidence rates of top ten
leading cancer sites in rural registration
areas of China,2018

图 4-9b 2018 年中国农村肿瘤登记地区
前 10 位癌症发病构成
Figure 4-9b Distribution of top ten leading
causes of new cancer cases in rural
registration areas of China,2018

3.6 中国农村肿瘤登记地区前 10 位癌症死亡情况

中国农村肿瘤登记地区合计癌症死亡第 1 位的是肺癌,其次为肝癌、胃癌、食管癌和结直肠癌。男性癌症死亡第 1 位的是肺癌,其次为肝癌、胃癌、食管癌和结直肠癌;女性癌症死亡第 1 位的是肺癌,其次为肝癌、胃癌、结直肠癌和食管癌(表 4-11,图 4-10a,图 4-10b)。

3.6 Top ten leading causes of cancer deaths in rural registration areas of China

Lung cancer was the leading cause of cancer death in rural areas of China, followed by cancers of liver, stomach, esophagus and colon-rectum. In males, lung cancer was the leading cause of cancer death, followed by liver cancer, stomach cancer, esophageal cancer and colorectal cancer. In females, lung cancer ranked as the leading cause of cancer death, followed by liver cancer, stomach cancer, colorectal cancer and esophageal cancer(Table 4-11, Figure 4-10a, Figure 4-10b).

表 4-11 2018 年中国农村肿瘤登记地区前 10 位癌症死亡率

Table 4-11 Mortality rates of top ten leading cancer sites in rural registration areas of China, 2018

单位:100 000^{-1}

顺位 Rank	合计 All				男性 Male				女性 Female			
	部位 Site	粗率 Crude rate	世标率 ASR World	中标率 ASR China	部位 Site	粗率 Crude rate	世标率 ASR World	中标率 ASR China	部位 Site	粗率 Crude rate	世标率 ASR World	中标率 ASR China
1	肺 Lung	47.44	27.65	27.71	肺 Lung	65.21	40.10	40.11	肺 Lung	28.81	15.65	15.75
2	肝 Liver	25.19	15.69	15.99	肝 Liver	36.36	23.71	24.23	肝 Liver	13.47	7.65	7.72
3	胃 Stomach	21.13	12.16	12.29	胃 Stomach	29.01	17.68	17.79	胃 Stomach	12.86	6.88	7.01
4	食管 Esophagus	16.66	9.45	9.44	食管 Esophagus	23.64	14.39	14.31	结直肠 Colon-rectum	10.46	5.60	5.67
5	结直肠 Colon-rectum	12.46	7.14	7.22	结直肠 Colon-rectum	14.36	8.77	8.86	食管 Esophagus	9.33	4.69	4.74
6	乳腺 Breast	8.44	5.29	5.48	胰腺 Pancreas	6.53	4.04	4.04	乳腺 Breast	8.44	5.29	5.48
7	子宫颈 Cervix	6.01	3.72	3.86	脑 Brain	4.70	3.35	3.37	子宫颈 Cervix	6.01	3.72	3.86
8	胰腺 Pancreas	5.67	3.31	3.32	白血病 Leukemia	4.23	3.17	3.20	胰腺 Pancreas	4.78	2.60	2.61
9	脑 Brain	4.37	3.00	3.00	前列腺 Prostate	4.07	2.30	2.27	脑 Brain	4.02	2.64	2.63
10	前列腺 Prostate	4.07	2.30	2.27	淋巴瘤 Lymphoma	3.93	2.57	2.60	白血病 Leukemia	3.15	2.27	2.26

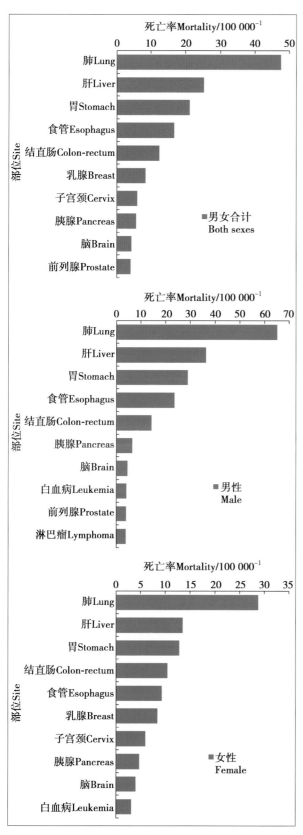

图 4-10a　2018 年中国农村肿瘤登记地区
前 10 位癌症死亡率
Figure 4-10a　Mortality rates of top ten
leading cancer sites in rural registration
areas of China, 2018

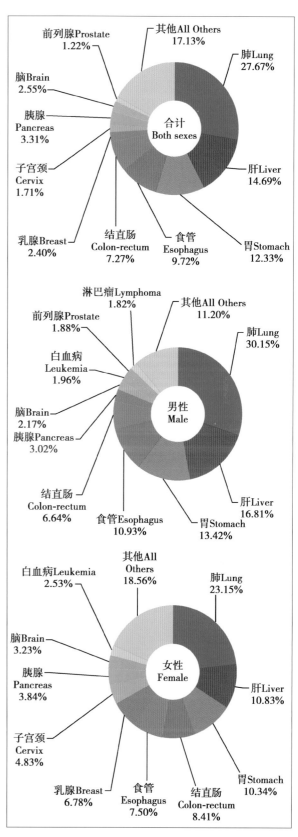

图 4-10b　2018 年中国农村肿瘤登记地区
前 10 位癌症死亡构成
Figure 4-10b　Distribution of top ten leading
causes of cancer deaths in rural
registration areas of China, 2018

3.7 中国东部肿瘤登记地区前10位癌症发病情况

中国东部肿瘤登记地区合计发病第1位癌症为肺癌,其次为女性乳腺癌、结直肠癌、胃癌和肝癌。男性发病第1位癌症为肺癌,其次为结直肠癌、胃癌、肝癌和食管癌;女性发病第1位癌症为肺癌,其次为乳腺癌、甲状腺癌、结直肠癌和胃癌(表4-12,图4-11a,图4-11b)。

3.7 Top ten leading causes of new cancer cases in eastern registration areas of China

Lung cancer was the most common cancer in eastern areas of China, followed by female breast cancer, colorectal cancer, stomach cancer and liver cancer. In males, lung cancer was the most common cancer, followed by colorectal cancer, stomach cancer, liver cancer and esophageal cancer. In females, lung cancer was the most common cancer, followed by breast cancer, thyroid cancer, colorectal cancer and stomach cancer (Table 4-12, Figure 4-11a, Figure 4-11b).

表4-12　2018年中国东部肿瘤登记地区前10位癌症发病率

Table 4-12　Incidence rates of top ten leading cancer sites in eastern registration areas of China, 2018

单位:100 000^{-1}

顺位 Rank	合计 All				男性 Male				女性 Female			
	部位 Site	粗率 Crude rate	世标率 ASR World	中标率 ASR China	部位 Site	粗率 Crude rate	世标率 ASR World	中标率 ASR China	部位 Site	粗率 Crude rate	世标率 ASR World	中标率 ASR China
1	肺 Lung	75.31	39.97	40.19	肺 Lung	92.65	50.68	50.58	肺 Lung	57.81	30.15	30.67
2	乳腺 Breast	55.53	34.62	36.99	结直肠 Colon-rectum	44.70	24.91	25.04	乳腺 Breast	55.53	34.62	36.99
3	结直肠 Colon-rectum	38.16	20.34	20.56	胃 Stomach	43.52	23.81	23.86	甲状腺 Thyroid	38.06	27.59	32.07
4	胃 Stomach	31.47	16.53	16.68	肝 Liver	37.57	22.08	22.36	结直肠 Colon-rectum	31.56	16.03	16.34
5	肝 Liver	25.69	14.35	14.50	食管 Esophagus	26.39	14.29	14.12	胃 Stomach	19.30	9.71	9.98
6	甲状腺 Thyroid	25.54	18.74	21.95	前列腺 Prostate	18.65	9.42	9.56	子宫颈 Cervix	15.96	10.15	11.00
7	前列腺 Prostate	18.65	9.42	9.56	甲状腺 Thyroid	13.13	9.89	11.81	肝 Liver	13.70	6.85	6.88
8	食管 Esophagus	18.06	9.18	9.12	膀胱 Bladder	11.70	6.26	6.31	子宫体 Uterus	12.49	7.55	7.79
9	子宫颈 Cervix	15.96	10.15	11.00	胰腺 Pancreas	10.56	5.73	5.72	脑 Brain	10.05	6.26	6.37
10	子宫体 Uterus	12.49	7.55	7.79	淋巴瘤 Lymphoma	9.67	5.93	6.04	食管 Esophagus	9.66	4.33	4.39

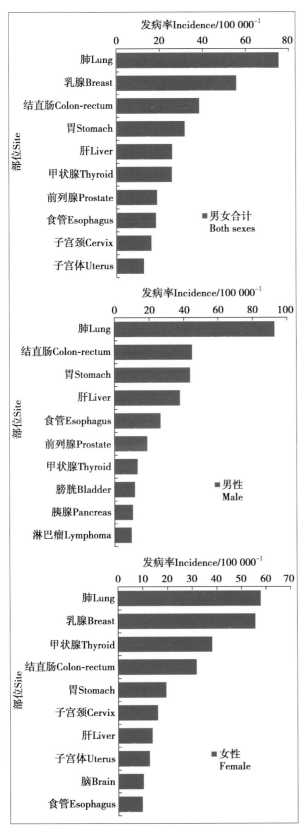

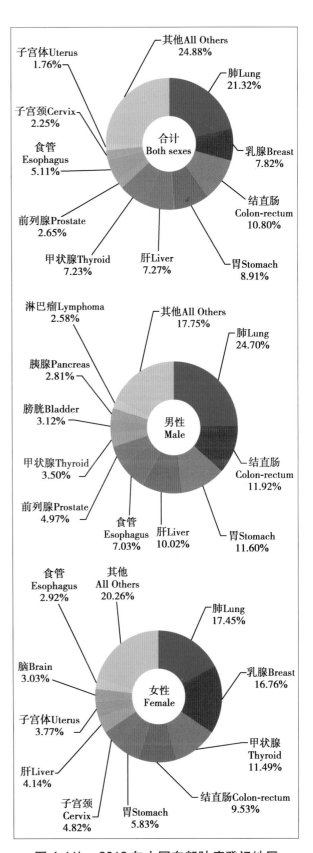

图 4-11a　2018 年中国东部肿瘤登记地区
前 10 位癌症发病率
Figure 4-11a　Incidence rates of top ten
leading cancer sites in eastern registration
areas of China,2018

图 4-11b　2018 年中国东部肿瘤登记地区
前 10 位癌症发病构成
Figure 4-11b　Distribution of top ten leading
causes of new cancer cases in eastern
registration areas of China,2018

3.8 中国东部肿瘤登记地区前 10 位癌症死亡情况

中国东部肿瘤登记地区男女合计癌症死亡第 1 位的为肺癌,其次为肝癌、胃癌、结直肠癌和食管癌;男性癌症死亡第 1 位的是肺癌,其次是肝癌、胃癌、食管癌和结直肠癌;女性癌症死亡第 1 位的是肺癌,其次为结直肠癌、胃癌、肝癌和乳腺癌(表 4-13,图 4-12a,图 4-12b)。

3.8 Top ten leading causes of cancer deaths in eastern registration areas of China

Lung cancer was the leading cause of cancer death in eastern areas of China, followed by liver cancer, stomach cancer, colorectal cancer and esophageal cancer. In males, lung cancer was the leading cause of cancer death, followed by liver cancer, stomach cancer, esophageal cancer and colorectal cancer. In females, lung cancer was still the leading cause of cancer death, followed by colorectal cancer, stomach cancer, liver cancer and breast cancer (Table 4-13, Figure 4-12a, Figure 4-12b).

表 4-13　2018 年中国东部肿瘤登记地区前 10 位癌症死亡率
Table 4-13　Mortality rates of top ten leading cancer sites in eastern registration areas of China,2018

单位:100 000⁻¹

单位:$100\ 000^{-1}$

顺位 Rank	合计 All				男性 Male				女性 Female			
	部位 Site	粗率 Crude rate	世标率 ASR World	中标率 ASR China	部位 Site	粗率 Crude rate	世标率 ASR World	中标率 ASR China	部位 Site	粗率 Crude rate	世标率 ASR World	中标率 ASR China
1	肺 Lung	52.76	26.02	26.13	肺 Lung	72.33	38.06	38.10	肺 Lung	33.02	14.94	15.12
2	肝 Liver	22.58	12.22	12.35	肝 Liver	32.56	18.73	18.92	结直肠 Colon-rectum	14.49	6.34	6.39
3	胃 Stomach	22.54	11.04	11.23	胃 Stomach	31.31	16.32	16.52	胃 Stomach	13.69	6.24	6.40
4	结直肠 Colon-rectum	17.35	8.29	8.32	食管 Esophagus	21.83	11.47	11.43	肝 Liver	12.51	5.96	6.01
5	食管 Esophagus	15.02	7.28	7.29	结直肠 Colon-rectum	20.20	10.47	10.45	乳腺 Breast	11.67	6.29	6.45
6	乳腺 Breast	11.67	6.29	6.45	胰腺 Pancreas	9.72	5.18	5.18	食管 Esophagus	8.15	3.36	3.43
7	胰腺 Pancreas	8.58	4.26	4.27	前列腺 Prostate	6.65	3.07	3.00	胰腺 Pancreas	7.44	3.39	3.42
8	前列腺 Prostate	6.65	3.07	3.00	淋巴瘤 Lymphoma	5.77	3.22	3.26	子宫颈 Cervix	4.81	2.73	2.85
9	淋巴瘤 Lymphoma	4.84	2.56	2.60	白血病 Leukemia	5.32	3.37	3.38	卵巢 Ovary	4.35	2.37	2.40
10	子宫颈 Cervix	4.81	2.73	2.85	膀胱 Bladder	4.99	2.39	2.33	脑 Brain	4.09	2.35	2.34

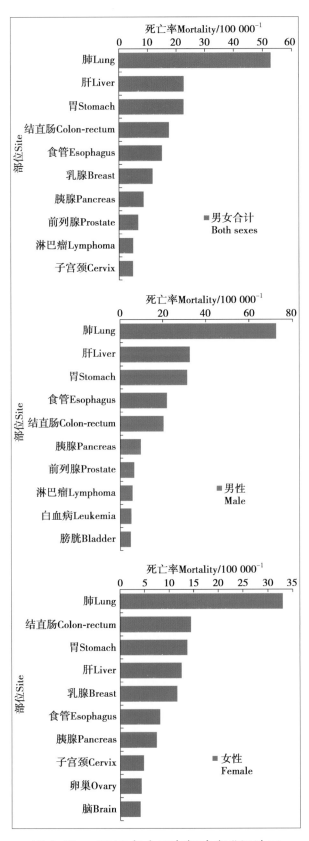

图 4-12a　2018 年中国东部肿瘤登记地区
前 10 位癌症死亡率
Figure 4-12a　Mortality rates of top ten
leading cancer sites in eastern registration
areas of China,2018

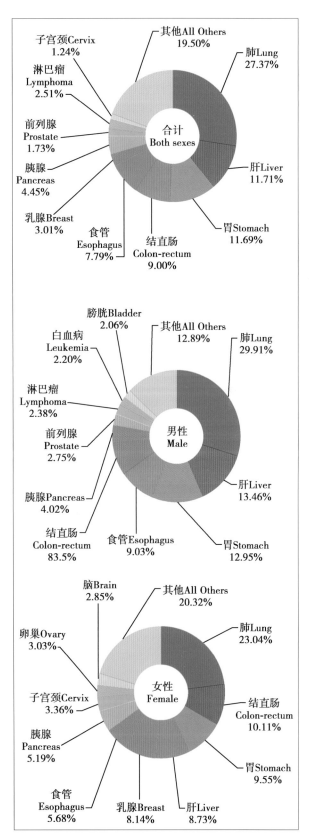

图 4-12b　2018 年中国东部肿瘤登记地区
前 10 位癌症死亡构成
Figure 4-12b　Distribution of top ten leading
causes of cancer deaths in eastern
registration areas of China,2018

3.9 中国中部肿瘤登记地区前 10 位癌症发病情况

中国中部肿瘤登记地区男女合计发病第 1 位癌症为肺癌，其次为女性乳腺癌、胃癌、肝癌和结直肠癌。男性发病第 1 位癌症为肺癌，其次为胃癌、肝癌、结直肠癌和食管癌；女性发病第 1 位癌症为乳腺癌，其次为肺癌、子宫颈癌、结直肠癌和甲状腺癌（表 4-14，图 4-13a，图 4-13b）。

3.9 Top ten leading causes of new cancer cases in central registration areas of China

Lung cancer was the most common cancer in the central areas of China, followed by female breast cancer, stomach cancer, liver cancer and colorectal cancer. In males, lung cancer was the most common cancer, followed by stomach cancer, liver cancer, colorectal cancer and esophageal cancer. In females, breast cancer was the most common cancer, followed by lung cancer, cervical cancer, colorectal cancer and thyroid cancer (Table 4-14, Figure 4-13a, Figure 4-13b).

表 4-14　2018 年中国中部肿瘤登记地区前 10 位癌症发病率

Table 4-14　Incidence rates of top ten leading cancer sites in central registration areas of China, 2018

单位：100 000^{-1}

顺位 Rank	合计 All				男性 Male				女性 Female			
	部位 Site	粗率 Crude rate	世标率 ASR World	中标率 ASR China	部位 Site	粗率 Crude rate	世标率 ASR World	中标率 ASR China	部位 Site	粗率 Crude rate	世标率 ASR World	中标率 ASR China
1	肺 Lung	57.54	37.04	36.94	肺 Lung	77.60	51.94	51.66	乳腺 Breast	40.49	28.17	30.17
2	乳腺 Breast	40.49	28.17	30.17	胃 Stomach	37.59	25.33	25.20	肺 Lung	36.58	22.53	22.61
3	胃 Stomach	27.58	17.89	17.90	肝 Liver	37.33	25.81	26.23	子宫颈 Cervix	21.74	15.03	16.11
4	肝 Liver	26.33	17.53	17.79	结直肠 Colon-rectum	27.73	18.84	18.92	结直肠 Colon-rectum	21.11	13.32	13.51
5	结直肠 Colon-rectum	24.49	16.05	16.19	食管 Esophagus	23.68	15.85	15.61	甲状腺 Thyroid	19.65	14.61	16.66
6	子宫颈 Cervix	21.74	15.03	16.11	前列腺 Prostate	8.13	5.07	5.12	胃 Stomach	17.12	10.59	10.76
7	食管 Esophagus	17.32	11.04	10.91	膀胱 Bladder	7.22	4.78	4.79	肝 Liver	14.82	9.23	9.32
8	甲状腺 Thyroid	12.52	9.41	10.78	脑 Brain	6.61	5.15	5.21	食管 Esophagus	10.67	6.32	6.31
9	子宫体 Uterus	9.54	6.54	6.75	淋巴瘤 Lymphoma	6.39	4.72	4.77	子宫体 Uterus	9.54	6.54	6.75
10	前列腺 Prostate	8.13	5.07	5.12	胰腺 Pancreas	6.30	4.21	4.22	卵巢 Ovary	7.54	5.37	5.65

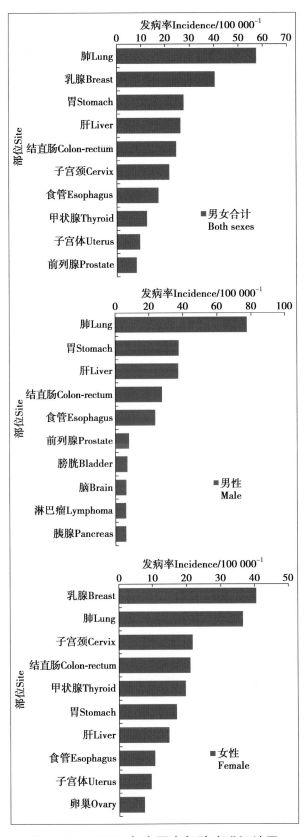

图 4-13a　2018 年中国中部肿瘤登记地区
前 10 位癌症发病率
Figure 4-13a　Incidence rates of top ten
leading cancer sites in central registration
areas of China, 2018

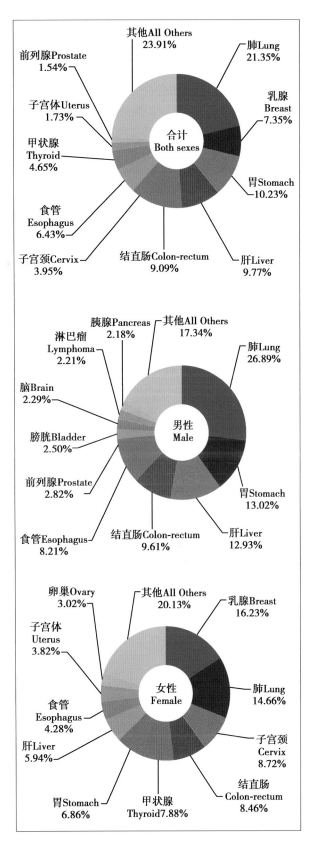

图 4-13b　2018 年中国中部肿瘤登记地区
前 10 位癌症发病构成
Figure 4-13b　Distribution of top ten leading
causes of new cancer cases in central
registration areas of China, 2018

3.10 中国中部肿瘤登记地区前 10 位癌症死亡情况

中国中部肿瘤登记地区癌症死亡第 1 位的是肺癌,其次为肝癌、胃癌、食管癌和结直肠癌。男性癌症死亡第 1 位的是肺癌,其次是肝癌、胃癌、食管癌和结直肠癌;女性癌症死亡第 1 位的是肺癌,其次为肝癌、胃癌、结直肠癌和乳腺癌(表 4-15,图 4-14a,图 4-14b)。

3.10 Top ten leading causes of cancer deaths in central registration areas of China

Lung cancer was the leading cause of cancer death in the central areas of China, followed by liver cancer, stomach cancer, esophageal cancer and colorectal cancer. In males, lung cancer was the leading cause of cancer death, followed by liver cancer, stomach cancer, esophageal cancer and colorectal cancer. In females, lung cancer was still the leading cause of cancer death, followed by liver cancer, stomach cancer, colorectal cancer and breast cancer (Table 4-15, Figure 4-14a, Figure 4-14b).

表 4-15　2018 年中国中部肿瘤登记地区前 10 位癌症死亡率

Table 4-15　Mortality rates of top ten leading cancer sites in central registration areas of China, 2018

单位:100 000^{-1}

顺位 Rank	合计 All				男性 Male				女性 Female			
	部位 Site	粗率 Crude rate	世标率 ASR World	中标率 ASR China	部位 Site	粗率 Crude rate	世标率 ASR World	中标率 ASR China	部位 Site	粗率 Crude rate	世标率 ASR World	中标率 ASR China
1	肺 Lung	45.41	28.30	28.27	肺 Lung	63.75	41.79	41.69	肺 Lung	26.24	15.25	15.30
2	肝 Liver	22.85	14.96	15.15	肝 Liver	32.44	22.19	22.51	肝 Liver	12.83	7.74	7.80
3	胃 Stomach	20.39	12.65	12.74	胃 Stomach	27.77	18.11	18.19	胃 Stomach	12.67	7.38	7.48
4	食管 Esophagus	13.49	8.25	8.22	食管 Esophagus	18.69	12.18	12.09	结直肠 Colon-rectum	10.00	5.81	5.90
5	结直肠 Colon-rectum	11.90	7.32	7.41	结直肠 Colon-rectum	13.72	8.92	8.98	乳腺 Breast	9.33	6.14	6.33
6	乳腺 Breast	9.33	6.14	6.33	胰腺 Pancreas	5.67	3.74	3.75	食管 Esophagus	8.05	4.44	4.46
7	子宫颈 Cervix	6.68	4.31	4.44	脑 Brain	4.62	3.42	3.44	子宫颈 Cervix	6.68	4.31	4.44
8	胰腺 Pancreas	4.94	3.10	3.10	白血病 Leukemia	4.08	3.17	3.19	胰腺 Pancreas	4.18	2.46	2.47
9	脑 Brain	4.24	3.04	3.04	淋巴瘤 Lymphoma	3.78	2.62	2.65	脑 Brain	3.84	2.65	2.64
10	前列腺 Prostate	3.78	2.25	2.25	前列腺 Prostate	3.78	2.25	2.25	卵巢 Ovary	3.41	2.27	2.29

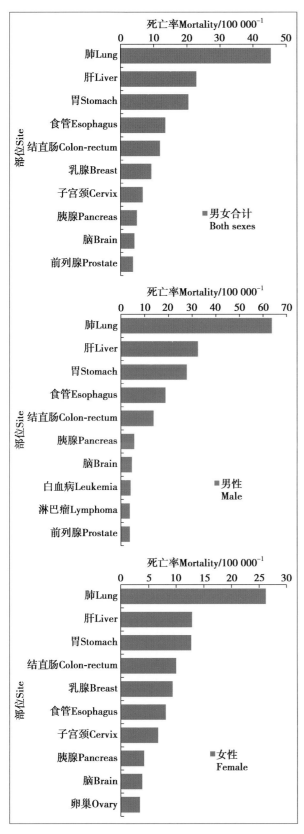

图 4-14a 2018 年中国中部肿瘤登记地区
前 10 位癌症死亡率
Figure 4-14a Mortality rates of top ten
leading cancer sites in central registration
areas of China,2018

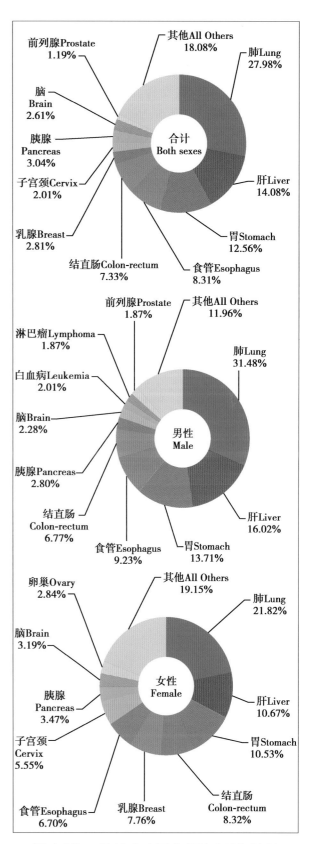

图 4-14b 2018 年中国中部肿瘤登记地区
前 10 位癌症死亡构成
Figure 4-14b Distribution of top ten leading
causes of cancer deaths in central
registration areas of China,2018

3.11 中国西部肿瘤登记地区前10位癌症发病情况

中国西部肿瘤登记地区合计发病第1位癌症为肺癌,其次为肝癌、女性乳腺癌、结直肠癌、胃癌。男性发病第1位癌症为肺癌,其次为肝癌、结直肠癌、胃癌和食管癌;女性发病第1位癌症为肺癌,其次为乳腺癌、结直肠癌、子宫颈癌和肝癌(表4-16,图4-15a,图4-15b)。

3.11 Top ten leading causes of new cancer cases in western registration areas of China

Lung cancer was the most common cancer in the western areas of China, followed by liver cancer, female breast cancer, colorectal cancer and stomach cancer. In males, lung cancer was the most common cancer, followed by liver cancer, colorectal cancer, stomach cancer and esophageal cancer. In females, lung cancer was the most common cancer, followed by breast cancer, colorectal cancer, cervical cancer and liver cancer (Table 4-16, Figure 4-15a, Figure 4-15b).

表 4-16 2018 年中国西部肿瘤登记地区前 10 位癌症发病率

Table 4-16 Incidence rates of top ten leading cancer sites in western registration areas of China, 2018

单位:100 000^{-1}

顺位 Rank	合计 All				男性 Male				女性 Female			
	部位 Site	粗率 Crude rate	世标率 ASR World	中标率 ASR China	部位 Site	粗率 Crude rate	世标率 ASR World	中标率 ASR China	部位 Site	粗率 Crude rate	世标率 ASR World	中标率 ASR China
1	肺 Lung	57.95	36.69	36.58	肺 Lung	76.62	50.01	49.60	肺 Lung	38.41	23.47	23.67
2	肝 Liver	30.35	20.01	20.54	肝 Liver	44.96	30.50	31.40	乳腺 Breast	29.21	20.12	21.61
3	乳腺 Breast	29.21	20.12	21.61	结直肠 Colon-rectum	29.55	19.31	19.46	结直肠 Colon-rectum	21.31	13.06	13.34
4	结直肠 Colon-rectum	25.52	16.16	16.38	胃 Stomach	29.02	18.96	18.87	子宫颈 Cervix	18.09	12.45	13.40
5	胃 Stomach	21.17	13.40	13.44	食管 Esophagus	28.11	18.27	17.96	肝 Liver	15.06	9.30	9.44
6	食管 Esophagus	18.30	11.43	11.28	前列腺 Prostate	9.02	5.35	5.43	胃 Stomach	12.95	7.85	8.04
7	子宫颈 Cervix	18.09	12.45	13.40	膀胱 Bladder	7.31	4.61	4.66	甲状腺 Thyroid	11.37	8.56	9.92
8	前列腺 Prostate	9.02	5.35	5.43	胰腺 Pancreas	6.52	4.24	4.25	子宫体 Uterus	8.90	6.06	6.31
9	子宫体 Uterus	8.90	6.06	6.31	脑 Brain	6.08	4.55	4.68	食管 Esophagus	8.02	4.62	4.63
10	甲状腺 Thyroid	7.32	5.52	6.41	鼻咽 Nasopharynx	6.03	4.25	4.53	卵巢 Ovary	7.03	4.97	5.25

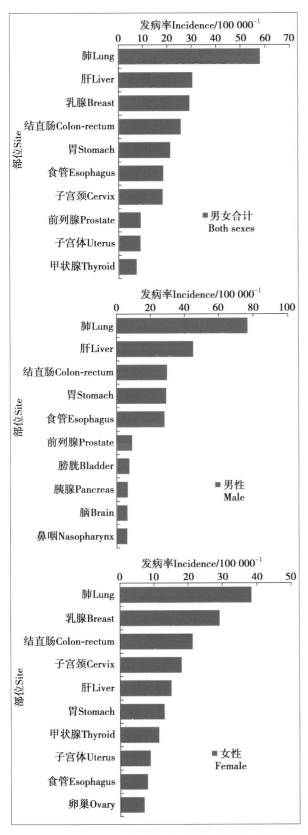

图 4-15a　2018 年中国西部肿瘤登记地区
前 10 位癌症发病率
Figure 4-15a　Incidence rates of top ten
leading cancer sites in western registration
areas of China,2018

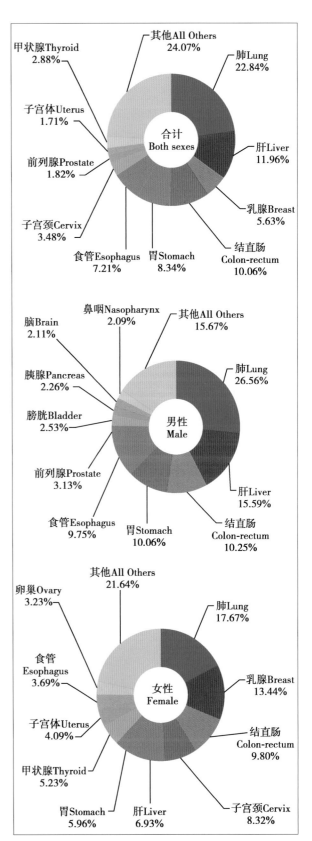

图 4-15b　2018 年中国西部肿瘤登记地区
前 10 位癌症发病构成
Figure 4-15b　Distribution of top ten leading
causes of new cancer cases in western
registration areas of China,2018

3.12 中国西部肿瘤登记地区前 10 位癌症死亡情况

中国西部肿瘤登记地区癌症死亡第 1 位的为肺癌,其次为肝癌、胃癌、食管癌和结直肠癌。男性癌症死亡第 1 位的是肺癌,其次是肝癌、胃癌、食管癌和结直肠癌;女性癌症死亡第 1 位的是肺癌,其次为肝癌、结直肠癌、胃癌和乳腺癌(表 4-17,图 4-16a,图 4-16b)。

3.12 Top ten leading causes of cancer deaths in western registration areas of China

Lung cancer was the leading cause of cancer death in the western areas of China, followed by liver cancer, stomach cancer, esophageal cancer and colorectal cancer. In males, lung cancer ranked as the leading cause of cancer death, followed by liver cancer, stomach cancer, esophageal cancer and colorectal cancer. In females, lung cancer was also the leading cause of cancer death, followed by liver cancer, colorectal cancer, stomach cancer and breast cancer(Table 4-17, Figure 4-16a, Figure 4-16b).

表 4-17　2018 年中国西部肿瘤登记地区前 10 位癌症死亡率

Table 4-17　Mortality rates of top ten leading cancer sites in western registration areas of China, 2018

单位:100 000^{-1}

顺位 Rank	合计 All				男性 Male				女性 Female			
	部位 Site	粗率 Crude rate	世标率 ASR World	中标率 ASR China	部位 Site	粗率 Crude rate	世标率 ASR World	中标率 ASR China	部位 Site	粗率 Crude rate	世标率 ASR World	中标率 ASR China
1	肺 Lung	45.50	28.00	27.91	肺 Lung	63.12	40.51	40.24	肺 Lung	27.07	15.66	15.73
2	肝 Liver	26.91	17.48	17.86	肝 Liver	39.81	26.75	27.42	肝 Liver	13.41	8.04	8.11
3	胃 Stomach	15.88	9.69	9.74	胃 Stomach	21.75	13.87	13.87	结直肠 Colon-rectum	10.41	5.92	6.03
4	食管 Esophagus	14.06	8.55	8.48	食管 Esophagus	21.57	13.78	13.61	胃 Stomach	9.74	5.55	5.65
5	结直肠 Colon-rectum	12.96	7.78	7.89	结直肠 Colon-rectum	15.39	9.70	9.80	乳腺 Breast	7.37	4.83	5.03
6	乳腺 Breast	7.37	4.83	5.03	胰腺 Pancreas	5.61	3.61	3.60	食管 Esophagus	6.20	3.38	3.40
7	子宫颈 Cervix	6.15	4.01	4.17	脑 Brain	4.18	3.07	3.11	子宫颈 Cervix	6.15	4.01	4.17
8	胰腺 Pancreas	4.77	2.93	2.94	前列腺 Prostate	4.10	2.37	2.36	胰腺 Pancreas	3.89	2.25	2.28
9	前列腺 Prostate	4.10	2.37	2.36	白血病 Leukemia	3.57	2.79	2.80	脑 Brain	3.54	2.46	2.43
10	脑 Brain	3.87	2.77	2.78	淋巴瘤 Lymphoma	3.28	2.24	2.27	卵巢 Ovary	2.95	1.93	1.97

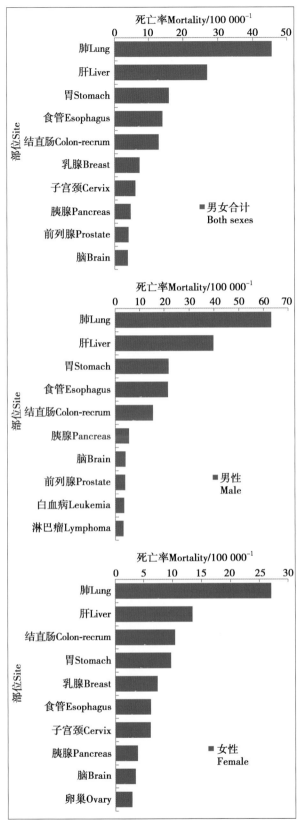

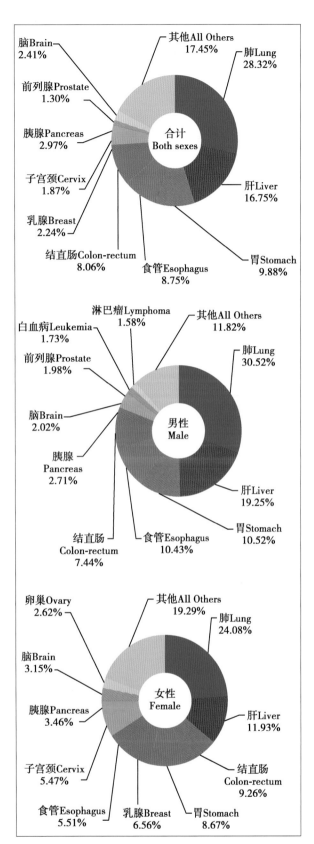

图 4-16a　2018 年中国西部肿瘤登记地区前 10 位癌症死亡率
Figure 4-16a　Mortality rates of top ten leading cancer sites in western registration areas of China, 2018

图 4-16b　2018 年中国西部肿瘤登记地区前 10 位癌症死亡构成
Figure 4-16b　Distribution of top ten leading causes of cancer death in western registration areas of China, 2018

第五章 各部位癌症的发病与死亡

1 口腔和咽(除外鼻咽)

2018 年口腔癌和咽癌位居中国肿瘤登记地区癌症发病谱第 19 位。新发病例数为 21 047 例,占全部癌症发病的 1.35%;其中男性 14 607 例,女性 6 440 例,城市地区 10 522 例,农村地区 10 525 例。发病率为 4.02/10 万,中标发病率为 2.58/10 万,世标发病率为 2.53/10 万;男性中标发病率为女性的 2.25 倍,城市中标发病率为农村的 1.13 倍。0~74 岁累积发病率为 0.30%(表 5-1a)。

口腔癌和咽癌位居中国肿瘤登记地区癌症死亡谱第 17 位。口腔癌和咽癌死亡病例 10 389 例,占全部癌症死亡数的 1.14%;其中男性 7 538 例,女性 2 851 例,城市地区 5 375 例,农村地区 5 014 例。死亡率为 1.99/10 万,中标和世标死亡率均为 1.15/10 万;男性中标死亡率为女性的 2.97 倍,城市中标死亡率为农村的 1.20 倍。0~74 岁累积死亡率为 0.13%(表 5-1b)。

口腔癌和咽癌的年龄别发病率和死亡率在 40 岁以前均处于较低水平,40 岁之后开始快速上升,男性上升速度快于女性。男性年龄别发病率在 70 岁组以后达到平台期,女性在 85 岁及以上年龄组达到高峰,年龄别死亡率均在 85 岁及以上年龄组达到高峰(图 5-1a)。

Chapter 5 Cancer incidence and mortality by site

1 Oral cavity & pharynx(except nasopharynx)

Oral cavity and pharyngeal cancer were the 19th most common cancer in the registration areas of China in 2018. There were 21 047 new cases diagnosed as oral cavity and pharyngeal cancer(14 607 males and 6 440 females,10 522 in urban areas and 10 525 in rural areas), accounting for 1.35% of all new cancer cases. The crude incidence rate was 4.02 per 100 000, with ASR China 2.58 per 100 000 and ASR World 2.53 per 100 000,respectively. The incidence of ASR China was 2.25 times in males as that in females,and was 1.13 times in urban areas as that in rural areas. The cumulative incidence rate for subjects aged 0 to 74 years was 0.30%(Table 5-1a).

Oral cavity and pharyngeal cancer were the 17th most common cause of cancer deaths in the registration areas of China. A total of 10 389 cases died of oral cavity and pharyngeal cancer(7 538 males and 2 851 females,5 375 in urban areas and 5 014 in rural areas),accounting for 1.14% of all cancer deaths. The crude mortality rate was 1.99 per 100 000,with ASR China 1.15 per 100 000 and the same as ASR World. The mortality of ASR China was 2.97 times in males as that in females,and was 1.20 times in urban areas as that in rural areas. The cumulative mortality rate for subjects aged 0 to 74 years was 0.13%(Table 5-1b).

The age-specific incidence and mortality rates for oral cavity and pharyngeal cancer were low before 40 years old,but increased sharply thereafter. The age-specific rates increased faster in males than that in females. The age-specific incidence rates of males reached its peak at 70 years old and remained stable thereafter. For females,the age-specific incidence rate was the highest in 85 + years age group. The age-specific mortality rates peaked at the age group of 85+ years for both sexes(Figure 5-1a).

城市地区口腔癌和咽癌的发病率和死亡率均略高于农村。男性中标发病率中部地区最高,西部地区 70~84 岁年龄组出现明显的高峰,中标死亡率西部地区最高。女性中标发病率东部地区最高,中标死亡率西部地区最高。在七大行政区中,男性和女性口腔癌和咽癌的中标发病率均在华南地区最高,中标死亡率男性在东北地区最高,女性在华南地区最高(表 5-1a,表 5-1b,图 5-1b)。

全部口腔癌和咽癌新发病例中,口腔是最常见的发病部位,占 28.26%;其次是舌、唾液腺和下咽,分别占全部口腔癌和咽癌的 21.93%、15.30% 和 12.60%(图 5-1c)。

The incidence and mortality rates of oral cavity and pharyngeal cancer were slightly higher in urban areas than that in rural areas. For males, the incidence rate (ASR China) was the highest in the central areas and showed an obvious peak at the age group of 70-84 years in the western areas, and the mortality rate (ASR China) was the highest in the western areas. For females, the incidence and mortality rates (ASR China) were the highest in the eastern areas and western areas, respectively. Among the seven administrative districts, the incidence rates (ASR China) were the highest in South China for both sexes, and the mortality rates (ASR China) were the highest in Northeast China in males and in South China in females, respectively (Table 5-1a, Table 5-1b, Figure 5-1b).

Mouth was the most common subsite of the oral cavity and pharyngeal cancer, accounting for 28.26% of the total cases, followed by tongue, salivary glands, and hypopharynx, with proportions of 21.93%, 15.30%, and 12.60%, respectively (Figure 5-1c).

表 5-1a 2018 年中国肿瘤登记地区口腔癌和咽癌发病情况

表 5-1a 2018 年中国肿瘤登记地区口腔癌和咽癌发病情况

Table 5-1a Incidence of oral cavity and pharyngeal cancer in the registration areas of China, 2018

地区 Area	性别 Sex	病例数 No. cases	粗率 Crude rate/ 100 000⁻¹	构成比 Freq. /%	中标率 ASR China/ 100 000⁻¹	世标率 ASR World/ 100 000⁻¹	累积率 Cum. rate 0~74/%	顺位 Rank
合计 All	合计 Both	21 047	4. 02	1. 35	2. 58	2. 53	0. 30	19
	男性 Male	14 607	5. 50	1. 70	3. 58	3. 55	0. 42	14
	女性 Female	6 440	2. 50	0. 92	1. 59	1. 53	0. 17	18
城市地区 Urban areas	合计 Both	10 522	4. 46	1. 39	2. 74	2. 70	0. 32	18
	男性 Male	7 324	6. 18	1. 80	3. 84	3. 83	0. 46	14
	女性 Female	3 198	2. 72	0. 91	1. 67	1. 60	0. 18	18
农村地区 Rural areas	合计 Both	10 525	3. 67	1. 30	2. 43	2. 39	0. 28	19
	男性 Male	7 283	4. 95	1. 60	3. 35	3. 30	0. 39	14
	女性 Female	3 242	2. 31	0. 92	1. 52	1. 47	0. 16	17
东部地区 Eastern areas	合计 Both	9 517	4. 38	1. 24	2. 56	2. 53	0. 30	19
	男性 Male	6 503	5. 96	1. 59	3. 52	3. 52	0. 42	14
	女性 Female	3 014	2. 79	0. 84	1. 64	1. 57	0. 17	18
中部地区 Central areas	合计 Both	4 870	3. 75	1. 39	2. 64	2. 59	0. 30	18
	男性 Male	3 426	5. 17	1. 79	3. 73	3. 66	0. 43	13
	女性 Female	1 444	2. 28	0. 91	1. 55	1. 50	0. 17	17
西部地区 Western areas	合计 Both	6 660	3. 78	1. 49	2. 55	2. 50	0. 30	18
	男性 Male	4 678	5. 19	1. 80	3. 52	3. 49	0. 42	12
	女性 Female	1 982	2. 30	1. 06	1. 57	1. 52	0. 17	18

表 5-1b 2018 年中国肿瘤登记地区口腔癌和咽癌死亡情况

Table 5-1b Mortality of oral cavity and pharyngeal cancer in the registration areas of China, 2018

地区 Area	性别 Sex	死亡数 No. deaths	粗率 Crude rate/ 100 000⁻¹	构成比 Freq. /%	中标率 ASR China/ 100 000⁻¹	世标率 ASR World/ 100 000⁻¹	累积率 Cum. rate 0~74/%	顺位 Rank
合计 All	合计 Both	10 389	1. 99	1. 14	1. 15	1. 15	0. 13	17
	男性 Male	7 538	2. 84	1. 29	1. 74	1. 74	0. 20	13
	女性 Female	2 851	1. 11	0. 87	0. 58	0. 58	0. 06	17
城市 Urban areas	合计 Both	5 375	2. 28	1. 28	1. 26	1. 27	0. 14	18
	男性 Male	3 897	3. 29	1. 46	1. 93	1. 94	0. 23	13
	女性 Female	1 478	1. 26	0. 96	0. 62	0. 61	0. 06	17
农村 Rural areas	合计 Both	5 014	1. 75	1. 02	1. 06	1. 05	0. 12	18
	男性 Male	3 641	2. 48	1. 15	1. 57	1. 57	0. 19	14
	女性 Female	1 373	0. 98	0. 79	0. 55	0. 54	0. 06	18
东部地区 Eastern areas	合计 Both	4 576	2. 11	1. 09	1. 09	1. 09	0. 12	18
	男性 Male	3 241	2. 97	1. 23	1. 63	1. 65	0. 19	14
	女性 Female	1 335	1. 24	0. 86	0. 56	0. 56	0. 06	17
中部地区 Central areas	合计 Both	2 362	1. 82	1. 12	1. 18	1. 17	0. 14	17
	男性 Male	1 752	2. 64	1. 31	1. 79	1. 79	0. 21	12
	女性 Female	610	0. 96	0. 80	0. 57	0. 56	0. 06	18
西部地区 Western areas	合计 Both	3 451	1. 96	1. 22	1. 23	1. 22	0. 14	18
	男性 Male	2 545	2. 82	1. 36	1. 83	1. 83	0. 22	13
	女性 Female	906	1. 05	0. 94	0. 63	0. 62	0. 07	17

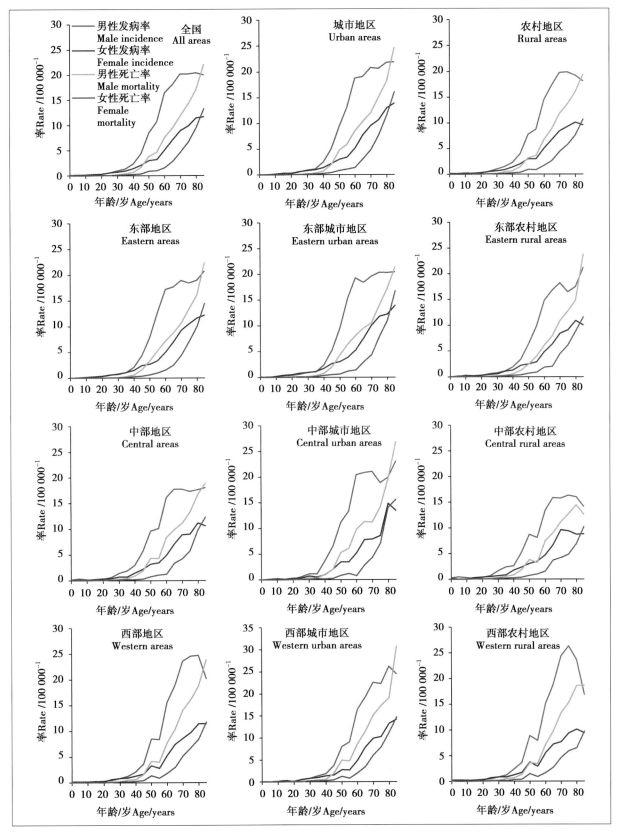

图 5-1a　2018 年中国肿瘤登记地区口腔癌和咽癌年龄别发病率和死亡率
Figure 5-1a　Age-specific incidence and mortality rates of oral cavity and
pharyngeal cancer in the registration areas of China,2018

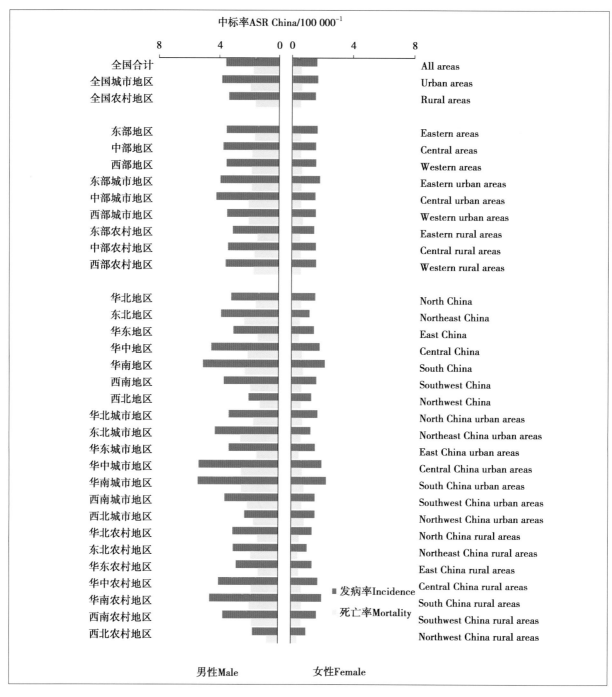

图 5-1b　2018 年中国肿瘤登记不同地区口腔癌和咽癌发病率和死亡率

Figure 5-1b　Incidence and mortality rates of oral cavity and pharyngeal cancer in different registration areas of China,2018

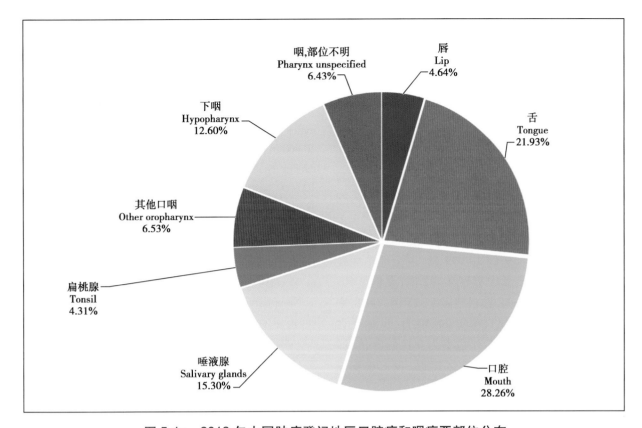

图 5-1c 2018 年中国肿瘤登记地区口腔癌和咽癌亚部位分布

Figure 5-1c Subsite distribution of oral cavity and pharyngeal cancer in the
registration areas of China, 2018

2 鼻咽

　　2018年鼻咽癌位居中国肿瘤登记地区癌症发病谱第20位。新发病例19 564例，占全部癌症发病的1.25%。其中男性13 912例，女性5 652例；城市地区9 104例，农村地区10 460例。发病率为3.74/10万，中标发病率为2.71/10万，世标发病率为2.53/10万；男性中标发病率为女性的2.42倍，城市地区中标发病率与农村地区接近。0~74岁累积发病率为0.28%（表5-2a）。

　　鼻咽癌位居中国肿瘤登记地区癌症死亡谱第18位。鼻咽癌死亡病例10 099例，占全部癌症死亡人数的1.11%。其中男性7 492例，女性2 607例；城市地区4 726例，农村地区5 373例。死亡率为1.93/10万，中标死亡率1.24/10万，世标死亡率1.21/10万；男性中标死亡率为女性的3倍，城市地区中标死亡率与农村地区接近。0~74岁累积死亡率为0.14%（表5-2b）。

　　鼻咽癌的年龄别发病率和死亡率男性明显高于女性。发病率在20岁之前处于较低水平，20岁以后开始快速上升，在55~59岁组有所下降，随后上升，男性和女性分别在60~69岁和70~74岁组出现最高峰，随后下降。鼻咽癌的年龄别死亡率男性和女性30岁之前均处于较低水平，随后快速上升，男性65~74岁组达到高峰，女性85+岁组达到高峰（图5-2a）。

　　城市鼻咽癌发病率和死亡率与农村接近。中标发病率和死亡率均是西部地区最高，东部和中部地区相似。在七大行政区中，华南地区中标发病率和死亡率均最高，华北地区最低（表5-2a，表5-2b，图5-2b）。

2 Nasopharynx

Nasopharyngeal cancer was the 20th most common cancer in the registration areas of China in 2018. There were 19 564 new cases of nasopharyngeal cancer (13 912 males and 5 652 females, 9 104 in urban areas and 10 460 in rural areas), accounting for 1.25% of all new cancer cases. The crude incidence rate was 3.74 per 100 000, with ASR China 2.71 per 100 000 and ASR World 2.53 per 100 000, respectively. The incidence of ASR China in males was 2.42 times as that in females, while the rate in urban areas was close to that in rural areas. The cumulative incidence rate for subjects aged 0 to 74 years was 0.28% (Table 5-2a).

Nasopharyngeal cancer was the 18th most common cause of cancer deaths. A total of 10 099 cases died of nasopharyngeal cancer(7 492 males and 2 607 females, 4 726 in urban areas and 5 373 in rural areas), accounting for 1.11% of all cancer deaths. The crude mortality rate was 1.93 per 100 000, with ASR China 1.24 per 100 000 and ASR World 1.21 per 100 000, respectively. The ASR China in males was 3 times as that in females, while the rate in urban areas was close to that in rural areas. The cumulative mortality rate for subjects aged 0 to 74 years was 0.14% (Table 5-2b).

The age-specific incidence and mortality rates of nasopharyngeal cancer were higher in males than that in females. For both sexes, the age-specific incidence rates were low before 20 years old but increased sharply thereafter. Then the incidence rates slightly decreased at the age group of 55-59 years, but increased to the peak age group of 60-69 years for males and 70-74 years for females. For both sexes, the age-specific mortality rates were low before 30 years old and increased fast thereafter, with a peak age group of 65-74 years in males and 85+ years in females(Figure 5-2a).

The incidence and mortality rates of nasopharyngeal cancer in urban areas were closed to that in rural areas. The incidence and mortality rates(ASR China) were the highest in the western areas, and were similar in the eastern areas and central areas. Among the seven administrative districts, the incidence and mortality rates (ASR China) were the highest in South China and the lowest in North China (Table 5-2a, Table 5-2b, Figure 5-2b).

表 5-2a　2018 年中国肿瘤登记地区鼻咽癌发病情况

Table 5-2a　Incidence of nasopharyngeal cancer in the registration areas of China,2018

地区 Area	性别 Sex	病例数 No. cases	粗率 Crude rate/ 100 000^{-1}	构成比 Freq./%	中标率 ASR China/ 100 000^{-1}	世标率 ASR World/ 100 000^{-1}	累积率 Cum. rate 0~74/%	顺位 Rank
合计	合计 Both	19 564	3.74	1.25	2.71	2.53	0.28	20
All	男性 Male	13 912	5.24	1.62	3.82	3.59	0.39	15
	女性 Female	5 652	2.19	0.80	1.58	1.46	0.16	19
城市地区	合计 Both	9 104	3.86	1.20	2.75	2.56	0.28	20
Urban areas	男性 Male	6 478	5.47	1.59	3.92	3.66	0.40	15
	女性 Female	2 626	2.23	0.75	1.59	1.46	0.15	19
农村地区	合计 Both	10 460	3.64	1.30	2.67	2.51	0.27	20
Rural areas	男性 Male	7 434	5.06	1.64	3.74	3.53	0.39	13
	女性 Female	3 026	2.16	0.86	1.57	1.47	0.16	18
东部地区	合计 Both	7 659	3.53	1.00	2.47	2.29	0.25	20
Eastern areas	男性 Male	5 537	5.08	1.35	3.58	3.33	0.36	16
	女性 Female	2 122	1.96	0.59	1.39	1.26	0.13	19
中部地区	合计 Both	4 164	3.21	1.19	2.38	2.28	0.25	20
Central areas	男性 Male	2 938	4.43	1.54	3.34	3.20	0.36	15
	女性 Female	1 226	1.93	0.77	1.41	1.34	0.15	19
西部地区	合计 Both	7 741	4.39	1.73	3.28	3.07	0.33	17
Western areas	男性 Male	5 437	6.03	2.09	4.53	4.25	0.46	10
	女性 Female	2 304	2.67	1.23	1.99	1.85	0.20	16

表 5-2b　2018 年中国肿瘤登记地区鼻咽癌死亡情况

Table 5-2b　Mortality of nasopharyngeal cancer in the registration areas of China,2018

地区 Area	性别 Sex	死亡数 No. deaths	粗率 Crude rate/ 100 000^{-1}	构成比 Freq./%	中标率 ASR China/ 100 000^{-1}	世标率 ASR World/ 100 000^{-1}	累积率 Cum. rate 0~74/%	顺位 Rank
合计	合计 Both	10 099	1.93	1.11	1.24	1.21	0.14	18
All	男性 Male	7 492	2.82	1.28	1.86	1.82	0.22	14
	女性 Female	2 607	1.01	0.79	0.62	0.60	0.07	19
城市地区	合计 Both	4 726	2.00	1.12	1.25	1.22	0.15	19
Urban areas	男性 Male	3 502	2.96	1.31	1.88	1.85	0.22	15
	女性 Female	1 224	1.04	0.80	0.62	0.60	0.07	18
农村地区	合计 Both	5 373	1.87	1.09	1.24	1.21	0.14	17
Rural areas	男性 Male	3 990	2.71	1.26	1.85	1.80	0.21	12
	女性 Female	1 383	0.99	0.79	0.62	0.60	0.07	17
东部地区	合计 Both	4 238	1.95	1.01	1.14	1.12	0.13	19
Eastern areas	男性 Male	3 159	2.90	1.20	1.75	1.72	0.21	15
	女性 Female	1 079	1.00	0.70	0.56	0.54	0.06	18
中部地区	合计 Both	2 111	1.63	1.00	1.12	1.10	0.13	18
Central areas	男性 Male	1 556	2.35	1.16	1.66	1.64	0.20	14
	女性 Female	555	0.88	0.73	0.57	0.56	0.07	19
西部地区	合计 Both	3 750	2.13	1.32	1.47	1.43	0.16	16
Western areas	男性 Male	2 777	3.08	1.49	2.16	2.10	0.24	12
	女性 Female	973	1.13	1.00	0.76	0.73	0.08	15

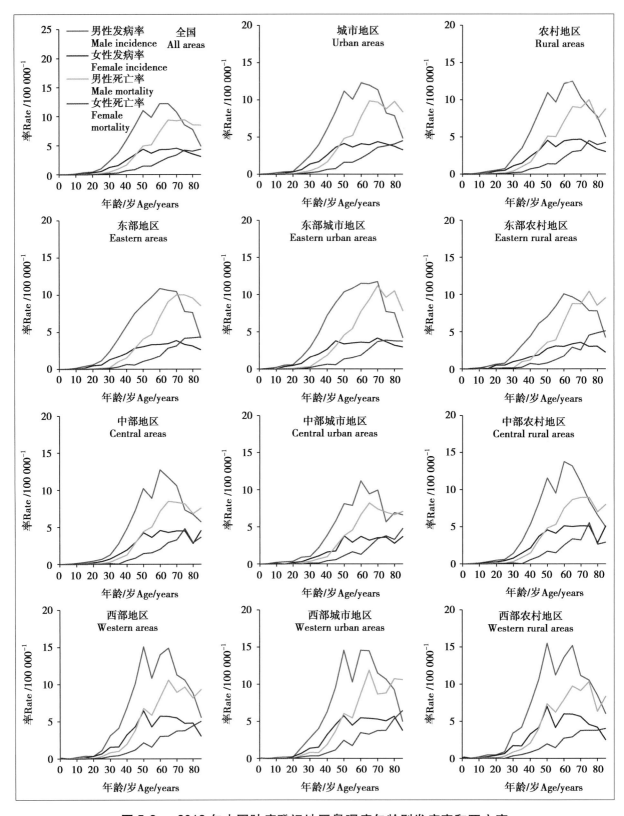

图 5-2a　2018 年中国肿瘤登记地区鼻咽癌年龄别发病率和死亡率

Figure 5-2a　Age-specific incidence and mortality rates of nasopharyngeal cancer in the registration areas of China,2018

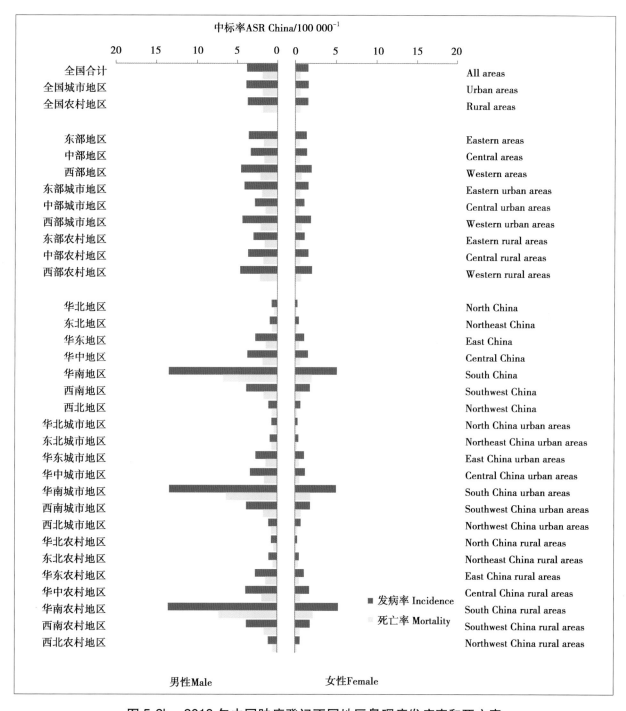

图 5-2b　2018 年中国肿瘤登记不同地区鼻咽癌发病率和死亡率

Figure 5-2b　Incidence and mortality rates of nasopharyngeal cancer in different registration areas of China,2018

3 食管

2018 年中国肿瘤登记地区食管癌位居癌症发病谱第 7 位。新发病例数为 93 945 例,占全部癌症发病的 6.01%;其中男性 69 821 例,女性 24 124 例,城市地区 33 601 例,农村地区 60 344 例。食管癌发病率为 17.96/10 万,中标发病率为 10.20/10 万,世标发病率为 10.29/10 万;男性中标发病率为女性的 3.20 倍,农村中标发病率为城市的 1.57 倍。0~74 岁累积发病率为 1.30%(表 5-3a)。

2018 年中国肿瘤登记地区食管癌位居癌症死亡谱第 5 位。食管癌死亡病例 74 902 例,占全部癌症死亡的 8.21%;其中男性 55 649 例,女性 19 253 例,城市地区 27 069 例,农村地区 47 833 例。食管癌死亡率为 14.32/10 万,中标死亡率 7.87/10 万,世标死亡率 7.89/10 万;男性中标死亡率为女性的 3.36 倍,农村中标死亡率为城市的 1.55 倍。0~74 岁累积死亡率为 0.94%(表 5-3b)。

食管癌的年龄别发病率和死亡率在 40 岁之前处于较低水平,自 40 岁之后快速上升。男女发病率均于 80~84 岁达到高峰,死亡率均在 85 岁之后达到高峰。男性各年龄别发病率和死亡率均明显高于女性(图 5-3a)。

3 Esophagus

Esophageal cancer was the 7th most common cancer in the registration areas of China in 2018. There were 93 945 new cases of esophageal cancer(69 821 males and 24 124 females,33 601 in urban areas and 60 344 in rural areas),accounting for 6.01% of new cases of all cancers. The crude incidence rate was 17.96 per 100 000,with ASR China 10.20 per 100 000 and ASR World 10.29 per 100 000,respectively. Subgroup analyses showed that the incidence of ASR China was 3.20 times in males as that in females,and was 1.57 times in rural areas as that in urban areas. The cumulative incidence rate for subjects aged 0 to 74 years was 1.30%(Table 5-3a).

Esophageal cancer was the 5th most common cause of cancer deaths in the registration areas of China in 2018. A total of 74 902 cases died of esophageal cancer(55 649 males and 19 253 females,27 069 in urban areas and 47 833 in rural areas),accounting for 8.21% of all cancer deaths. The crude mortality rate was 14.32 per 100 000,with ASR China 7.87 per 100 000 and ASR World 7.89 per 100 000,respectively. Subgroup analyses showed that the mortality of ASR China was 3.36 times in males as that in females,and was 1.55 times in rural areas as that in urban areas. The cumulative mortality rate for subjects aged 0 to 74 years was 0.94%(Table 5-3b).

The age-specific incidence and mortality rates of esophageal cancer were relatively low before 40 years old and increased dramatically since then. The age-specific incidence rates were the highest in the age group of 80-84 years for both sexes. The mortality rates peaked in age group of 85+ years for both sexes. The age-specific incidence and mortality rates were generally higher in males than those in females (Figure 5-3a).

农村食管癌的发病率和死亡率均高于城市。男性中标发病率和死亡率西部地区最高,东部地区最低。女性中标发病率和死亡率在中部地区最高,中标发病率东部地区最低,中标死亡率西部地区最低。七大行政区中,男性中标发病率和死亡率在西南地区最高,中标发病率在东北地区最低,中标死亡率在华南地区最低;女性中标发病率和死亡率在华中地区最高,东北地区最低(表5-3a,表5-3b,图5-3b)。

食管癌病例中有明确亚部位信息的占31.60%,其中47.23%的病例发生在食管中段,其次是食管上段占23.29%,食管下段占20.90%,交搭跨越占8.58%(图5-3c)。

全部食管癌病例中有明确组织学类型的病例占66.04%,其中鳞状细胞癌是最主要的病理类型,占85.17%;其次是腺癌,占10.52%;腺鳞癌占1.12%(图5-3d)。

The incidence and mortality rates of esophageal cancer were higher in rural areas than those in urban areas. The incidence and mortality rates (ASR China) in males were the highest in the western areas and the lowest in eastern areas. The incidence and mortality rates (ASR China) in females were the highest in the central areas, and the lowest in the eastern and western areas, respectively. Among the seven administrative districts, the incidence and mortality rates (ASR China) in males were the highest in Southwest China, and the lowest in Northeast China and South China, respectively. The incidence and mortality rates (ASR China) in females were the highest in Central China and the lowest in Northeast China (Table 5-3a, Table 5-3b, Figure 5-3b).

There were 31.60% of the esophageal cancer cases having specific subsite information. Esophageal cancer occurred the most frequently in the middle third of the esophagus (47.23%), followed by upper third (23.29%), lower third (20.90%) and overlapping esophagus (8.58%) (Figure 5-3c).

About 66.04% of the esophageal cancer cases had morphological verification. Among those, esophageal squamous cell carcinoma was the most common type, accounting for 85.17% of all cases, followed by adenocarcinoma (10.52%) and adenosquamous carcinoma (1.12%) (Figure 5-3d).

表 5-3a　2018 年中国肿瘤登记地区食管癌发病情况

Table 5-3a　Incidence of esophageal cancer in the registration areas of China, 2018

地区 Area	性别 Sex	病例数 No. cases	粗率 Crude rate/ $100\ 000^{-1}$	构成比 Freq./%	中标率 ASR China/ $100\ 000^{-1}$	世标率 ASR World/ $100\ 000^{-1}$	累积率 Cum. rate 0~74/%	顺位 Rank
合计	合计 Both	93 945	17.96	6.01	10.20	10.29	1.30	7
All	男性 Male	69 821	26.30	8.11	15.67	15.90	2.03	5
	女性 Female	24 124	9.36	3.43	4.89	4.86	0.58	9
城市地区	合计 Both	33 601	14.23	4.44	7.81	7.91	0.99	9
Urban areas	男性 Male	25 809	21.78	6.35	12.50	12.72	1.62	5
	女性 Female	7 792	6.63	2.22	3.33	3.29	0.39	13
农村地区	合计 Both	60 344	21.02	7.48	12.28	12.39	1.57	6
Rural areas	男性 Male	44 012	29.94	9.69	18.41	18.65	2.38	4
	女性 Female	16 332	11.66	4.63	6.29	6.26	0.76	8
东部地区	合计 Both	39 219	18.06	5.11	9.12	9.18	1.15	8
Eastern areas	男性 Male	28 777	26.39	7.03	14.12	14.29	1.80	5
	女性 Female	10 442	9.66	2.92	4.39	4.33	0.51	10
中部地区	合计 Both	22 464	17.32	6.43	10.91	11.04	1.42	7
Central areas	男性 Male	15 696	23.68	8.21	15.61	15.85	2.03	5
	女性 Female	6 768	10.67	4.28	6.31	6.32	0.79	8
西部地区	合计 Both	32 262	18.30	7.21	11.28	11.43	1.46	6
Western areas	男性 Male	25 348	28.11	9.75	17.96	18.27	2.35	5
	女性 Female	6 914	8.02	3.69	4.63	4.62	0.55	9

表 5-3b　2018 年中国肿瘤登记地区食管癌死亡情况

Table 5-3b　Mortality of esophageal cancer in the registration areas of China, 2018

地区 Area	性别 Sex	死亡数 No. deaths	粗率 Crude rate/ $100\ 000^{-1}$	构成比 Freq./%	中标率 ASR China/ $100\ 000^{-1}$	世标率 ASR World/ $100\ 000^{-1}$	累积率 Cum. rate 0~74/%	顺位 Rank
合计	合计 Both	74 902	14.32	8.21	7.87	7.89	0.94	5
All	男性 Male	55 649	20.96	9.52	12.27	12.36	1.50	4
	女性 Female	19 253	7.47	5.87	3.65	3.60	0.38	6
城市地区	合计 Both	27 069	11.47	6.44	6.08	6.12	0.72	5
Urban areas	男性 Male	20 894	17.63	7.84	9.93	10.05	1.22	5
	女性 Female	6 175	5.25	4.02	2.42	2.39	0.24	8
农村地区	合计 Both	47 833	16.66	9.72	9.44	9.45	1.12	4
Rural areas	男性 Male	34 755	23.64	10.93	14.31	14.39	1.74	4
	女性 Female	13 078	9.33	7.50	4.74	4.69	0.51	5
东部地区	合计 Both	32 616	15.02	7.79	7.29	7.28	0.84	5
Eastern areas	男性 Male	23 810	21.83	9.03	11.43	11.47	1.36	4
	女性 Female	8 806	8.15	5.68	3.43	3.36	0.34	6
中部地区	合计 Both	17 494	13.49	8.31	8.22	8.25	0.99	4
Central areas	男性 Male	12 387	18.69	9.23	12.09	12.18	1.49	4
	女性 Female	5 107	8.05	6.70	4.46	4.44	0.50	6
西部地区	合计 Both	24 792	14.06	8.75	8.48	8.55	1.04	4
Western areas	男性 Male	19 452	21.57	10.43	13.61	13.78	1.71	4
	女性 Female	5 340	6.20	5.51	3.40	3.38	0.37	6

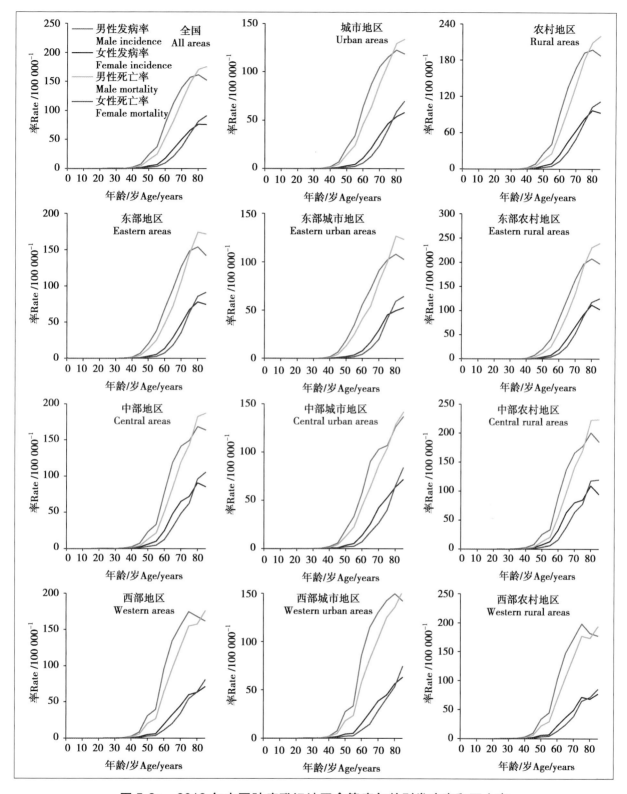

图 5-3a 2018 年中国肿瘤登记地区食管癌年龄别发病率和死亡率

Figure 5-3a Age-specific incidence and mortality rates of esophageal cancer in the registration areas of China, 2018

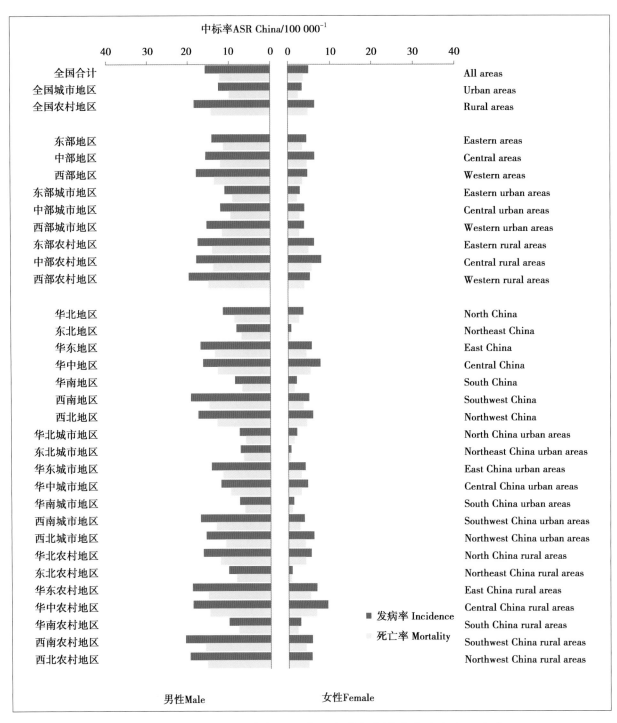

图 5-3b　2018 年中国肿瘤登记地区分城乡食管癌发病率和死亡率

Figure 5-3b　Incidence and mortality rates of esophageal cancer in different registration areas of China,2018

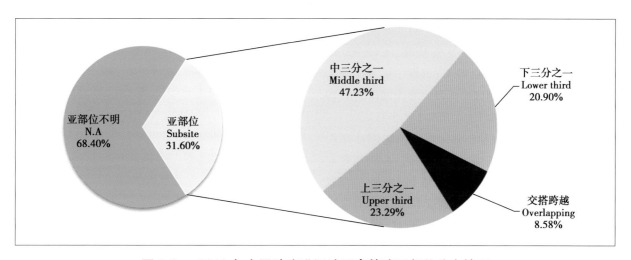

图 5-3c　2018 年中国肿瘤登记地区食管癌亚部位分布情况

Figure 5-3c　Subsite distribution of esophageal cancer in the registration areas of China,2018

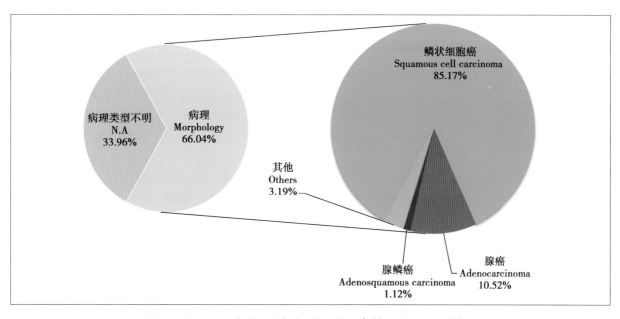

图 5-3d　2018 年中国肿瘤登记地区食管癌病理分型情况

Figure 5-3d　Morphological distribution of esophageal cancer in the registration areas of China,2018

4 胃

2018 年中国肿瘤登记地区胃癌位居癌症发病谱第 5 位。新发病例数为 141 415 例,占全部癌症发病的 9.04%;其中男性 98 542 例,女性 42 873 例,城市地区 59 979 例,农村地区 81 436 例。胃癌发病率为 27.03/10 万,中标发病率为 15.92/10 万,世标发病率为 15.84/10 万;男性中标发病率为女性的 2.36 倍,农村地区中标发病率为城市的 1.19 倍。0~74 岁累积发病率为 1.95%(表 5-4a)。

2018 年中国肿瘤登记地区胃癌位居癌症死亡谱第 3 位。胃癌死亡病例 103 378 例,占全部癌症死亡的 11.33%;其中男性 72 156 例,女性 31 222 例,城市地区 42 711 例,农村地区 60 667 例。胃癌死亡率为 19.76/10 万,中标死亡率 11.09/10 万,世标死亡率 10.98/10 万;男性中标死亡率为女性的 2.51 倍,农村地区中标死亡率为城市的 1.26 倍。0~74 岁累积死亡率为 1.27%(表 5-4b)。

胃癌的年龄别发病率和死亡率在 40 岁之前处于较低水平,40 岁后快速上升,男女发病率均于 80~84 岁组达到高峰,男性死亡率在 80~84 岁组达到高峰,女性死亡率在 85 岁之后达到高峰。男性各年龄别发病率和死亡率均高于女性(图 5-4a)。

4　Stomach

Stomach cancer was the 5th most common cancer in the registration areas of China in 2018. There were 141 415 new cases of stomach cancer(98 542 males and 42 873 females,59 979 in urban areas and 81 436 in rural areas),accounting for 9.04% of new cases of all cancers. The crude incidence rate was 27.03 per 100 000,with ASR China 15.92 per 100 000 and ASR World 15.84 per 100 000,respectively. Subgroup analyses showed that the incidence of ASR China was 2.36 times in males as that in females,and was 1.19 times in rural areas as that in urban areas. The cumulative incidence rate for subjects aged 0 to 74 years was 1.95%(Table 5-4a).

Stomach cancer was the 3rd most common cause of cancer deaths in 2018. A total of 103 378 cases died of stomach cancer in 2018(72 156 males and 31 222 females,42 711 in urban areas and 60 667 in rural areas),accounting for 11.33% of all cancer deaths. The crude mortality rate was 19.76 per 100 000,with ASR China 11.09 per 100 000 and ASR World 10.98 per 100 000,respectively. Subgroup analyses showed that the mortality of ASR China was 2.51 times in males as that in females,and was 1.26 times in rural areas as that in urban areas. The cumulative mortality rate for subjects aged 0 to 74 years was 1.27%(Table 5-4b).

The age-specific incidence and mortality rates of stomach cancer were relatively low before 40 years old and increased rapidly since then. The incidence rates in age group of 80-84 years were the highest in both sexes. The mortality rates peaked at age group of 80-84 years in males and 85+ years in females. Age-specific incidence and mortality rates in males were generally higher than those in females across all age groups(Figure 5-4a).

农村胃癌的发病率和死亡率均高于城市。中标发病率和死亡率均以中部地区最高，其次是东部地区，西部地区最低。七大行政区中，西北地区男性和女性中标发病率和死亡率最高，华南地区最低（表 5-4a，表 5-4b，图 5-4b）。

全部胃癌病例中有明确亚部位信息的病例占 40.95%。其中贲门病例最多，占 38.31%，其次是幽门窦（20.96%）、胃体（17.12%）、胃底（8.18%）、胃小弯（7.28%）、交搭跨越（5.31%）、幽门（1.52%）和胃大弯（1.32%）（图 5-4c）。

全部胃癌病例中有明确组织学类型的病例占 66.46%，其中腺癌是最主要的病理类型，占 90.26%；其次是鳞状细胞癌（4.01%），其他类型（4.90%），类癌（0.55%）和腺鳞癌（0.28%）（图 5-4d）。

The incidence and mortality rates of stomach cancer were higher in rural areas than those in urban areas. The incidence and mortality rates (ASR China) were the highest in the central areas, followed by the eastern areas and western areas. Among the seven administrative districts, the incidence and mortality rates (ASR China) were the highest in Northwest China and the lowest in South China for both sexes (Table 5-4a, Table 5-4b, Figure 5-4b).

About 40.95% of the stomach cancer cases had complete information onsubsite. Among those, cardia was the most common subsite and accounted for 38.31% of the total cases, followed by pyloric antrum (20.96%), body(17.12%), fundus(8.18%), lesser curvature(7.28%), overlapping(5.31%), pylorus(1.52%) and greater curvature(1.32%) (Figure 5-4c).

About 66.22% of the stomach cancer cases had morphological verification. Among those, adenocarcinoma was the most common histological type, accounting for 90.26% of all cases, followed by squamous cell carcinoma(4.01%), other type(3.82%), carcinoid (0.55%) and adenosquamous carcinoma (0.28%) (Figure 5-4d).

表 5-4a 2018 年中国肿瘤登记地区胃癌发病情况

Table 5-4a Incidence of stomach cancer in the registration areas of China, 2018

地区 Area	性别 Sex	病例数 No. cases	粗率 Crude rate/ 100 000⁻¹	构成比 Freq./%	中标率 ASR China/ 100 000⁻¹	世标率 ASR World/ 100 000⁻¹	累积率 Cum. rate 0~74/%	顺位 Rank
合计 All	合计 Both	141 415	27.03	9.04	15.92	15.84	1.95	5
	男性 Male	98 542	37.12	11.45	22.55	22.60	2.84	3
	女性 Female	42 873	16.64	6.09	9.54	9.32	1.07	6
城市地区 Urban areas	合计 Both	59 979	25.41	7.92	14.42	14.33	1.74	5
	男性 Male	41 142	34.72	10.12	20.23	20.28	2.52	4
	女性 Female	18 837	16.02	5.37	8.92	8.70	0.99	6
农村地区 Rural areas	合计 Both	81 436	28.36	10.10	17.22	17.14	2.13	3
	男性 Male	57 400	39.05	12.64	24.53	24.57	3.10	3
	女性 Female	24 036	17.15	6.82	10.08	9.87	1.15	6
东部地区 Eastern areas	合计 Both	68 325	31.47	8.91	16.68	16.53	2.03	4
	男性 Male	47 463	43.52	11.60	23.86	23.81	2.97	3
	女性 Female	20 862	19.30	5.83	9.98	9.71	1.12	5
中部地区 Central areas	合计 Both	35 768	27.58	10.23	17.90	17.89	2.24	3
	男性 Male	24 911	37.59	13.02	25.20	25.33	3.24	2
	女性 Female	10 857	17.12	6.86	10.76	10.59	1.24	6
西部地区 Western areas	合计 Both	37 322	21.17	8.34	13.44	13.40	1.64	5
	男性 Male	26 168	29.02	10.06	18.87	18.96	2.37	4
	女性 Female	11 154	12.95	5.96	8.04	7.85	0.90	6

表 5-4b 2018 年中国肿瘤登记地区胃癌死亡情况

Table 5-4b Mortality of stomach cancer in the registration areas of China, 2018

地区 Area	性别 Sex	死亡数 No. deaths	粗率 Crude rate/ 100 000⁻¹	构成比 Freq./%	中标率 ASR China/ 100 000⁻¹	世标率 ASR World/ 100 000⁻¹	累积率 Cum. rate 0~74/%	顺位 Rank
合计 All	合计 Both	103 378	19.76	11.33	11.09	10.98	1.27	3
	男性 Male	72 156	27.18	12.35	16.05	15.95	1.87	3
	女性 Female	31 222	12.12	9.52	6.40	6.28	0.67	3
城市地区 Urban areas	合计 Both	42 711	18.09	10.16	9.72	9.61	1.08	3
	男性 Male	29 507	24.90	11.07	14.02	13.93	1.60	3
	女性 Female	13 204	11.23	8.59	5.72	5.60	0.58	4
农村地区 Rural areas	合计 Both	60 667	21.13	12.33	12.29	12.16	1.42	3
	男性 Male	42 649	29.01	13.42	17.79	17.68	2.10	3
	女性 Female	18 018	12.86	10.34	7.01	6.88	0.74	3
东部地区 Eastern areas	合计 Both	48 939	22.54	11.69	11.23	11.04	1.24	3
	男性 Male	34 141	31.31	12.95	16.52	16.32	1.86	3
	女性 Female	14 798	13.69	9.55	6.40	6.24	0.65	3
中部地区 Central areas	合计 Both	26 440	20.39	12.56	12.74	12.65	1.50	3
	男性 Male	18 407	27.77	13.71	18.19	18.11	2.19	3
	女性 Female	8 033	12.67	10.53	7.48	7.38	0.81	3
西部地区 Western areas	合计 Both	27 999	15.88	9.88	9.74	9.69	1.14	3
	男性 Male	19 608	21.75	10.52	13.87	13.87	1.67	3
	女性 Female	8 391	9.74	8.67	5.65	5.55	0.60	4

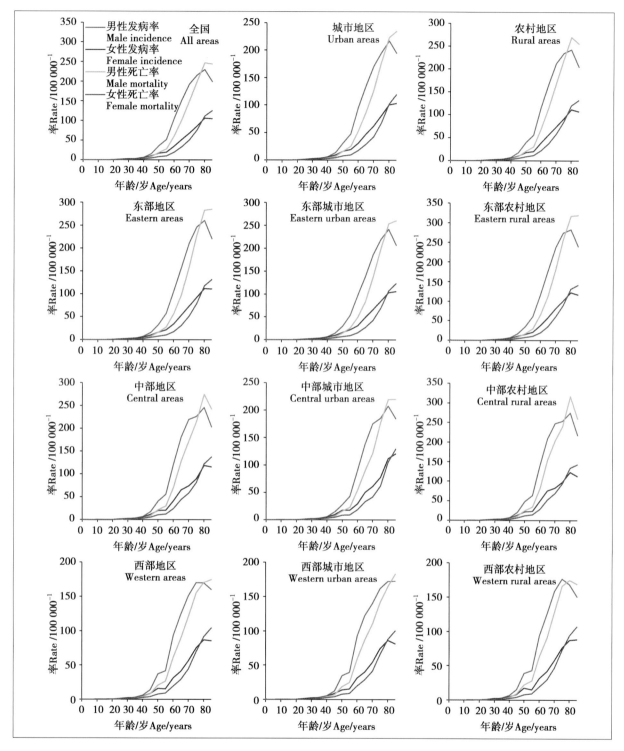

图 5-4a　2018 年中国肿瘤登记地区胃癌年龄别发病率和死亡率

Figure 5-4a　Age-specific incidence and mortality rates of stomach cancer in the registration areas of China, 2018

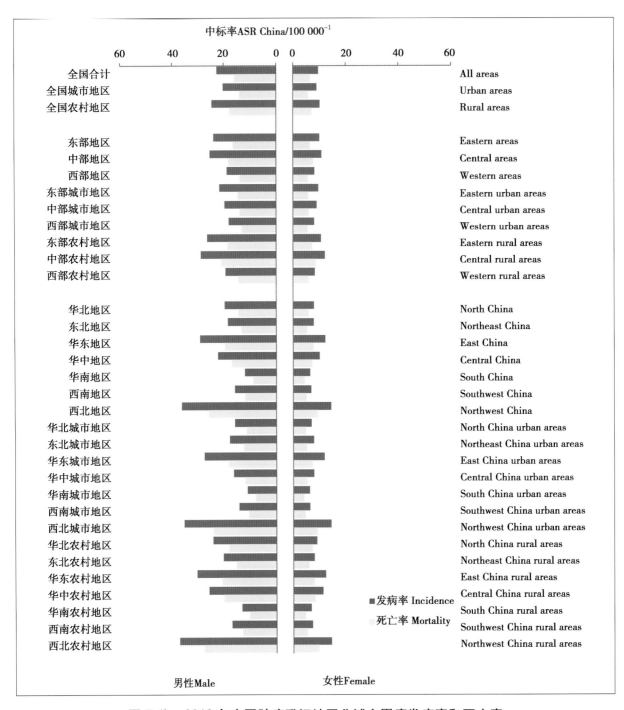

图 5-4b 2018 年中国肿瘤登记地区分城乡胃癌发病率和死亡率

Figure 5-4b Incidence and mortality rates of stomach cancer in different registration areas of China, 2018

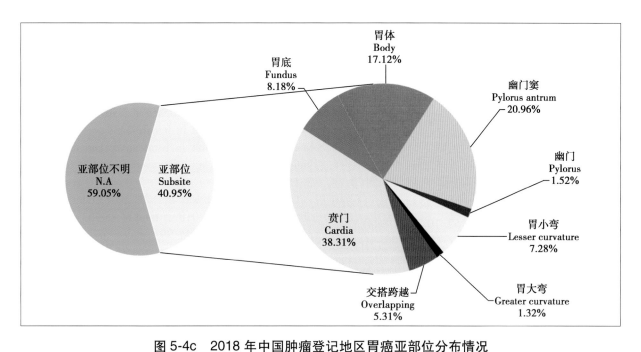

图 5-4c　2018 年中国肿瘤登记地区胃癌亚部位分布情况

Figure 5-4c　Subsite distribution of stomach cancer in the registration areas of China,2018

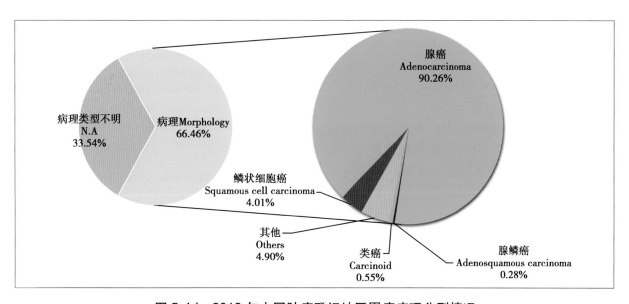

图 5-4d　2018 年中国肿瘤登记地区胃癌病理分型情况

Figure 5-4d　Morphological distribution of stomach cancer in the registration
areas of China,2018

5 结直肠

2018年中国肿瘤登记地区结直肠癌位居癌症发病谱第3位。新发病例数为159 635例,占全部癌症发病的10.21%;其中男性93 765例,女性65 870例,城市地区84 967例,农村地区74 668例。发病率为30.51/10万,中标发病率为18.23/10万,世标发病率18.05/10万;男性中标发病率为女性的1.48倍,城市中标发病率为农村的1.27倍。0~74岁累积发病率为2.16%(表5-5a)。

2018年中国肿瘤登记地区结直肠癌位居癌症死亡谱第4位。结直肠癌死亡病例75 963例,占全部癌症死亡的8.33%;其中男性44 991例,女性30 972例,城市地区40 194例,农村地区35 769例。结直肠癌死亡率为14.52/10万,中标死亡率8.00/10万,世标死亡率7.94/10万;男性中标死亡率为女性的1.60倍,城市中标死亡率为农村的1.23倍。0~74岁累积死亡率为0.83%(表5-5b)。

结肠癌新发病例数为78 460例,占全部癌症发病的5.02%,发病率为15.00/10万,中标发病率为8.94/10万,世标发病率8.83/10万;其中男性44 282例,女性34 178例,男性中标发病率为女性的1.36倍;城市地区45 051例,农村地区33 409例,城市中标发病率为农村的1.49倍(表5-5c)。结肠癌死亡病例数为34 571例,占全部癌症死亡的3.79%,死亡率为6.61/10万,中标死亡率为3.60/10万,世标死亡率3.58/10万;其中男性19 393例,女性15 178例,男性中标死亡率为女性的1.42倍;城市地区20 288例,农村地区14 283例,城市中标死亡率为农村的1.54倍(表5-5d)。

5 Colon-rectum

Colorectal cancer was the 3rd most common cancer in the registration areas of China in 2018. There were 159 635 new cases of colorectal cancer(93 765 males and 65 870 females, 84 967 in urban areas and 74 668 in rural areas), accounting for 10.21% of new cases of all cancers. The crude incidence rate was 30.51 per 100 000, with ASR China 18.23 per 100 000 and ASR World 18.05 per 100 000, respectively. Subgroup analyses showed that the incidence of ASR China in males was 1.48 times as that in females, and was 1.27 times in urban areas as that in rural areas. The cumulative incidence rate for subjects aged 0 to 74 years was 2.16% (Table 5-5a).

Colorectal cancer was the 4th most common cause of cancer deaths in 2018. A total of 75 963 cases died of colorectal cancer(44 991 males and 30 972 females, 40 194 in urban areas and 35 769 in rural areas), accounting for 8.33% of all cancer deaths. The crude mortality rate was 14.52 per 100 000, with ASR China 8.00 per 100 000 and ASR World 7.94 per 100 000, respectively. Subgroup analyses showed that the mortality of ASR China was 1.60 times in males as that in females, and was 1.23 times in urban areas as that in rural areas. The cumulative mortality rate for subjects aged 0 to 74 years was 0.83% (Table 5-5b).

There were 78 460 new cases of colon cancer in 2018(44 282 males and 34 178 females, 45 051 in urban areas and 33 409 in rural areas), accounting for 5.02% of new cases of all cancers. The crude incidence rate was 15.00 per 100 000, with ASR China 8.94 per 100 000 and ASR World 8.83 per 100 000, respectively. Subgroup analyses showed that the incidence of ASR China was 1.36 times in males of in females, and was 1.49 times in urban areas of in rural areas(Table 5-5c). A total of 34 571 cases died of colon cancer(19 393 males and 15 178 in females, 20 288 in urban areas and 14 283 in rural areas), accounting for 3.79% of all cancer deaths. The crude mortality rate was 6.61 per 100 000, with ASR China 3.60 per 100 000 and ASR World 3.58 per 100 000, respectively. Subgroup analyses showed that the mortality of ASR China was 1.42 times in males as that in females, and was 1.54 times in urban areas as that in rural areas(Table 5-5d).

直肠癌新发病例数为 79 281 例,占全部癌症发病的 5.07%,发病率为 15.15/10 万,中标发病率为 9.07/10 万,世标发病率 9.00/10 万;其中男性 48 406 例,女性 30 875 例,男性中标发病率为女性的 1.62 倍;城市地区 39 053 例,农村地区 40 228 例,城市中标发病率为农村的 1.10 倍(表 5-5e)。直肠癌死亡病例数为 40 124 例,占全部癌症死亡的 4.40%,死亡率为 7.67/10 万,中标死亡率为 4.26/10 万,世标死亡率 4.22/10 万;其中男性 24 861 例,女性 15 263 例,男性中标死亡率为女性的 1.79 倍;城市地区 19 364 例,农村地区 20 760 例,城市中标死亡率和农村接近(表 5-5f)。

结直肠癌年龄别发病率和死亡率在男性和女性中均随年龄呈上升趋势,40~44 岁组开始上升明显,发病率在 80~84 岁组达高峰,死亡率在 85 岁及以上组达到高峰,男性各年龄别发病率和死亡率均明显高于女性(图 5-5a)。

城市地区结直肠癌的发病率和死亡率均高于农村地区,中标发病率和死亡率东部地区高于西部和中部地区(表 5-5a,表 5-5b,图 5-5a)。七大行政区中,男性和女性发病率分别在东北地区和华南地区最高,西北地区最低。死亡率男性和女性均东北地区最高,西北地区最低(图 5-5b)。

在全部结肠癌病例中,有明确亚部位的病例占 59.10%,其中乙状结肠发生癌症的比例最高,占 41.55%,其次是升结肠、横结肠和降结肠,分别占 23.79%、9.10% 和 8.34%(图 5-5c)。

There were 79 281 new cases of rectal cancer in 2018(48 406 males and 30 875 females,39 053 in urban areas and 40 228 in rural areas),accounting for 5.07% of new cases of all cancers. The crude incidence rate was 15.15 per 100 000,with ASR China 9.07 per 100 000 and ASR World 9.00 per 100 000,respectively. Subgroup analyses showed that the incidence of ASR China was 1.62 times in males as that in females,and was 1.10 times in urban areas as that in rural areas(Table 5-5e). A total of 40 124 cases died of rectal cancer(24 861 males and 15 263 females,19 364 in urban areas and 20 760 in rural areas),accounting for 4.40% of all cancer deaths. The crude mortality rate was 7.67 per 100 000,with ASR China 4.26 per 100 000 and ASR World 4.22 per 100 000,respectively. Subgroup analyses showed that the mortality of ASR China was 1.79 times in males as that in females,and that was similar in urban and rural areas(Table 5-5f).

The age-specific incidence and mortality rates of colorectal cancer increased with age in both sexes,especially after age of 40 years,and reached the peak at the age group of 80-84 years for the incidence rates and at the age group of 85+ years for the mortality rates in both sexes. Age-specific incidence and mortality rates in males were generally higher than those in females across all age groups(Figure 5-5a).

The incidence and mortality rates of colorectal cancer were higher in urban areas than those in rural areas. The incidence and mortality rates(ASR China) were higher in eastern areas than in western and central areas(Table 5-5a,Table 5-5b,Figure 5-5a). Among the seven administrative districts,the incidence rates(ASR China) were the highest in Northeast and South China for males and females,respectively,and the lowest in Northwest China for both sexes. The mortality rates(ASR China)were the highest in Northeast China and the lowest in Northwest China for both sexes(Figure 5-5b).

Approximately 59.10% of the colon cancer cases had complete information on subsite. Among those,sigmoid colon was the most common subsite(41.55%),followed by ascending colon(23.79%),transverse colon(9.10%) and descending colon(8.34%)(Figure 5-5c).

表 5-5a　2018 年中国肿瘤登记地区结直肠癌发病情况

表 5-5a　2018 年中国肿瘤登记地区结直肠癌发病情况
Table 5-5a　Incidence of colorectal cancer in the registration areas of China,2018

地区 Area	性别 Sex	病例数 No. cases	粗率 Crude rate/ 100 000^{-1}	构成比 Freq./%	中标率 ASR China/ 100 000^{-1}	世标率 ASR World/ 100 000^{-1}	累积率 Cum. rate 0~74/%	顺位 Rank
合计 All	合计 Both	159 635	30.51	10.21	18.23	18.05	2.16	3
	男性 Male	93 765	35.32	10.90	21.84	21.74	2.62	4
	女性 Female	65 870	25.56	9.36	14.75	14.49	1.70	3
城市地区 Urban areas	合计 Both	84 967	36.00	11.22	20.57	20.42	2.43	3
	男性 Male	49 890	42.10	12.27	24.85	24.82	2.99	2
	女性 Female	35 077	29.84	10.00	16.51	16.23	1.88	4
农村地区 Rural areas	合计 Both	74 668	26.01	9.26	16.18	15.95	1.92	5
	男性 Male	43 875	29.85	9.66	19.24	19.05	2.30	5
	女性 Female	30 793	21.98	8.73	13.18	12.94	1.54	3
东部地区 Eastern areas	合计 Both	82 863	38.16	10.80	20.56	20.34	2.43	3
	男性 Male	48 744	44.70	11.92	25.04	24.91	3.01	2
	女性 Female	34 119	31.56	9.53	16.34	16.03	1.87	4
中部地区 Central areas	合计 Both	31 767	24.49	9.09	16.19	16.05	1.93	5
	男性 Male	18 376	27.73	9.61	18.92	18.84	2.28	4
	女性 Female	13 391	21.11	8.46	13.51	13.32	1.58	4
西部地区 Western areas	合计 Both	45 005	25.52	10.06	16.38	16.16	1.92	4
	男性 Male	26 645	29.55	10.25	19.46	19.31	2.30	3
	女性 Female	18 360	21.31	9.80	13.34	13.06	1.53	3

表 5-5b　2018 年中国肿瘤登记地区结直肠癌死亡情况
Table 5-5b　Mortality of colorectal cancer in the registration areas of China,2018

地区 Area	性别 Sex	死亡数 No. deaths	粗率 Crude rate/ 100 000^{-1}	构成比 Freq./%	中标率 ASR China/ 100 000^{-1}	世标率 ASR World/ 100 000^{-1}	累积率 Cum. rate 0~74/%	顺位 Rank
合计 All	合计 Both	75 963	14.52	8.33	8.00	7.94	0.83	4
	男性 Male	44 991	16.95	7.70	9.93	9.90	1.05	5
	女性 Female	30 972	12.02	9.44	6.19	6.12	0.62	4
城市地区 Urban areas	合计 Both	40 194	17.03	9.57	8.86	8.82	0.91	4
	男性 Male	23 877	20.15	8.96	11.13	11.15	1.17	4
	女性 Female	16 317	13.88	10.62	6.76	6.68	0.66	2
农村地区 Rural areas	合计 Both	35 769	12.46	7.27	7.22	7.14	0.77	5
	男性 Male	21 114	14.36	6.64	8.86	8.77	0.94	5
	女性 Female	14 655	10.46	8.41	5.67	5.60	0.59	4
东部地区 Eastern areas	合计 Both	37 682	17.35	9.00	8.32	8.29	0.84	4
	男性 Male	22 024	20.20	8.35	10.45	10.47	1.07	5
	女性 Female	15 658	14.49	10.11	6.39	6.34	0.62	2
中部地区 Central areas	合计 Both	15 436	11.90	7.33	7.41	7.32	0.81	5
	男性 Male	9 091	13.72	6.77	8.98	8.92	0.98	5
	女性 Female	6 345	10.00	8.32	5.90	5.81	0.63	4
西部地区 Western areas	合计 Both	22 845	12.96	8.06	7.89	7.78	0.84	5
	男性 Male	13 876	15.39	7.44	9.80	9.70	1.06	5
	女性 Female	8 969	10.41	9.26	6.03	5.92	0.63	3

表 5-5c　2018 年中国肿瘤登记地区结肠癌发病情况

地区 Area	性别 Sex	病例数 No. cases	粗率 Crude rate/ 100 000^{-1}	构成比 Freq./%	中标率 ASR China/ 100 000^{-1}	世标率 ASR World/ 100 000^{-1}	累积率 Cum. rate 0~74/%
合计	合计 Both	78 460	15.00	5.02	8.94	8.83	1.04
All	男性 Male	44 282	16.68	5.15	10.33	10.24	1.21
	女性 Female	34 178	13.26	4.86	7.61	7.47	0.87
城市地区	合计 Both	45 051	19.09	5.95	10.84	10.73	1.26
Urban areas	男性 Male	25 384	21.42	6.25	12.60	12.54	1.48
	女性 Female	19 667	16.73	5.61	9.17	9.01	1.04
农村地区	合计 Both	33 409	11.64	4.14	7.28	7.15	0.85
Rural areas	男性 Male	18 898	12.86	4.16	8.37	8.24	0.98
	女性 Female	14 511	10.36	4.11	6.21	6.09	0.72
东部地区	合计 Both	45 067	20.75	5.88	11.12	10.97	1.29
Eastern areas	男性 Male	25 465	23.35	6.23	13.06	12.95	1.54
	女性 Female	19 602	18.13	5.48	9.30	9.11	1.05
中部地区	合计 Both	15 225	11.74	4.36	7.78	7.69	0.92
Central areas	男性 Male	8 516	12.85	4.45	8.83	8.75	1.05
	女性 Female	6 709	10.58	4.24	6.76	6.66	0.79
西部地区	合计 Both	18 168	10.30	4.06	6.67	6.54	0.76
Western areas	男性 Male	10 301	11.42	3.96	7.59	7.48	0.86
	女性 Female	7 867	9.13	4.20	5.75	5.61	0.66

表 5-5d　2018 年中国肿瘤登记地区结肠癌死亡情况

地区 Area	性别 Sex	死亡数 No. deaths	粗率 Crude rate/ 100 000^{-1}	构成比 Freq./%	中标率 ASR China/ 100 000^{-1}	世标率 ASR World/ 100 000^{-1}	累积率 Cum. rate 0~74/%
合计	合计 Both	34 571	6.61	3.79	3.60	3.58	0.37
All	男性 Male	19 393	7.30	3.32	4.26	4.25	0.44
	女性 Female	15 178	5.89	4.63	2.99	2.97	0.30
城市地区	合计 Both	20 288	8.59	4.83	4.42	4.40	0.44
Urban areas	男性 Male	11 487	9.69	4.31	5.31	5.33	0.55
	女性 Female	8 801	7.49	5.73	3.59	3.56	0.34
农村地区	合计 Both	14 283	4.97	2.90	2.88	2.85	0.30
Rural areas	男性 Male	7 906	5.38	2.49	3.32	3.29	0.34
	女性 Female	6 377	4.55	3.66	2.46	2.43	0.25
东部地区	合计 Both	19 842	9.14	4.74	4.34	4.33	0.43
Eastern areas	男性 Male	11 003	10.09	4.17	5.20	5.21	0.52
	女性 Female	8 839	8.18	5.70	3.56	3.54	0.34
中部地区	合计 Both	6 942	5.35	3.30	3.32	3.29	0.36
Central areas	男性 Male	3 897	5.88	2.90	3.84	3.83	0.41
	女性 Female	3 045	4.80	3.99	2.84	2.79	0.30
西部地区	合计 Both	7 787	4.42	2.75	2.70	2.65	0.28
Western areas	男性 Male	4 493	4.98	2.41	3.18	3.13	0.33
	女性 Female	3 294	3.82	3.40	2.23	2.18	0.23

表 5-5e　2018 年中国肿瘤登记地区直肠癌发病情况

Table 5-5e　Incidence of rectal cancer in the registration areas of China,2018

地区 Arca	性别 Sex	病例数 No. cases	粗率 Crude rate/ 100 000⁻¹	构成比 Freq. /%	中标率 ASR China/ 100 000⁻¹	世标率 ASR World/ 100 000⁻¹	累积率 Cum. rate 0~74/%
合计 All	合计 Both	79 281	15. 15	5. 07	9. 07	9. 00	1. 09
	男性 Male	48 406	18. 23	5. 63	11. 26	11. 24	1. 38
	女性 Female	30 875	11. 98	4. 39	6. 96	6. 84	0. 81
城市地区 Urban areas	合计 Both	39 053	16. 54	5. 16	9. 52	9. 48	1. 15
	男性 Male	24 028	20. 28	5. 91	12. 01	12. 03	1. 48
	女性 Female	15 025	12. 78	4. 28	7. 15	7. 04	0. 83
农村地区 Rural areas	合计 Both	40 228	14. 01	4. 99	8. 67	8. 58	1. 04
	男性 Male	24 378	16. 58	5. 37	10. 61	10. 55	1. 29
	女性 Female	15 850	11. 31	4. 49	6. 78	6. 66	0. 80
东部地区 Eastern areas	合计 Both	37 128	17. 10	4. 84	9. 28	9. 21	1. 12
	男性 Male	22 913	21. 01	5. 60	11. 79	11. 77	1. 45
	女性 Female	14 215	13. 15	3. 97	6. 90	6. 78	0. 81
中部地区 Central areas	合计 Both	16 100	12. 41	4. 61	8. 18	8. 14	0. 99
	男性 Male	9 621	14. 52	5. 03	9. 85	9. 84	1. 20
	女性 Female	6 479	10. 22	4. 10	6. 54	6. 47	0. 77
西部地区 Western areas	合计 Both	26 053	14. 78	5. 82	9. 43	9. 34	1. 13
	男性 Male	15 872	17. 60	6. 10	11. 53	11. 49	1. 40
	女性 Female	10 181	11. 82	5. 44	7. 35	7. 22	0. 85

表 5-5f　2018 年中国肿瘤登记地区直肠癌死亡情况

Table 5-5f　Mortality of rectal cancer in the registration areas of China,2018

地区 Area	性别 Sex	死亡数 No. deaths	粗率 Crude rate/ 100 000⁻¹	构成比 Freq. /%	中标率 ASR China/ 100 000⁻¹	世标率 ASR World/ 100 000⁻¹	累积率 Cum. rate 0~74/%
合计 All	合计 Both	40 124	7. 67	4. 40	4. 26	4. 22	0. 45
	男性 Male	24 861	9. 36	4. 25	5. 51	5. 48	0. 59
	女性 Female	15 263	5. 92	4. 65	3. 09	3. 04	0. 32
城市地区 Urban areas	合计 Both	19 364	8. 20	4. 61	4. 32	4. 30	0. 46
	男性 Male	12 073	10. 19	4. 53	5. 66	5. 67	0. 61
	女性 Female	7 291	6. 20	4. 74	3. 07	3. 03	0. 31
农村地区 Rural areas	合计 Both	20 760	7. 23	4. 22	4. 20	4. 14	0. 45
	男性 Male	12 788	8. 70	4. 02	5. 36	5. 30	0. 58
	女性 Female	7 972	5. 69	4. 57	3. 09	3. 05	0. 33
东部地区 Eastern areas	合计 Both	17 496	8. 06	4. 18	3. 90	3. 89	0. 41
	男性 Male	10 835	9. 94	4. 11	5. 16	5. 17	0. 54
	女性 Female	6 661	6. 16	4. 30	2. 76	2. 74	0. 28
中部地区 Central areas	合计 Both	8 181	6. 31	3. 89	3. 93	3. 88	0. 43
	男性 Male	5 005	7. 55	3. 73	4. 95	4. 91	0. 55
	女性 Female	3 176	5. 01	4. 16	2. 95	2. 90	0. 32
西部地区 Western areas	合计 Both	14 447	8. 19	5. 10	4. 98	4. 92	0. 54
	男性 Male	9 021	10. 01	4. 84	6. 35	6. 30	0. 70
	女性 Female	5 426	6. 30	5. 60	3. 64	3. 57	0. 38

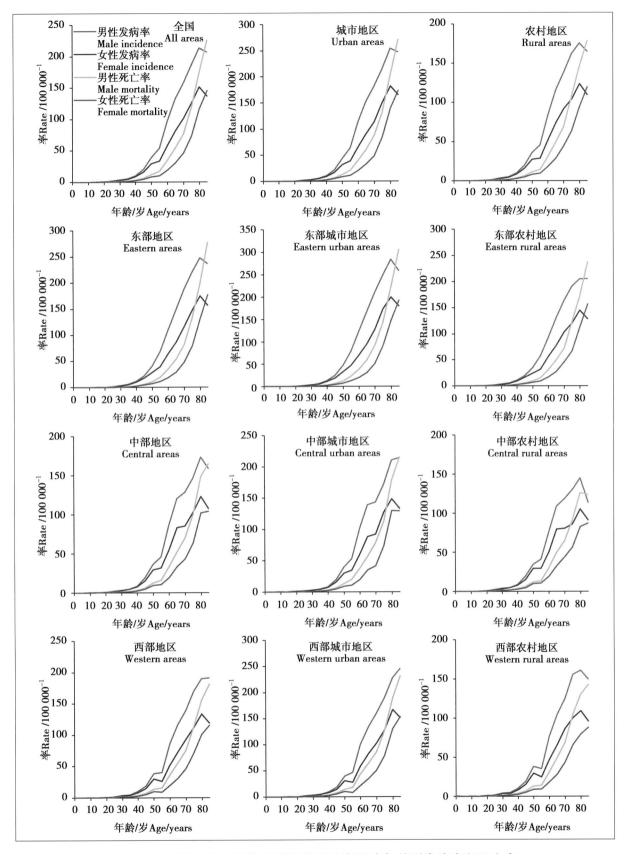

图 5-5a　2018 年中国肿瘤登记地区结直肠癌年龄别发病率和死亡率

Figure 5-5a　Age-specific incidence and mortality rates of colorectal cancer in the registration areas of China,2018

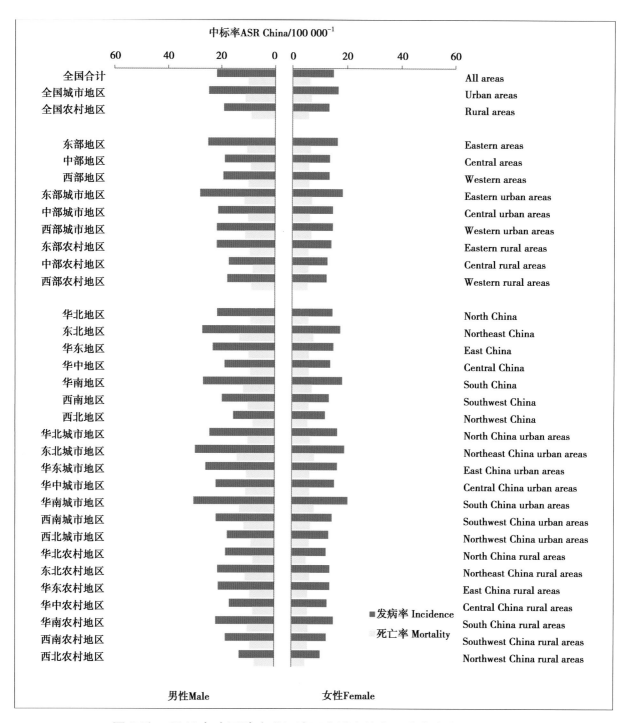

中标率ASR China/100 000⁻¹

全国合计		All areas
全国城市地区		Urban areas
全国农村地区		Rural areas
东部地区		Eastern areas
中部地区		Central areas
西部地区		Western areas
东部城市地区		Eastern urban areas
中部城市地区		Central urban areas
西部城市地区		Western urban areas
东部农村地区		Eastern rural areas
中部农村地区		Central rural areas
西部农村地区		Western rural areas
华北地区		North China
东北地区		Northeast China
华东地区		East China
华中地区		Central China
华南地区		South China
西南地区		Southwest China
西北地区		Northwest China
华北城市地区		North China urban areas
东北城市地区		Northeast China urban areas
华东城市地区		East China urban areas
华中城市地区		Central China urban areas
华南城市地区		South China urban areas
西南城市地区		Southwest China urban areas
西北城市地区		Northwest China urban areas
华北农村地区		North China rural areas
东北农村地区		Northeast China rural areas
华东农村地区		East China rural areas
华中农村地区		Central China rural areas
华南农村地区		South China rural areas
西南农村地区		Southwest China rural areas
西北农村地区		Northwest China rural areas

■发病率 Incidence
死亡率 Mortality

男性Male   女性Female

图 5-5b   2018 年中国肿瘤登记地区分城乡结直肠癌发病率和死亡率
Figure 5-5b   Incidence and mortality rates of colorectal cancer in different registration areas of China,2018

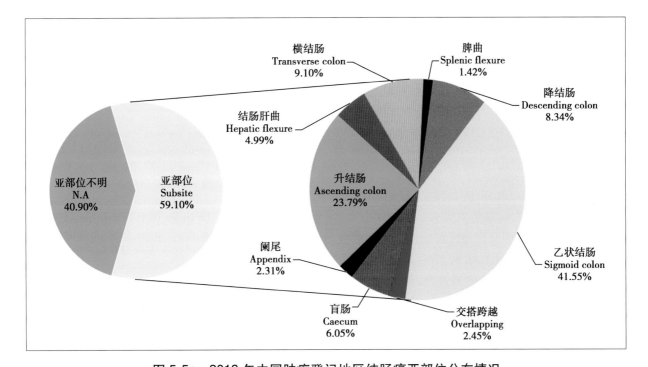

图 5-5c　2018 年中国肿瘤登记地区结肠癌亚部位分布情况

Figure 5-5c　Subsite distribution of colon cancer in the registration areas of China, 2018

6 肝

2018年中国肿瘤登记地区肝癌发病位居癌症发病谱第4位。新发病例数为143 438例，占全部癌症发病的9.17%；其中男性106 248例，女性37 190例，城市地区62 003例，农村地区81 435例。肝癌发病率为27.42/10万，中标发病率为17.21/10万，世标发病率为16.90/10万。中标发病率男性为女性的3.18倍，农村为城市的1.16倍。0~74岁累积发病率为1.97%（表5-6a）。

2018年中国肿瘤登记地区肝癌死亡位居癌症死亡谱第2位。肝癌死亡病例126 122例，占全部癌症死亡的13.82%；其中男性92 906例，女性33 216例，城市地区53 793例，农村地区72 329例。死亡率为24.11/10万，中标死亡率14.77/10万，世标死亡率14.54/10万。中标死亡率男性为女性的3.18倍，农村为城市的1.20倍。0~74岁累积死亡率为1.68%（表5-6b）。

肝癌的年龄别发病率和死亡率呈明显的性别差异，男性均高于女性。男性、女性发病率分别自30~34岁和40~44岁组开始上升，并分别在80~84岁年龄组和85岁及以上年龄组达到高峰，死亡率均在85岁及以上年龄组达到高峰。男性、女性死亡率曲线趋势分别与男女性发病率趋势相似（图5-6a）。

肝癌的发病率和死亡率呈现地域差异。农村地区发病率和死亡率高于城市地区，西部地区高于中部和东部地区。七大行政区中，发病率和死亡率男性在华南地区为最高，女性在西北地区为最高。华北地区的男性和女性的发病率和死亡率均为最低（表5-6a，表5-6b，图5-6a，图5-6b）。

6 Liver

Liver cancer was the 4th most common cancer in the registration areas of China in 2018. There were 143 438 new cases of liver cancer(106 248 males and 37 190 females,62 003 in urban areas and 81 435 in rural areas), accounting for 9.17% of all new cancer cases. The crude incidence rate was 27.42 per 100 000, with ASR China of 17.21 per 100 000 and ASR World of 16.90 per 100 000, respectively. Subgroup analyses showed that the incidence of ASR China in males was 3.18 times than that in females, and it was 1.16 times in rural areas than in urban areas. The cumulative incidence rate of 0 to 74 years old was 1.97% (Table 5-6a).

Liver cancer was the second most common cause of cancer death in the registration areas of China in 2018. A total of 126 122 cases died of liver cancer(92 906 males and 33 216 females,53 793 in urban areas and 72 329 in rural areas), accounting for 13.82% of all cancer deaths. The crude mortality rate was 24.11 per 100 000, with ASR China of 14.77 per 100 000 and ASR World of 14.54 per 100 000, respectively. Subgroup analyses showed that the mortality of ASR China in males was 3.18 times than that in females, and it was 1.20 times in rural areas than in urban areas. The cumulative mortality rate of 0 to 74 years old was 1.68% (Table 5-6b).

Trends of age-specific incidence and mortality rates showed significant differences between males and females, with males were higher than females. The age-specific incidence rates increased rapidly since 30-34 in males and 40-44 years in females, the incidence rate peaked at the age group of 80-84 years old for males and 85 + years old for females, the mortality rate reached peak both at the age group of 85 + years. The curve trends of age-specific mortality rate in males and females were similar as that of age-specific incidence (Figure 5-6a).

The incidence and mortality rates of liver cancer varied by geographical areas. Both incidence and mortality rates were higher in rural areas than in urban areas. Western areas had the higher rates of incidence and mortality(ASR China). Among the seven administrative districts, South China had the highest incidence and mortality rate (ASR China) for males, and Northwest had the highest incidence and mortality rates for females. North China had the lowest incidence and mortality rates both for males and females(Table 5-6a, Table 5-6b, Figure 5-6a, Figure 5-6b).

表 5-6a 2018 年中国肿瘤登记地区肝癌发病情况
表 5-6a 2018 年中国肿瘤登记地区肝癌发病情况

Table 5-6a Incidence of liver cancer in registration areas of China,2018

地区 Area	性别 Sex	病例数 No. cases	粗率 Crude rate/ 100 000^{-1}	构成比 Freq./%	中标率 ASR China/ 100 000^{-1}	世标率 ASR World/ 100 000^{-1}	累积率 Cum. rate 0~74/%	顺位 Rank
合计 All	合计 Both	143 438	27.42	9.17	17.21	16.90	1.97	4
	男性 Male	106 248	40.02	12.35	26.22	25.68	2.98	2
	女性 Female	37 190	14.43	5.29	8.25	8.17	0.95	7
城市地区 Urban areas	合计 Both	62 003	26.27	8.19	15.84	15.61	1.81	4
	男性 Male	45 830	38.68	11.28	24.33	23.95	2.78	3
	女性 Female	16 173	13.76	4.61	7.53	7.44	0.85	7
农村地区 Rural areas	合计 Both	81 435	28.36	10.10	18.39	18.00	2.10	4
	男性 Male	60 418	41.10	13.31	27.80	27.14	3.15	2
	女性 Female	21 017	15.00	5.96	8.89	8.80	1.04	7
东部地区 Eastern areas	合计 Both	55 780	25.69	7.27	14.50	14.35	1.67	5
	男性 Male	40 969	37.57	10.02	22.36	22.08	2.56	4
	女性 Female	14 811	13.70	4.14	6.88	6.85	0.79	7
中部地区 Central areas	合计 Both	34 143	26.33	9.77	17.79	17.53	2.07	4
	男性 Male	24 743	37.33	12.93	26.23	25.81	3.04	3
	女性 Female	9 400	14.82	5.94	9.32	9.23	1.09	7
西部地区 Western areas	合计 Both	53 515	30.35	11.96	20.54	20.01	2.32	2
	男性 Male	40 536	44.96	15.59	31.40	30.50	3.52	2
	女性 Female	12 979	15.06	6.93	9.44	9.30	1.08	5

表 5-6b 2018 年中国肿瘤登记地区肝癌死亡情况

Table 5-6b Mortality of liver cancer in registration areas of China,2018

地区 Area	性别 Sex	死亡数 No. deaths	粗率 Crude rate/ 100 000^{-1}	构成比 Freq./%	中标率 ASR China/ 100 000^{-1}	世标率 ASR World/ 100 000^{-1}	累积率 Cum. rate 0~74/%	顺位 Rank
合计地区 All	合计 Both	126 122	24.11	13.82	14.77	14.54	1.68	2
	男性 Male	92 906	34.99	15.90	22.54	22.15	2.56	2
	女性 Female	33 216	12.89	10.13	7.08	7.01	0.79	2
城市地区 Urban areas	合计 Both	53 793	22.79	12.80	13.35	13.19	1.51	2
	男性 Male	39 457	33.30	14.81	20.54	20.29	2.35	2
	女性 Female	14 336	12.20	9.33	6.34	6.28	0.69	3
农村地区 Rural areas	合计 Both	72 329	25.19	14.69	15.99	15.69	1.82	2
	男性 Male	53 449	36.36	16.81	24.23	23.71	2.74	2
	女性 Female	18 880	13.47	10.83	7.72	7.65	0.88	2
东部地区 Eastern areas	合计 Both	49 032	22.58	11.71	12.35	12.22	1.41	2
	男性 Male	35 506	32.56	13.46	18.92	18.73	2.17	2
	女性 Female	13 526	12.51	8.73	6.01	5.96	0.66	4
中部地区 Central areas	合计 Both	29 636	22.85	14.08	15.15	14.96	1.76	2
	男性 Male	21 502	32.44	16.02	22.51	22.19	2.60	2
	女性 Female	8 134	12.83	10.67	7.80	7.74	0.90	2
西部地区 Western areas	合计 Both	47 454	26.91	16.75	17.86	17.48	2.01	2
	男性 Male	35 898	39.81	19.25	27.42	26.75	3.08	2
	女性 Female	11 556	13.41	11.93	8.11	8.04	0.91	2

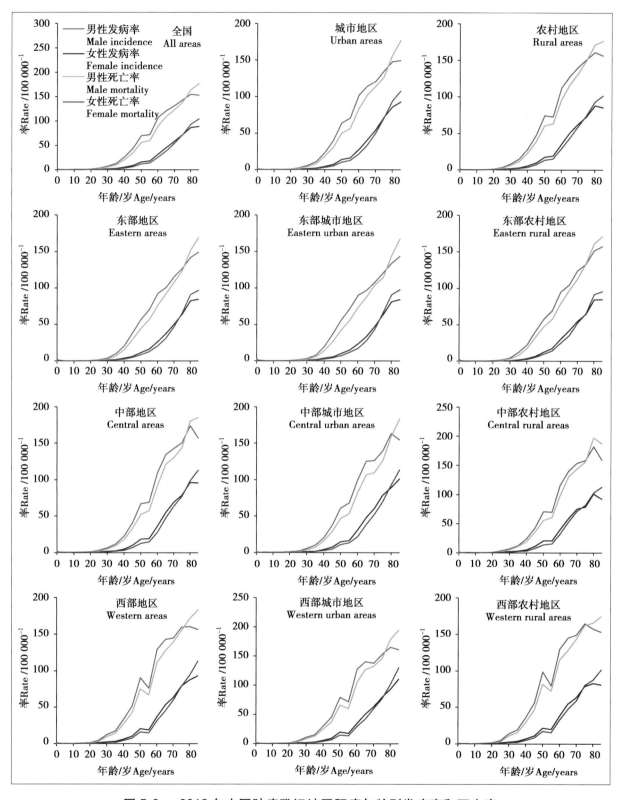

图 5-6a 2018 年中国肿瘤登记地区肝癌年龄别发病率和死亡率

Figure 5-6a Age-specific incidence and mortality rates of liver cancer in registration areas of China, 2018

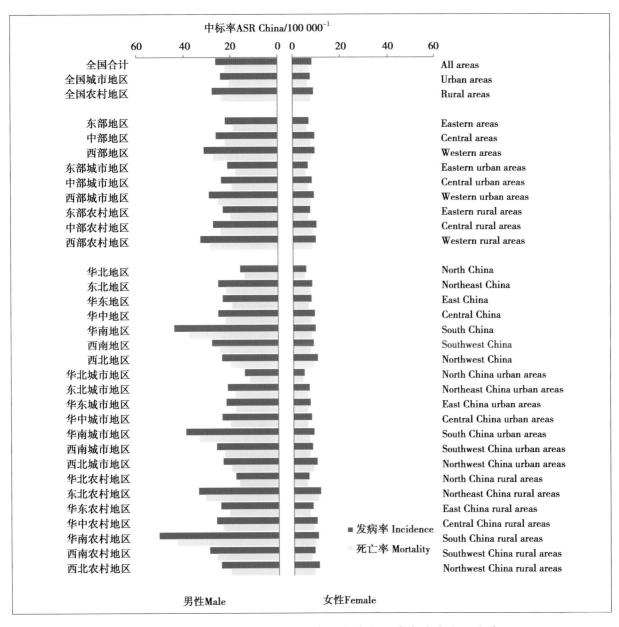

中标率ASR China/100 000⁻¹

全国合计	All areas
全国城市地区	Urban areas
全国农村地区	Rural areas
东部地区	Eastern areas
中部地区	Central areas
西部地区	Western areas
东部城市地区	Eastern urban areas
中部城市地区	Central urban areas
西部城市地区	Western urban areas
东部农村地区	Eastern rural areas
中部农村地区	Central rural areas
西部农村地区	Western rural areas
华北地区	North China
东北地区	Northeast China
华东地区	East China
华中地区	Central China
华南地区	South China
西南地区	Southwest China
西北地区	Northwest China
华北城市地区	North China urban areas
东北城市地区	Northeast China urban areas
华东城市地区	East China urban areas
华中城市地区	Central China urban areas
华南城市地区	South China urban areas
西南城市地区	Southwest China urban areas
西北城市地区	Northwest China urban areas
华北农村地区	North China rural areas
东北农村地区	Northeast China rural areas
华东农村地区	East China rural areas
华中农村地区	Central China rural areas
华南农村地区	South China rural areas
西南农村地区	Southwest China rural areas
西北农村地区	Northwest China rural areas

■ 发病率 Incidence
死亡率 Mortality

男性Male　　　女性Female

图 5-6b　2018 年中国肿瘤登记地区分城乡肝癌发病率和死亡率
Figure 5-6b　Incidence and mortality rates of liver cancer in different
registration areas of China,2018

7 胆囊

2018 年中国肿瘤登记地区胆囊癌位居癌症发病谱第 18 位。新发病例数为 21 260 例，占全部癌症发病的 1.36%；其中男性 10 293 例，女性 10 967 例，城市地区 10 363 例，农村地区 10 897 例。发病率为 4.06/10 万，中标发病率为 2.30/10 万，世标发病率为 2.30/10 万。中标发病率男性与女性基本相同，城市与农村接近。0~74 岁累积发病率为 0.27%（表 5-7a）。

2018 年中国肿瘤登记地区胆囊癌位居癌症死亡谱第 14 位。胆囊癌死亡病例为 16 140 例，占全部癌症死亡的 1.77%；其中男性 7 601 例，女性 8 539 例，城市地区 8 142 例，农村地区 7 998 例。胆囊癌死亡率为 3.09/10 万，中标死亡率为 1.69/10 万，世标死亡率为 1.69/10 万；女性中标死亡率与男性接近，城市地区中标死亡率为农村地区的 1.13 倍，0~74 岁累积死亡率为 0.19%（表 5-7b）。

中国肿瘤登记地区胆囊癌年龄别发病率和死亡率在 40 岁之前处于较低水平，40~44 岁年龄组开始呈显著上升趋势。男性发病率于 85 岁及以上年龄组达到高峰，女性发病率于 80~84 岁组达到高峰，男女死亡率均于 85 岁及以上年龄组达到高峰。男性与女性年龄别发病率和死亡率差别不大（图 5-7a）。

城市地区胆囊癌发病和死亡率高于农村地区，东部地区高于中部和西部地区。在七大行政区中，男性和女性发病率分别在华北地区和西北地区最高，死亡率均在西北地区最高，男性在西南地区最低，女性在华南地区最低（表 5-7a，表 5-7b，图 5-7b）。

7 Gallbladder

The incidence of gallbladder cancer ranked 18th among all cancer types in the registration areas of China in 2018. There were 21 260 new cases of gallbladder cancer (10 293 males and 10 967 females, 10 363 in urban areas and 10 897 in rural areas), accounting for 1.36% of all new cancer cases. The crude incidence rate was 4.06 per 100 000, with ASR China 2.30 per 100 000 and ASR World 2.30 per 100 000, respectively. Subgroup analyses showed that the incidence of ASR China in males was similar to that in females, the urban and rural was similar. The cumulative incidence rate of 0 to 74 years old was 0.27% (Table 5-7a).

The mortality rate of gallbladder cancer ranked 14th among different causes of cancer death in the registration areas of China in 2018. There were 16 140 cases dying of gallbladder cancer in 2018 (7 601 males and 8 539 females, 8 142 in urban areas and 7 998 in rural areas), accounting for 1.77% of all cancer deaths. The crude mortality rate was 3.09 per 100 000, with ASR China 1.69 per 100 000 and ASR World 1.69 per 100 000, respectively. Subgroup analyses showed that the mortality of ASR China in males and females were similar, and it was 1.13 times in urban areas as that in rural areas. The cumulative mortality rate of 0 to 74 years old was 0.19% (Table 5-7b).

The age-specific incidence and mortality rates were relatively low before 40 years old, and increased rapidly since then. The age-specific incidence rates peaked at the age group of 85+ years in males and 80-84 years in females, the mortality peaked at the age group of 85+ years both in males and females. Both for males and females, the age-specific incidence and mortality rate were similar (Figure 5-7a).

The incidence and mortality rates of gallbladder cancer were higher in urban areas than those in rural areas. Eastern areas had the highest incidence and mortality rates (ASR China), followed by central and the western areas. Among seven administrative districts, the incidence rate was highest in North China for males and Northwest for females, and the mortality rate was highest in Northwest both for males and females, and lowest in Southwest for males and South China for females (Table 5-7a, Table 5-7b, Figure 5-7b).

表 5-7a 2018 年中国肿瘤登记地区胆囊癌发病情况

Table 5-7a Incidence of gallbladder cancer in registration areas of China,2018

地区 Area	性别 Sex	病例数 No. cases	粗率 Crude rate/ 100 000⁻¹	构成比 Freq./%	中标率 ASR China/ 100 000⁻¹	世标率 ASR World/ 100 000⁻¹	累积率 Cum. rate 0~74/%	顺位 Rank
合计 All	合计 Both	21 260	4.06	1.36	2.30	2.30	0.27	18
	男性 Male	10 293	3.88	1.20	2.31	2.32	0.28	16
	女性 Female	10 967	4.26	1.56	2.29	2.28	0.27	15
城市地区 Urban areas	合计 Both	10 363	4.39	1.37	2.36	2.36	0.27	19
	男性 Male	5 084	4.29	1.25	2.43	2.44	0.28	16
	女性 Female	5 279	4.49	1.50	2.30	2.28	0.26	16
农村地区 Rural areas	合计 Both	10 897	3.80	1.35	2.24	2.24	0.27	18
	男性 Male	5 209	3.54	1.15	2.20	2.21	0.27	16
	女性 Female	5 688	4.06	1.61	2.28	2.27	0.27	15
东部地区 Eastern areas	合计 Both	11 186	5.15	1.46	2.59	2.58	0.30	18
	男性 Male	5 678	5.21	1.39	2.77	2.79	0.33	15
	女性 Female	5 508	5.10	1.54	2.41	2.39	0.28	16
中部地区 Central areas	合计 Both	4 560	3.52	1.30	2.22	2.23	0.27	19
	男性 Male	2 051	3.09	1.07	2.06	2.07	0.25	17
	女性 Female	2 509	3.96	1.59	2.37	2.38	0.29	15
西部地区 Western areas	合计 Both	5 514	3.13	1.23	1.94	1.92	0.23	19
	男性 Male	2 564	2.84	0.99	1.83	1.82	0.21	16
	女性 Female	2 950	3.42	1.58	2.04	2.02	0.24	15

表 5-7b 2018 年中国肿瘤登记地区胆囊癌死亡情况

Table 5-7b Mortality of gallbladder cancer inregistration areas of China,2018

地区 Area	性别 Sex	死亡数 No. deaths	粗率 Crude rate/ 100 000⁻¹	构成比 Freq./%	中标率 ASR China/ 100 000⁻¹	世标率 ASR World/ 100 000⁻¹	累积率 Cum. rate 0~74/%	顺位 Rank
合计 All	合计 Both	16 140	3.09	1.77	1.69	1.69	0.19	14
	男性 Male	7 601	2.86	1.30	1.67	1.68	0.19	12
	女性 Female	8 539	3.31	2.60	1.71	1.69	0.19	11
城市地区 Urban areas	合计 Both	8 142	3.45	1.94	1.79	1.78	0.19	14
	男性 Male	3 919	3.31	1.47	1.82	1.84	0.20	12
	女性 Female	4 223	3.59	2.75	1.75	1.74	0.18	11
农村地区 Rural areas	合计 Both	7 998	2.79	1.62	1.59	1.59	0.18	14
	男性 Male	3 682	2.50	1.16	1.53	1.53	0.18	13
	女性 Female	4 316	3.08	2.48	1.66	1.65	0.19	11
东部地区 Eastern areas	合计 Both	8 552	3.94	2.04	1.89	1.88	0.21	14
	男性 Male	4 201	3.85	1.59	1.99	2.00	0.22	12
	女性 Female	4 351	4.03	2.81	1.80	1.78	0.19	11
中部地区 Central areas	合计 Both	3 543	2.73	1.68	1.68	1.69	0.20	14
	男性 Male	1 573	2.37	1.17	1.55	1.56	0.18	13
	女性 Female	1 970	3.11	2.58	1.80	1.81	0.21	11
西部地区 Western areas	合计 Both	4 045	2.29	1.43	1.39	1.38	0.16	15
	男性 Male	1 827	2.03	0.98	1.29	1.29	0.15	14
	女性 Female	2 218	2.57	2.29	1.49	1.48	0.17	13

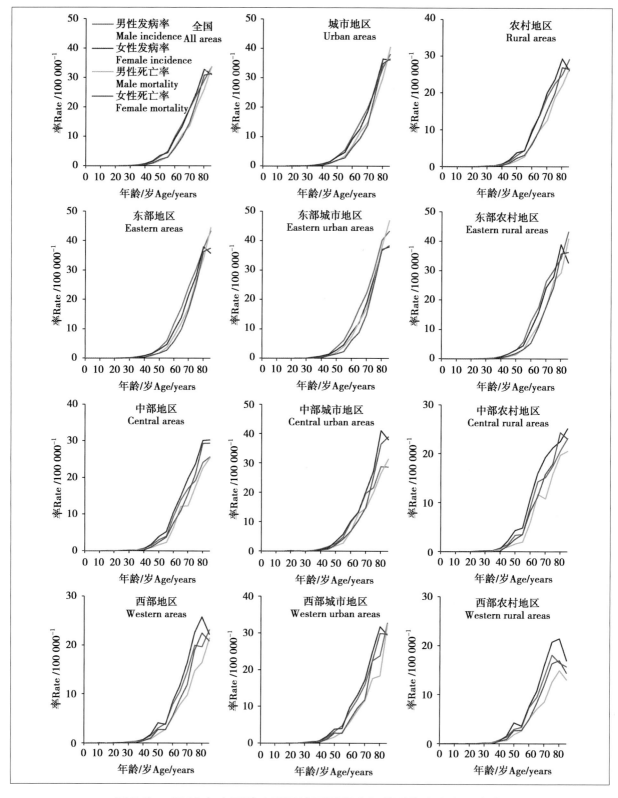

图 5-7a 2018 年中国肿瘤登记地区胆囊癌年龄别发病率和死亡率

Figure 5-7a Age-specific incidence and mortality rates of gallbladder cancer in registration areas of China, 2018

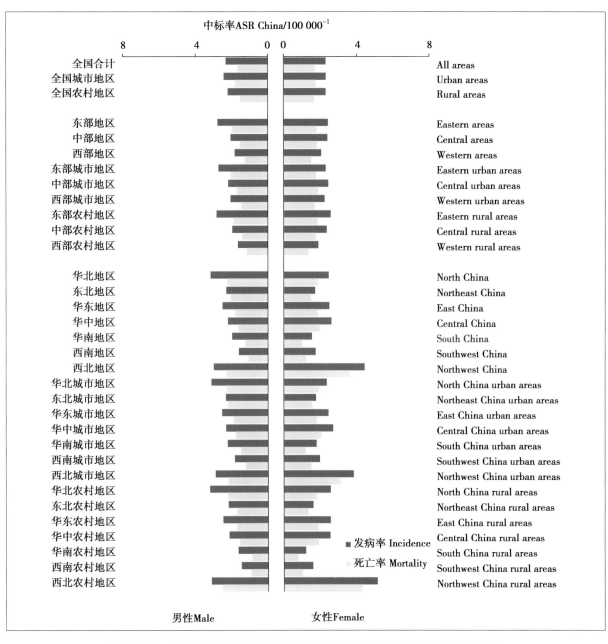

图 5-7b 2018 年中国肿瘤登记地区分城乡胆囊癌发病率和死亡率

Figure 5-7b Incidence and mortality rates of gallbladder cancer in different registration areas of China,2018

8 胰腺

2018 年中国肿瘤登记地区胰腺癌位居癌症发病谱第 13 位。新发病例数为 37 617 例,占全部癌症发病的 2.41%;其中男性 21 565 例,女性 16 052 例,城市地区 18 932 例,农村地区 18 685 例。发病率为 7.19/10 万,中标发病率为 4.13/10 万,世标发病率为 4.12/10 万。男性中标发病率为女性的 1.45 倍,城市中标发病率为农村的 1.13 倍。0 ~ 74 岁累积发病率为 0.49%(表 5-8a)。

2018 年中国肿瘤登记地区胰腺癌位居癌症死亡谱第 7 位。因胰腺癌死亡病例 33 455 例,占全部癌症死亡的 3.67%;其中男性 19 409 例,女性 14 046 例,城市地区 17 165 例,农村地区 16 290 例。胰腺癌死亡率为 6.39/10 万,中标死亡率 3.59/10 万,世标死亡率 3.58/10 万。男性中标死亡率为女性的 1.53 倍,城市中标死亡率为农村的 1.17 倍。0 ~ 74 岁累积死亡率为 0.42%(表 5-8b)。

胰腺癌年龄别发病率和死亡率在 44 岁之前均处于较低水平,自 45 ~ 49 岁组快速上升。男性和女性发病率分别在 85 岁及以上和 80 ~ 84 岁年龄组达到顶峰,死亡率均在 85 岁及以上达到顶峰,男性的发病率和死亡率均高于女性(图 5-8a)。

城市地区胰腺癌的发病率和死亡率均高于农村地区。东部地区中标发病率和死亡率高于中部和西部地区。七大行政区中,东北地区最高,华南地区最低(表 5-8a,表 5-8b,图 5-8b)。

33.28% 的胰腺癌病例报告了明确亚部位信息。各亚部位的胰腺癌比例构成如下:胰头占 55.32%、胰岛(朗格汉斯岛)占 17.64%、胰体占 10.46%、胰尾占 8.97%、交搭跨越占 4.54%,胰管占 0.99%(图 5-8c)。

8 Pancreas

The incidence of pancreatic cancer ranked 13th among all cancer types in the registration areas of China in 2018. There were 37 617 new cases of pancreatic cancer(21 565 males and 16 052 females, 18 932 in urban areas and 18 685 in rural areas), accounting for 2.41% of new cases. The crude incidence rate was 7.19 per 100 000, with ASR China 4.13 per 100 000 and ASR World 4.12 per 100 000, respectively. Subgroup analyses showed that the incidence of ASR China was 1.45 times in males as high as that in females, and it was 1.13 times in urban areas as high as that in rural areas. The cumulative incidence rate for subjects aged from 0 to 74 years old was 0.49%(Table 5-8a).

Pancreatic cancer was the 7th leading cause of cancer death in the registration areas of China in 2018. A total of 33 455 cases died of pancreatic cancer(19 409 males and 14 046 females, 17 165 in urban areas and 16 290 in rural areas), accounting for 3.67% of all cancer deaths. The crude mortality rate was 6.39 per 100 000, with ASR China 3.59 per 100 000 and ASR World 3.58 per 100 000, respectively. Subgroup analyses showed that the mortality of ASR China was 1.53 times in males as high as that in females, and it was 1.17 times in urban areas as high as that in rural areas. The cumulative mortality rate for subjects aged from 0 to 74 years old was 0.42% (Table 5-8b).

The age-specific incidence and mortality rates were relatively low before 44 years old and increased rapidly from the age group of 45-49 years old. The incidence rate of males and females peaked at the age group of 85+ and 80-84 years old, respectively. The incidence and mortality rates in males were generally higher than those in females(Figure 5-8a).

The incidence and mortality rates of pancreatic cancer were higher in urban areas than those in rural areas. Eastern areas had the higher incidence and mortality rates(ASR China) than central and western areas. Among the seven administrative districts, the highest pancreatic cancer incidence and mortality (ASR China) were shown in Northeast, and the lowest in South China(Table 5-8a, Table 5-8b, Figure 5-8b).

There were 33.28% of pancreatic cancer cases with specificsubsite information. Among those, 55.32% of cases occurred in head, followed by islets of Langerhans(17.64%), body(10.46%), tail(8.97%), overlapping(4.54%) and pancreatic duct(0.99%) (Figure 5-8c).

表 5-8a 2018 年中国肿瘤登记地区胰腺癌发病情况
Table 5-8a Incidence of pancreatic cancer in the registration areas of China,2018

地区 Area	性别 Sex	病例数 No. cases	粗率 Crude rate/ 100 000⁻¹	构成比 Freq./%	中标率 ASR China/ 100 000⁻¹	世标率 ASR World/ 100 000⁻¹	累积率 Cum. rate 0~74/%	顺位 Rank
合计 All	合计 Both	37 617	7.19	2.41	4.13	4.12	0.49	13
	男性 Male	21 565	8.12	2.51	4.91	4.92	0.58	8
	女性 Female	16 052	6.23	2.28	3.38	3.35	0.39	12
城市地区 Urban areas	合计 Both	18 932	8.02	2.50	4.41	4.40	0.51	12
	男性 Male	10 711	9.04	2.64	5.22	5.24	0.62	9
	女性 Female	8 221	6.99	2.34	3.63	3.59	0.41	11
农村地区 Rural areas	合计 Both	18 685	6.51	2.32	3.89	3.88	0.46	13
	男性 Male	10 854	7.38	2.39	4.64	4.63	0.56	8
	女性 Female	7 831	5.59	2.22	3.16	3.13	0.37	12
东部地区 Eastern areas	合计 Both	20 426	9.41	2.66	4.80	4.79	0.56	11
	男性 Male	11 514	10.56	2.81	5.72	5.73	0.68	9
	女性 Female	8 912	8.24	2.49	3.93	3.89	0.45	12
中部地区 Central areas	合计 Both	7 264	5.60	2.08	3.59	3.58	0.43	13
	男性 Male	4 174	6.30	2.18	4.22	4.21	0.50	10
	女性 Female	3 090	4.87	1.95	2.97	2.96	0.35	12
西部地区 Western areas	合计 Both	9 927	5.63	2.22	3.55	3.52	0.42	13
	男性 Male	5 877	6.52	2.26	4.25	4.24	0.51	8
	女性 Female	4 050	4.70	2.16	2.84	2.80	0.33	12

表 5-8b 2018 年中国肿瘤登记地区胰腺癌死亡情况
Table 5-8b Mortality of pancreatic cancer in the registration areas of China,2018

地区 Area	性别 Sex	死亡数 No. deaths	粗率 Crude rate/ 100 000⁻¹	构成比 Freq./%	中标率 ASR China/ 100 000⁻¹	世标率 ASR World/ 100 000⁻¹	累积率 Cum. rate 0~74/%	顺位 Rank
合计地区 All	合计 Both	33 455	6.39	3.67	3.59	3.58	0.42	7
	男性 Male	19 409	7.31	3.32	4.35	4.36	0.51	6
	女性 Female	14 046	5.45	4.28	2.85	2.83	0.32	8
城市地区 Urban areas	合计 Both	17 165	7.27	4.08	3.89	3.89	0.44	7
	男性 Male	9 817	8.28	3.68	4.70	4.71	0.54	6
	女性 Female	7 348	6.25	4.78	3.12	3.09	0.34	6
农村地区 Rural areas	合计 Both	16 290	5.67	3.31	3.32	3.31	0.40	8
	男性 Male	9 592	6.53	3.02	4.04	4.04	0.49	6
	女性 Female	6 698	4.78	3.84	2.61	2.60	0.30	8
东部地区 Eastern areas	合计 Both	18 638	8.58	4.45	4.27	4.26	0.49	7
	男性 Male	10 596	9.72	4.02	5.18	5.18	0.60	6
	女性 Female	8 042	7.44	5.19	3.42	3.39	0.38	7
中部地区 Central areas	合计 Both	6 406	4.94	3.04	3.10	3.10	0.36	8
	男性 Male	3 757	5.67	2.80	3.75	3.74	0.44	6
	女性 Female	2 649	4.18	3.47	2.47	2.46	0.28	8
西部地区 Western areas	合计 Both	8 411	4.77	2.97	2.94	2.93	0.35	8
	男性 Male	5 056	5.61	2.71	3.60	3.61	0.43	6
	女性 Female	3 355	3.89	3.46	2.28	2.25	0.26	8

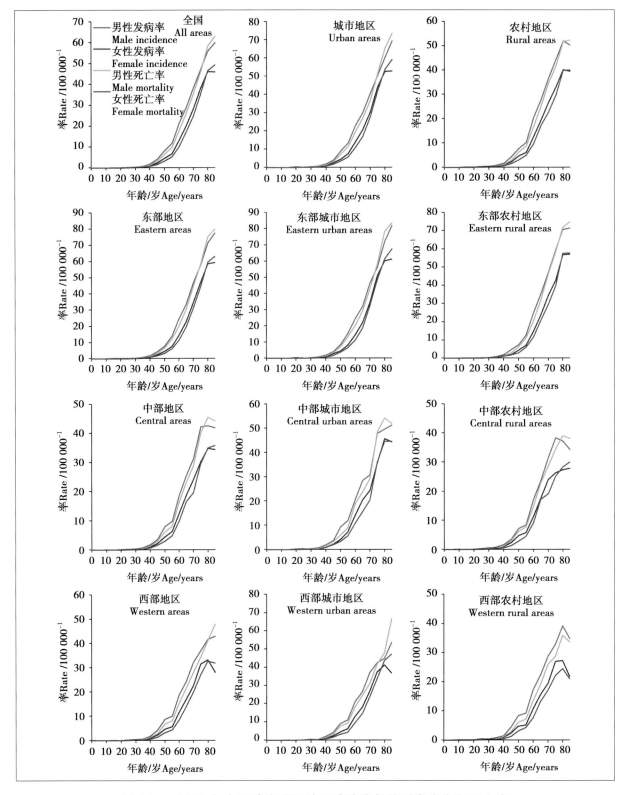

图 5-8a　2018 年中国肿瘤登记地区胰腺癌年龄别发病率和死亡率

Figure 5-8a　Age-specific incidence and mortality rates of pancreatic cancer in the registration areas of China, 2018

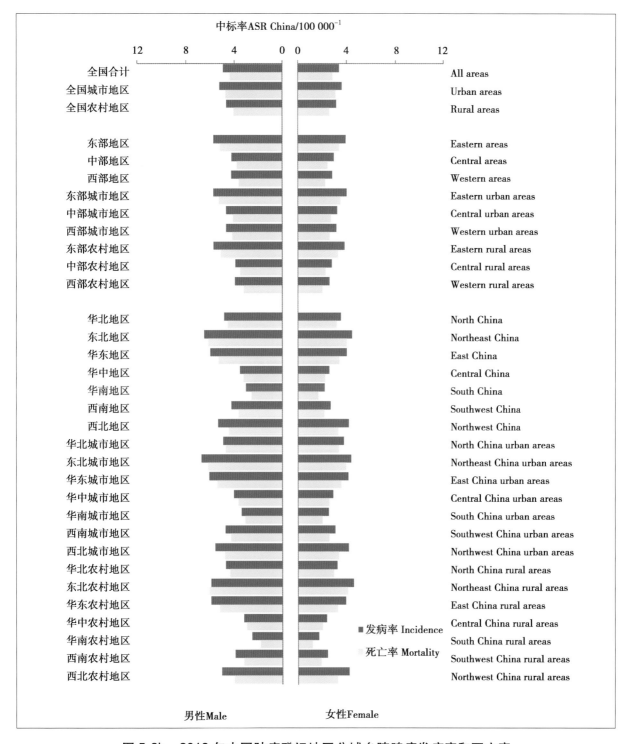

图 5-8b　2018 年中国肿瘤登记地区分城乡胰腺癌发病率和死亡率

Figure 5-8b　Incidence and mortality rates of pancreatic cancer in different registration areas of China, 2018

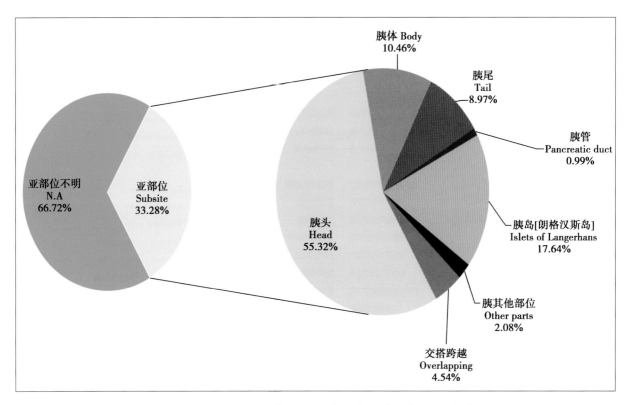

图 5-8c　2018 年中国肿瘤登记地区胰腺癌亚部位分布情况

Figure 5-8c　Subsite distribution of pancreatic cancer in the
registration areas of China,2018

9 喉

2018 年,中国肿瘤登记地区喉癌位居癌症发病谱第 21 位。新发病例数为 9 898 例,占全部癌症发病的 0.63%;其中男性 8 994 例,女性 904 例,城市地区 5 117 例,农村地区 4 781 例。喉癌发病率为 1.89/10 万,中标发病率为 1.12/10 万,世标发病率为 1.14/10 万;男性中标发病率为女性的 10.35 倍,城市中标发病率为农村的 1.22 倍。0~74 岁累积发病率为 0.15%(表 5-9a)。

2018 年,中国肿瘤登记地区喉癌位居癌症死亡谱第 21 位。喉癌死亡病例 5 652 例,占全部癌症死亡的 0.62%;其中男性 4 993 例,女性 659 例,城市地区 2 811 例,农村地区 2 841 例。喉癌死亡率为 1.08/10 万,中标死亡率和世标死亡率均为 0.61/10 万;男性中标死亡率为女性的 8.55 倍,城市中标死亡率稍高于农村。0~74 岁累积死亡率为 0.07%(表 5-9b)。

喉癌年龄别发病率、年龄别死亡率呈现性别差异。男性年龄别发病率和死亡率在 0~39 岁处于较低水平,40~44 岁组后显著上升;女性在 0~49 岁处于较低水平,50~54 岁组后上升。各年龄组男性发病率和死亡率一般高于女性(图 5-9a)。

城市地区喉癌发病率和死亡率均高于农村地区。中部地区中标发病率最高。七大行政区中,男性喉癌的发病率和死亡率最高的是东北地区和华南地区,西北地区最低;女性发病率和死亡率最高的是东北地区;发病率和死亡率西北地区最低(表 5-9a、表 5-9b、图 5-9b)。

9 Larynx

In 2018, the incidence of laryngeal cancer ranked 21st among all cancer types in cancer registration areas of China. There were 9 898 new cases diagnosed with laryngeal cancer(8 994 males and 904 females, 5 117 in urban areas and 4 781 in rural areas), accounting for 0.63% of new cancer cases. The crude incidence rate was 1.89 per 100 000, with ASR China and ASR World 1.12 per 100 000 and 1.14 per 100 000, respectively. The incidence rate of ASR China in males was 10.35 times as high as that in females. The incidence rate of ASR China in urban areas was 1.22 folds as high as that in rural areas. The cumulative incidence rate for subjects aged 0 to 74 years was 0.15%(Table 5-9a).

Laryngeal cancer ranked 21st among all causes of cancer death in 2018. A total of 5 652 cases died of laryngeal cancer(4 993 males and 659 females, 2 811 in urban areas and 2 841 in rural areas), accounting for 0.62% of all cancer deaths. The crude mortality rate was 1.08 per 100 000. The ASR China and ASR World were both 0.61 per 100 000. The mortality rate of ASR China in males was 8.55 times as high as that in females. The mortality rate of ASR China in urban areas was slightly higher than that in rural areas. The cumulative mortality rate for subjects aged 0 to 74 years was 0.07%(Table 5-9b).

The age-specific incidence and mortality rates showed differences between males and females. The incidence and mortality rates for males were relatively low in 0-39 years old, but increased sharply since then. For females, the age-specific rates were relatively low in 0-49 years old and increased since then. Age-specific incidence and mortality rates in males were generally higher than those in females(Figure 5-9a).

The incidence and mortality rates of laryngeal cancer in urban areas were higher than those in rural areas. Central areas had the highest incidence rate of ASR China. Among the seven administrative districts, for males, Northeast China and South China had the highest incidence and mortality rates, while Northwest China had the lowest rates. For females, the highest incidence and mortality rate was in Northeast China; the lowest incidence and mortality rate was in Northwest China(Table 5-9a, Table 5-9b, Figure 5-9b).

表 5-9a 2018 年中国肿瘤登记地区喉癌发病情况

表 5-9a 2018 年中国肿瘤登记地区喉癌发病情况
Table 5-9a Incidence of laryngeal cancer in registration areas of China, 2018

地区 Area	性别 Sex	病例数 No. cases	粗率 Crude rate/ 100 000⁻¹	构成比 Freq./%	中标率 ASR China/ 100 000⁻¹	世标率 ASR World/ 100 000⁻¹	累积率 Cum. rate 0~74/%	顺位 Rank
合计 All	合计 Both	9 898	1.89	0.63	1.12	1.14	0.15	21
	男性 Male	8 994	3.39	1.05	2.06	2.10	0.27	17
	女性 Female	904	0.35	0.13	0.20	0.20	0.02	23
城市地区 Urban areas	合计 Both	5 117	2.17	0.68	1.24	1.26	0.16	21
	男性 Male	4 662	3.93	1.15	2.30	2.36	0.30	17
	女性 Female	455	0.39	0.13	0.21	0.21	0.02	23
农村地区 Rural areas	合计 Both	4 781	1.67	0.59	1.02	1.03	0.13	22
	男性 Male	4 332	2.95	0.95	1.85	1.88	0.24	17
	女性 Female	449	0.32	0.13	0.19	0.19	0.02	23
东部地区 Eastern areas	合计 Both	4 718	2.17	0.62	1.16	1.19	0.15	21
	男性 Male	4 374	4.01	1.07	2.21	2.26	0.29	17
	女性 Female	344	0.32	0.10	0.16	0.16	0.02	23
中部地区 Central areas	合计 Both	2 392	1.84	0.68	1.19	1.21	0.15	22
	男性 Male	2 115	3.19	1.11	2.13	2.17	0.28	16
	女性 Female	277	0.44	0.18	0.27	0.27	0.03	22
西部地区 Western areas	合计 Both	2 788	1.58	0.62	1.00	1.02	0.13	22
	男性 Male	2 505	2.78	0.96	1.80	1.83	0.23	17
	女性 Female	283	0.33	0.15	0.20	0.20	0.02	23

表 5-9b 2018 年中国肿瘤登记地区喉癌死亡情况
Table 5-9b Mortality of laryngeal cancer in registration areas of China, 2018

地区 Area	性别 Sex	死亡数 No. deaths	粗率 Crude rate/ 100 000⁻¹	构成比 Freq./%	中标率 ASR China/ 100 000⁻¹	世标率 ASR World/ 100 000⁻¹	累积率 Cum. rate 0~74/%	顺位 Rank
合计 All	合计 Both	5 652	1.08	0.62	0.61	0.61	0.07	21
	男性 Male	4 993	1.88	0.85	1.11	1.11	0.13	16
	女性 Female	659	0.26	0.20	0.13	0.12	0.01	23
城市地区 Urban areas	合计 Both	2 811	1.19	0.67	0.64	0.64	0.07	20
	男性 Male	2 494	2.10	0.94	1.18	1.19	0.14	16
	女性 Female	317	0.27	0.21	0.13	0.12	0.01	23
农村地区 Rural areas	合计 Both	2 841	0.99	0.58	0.58	0.58	0.07	21
	男性 Male	2 499	1.70	0.79	1.04	1.04	0.13	16
	女性 Female	342	0.24	0.20	0.13	0.13	0.01	22
东部地区 Eastern areas	合计 Both	2 409	1.11	0.58	0.55	0.55	0.06	21
	男性 Male	2 132	1.96	0.81	1.03	1.03	0.12	16
	女性 Female	277	0.26	0.18	0.11	0.11	0.01	23
中部地区 Central areas	合计 Both	1 448	1.12	0.69	0.69	0.70	0.08	21
	男性 Male	1 278	1.93	0.95	1.25	1.26	0.15	16
	女性 Female	170	0.27	0.22	0.15	0.15	0.02	22
西部地区 Western areas	合计 Both	1 795	1.02	0.63	0.62	0.63	0.07	21
	男性 Male	1 583	1.76	0.85	1.11	1.12	0.14	15
	女性 Female	212	0.25	0.22	0.14	0.14	0.01	22

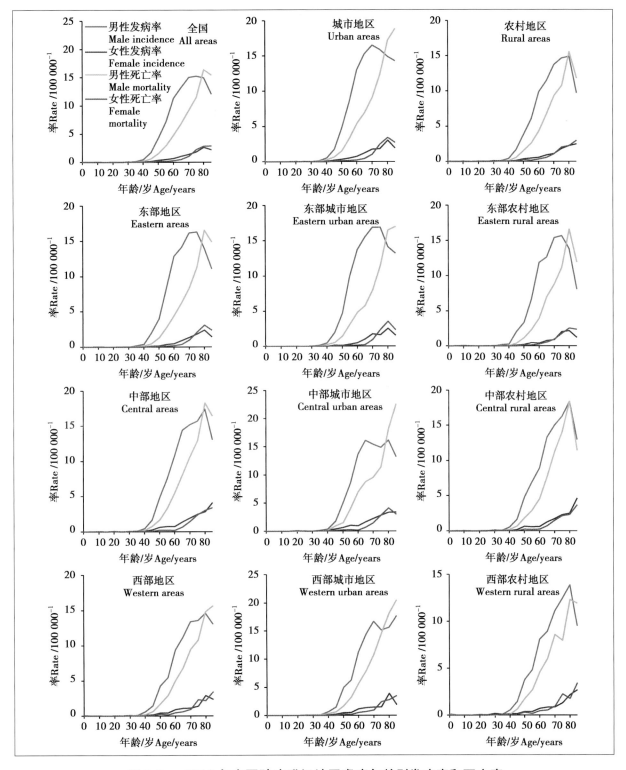

图 5-9a　2018 年中国肿瘤登记地区喉癌年龄别发病率和死亡率

Figure 5-9a　Age-specific incidence and mortality rates of laryngeal cancer in registration areas of China,2018

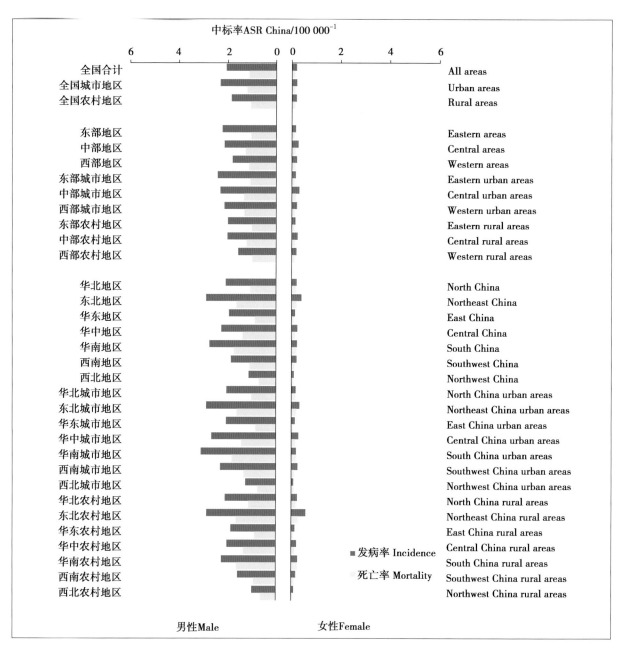

图 5-9b 2018 年中国肿瘤登记不同地区喉癌发病率和死亡率

Figure 5-9b Incidence and mortality rates of laryngeal cancer in different registration areas of China,2018

10 肺

2018 年,中国肿瘤登记地区肺癌位居癌症发病谱第 1 位。新发病例数为 340 332 例,占全部癌症发病的 21.76%;其中男性 221 553 例,女性 118 779 例,城市地区 161 972 例,农村地区 178 360 例。肺癌发病率为 65.05/10 万,中标发病率为 38.23/10 万,世标发病率为 38.20/10 万;男性中标发病率为女性的 1.90 倍,城市中标发病率为农村的 1.03 倍。0~74 岁累积发病率为 4.70%(表 5-10a)。

2018 年,中国肿瘤登记地区肺癌位居癌症死亡谱第 1 位。肺癌死亡病例 253 701 例,占全部癌症死亡的 27.81%;其中男性 178 041 例,女性 75 660 例,城市地区 117 482 例,农村地区 136 219 例。肺癌死亡率为 48.49/10 万,中标死亡率为 27.18/10 万,世标死亡率为 27.16/10 万;男性中标死亡率为女性的 2.58 倍,城市中标死亡率与农村接近。0~74 岁累积死亡率为 3.20%(表 5-10b)。

肺癌年龄别发病率和死亡率在 40 岁之前均处于较低水平,自 40~44 岁组开始快速上升,男性和女性发病率均在 80~84 岁组达到高峰,男性死亡率在 85 岁及以上组达到高峰,女性死亡率在 85 岁及以上组达到高峰,男性上升速度快于女性。40~44 岁组后,男性各年龄别发病率和死亡率均明显高于女性(图 5-10a)。

10 Lung

In 2018, lung cancer was the most frequently diagnosed cancer in registration areas of China. There were 340 332 new cases diagnosed as lung cancer (221 553 males and 118 779 females, 161 972 in urban areas and 178 360 in rural areas), accounting for 21.76% of new cases of all cancers. The crude incidence rate was 65.05 per 100 000, with the ASR China and ASR World were 38.23 and 38.20 per 100 000, respectively. The incidence rate of ASR China was 1.90 and 1.03 folds in males and in urban areas as those in females and in rural areas, respectively. The cumulative incidence rate for subjects aged 0 to 74 years was 4.70% (Table 5-10a).

Lung cancer was the leading cause of cancer death in 2018. A total of 253 701 cases died of lung cancer (178 041 males and 75 660 females, 117 482 in urban areas and 136 219 in rural areas), accounting for 27.81% of all cancer deaths. The crude mortality rate was 48.49 per 100 000, with the ASR China and ASR World were 27.18 and 27.16 per 100 000, respectively. The mortality rate of ASR China was 2.58 folds in males as that in females, while the ASR China in urban areas was similar to that in rural areas. The cumulative mortality rate for subjects aged 0 to 74 years was 3.20% (Table 5-10b).

The age-specific incidence and mortality rates of lung cancer were relatively low before 40 years old and increased dramatically since then. The age-specific incidence rate for both males and females peaked at age group of 80-84 years, while the age-specific mortality rate peaked at age group of 85+ years for males and females, respectively. Incidence and mortality rates in males increased faster than those in females. Age-specific incidence and mortality rates in males were generally higher than those in females since the age group of 40-44 years (Figure 5-10a).

城市地区肺癌的发病率和死亡率略高于农村地区。东部地区中标发病率略高于中部地区和西部地区；中标死亡率以中部地区最高，其次是西部地区，东部地区最低。在七大行政区中，男性发病率和死亡率华中地区最高，西北地区男性发病率和死亡率均最低，女性发病率和死亡率均是东北地区最高，西北地区女性发病率和死亡率最低（表5-10a，表5-10b，图5-10b）。

全部肺癌病例中有明确亚部位的病例占31.13%，其中主要在肺上叶，占50.07%，其次是肺下叶（30.56%）和肺中叶（10.10%），主支气管仅占6.03%（图5-10c）。

全部肺癌病例中有明确组织学类型的病例占54.81%，其中腺癌是主要的病理类型，占58.66%，其次是鳞状细胞癌（24.87%）和小细胞癌（10.94%）（图5-10d）。

The incidence and mortality rates of lung cancer in urban areas were slightly higher than those in rural areas. The incidence rate of ASR China in eastern areas was slightly higher than the central areas and western areas. Central areas had the highest mortality rate of ASR China, followed by western areas and eastern areas. While Central China had the highest incidence and mortality rate of ASR China for males, but the lowest incidence and mortality rate of ASR China for lung cancer of males was in Northwest China. Among the seven administrative districts, the incidence and mortality rates of lung cancer for females were highest in Northeast China and the lowest incidence and mortality rate of ASR China for females was in Northwest China (Table 5-10a, Table 5-10b, Figure 5-10b).

About 31.13% cases of lung cancer had specified subsite. Among those, lung cancer occurred more frequently in upper lobe (50.07%), followed by lower lobe (30.56%), middle lobe (10.10%) and main bronchus (6.03%) (Figure 5-10c).

About 54.81% cases of lung cancer had morphological verification. Among those, adenocarcinoma was the most common histological type, accounting for 58.66% of all cases, followed by squamous cell carcinoma (24.87%) and small cell carcinoma (10.94%) (Figure 5-10d).

表 5-10a 2018 年中国肿瘤登记地区肺癌发病情况
Table 5-10a Incidence of lung cancer in the registration areas of China, 2018

地区 Area	性别 Sex	病例数 No. cases	粗率 Crude rate/ $100\ 000^{-1}$	构成比 Freq./%	中标率 ASR China/ $100\ 000^{-1}$	世标率 ASR World/ $100\ 000^{-1}$	累积率 Cum. rate 0~74/%	顺位 Rank
合计	合计 Both	340 332	65.05	21.76	38.23	38.20	4.70	1
All	男性 Male	221 553	83.45	25.75	50.48	50.72	6.30	1
	女性 Female	118 779	46.10	16.88	26.54	26.25	3.12	1
城市地区	合计 Both	161 972	68.62	21.39	38.83	38.84	4.75	1
Urban areas	男性 Male	103 359	87.23	25.43	50.53	50.89	6.31	1
	女性 Female	58 613	49.86	16.71	27.86	27.53	3.24	2
农村地区	合计 Both	178 360	62.12	22.11	37.68	37.62	4.65	1
Rural areas	男性 Male	118 194	80.41	26.04	50.40	50.53	6.29	1
	女性 Female	60 166	42.94	17.06	25.36	25.11	3.01	1
东部地区	合计 Both	163 529	75.31	21.32	40.19	39.97	4.91	1
Eastern areas	男性 Male	101 041	92.65	24.70	50.58	50.68	6.31	1
	女性 Female	62 488	57.81	17.45	30.67	30.15	3.57	1
中部地区	合计 Both	74 629	57.54	21.35	36.94	37.04	4.60	1
Central areas	男性 Male	51 430	77.60	26.89	51.66	51.94	6.52	1
	女性 Female	23 199	36.58	14.66	22.61	22.53	2.68	2
西部地区	合计 Both	102 174	57.95	22.84	36.58	36.69	4.48	1
Western areas	男性 Male	69 082	76.62	26.56	49.60	50.01	6.16	1
	女性 Female	33 092	38.41	17.67	23.67	23.47	2.78	1

表 5-10b 2018 年中国肿瘤登记地区肺癌死亡情况
Table 5-10b Mortality of lung cancer in the registration areas of China, 2018

地区 Area	性别 Sex	死亡数 No. deaths	粗率 Crude rate/ $100\ 000^{-1}$	构成比 Freq./%	中标率 ASR China/ $100\ 000^{-1}$	世标率 ASR World/ $100\ 000^{-1}$	累积率 Cum. rate 0~74/%	顺位 Rank
合计	合计 Both	253 701	48.49	27.81	27.18	27.16	3.20	1
All	男性 Male	178 041	67.06	30.47	39.61	39.69	4.73	1
	女性 Female	75 660	29.36	23.07	15.35	15.24	1.68	1
城市地区	合计 Both	117 482	49.77	27.96	26.54	26.56	3.07	1
Urban areas	男性 Male	82 183	69.36	30.84	38.97	39.15	4.62	1
	女性 Female	35 299	30.03	22.97	14.89	14.75	1.56	1
农村地区	合计 Both	136 219	47.44	27.67	27.71	27.65	3.31	1
Rural areas	男性 Male	95 858	65.21	30.15	40.11	40.10	4.82	1
	女性 Female	40 361	28.81	23.15	15.75	15.65	1.79	1
东部地区	合计 Both	114 574	52.76	27.37	26.13	26.02	3.03	1
Eastern areas	男性 Male	78 878	72.33	29.91	38.10	38.06	4.50	1
	女性 Female	35 696	33.02	23.04	15.12	14.94	1.61	1
中部地区	合计 Both	58 894	45.41	27.98	28.27	28.30	3.40	1
Central areas	男性 Male	42 251	63.75	31.48	41.69	41.79	5.08	1
	女性 Female	16 643	26.24	21.82	15.30	15.25	1.72	1
西部地区	合计 Both	80 233	45.50	28.32	27.91	28.00	3.31	1
Western areas	男性 Male	56 912	63.12	30.52	40.24	40.51	4.84	1
	女性 Female	23 321	27.07	24.08	15.73	15.66	1.76	1

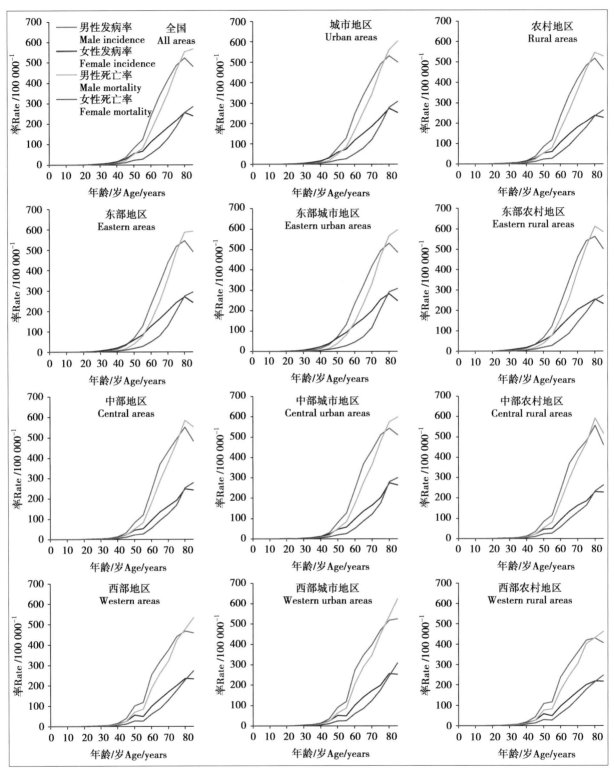

图 5-10a 2018 年中国肿瘤登记地区肺癌年龄别发病率和死亡率

Figure 5-10a Age-specific incidence and mortality rates of lung cancer in the registration areas of China, 2018

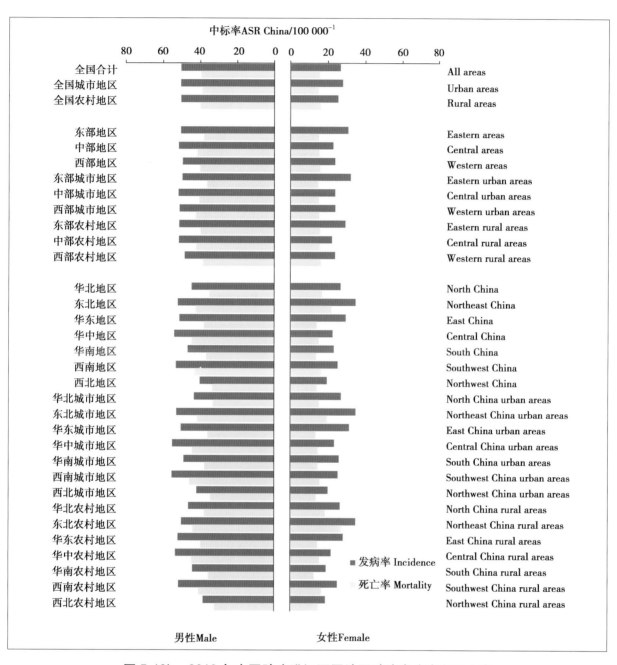

中标率ASR China/100 000⁻¹

	男性Male		女性Female	

全国合计　All areas
全国城市地区　Urban areas
全国农村地区　Rural areas

东部地区　Eastern areas
中部地区　Central areas
西部地区　Western areas
东部城市地区　Eastern urban areas
中部城市地区　Central urban areas
西部城市地区　Western urban areas
东部农村地区　Eastern rural areas
中部农村地区　Central rural areas
西部农村地区　Western rural areas

华北地区　North China
东北地区　Northeast China
华东地区　East China
华中地区　Central China
华南地区　South China
西南地区　Southwest China
西北地区　Northwest China
华北城市地区　North China urban areas
东北城市地区　Northeast China urban areas
华东城市地区　East China urban areas
华中城市地区　Central China urban areas
华南城市地区　South China urban areas
西南城市地区　Southwest China urban areas
西北城市地区　Northwest China urban areas
华北农村地区　North China rural areas
东北农村地区　Northeast China rural areas
华东农村地区　East China rural areas
华中农村地区　Central China rural areas
华南农村地区　South China rural areas
西南农村地区　Southwest China rural areas
西北农村地区　Northwest China rural areas

■ 发病率 Incidence
　死亡率 Mortality

图 5-10b　2018 年中国肿瘤登记不同地区肺癌发病率和死亡率

Figure 5-10b　Incidence and mortality rates of lung cancer in the different registration areas of China，2018

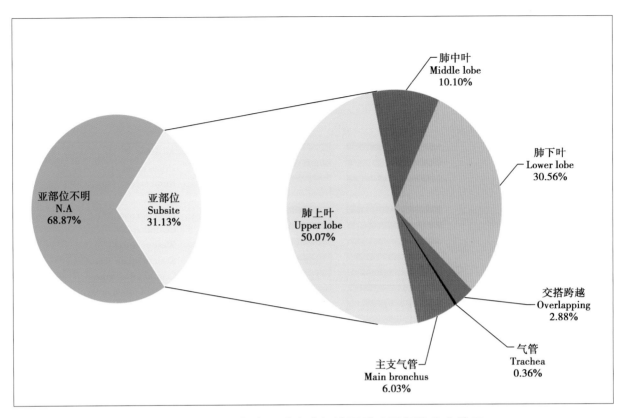

图 5-10c　2018 年中国肿瘤登记地区肺癌亚部位分布情况

Figure 5-10c　Subsite distribution of lung cancer in the registration areas of China,2018

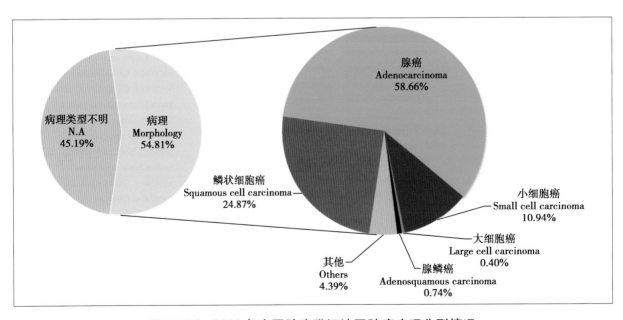

图 5-10d　2018 年中国肿瘤登记地区肺癌病理分型情况

Figure 5-10d　Morphological distribution of lung cancer in the registration areas of China,2018

11 骨

2018 年,中国肿瘤登记地区骨癌位居癌症发病谱第 22 位。新发病例数为 9 208 例,占全部癌症发病的 0.59%;其中男性 5 381 例,女性 3 827 例,城市地区 3 598 例,农村地区 5 610 例。骨癌发病率为 1.76/10 万,中标发病率为 1.30/10 万,世标发病率为 1.27/10 万;男性中标发病率为女性的 1.44 倍,农村中标发病率为城市的 1.34 倍。0~74 岁累积发病率为 0.13%(表 5-11a)。

2018 年,中国肿瘤登记地区骨癌位居癌症死亡谱第 20 位。骨癌死亡病例 6 593 例,占全部癌症死亡的 0.72%;其中男性 3 983 例,女性 2 610 例,城市地区 2 696 例,农村地区 3 897 例。骨癌死亡率为 1.26/10 万,中标死亡率为 0.81/10 万,世标死亡率为 0.80/10 万;男性中标死亡率为女性的 1.64 倍,农村中标死亡率为城市的 1.27 倍。0~74 岁累积死亡率为 0.08%(表 5-11b)。

骨癌年龄别发病率和死亡率均在 10~19 岁组出现一个小高峰,但总体看骨癌年龄别发病率和死亡率在 45 岁之前处于较低水平,45 岁之后迅速上升,呈现男性高于女性的分布特征,城乡和不同地区年龄别发病率、死亡率总体趋势基本相同(图 5-11a)。

农村地区骨癌发病率和死亡率高于城市。中标发病率中部地区最高。中标死亡率西部地区最高,其次是中部地区,东部地区最低。在七大行政区中,东北地区发病率最低、华北地区死亡率最低(表 5-11a,表 5-11b,图 5-11b)。

分亚部位比较,41.59% 的骨癌发生在四肢的骨和关节软骨,58.41% 发生在其他及未特指部位的骨和关节软骨(图 5-11c)。

11 Bone

In 2018, the incidence of bone cancer ranked 22nd among all cancer types in cancer registration areas of China. There were 9 208 new cases diagnosed with bone cancer(5 381 males and 3 827 females, 3 598 in urban areas and 5 610 in rural areas), accounting for 0.59% of all new cancer cases. The crude incidence rate was 1.76 per 100 000, with ASR China 1.30 per 100 000 and ASR World 1.27 per 100 000, respectively. The incidence rate of ASR China in males was 1.44 folds as high as that in females. It was 1.34 folds in rural areas as high as that in urban areas. The cumulative incidence rate for subjects aged 0 to 74 years was 0.13% (Table 5-11a).

In 2018, the mortality of bone cancer ranked 20th among all causes of cancer death in cancer registration areas of China. A total of 6 593 cases died of bone cancer(3 983 males and 2 610 females, 2 696 in urban areas and 3 897 in rural areas), accounting for 0.72% of all cancer deaths. The crude mortality rate was 1.26 per 100 000, with ASR China 0.81 per 100 000 and ASR World 0.80 per 100 000, respectively. The mortality rate of ASR China in males was 1.64 folds as high as that in females, and it was 1.27 folds in rural areas as high as that in urban areas. The cumulative mortality rate for subjects aged 0 to 74 years was 0.08% (Table 5-11b).

Both the age-specific incidence and mortality of bone cancer showed a small peak in the age group of 10-19 years. The age-specific incidence and mortality rate of bone cancer were relatively low before 45 years old, but dramatically increased after then. The incidence and mortality rates in males were higher than those in females across all age groups. The age specific incidence and mortality rates had slight variation among different areas, but showed similar trends(Figure 5-11a).

The incidence and mortality rates of bone cancer were higher in rural areas than those in urban areas. Central areas had the highest incidence of ASR China. Western areas had the highest mortality of ASR China, followed by central areas and eastern areas. Among the seven administrative districts, Northeast China had the lowest incidence and North China had the lowest mortality rate (Table 5-11a, Table 5-11b, Figure 5-11b).

By subsite, 41.59% of bone cancer occurred in bone and articular cartilage of limbs, whereas others occurred in other unspecific bone and articular cartilage sites(Figure 5-11c).

表 5-11a　2018 年中国肿瘤登记地区骨癌发病情况

表 5-11a　2018 年中国肿瘤登记地区骨癌发病情况
Table 5-11a　Incidence of bone cancer in registration areas of China, 2018

地区 Area	性别 Sex	病例数 No. cases	粗率 Crude rate/ 100 000^{-1}	构成比 Freq./%	中标率 ASR China/ 100 000^{-1}	世标率 ASR World/ 100 000^{-1}	累积率 Cum. rate 0~74/%	顺位 Rank
合计 All	合计 Both	9 208	1.76	0.59	1.30	1.27	0.13	22
	男性 Male	5 381	2.03	0.63	1.53	1.49	0.15	18
	女性 Female	3 827	1.49	0.54	1.07	1.04	0.10	20
城市地区 Urban areas	合计 Both	3 598	1.52	0.48	1.10	1.07	0.10	22
	男性 Male	2 099	1.77	0.52	1.31	1.27	0.12	18
	女性 Female	1 499	1.28	0.43	0.89	0.87	0.09	20
农村地区 Rural areas	合计 Both	5 610	1.95	0.70	1.47	1.43	0.15	21
	男性 Male	3 282	2.23	0.72	1.72	1.67	0.18	18
	女性 Female	2 328	1.66	0.66	1.22	1.19	0.12	20
东部地区 Eastern areas	合计 Both	3 293	1.52	0.43	1.07	1.04	0.10	22
	男性 Male	1 868	1.71	0.46	1.26	1.21	0.12	18
	女性 Female	1 425	1.32	0.40	0.88	0.86	0.08	20
中部地区 Central areas	合计 Both	2 489	1.92	0.71	1.53	1.49	0.16	21
	男性 Male	1 494	2.25	0.78	1.83	1.80	0.19	18
	女性 Female	995	1.57	0.63	1.21	1.18	0.12	20
西部地区 Western areas	合计 Both	3 426	1.94	0.77	1.46	1.42	0.15	21
	男性 Male	2 019	2.24	0.78	1.69	1.65	0.17	18
	女性 Female	1 070	1.77	0.82	1.31	1.29	0.13	20

表 5-11b　2018 年中国肿瘤登记地区骨癌死亡情况
Table 5-11b　Mortality of laryngeal cancer in registration areas of China, 2018

地区 Area	性别 Sex	死亡数 No. deaths	粗率 Crude rate/ 100 000^{-1}	构成比 Freq./%	中标率 ASR China/ 100 000^{-1}	世标率 ASR World/ 100 000^{-1}	累积率 Cum. rate 0~74/%	顺位 Rank
合计 All	合计 Both	6 593	1.26	0.72	0.81	0.80	0.08	20
	男性 Male	3 983	1.50	0.68	1.01	0.99	0.10	17
	女性 Female	2 610	1.01	0.80	0.62	0.61	0.06	18
城市地区 Urban areas	合计 Both	2 696	1.14	0.64	0.71	0.69	0.07	21
	男性 Male	1 606	1.36	0.60	0.88	0.86	0.09	17
	女性 Female	1 090	0.93	0.71	0.54	0.53	0.05	19
农村地区 Rural areas	合计 Both	3 897	1.36	0.79	0.90	0.88	0.10	20
	男性 Male	2 377	1.62	0.75	1.12	1.09	0.12	17
	女性 Female	1 520	1.08	0.87	0.68	0.67	0.07	15
东部地区 Eastern areas	合计 Both	2 573	1.18	0.61	0.71	0.69	0.07	20
	男性 Male	1 520	1.39	0.58	0.87	0.85	0.08	17
	女性 Female	1 053	0.97	0.68	0.55	0.54	0.05	19
中部地区 Central areas	合计 Both	1 536	1.18	0.73	0.83	0.81	0.09	20
	男性 Male	905	1.37	0.67	1.00	0.98	0.10	17
	女性 Female	631	0.99	0.83	0.65	0.64	0.07	16
西部地区 Western areas	合计 Both	2 484	1.41	0.88	0.96	0.94	0.11	19
	男性 Male	1 558	1.73	0.84	1.21	1.19	0.13	16
	女性 Female	926	1.07	0.96	0.70	0.70	0.08	16

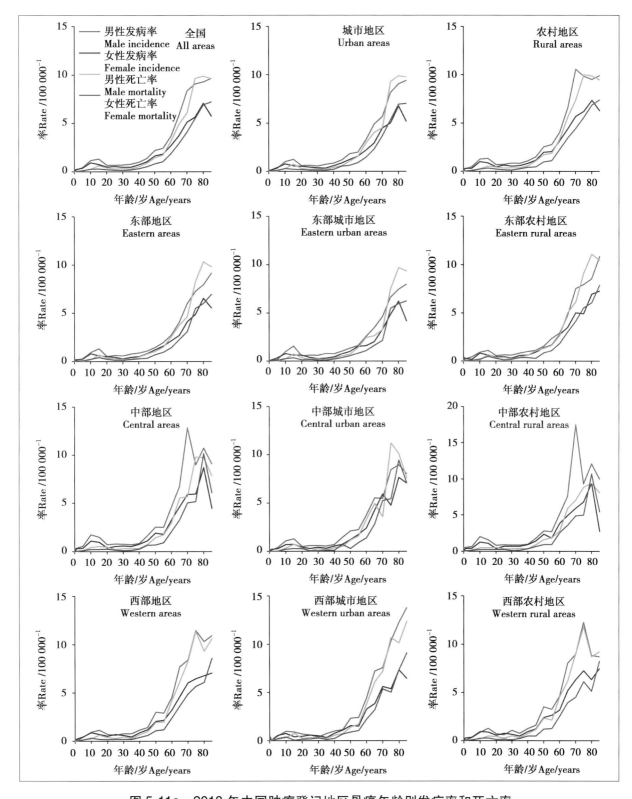

图 5-11a　2018 年中国肿瘤登记地区骨癌年龄别发病率和死亡率

Figure 5-11a　Age-specific incidence and mortality rates of bone cancer
in registration areas of China,2018

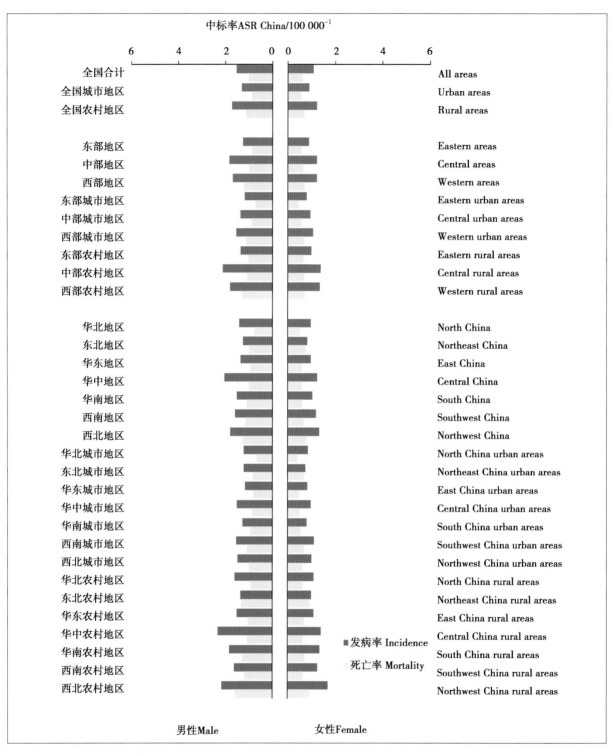

图 5-11b　2018 年中国肿瘤登记不同地区骨癌发病率和死亡率

Figure 5-11b　Incidence and mortality rates of bone cancer in different registration areas of China, 2018

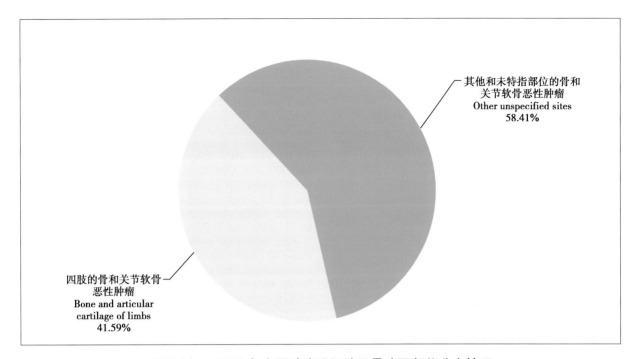

图 5-11c　2018 年中国肿瘤登记地区骨癌亚部位分布情况

Figure 5-11c　Subsite distribution of bone cancer in registration areas of China,2018

12 女性乳腺

中国肿瘤登记地区女性乳腺癌位居女性癌症发病谱第 2 位。新发病例数为 110 863 例，占全部女性癌症发病的 15.76%；城市地区 60 395 例，农村地区 50 468 例。发病率为 43.02/10 万，中标发病率为 30.35/10 万，世标发病率为 28.39/10 万；城市中标发病率为农村的 1.33 倍。0~74 岁累积发病率为 3.07%（表 5-12a）。

中国肿瘤登记地区女性乳腺癌位居女性癌症死亡谱第 5 位。女性乳腺癌死亡 24 883 例，占全部女性癌症死亡的 7.59%；城市地区 13 055 例，农村地区 11 828 例。女性乳腺癌死亡率为 9.66/10 万，中标死亡率 5.98/10 万，世标死亡率 5.81/10 万；城市中标死亡率为农村的 1.20 倍。0~74 岁累积死亡率为 0.64%（表 5-12b）。

城市和农村女性乳腺癌年龄别发病率特征相似。女性乳腺癌发病率均自 20~24 岁组开始快速上升，城市地区至 60~64 岁组达到高峰，而农村地区至 50~54 岁组达到高峰，随后快速下降；女性乳腺癌死亡率从 25~29 岁组开始缓慢上升（图 5-12a）。

城市女性乳腺癌的发病率和死亡率均高于农村。东部地区中标发病率最高，其次是中部地区，西部地区最低；七大行政区中，东北地区、华北地区和华南地区中标发病率依次显著高于全国平均水平，西南地区中标发病率最低；东部地区中标死亡率最高，其次是中部地区，西部地区最低；七大行政区中，东北地区、华北地区和华南地区中标死亡率依次高于全国平均水平，西南地区中标死亡率最低（表 5-12a，表 5-12b，图 5-12b）。

全部女性乳腺癌病例中，31.46% 的病例报告了明确的亚部位，其中上外象限是最主要的亚部位，占 35.93%；其次是交搭跨越，占 21.23%；上内象限，占 17.15%；下外象限，占 8.24%；下内象限，占 6.65%；中央部，占 5.69%；乳头和乳晕，占 4.54%；腋尾部，占 0.57%（图 5-12c）。

全部女性乳腺癌病例中有明确组织学类型的病例占 77.78%，其中导管癌是最主要的病理类型，占 79.58%；其次是小叶性癌，占 4.20%；佩吉特病，占 1.57%；髓样癌，占 0.30%（图 5-12d）。

12 Female breast

Female breast cancer was the 2nd common cancer among females in the registration areas of China. There were 110 683 new cases of female breast cancer(60 395 in urban areas and 50 468 in rural areas), accounting for 15.76% of new cases of all cancers among females. The crude incidence rate was 43.02 per 100 000, with ASR China 30.35 per 100 000 and ASR World 28.39 per 100 000, respectively. Subgroup analyses showed that the ASR China was 1.33 times in urban areas as that in rural areas. The cumulative incidence rate for subjects aged 0 to 74 years was 3.07% (Table 5-12a).

Female breast cancer was the 5th most common cause of cancer deaths among females in the registration areas of China. A total of 24 883 women died of breast cancer in 2018(13 055 in urban areas and 11 828 in rural areas), accounting for 7.59% of all cancer deaths among females. The crude mortality rate was 9.66 per 100 000, with ASR China 5.98 per 100 000 and ASR World 5.81 per 100 000, respectively. Subgroup analyses showed that the mortality of ASR China was 1.20 times in urban areas as that in rural areas. The cumulative mortality rate for subjects aged 0 to 74 years was 0.64% (Table 5-12b).

Age-specific incidence rates took on almost the same pattern between urban areas and rural areas. The incidence rate increased rapidly from the age group of 20-24 years with the peak occurring in the age group of 60-64 years in urban areas and 50-54 years in rural areas, thereafter began to drop quickly. Age-specific mortality rates increased slowly from the age group of 25-29 years(Figure 5-12a).

Both the incidence and mortality rates of female breast cancer were higher in urban areas than those in rural areas. Eastern areas had the highest incidence rate, followed by central and western areas. Among the seven administrative districts, Northeast China, North China and South China had the top three incidence rates, all higher than the national average, and Southwest China had the lowest incidence rate. Eastern areas had the highest mortality rate, followed by central and western areas. Among the seven administrative districts, Northeast China, North China, and South China had the top three mortality rates, all higher than the national average, and Southwest China had the lowest mortality rate(Table 5-12a, Table 5-12b, Figure 5-12b).

About 31.46% of female breast cancer cases with specific subsites were reported. Among them, 35.93% occurred in upper outer, 21.23% at overlapping, 17.15% in upper inner, 8.24% in lower outer, 6.65% in lower inner, 5.69% in central portion, 4.54% in nipple and areola, and 0.57% in axillary tail(Figure 5-12c).

About 77.78% cases of female breast cancer had morphological verification. Among them, ductal cancer was the most common histological type, accounting for 79.58%, followed by lobular carcinoma(4.20%), Paget's disease(1.57%), medullary carcinoma(0.30%)(Figure 5-12d).

表 5-12a 2018 年中国肿瘤登记地区女性乳腺癌发病情况
Table 5-12a Incidence of female breast cancer in the registration areas of China, 2018

地区 Area	病例数 No. cases	粗率 Crude rate/ 100 000^{-1}	构成比 Freq./%	中标率 ASR China/ 100 000^{-1}	世标率 ASR World/ 100 000^{-1}	累积率 Cum. rate 0~74/%	顺位 Rank
合计 All	110 863	43.02	15.76	30.35	28.39	3.07	2
城市地区 Urban areas	60 395	51.38	17.21	34.95	32.87	3.59	1
农村地区 Rural areas	50 468	36.02	14.31	26.30	24.44	2.60	2
东部地区 Eastern areas	60 022	55.53	16.76	36.99	34.62	3.77	2
中部地区 Central areas	25 677	40.49	16.23	30.17	28.17	3.02	1
西部地区 Western areas	25 164	29.21	13.44	21.61	20.12	2.12	2

表 5-12b 2018 年中国肿瘤登记地区女性乳腺癌死亡情况
Table 5-12b Mortality of female breast cancer in the registration areas of China, 2018

地区 Area	死亡数 No. deaths	粗率 Crude rate/ 100 000^{-1}	构成比 Freq./%	中标率 ASR China/ 100 000^{-1}	世标率 ASR World/ 100 000^{-1}	累积率 Cum. rate 0~74/%	顺位 Rank
合计 All	24 883	9.66	7.59	5.98	5.81	0.64	5
城市地区 Urban areas	13 055	11.11	8.49	6.56	6.39	0.70	5
农村地区 Rural areas	11 828	8.44	6.78	5.48	5.29	0.59	6
东部地区 Eastern areas	12 618	11.67	8.14	6.45	6.29	0.69	5
中部地区 Central areas	5 917	9.33	7.76	6.33	6.14	0.69	5
西部地区 Western areas	6 348	7.37	6.56	5.03	4.83	0.53	5

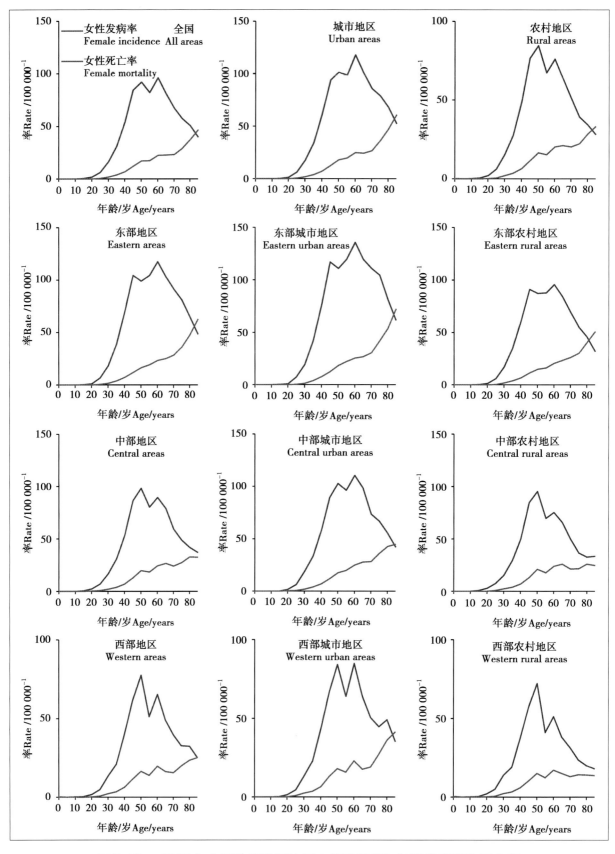

图 5-12a　2018 年中国肿瘤登记地区女性乳腺癌年龄别发病率和死亡率
Figure 5-12a　Age-specific incidence and mortality rates of female breast cancer in the registration areas of China, 2018

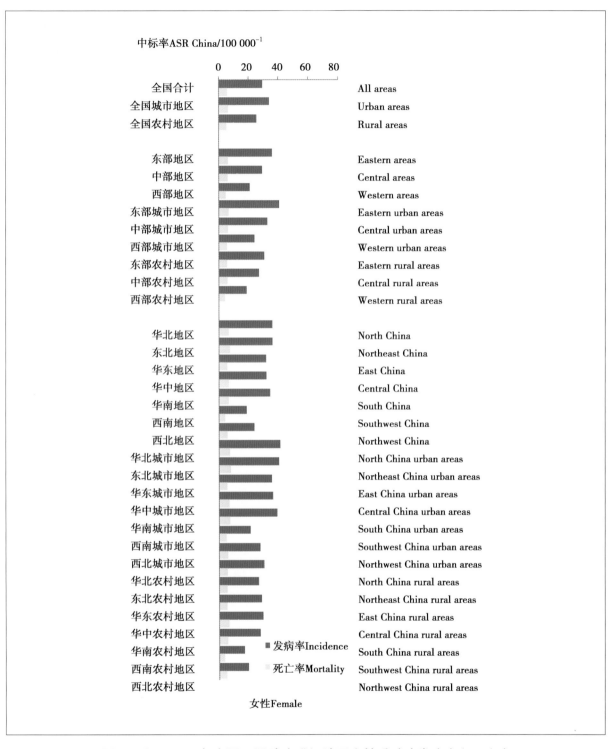

中标率ASR China/100 000⁻¹

| | 发病率Incidence | 死亡率Mortality |

全国合计 — All areas
全国城市地区 — Urban areas
全国农村地区 — Rural areas

东部地区 — Eastern areas
中部地区 — Central areas
西部地区 — Western areas
东部城市地区 — Eastern urban areas
中部城市地区 — Central urban areas
西部城市地区 — Western urban areas
东部农村地区 — Eastern rural areas
中部农村地区 — Central rural areas
西部农村地区 — Western rural areas

华北地区 — North China
东北地区 — Northeast China
华东地区 — East China
华中地区 — Central China
华南地区 — South China
西南地区 — Southwest China
西北地区 — Northwest China
华北城市地区 — North China urban areas
东北城市地区 — Northeast China urban areas
华东城市地区 — East China urban areas
华中城市地区 — Central China urban areas
华南城市地区 — South China urban areas
西南城市地区 — Southwest China urban areas
西北城市地区 — Northwest China urban areas
华北农村地区 — North China rural areas
东北农村地区 — Northeast China rural areas
华东农村地区 — East China rural areas
华中农村地区 — Central China rural areas
华南农村地区 — South China rural areas
西南农村地区 — Southwest China rural areas
西北农村地区 — Northwest China rural areas

女性Female

图 5-12b　2018 年中国不同肿瘤登记地区女性乳腺癌发病率和死亡率

Figure 5-12b　Incidence and mortality rates of female breast cancer in different registration areas of China,2018

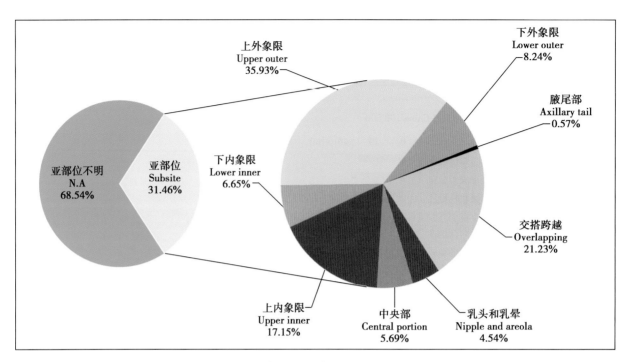

图 5-12c　2018 年中国肿瘤登记地区女性乳腺癌亚部位分布情况
Figure 5-12c　Subsite Distribution of female breast cancer in the registration areas of China,2018

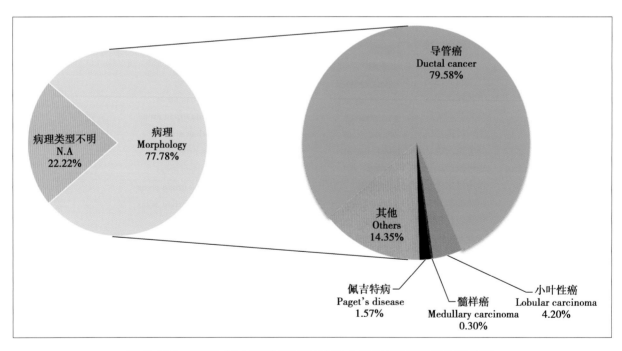

图 5-12d　2018 年中国肿瘤登记地区女性乳腺癌病理分型情况
Figure 5-12d　Morphological distribution of female breast cancer in the registration areas of China,2018

13 子宫颈

2018 年中国肿瘤登记地区子宫颈癌位居女性癌症发病谱第 5 位。新发病例数为 46 626 例，占女性全部癌症发病的 6.63%；其中城市地区 20 109 例，农村地区 26 517 例。发病率为 18.10/10 万，中标发病率为 12.95/10 万，世标发病率为 12.00/10 万；农村中标发病率是城市的 1.15 倍。0~74 岁累积发病率为 1.28%（表 5-13a）。

2018 年中国肿瘤登记地区子宫颈癌位居女性癌症死亡谱第 7 位。死亡病例数为 14 737 例，占女性全部癌症死亡的 4.49%。其中城市地区 6 318 例，农村地区 8 419 例。子宫颈癌死亡率为 5.72/10 万，中标死亡率 3.62/10 万，世标死亡率 3.49/10 万；农村中标死亡率为城市的 1.15 倍。0~74 岁累积死亡率为 0.39%（表 5-13b）。

子宫颈癌年龄别发病率在 20 岁之前处于较低水平，自 20 岁以后快速上升，至 50~54 岁年龄组达高峰，之后逐渐下降。年龄别死亡率在 25 岁之前处于较低水平，25 岁以后随年龄增加逐渐升高，在 80~84 岁组达到高峰（图 5-13a）。

农村地区子宫颈癌的发病率和死亡率均高于城市。中标发病率及中标死亡率均以中部地区最高，其次是西部地区，东部地区最低。在七大行政区中，华中地区和西北地区发病率和死亡率显著高于全国平均水平，华北地区发病率和死亡率明显低于全国平均水平（表 5-13a、表 5-13b、图 5-13b）。

全部子宫颈癌病例中，11.03% 的病例报告了明确的亚部位，其中宫颈内膜癌、外宫颈癌和宫颈交界部位癌分别占 51.72%、35.74%、12.54%（图 5-13c）。

13 Cervix

In 2018, cervical cancer was the 5th most common female cancer in the registration areas of China. There were 46 626 new cases of cervical cancer (20 109 in urban areas and 26 517 in rural areas), accounting for 6.63% of new cases of all female cancers. The crude incidence rate was 18.10 per 100 000, with ASR China 12.95 per 100 000 and ASR World 12.00 per 100 000, respectively. Subgroup analyses showed that the incidence of ASR China was 1.15 times in rural areas as that in urban areas. The cumulative incidence rate for subjects aged 0 to 74 years was 1.28% (Table 5-13a).

In 2018, cervical cancer was the 7th common cause of cancer deaths among females in the registration areas of China. A total of 14 737 women died of cervical cancer (6 318 in urban areas and 8 419 in rural areas), accounting for 4.49% of all female cancer deaths. The crude mortality rate was 5.72 per 100 000, with ASR China 3.62 per 100 000 and ASR World 3.49 per 100 000, respectively. Subgroup analyses showed that the mortality of ASR China was 1.15 times in rural areas as that in urban areas. The cumulative mortality rate for subjects aged 0 to 74 years was 0.39% (Table 5-13b).

The age-specific incidence rate was low before age 20. It went up rapidly thereafter, with the peak occurring in age group 50-54 years and then decreased gradually. The age-specific mortality was low before age 25 and increased with age gradually, reaching the peak in age group 80-84 years (Figure 5-13a).

Both the incidence and mortality rates of cervical cancer were higher in rural areas than in urban areas. Central areas had both the highest incidence and mortality rates while eastern areas had both the lowest incidence and mortality rates, leaving western areas in between. Among the seven administrative districts, both the incidence and mortality rates of cervical cancer in Central China and Northwest China were markedly higher than the national average whereas both the incidence and mortality rates in North China were lower than the national average (Table 5-13a, Table 5-13b, Figure 5-13b).

There were 11.03% cases of cervical cancers reported to have occurred in specific subsites, with endocervix, exocervix and overlapping parts comprising 51.72%, 35.74% and 12.54%, respectively (Figure 5-13c).

表 5-13a　2018 年中国肿瘤登记地区子宫颈癌发病情况

Table 5-13a　Incidence of cervical cancer in the registration areas of China,2018

地区 Area	病例数 No. cases	粗率 Crude rate/ 100 000^{-1}	构成比 Freq./%	中标率 ASR China/ 100 000^{-1}	世标率 ASR World/ 100 000^{-1}	累积率 Cum. rate 0~74/%	顺位 Rank
合计 All	46 626	18.10	6.63	12.95	12.00	1.28	5
城市地区 Urban areas	20 109	17.11	5.73	12.02	11.15	1.19	5
农村地区 Rural areas	26 517	18.92	7.52	13.76	12.75	1.36	4
东部地区 Eastern areas	17 253	15.96	4.82	11.00	10.15	1.07	6
中部地区 Central areas	13 790	21.74	8.72	16.11	15.03	1.63	3
西部地区 Western areas	15 583	18.09	8.32	13.40	12.45	1.34	4

表 5-13b　2018 年中国肿瘤登记地区子宫颈癌死亡情况

Table 5-13b　Mortality of cervical cancer in the registration areas of China,2018

地区 Area	死亡数 No. deaths	粗率 Crude rate/ 100 000^{-1}	构成比 Freq./%	中标率 ASR China/ 100 000^{-1}	世标率 ASR World/ 100 000^{-1}	累积率 Cum. rate 0~74/%	顺位 Rank
合计 All	14 737	5.72	4.49	3.62	3.49	0.39	7
城市地区 Urban areas	6 318	5.37	4.11	3.36	3.22	0.36	7
农村地区 Rural areas	8 419	6.01	4.83	3.86	3.72	0.43	7
东部地区 Eastern areas	5 202	4.81	3.36	2.85	2.73	0.30	8
中部地区 Central areas	4 235	6.68	5.55	4.44	4.31	0.50	7
西部地区 Western areas	5 300	6.15	5.47	4.17	4.01	0.46	7

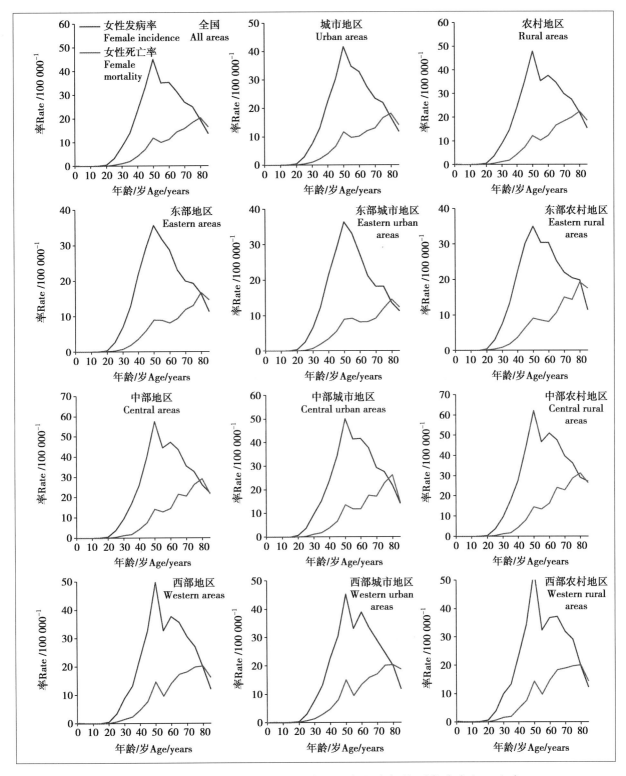

图 5-13a   2018 年中国肿瘤登记地区子宫颈癌年龄别发病率和死亡率

Figure 5-13a   Age-specific incidence and mortality rates of cervical cancer in the registration areas of China, 2018

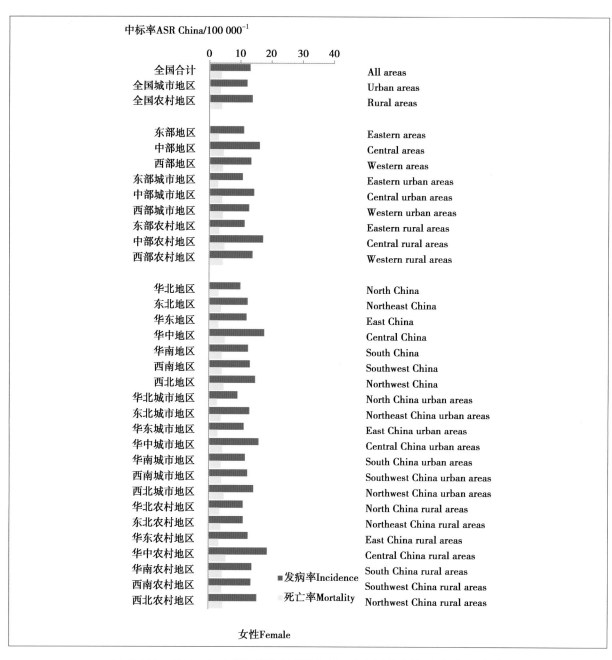

图 5-13b　2018 年中国不同肿瘤登记地区子宫颈癌发病率和死亡率

Figure 5-13b　Incidence and mortality rates of cervical cancer in different registration areas of China,2018

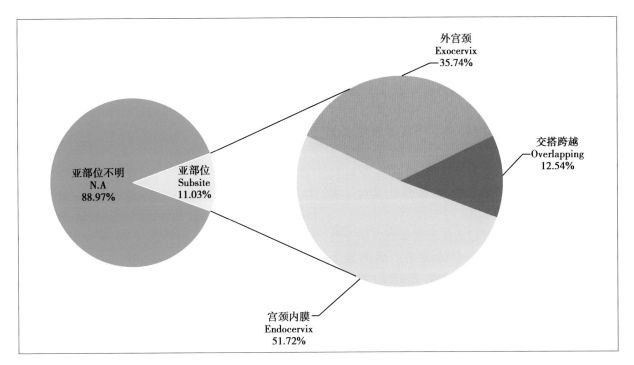

图 5-13c 2018 年中国肿瘤登记地区子宫颈癌亚部位分布情况

Figure 5-13c Subsite distribution of cervical cancer in the registration
areas of China, 2018

14 子宫体

2018 年中国肿瘤登记地区子宫体癌位居女性癌症发病谱第 8 位。新发病例数为 27 217 例，占女性全部癌症发病的 3.87%；其中城市地区 13 368 例，农村地区 13 849 例。子宫体癌发病率为 10.56/10 万，中标发病率为 7.08/10 万，世标发病率为 6.85/10 万；城市中标发病率为农村的 1.09 倍。0～74 岁累积发病率为 0.77%（表 5-14a）。

2018 年中国肿瘤登记地区子宫体癌位居女性癌症死亡谱第 14 位。子宫体癌死亡病例数为 6 796 例，占女性全部癌症死亡的 2.07%；其中城市地区 3 087 例，农村地区 3 709 例。子宫体癌死亡率为 2.66/10 万，中标死亡率 1.56/10 万，世标死亡率 1.54/10 万；农村中标死亡率为城市的 1.07 倍。0～74 岁累积死亡率为 0.18%（表 5-14b）。

子宫体癌年龄别发病率在 20 岁前处于较低水平，20 岁以后快速上升，至 50～54 岁组达高峰，之后逐渐下降。年龄别死亡率 30 岁前处于较低水平，30 岁以后迅速上升（图 5-14a）。

东部地区中标发病率最高，其次是中部地区，西部地区最低；西部地区中标死亡率最高，其次是中部地区，东部地区最低。在七大行政区中，华南、华北地区子宫体癌发病率明显高于全国平均水平（表 5-14a，表 5-14b，图 5-14b）。

14 Uterus

In 2018, uterus cancer was the 8th most common female cancer in the registration areas of China. There were 27 217 new cases of uterus cancer (13 368 in urban areas and 13 849 in rural areas), accounting for 3.87% of all female cancer cases. The crude incidence rate was 10.56 per 100 000, with ASR China 7.08 per 100 000 and ASR World 6.85 per 100 000, respectively. Subgroup analyses showed that the incidence of ASR China was 1.09 times in urban areas as that in rural areas. The cumulative incidence rate for persons aged 0-74 years was 0.77% (Table 5-14a).

In 2018, uterus cancer was the 14th most common cause of female cancer deaths in the registration areas of China. A total of 6 796 women died of uterus cancer (3 087 in urban areas and 3 709 in rural areas), accounting for 2.07% of all female cancer deaths. The crude mortality rate was 2.66 per 100 000, with ASR China 1.56 per 100 000 and ASR World 1.54 per 100 000, respectively. Subgroup analyses showed that the mortality of ASR China was 1.07 times in rural areas as that in urban areas. The cumulative mortality rate for persons aged 0-74 years was 0.18% (Table 5-14b).

The age-specific incidence rate was low before age 20. It went up rapidly thereafter and reached the peak at age group 50-54, then started to go down gradually from age 55. The age-specific mortality was low before age 30, then gradually went up thereafter (Figure 5-14a).

Eastern areas had the highest incidence rate, followed by central and western areas. Western areas had the highest mortality rate, followed by central and eastern areas. Among the seven administrative districts, the incidence rates of uterus cancer in South China and North China were obviously higher than the national average (Table 5-14a, Table 5-14b, Figure 5-14b).

表 5-14a　2018 年中国肿瘤登记地区子宫体癌发病情况

Table 5-14a　Incidence of uterus cancer in the registration areas of China,2018

地区 Area	病例数 No. cases	粗率 Crude rate/ 100 000⁻¹	构成比 Freq. /%	中标率 ASR China/ 100 000⁻¹	世标率 ASR World/ 100 000⁻¹	累积率 Cum. rate 0~74/%	顺位 Rank
合计 All	27 217	10. 56	3. 87	7. 08	6. 85	0. 77	8
城市地区 Urban areas	13 368	11. 37	3. 81	7. 42	7. 21	0. 82	8
农村地区 Rural areas	13 849	9. 88	3. 93	6. 78	6. 53	0. 73	9
东部地区 Eastern areas	13 500	12. 49	3. 77	7. 79	7. 55	0. 86	8
中部地区 Central areas	6 049	9. 54	3. 82	6. 75	6. 54	0. 73	9
西部地区 Western areas	7 668	8. 90	4. 09	6. 31	6. 06	0. 67	8

表 5-14b　2018 年中国肿瘤登记地区子宫体癌死亡情况

Table 5-14b　Mortality of uterus cancer in the registration areas of China,2018

地区 Area	死亡数 No. deaths	粗率 Crude rate/ 100 000⁻¹	构成比 Freq. /%	中标率 ASR China/ 100 000⁻¹	世标率 ASR World/ 100 000⁻¹	累积率 Cum. rate 0~74/%	顺位 Rank
合计 All	6 796	2. 66	2. 07	1. 56	1. 54	0. 18	14
城市地区 Urban areas	3 087	2. 63	2. 01	1. 50	1. 48	0. 17	14
农村地区 Rural areas	3 709	2. 65	2. 13	1. 61	1. 59	0. 19	14
东部地区 Eastern areas	2 859	2. 64	1. 85	1. 38	1. 36	0. 16	14
中部地区 Central areas	1 581	2. 49	2. 07	1. 62	1. 61	0. 19	14
西部地区 Western areas	2 356	2. 73	2. 43	1. 78	1. 75	0. 20	12

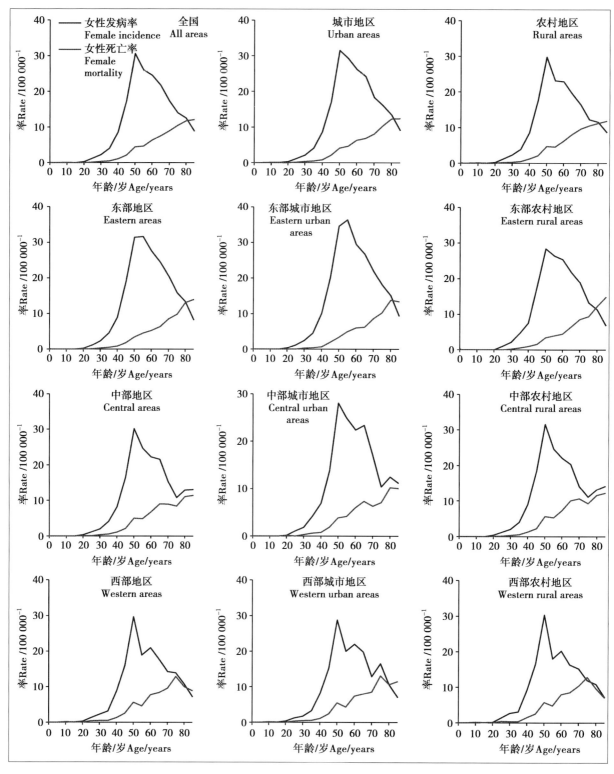

图 5-14a 2018 年中国肿瘤登记地区子宫体癌年龄别发病率和死亡率

Figure 5-14a Age-specific incidence and mortality rates of uterus cancer in the registration areas of China,2018

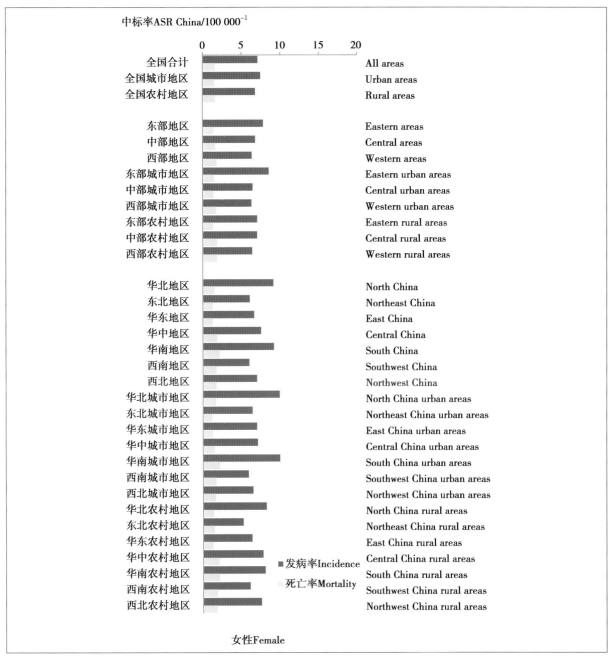

中标率ASR China/100 000⁻¹

全国合计	All areas
全国城市地区	Urban areas
全国农村地区	Rural areas
东部地区	Eastern areas
中部地区	Central areas
西部地区	Western areas
东部城市地区	Eastern urban areas
中部城市地区	Central urban areas
西部城市地区	Western urban areas
东部农村地区	Eastern rural areas
中部农村地区	Central rural areas
西部农村地区	Western rural areas
华北地区	North China
东北地区	Northeast China
华东地区	East China
华中地区	Central China
华南地区	South China
西南地区	Southwest China
西北地区	Northwest China
华北城市地区	North China urban areas
东北城市地区	Northeast China urban areas
华东城市地区	East China urban areas
华中城市地区	Central China urban areas
华南城市地区	South China urban areas
西南城市地区	Southwest China urban areas
西北城市地区	Northwest China urban areas
华北农村地区	North China rural areas
东北农村地区	Northeast China rural areas
华东农村地区	East China rural areas
华中农村地区	Central China rural areas
华南农村地区	South China rural areas
西南农村地区	Southwest China rural areas
西北农村地区	Northwest China rural areas

■发病率Incidence
死亡率Mortality

女性Female

图 5-14b 2018 年中国不同肿瘤登记地区子宫体癌发病率和死亡率
Figure 5-14b Incidence and mortality rates of uterus cancer in different registration areas of China,2018

15 卵巢

2018 年,中国肿瘤登记地区卵巢癌位居女性癌症发病谱第 11 位。新发病例数为 20 193 例,占女性癌症发病的 2.87%;其中城市地区 10 381 例,农村地区 9 812 例。发病率为 7.84/10 万,中标发病率为 5.54/10 万,世标发病率为 5.27/10 万;城市中标发病率为农村的 1.20 倍。0~74 岁累积发病率为 0.57%(表 5-15a)。

2018 年,中国肿瘤登记地区卵巢癌位居女性癌症死亡谱第 10 位。死亡病例数为 9 404 例,占女性癌症死亡的 2.87%;其中城市地区 5 100 例,农村地区 4 304 例。死亡率为 3.65/10 万,中标死亡率为 2.24/10 万,世标死亡率为 2.21/10 万;城市中标死亡率为农村的 1.31 倍。0~74 岁累积死亡率为 0.26%(表 5-15b)。

卵巢癌年龄别发病率从 35~39 岁组开始快速上升,至 60~64 岁组达高峰。卵巢癌年龄别死亡率从 35~39 岁组开始逐渐上升,至 75~79 岁组达高峰(图 5-15a)。

城市卵巢癌的发病率和死亡率均高于农村。中标发病率和中标死亡率均以东部地区最高,其次是中部地区,西部地区最低。在七大行政区中,中标发病率以东北地区最高,其次是华北地区和华中地区,华东地区最低;中标死亡率以东北地区最高,其次是华北地区和华中地区,西南地区最低(表 5-15a,表 5-15b,图 5-15b)。

15 Ovary

Ovarian cancer was the 11th most common female cancer in the registration areas of China in 2018. There were 20 193 new ovarian cancer cases(10 381 in urban areas and 9 812 in rural areas), accounting for 2.87% of new female cancer cases of all sites. The crude incidence rate was 7.84 per 100 000, with ASR China 5.54 per 100 000 and ASR World 5.27 per 100 000, respectively. Subgroup analyses showed that the incidence of ASR China was 1.20 times in urban areas as that in rural areas. The cumulative incidence rate for subjects aged 0 to 74 years was 0.57%(Table 5-15a).

Ovarian cancer was the 10th most common female cause of cancer deaths. A total of 9 404 cases died of ovary cancer in 2018(5 100 in urban areas and 4 304 in rural areas), accounting for 2.87% of all female cancer deaths. The crude mortality rate was 3.65 per 100 000, with ASR China 2.24 per 100 000 and ASR World 2.21 per 100 000, respectively. Subgroup analyses showed that the mortality of ASR China was 1.31 times in urban areas as that in rural areas. The cumulative mortality rate for subjects aged 0 to 74 years was 0.26%(Table 5-15b).

The age-specific incidence rates increased rapidly from the age group of 35-39 years and peaked at the age group of 60-64 years. The age-specific mortality rates increased from the age group of 35-39 years and peaked at the age group of 75-79 years(Figure 5-15a).

The incidence and mortality rates of ovarian cancer were higher in urban areas than in rural areas. Eastern areas had the highest incidence rate and mortality rate(ASR China), followed by central and western areas. Among the seven administrative districts, Northeast China had the highest incidence rate(ASR China), followed by North China and Central China, while the East China had the lowest incidence rate. Northeast China had the highest mortality rate, followed by North China and Central China, Southwest China had the lowest mortality rate(Table 5-15a, Table 5-15b, Figure 5-15b).

表 5-15a 2018 年中国肿瘤登记地区卵巢癌发病情况
Table 5-15a Incidence of ovarian cancer in the registration areas of China, 2018

地区 Area	病例数 No. cases	粗率 Crude rate/ 100 000⁻¹	构成比 Freq./%	中标率 ASR China/ 100 000⁻¹	世标率 ASR World/ 100 000⁻¹	累积率 Cum. rate 0~74/%	顺位 Rank
合计 All	20 193	7.84	2.87	5.54	5.27	0.57	11
城市地区 Urban areas	10 381	8.83	2.96	6.09	5.80	0.63	9
农村地区 Rural areas	9 812	7.00	2.78	5.06	4.81	0.52	11
东部地区 Eastern areas	9 360	8.66	2.61	5.70	5.43	0.59	11
中部地区 Central areas	4 780	7.54	3.02	5.65	5.37	0.58	10
西部地区 Western areas	6 053	7.03	3.23	5.25	4.97	0.53	10

表 5-15b 2018 年中国肿瘤登记地区卵巢癌死亡情况
Table 5-15b Mortality of ovarian cancer in the registration areas of China, 2018

地区 Area	死亡数 No. deaths	粗率 Crude rate/ 100 000⁻¹	构成比 Freq./%	中标率 ASR China/ 100 000⁻¹	世标率 ASR world/ 100 000⁻¹	累积率 Cum. rate 0~74/%	顺位 Rank
合计 All	9 404	3.65	2.87	2.24	2.21	0.26	10
城市地区 Urban areas	5 100	4.34	3.32	2.56	2.53	0.30	9
农村地区 Rural areas	4 304	3.07	2.47	1.96	1.93	0.23	12
东部地区 Eastern areas	4 698	4.35	3.03	2.40	2.37	0.28	9
中部地区 Central areas	2 165	3.41	2.84	2.29	2.27	0.27	10
西部地区 Western areas	2 541	2.95	2.62	1.97	1.93	0.23	10

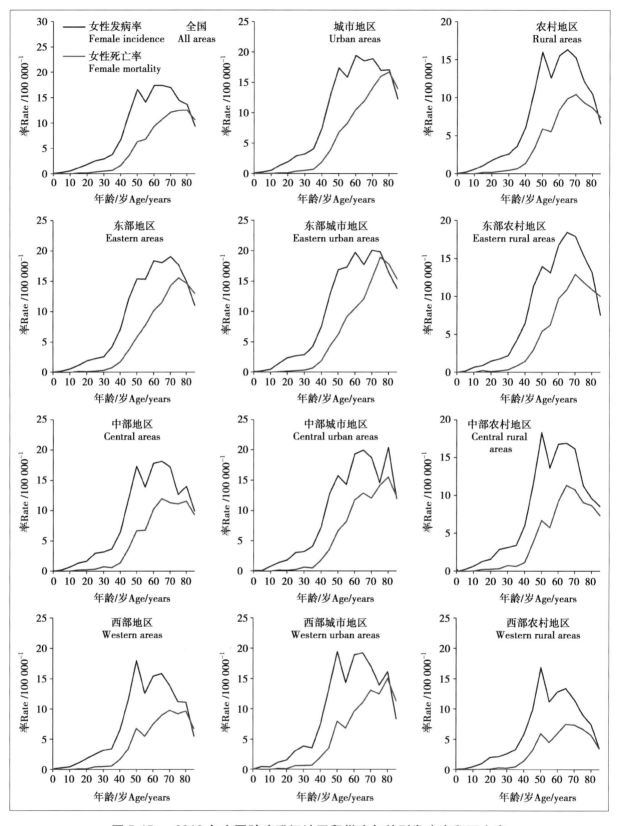

图 5-15a　2018 年中国肿瘤登记地区卵巢癌年龄别发病率和死亡率

Figure 5-15a　Age-specific incidence and mortality rates of ovarian cancer
in the registration areas of China,2018

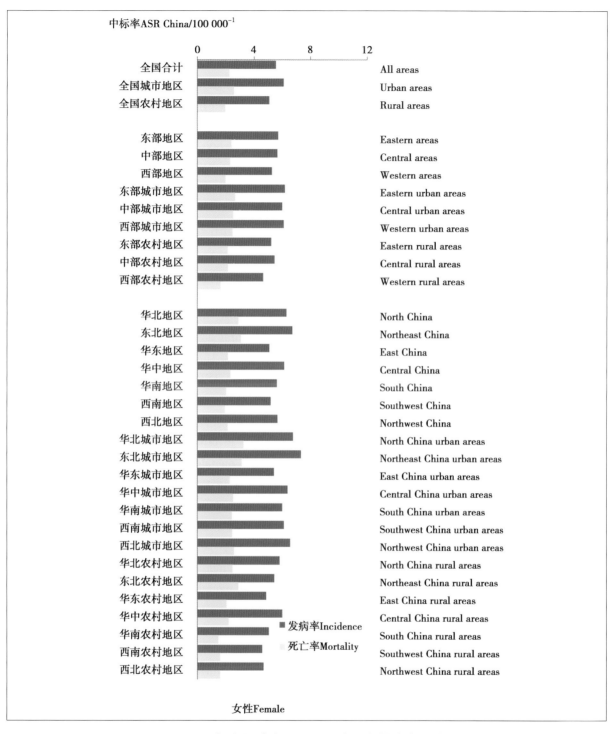

中标率ASR China/100 000⁻¹

全国合计	All areas
全国城市地区	Urban areas
全国农村地区	Rural areas
东部地区	Eastern areas
中部地区	Central areas
西部地区	Western areas
东部城市地区	Eastern urban areas
中部城市地区	Central urban areas
西部城市地区	Western urban areas
东部农村地区	Eastern rural areas
中部农村地区	Central rural areas
西部农村地区	Western rural areas
华北地区	North China
东北地区	Northeast China
华东地区	East China
华中地区	Central China
华南地区	South China
西南地区	Southwest China
西北地区	Northwest China
华北城市地区	North China urban areas
东北城市地区	Northeast China urban areas
华东城市地区	East China urban areas
华中城市地区	Central China urban areas
华南城市地区	South China urban areas
西南城市地区	Southwest China urban areas
西北城市地区	Northwest China urban areas
华北农村地区	North China rural areas
东北农村地区	Northeast China rural areas
华东农村地区	East China rural areas
华中农村地区	Central China rural areas
华南农村地区	South China rural areas
西南农村地区	Southwest China rural areas
西北农村地区	Northwest China rural areas

■ 发病率Incidence
死亡率Mortality

女性Female

图 5-15b　2018 年中国肿瘤登记不同地区卵巢癌发病率和死亡率
Figure 5-15b　Incidence and mortality rates of ovarian cancer in different registration areas of China, 2018

16 前列腺

2018 年,中国肿瘤登记地区前列腺癌位居男性癌症发病谱第 6 位。新发病例数为 33 856 例,占全部癌症发病的 3.93%;其中城市地区 19 448 例,农村地区 14 408 例。发病率为 12.75/10 万,中标发病率为 7.24/10 万,世标发病率为 7.14/10 万;城市中标发病率为农村的 1.53 倍。0~74 岁累积发病率为 0.80%(表 5-16a)。

2018 年,中国肿瘤登记地区前列腺癌位居男性癌症死亡谱第 7 位。死亡病例数为 13 451 例,占全部癌症死亡的 2.30%;其中城市地区 7 461 例,农村地区 5 990 例。前列腺癌死亡率为 5.07/10 万,中标死亡率 2.64/10 万,世标死亡率 2.68/10 万;城市中标死亡率为农村的 1.34 倍。0~74 岁累积死亡率为 0.19%(表 5-16b)。

前列腺癌年龄别发病率和死亡率在 55 岁之前处于较低水平,55 岁开始呈上升趋势,60 岁以后快速上升,在 85 岁及以上年龄组达到峰值(图 5-16a)。

城市前列腺癌的发病率和死亡率均高于农村。中标发病率和中标死亡率均以东部地区最高,其次是西部地区,中部地区最低。在七大行政区中,华东地区前列腺癌发病率最高,其次是华南地区和华北地区,东北地区最低;死亡率是华南地区最高,其次为华东地区和华北地区(表 5-16a,表 5-16b,图 5-16b)。

16 Prostate

Prostate cancer was the 6th most common male cancer in the registration areas of China in 2018. There were 33 856 new cases of prostate cancer(19 448 in urban areas and 14 408 in rural areas), accounting for 3.93% of new cancer cases of all sites. The crude incidence rate was 12.75 per 100 000, with ASR China 7.24 per 100 000 and ASR World 7.14 per 100 000, respectively. Subgroup analyses showed that the incidence of ASR China was 1.53 times in urban areas as that in rural areas. The cumulative incidence rate for subjects aged 0 to 74 years was 0.80% (Table 5-16a).

Prostate cancer was the 7th most common male cause of cancer deaths. A total of 13 451 cases died of prostate cancer in 2018 (7 461 in urban areas and 5 990 in rural areas), accounting for 2.30% of all cancer deaths. The crude mortality rate was 5.07 per 100 000, with ASR China 2.64 per 100 000 and ASR World 2.68 per 100 000, respectively. Subgroup analyses showed that the mortality of ASR China was 1.34 times in urban areas as that in rural areas. The cumulative mortality rate for subjects aged 0 to 74 years was 0.19% (Table 5-16b).

The age-specific incidence and mortality rates were low before 55 years old and increased constantly since then. The age-specific incidence and mortality rates dramatically increased over 60 years old. The incidence and mortality rate reached peak at the age group of 85+ years, respectively (Figure 5-16a).

The prostate cancer incidence rate and mortality rate were higher in urban areas than that in rural areas. Age-standardized incidence and mortality rates were highest in eastern areas, and followed by western areas and central areas. Among the seven administrative districts, the incidence rate was highest in East China, followed by South China and North China, and was lowest in Northeast China. Mortality rate was also highest in South China, followed by East China and North China (Table 5-16a, Table 5-16b, Figure 5-16b).

表 5-16a　2018 年中国肿瘤登记地区前列腺癌发病情况

Table 5-16a　Incidence of prostate cancer in the registration areas of China,2018

地区 Area	病例数 No. cases	粗率 Crude rate/ 100 000^{-1}	构成比 Freq./%	中标率 ASR China/ 100 000^{-1}	世标率 ASR World/ 100 000^{-1}	累积率 Cum. rate 0~74/%	顺位 Rank
合计 All	33 856	12.75	3.93	7.24	7.14	0.80	6
城市地区 Urban areas	19 448	16.41	4.78	8.87	8.74	0.98	6
农村地区 Rural areas	14 408	9.80	3.17	5.81	5.73	0.65	6
东部地区 Eastern areas	20 336	18.65	4.97	9.56	9.42	1.09	6
中部地区 Central areas	5 388	8.13	2.82	5.12	5.07	0.56	6
西部地区 Western areas	8 132	9.02	3.13	5.43	5.35	0.56	6

表 5-16b　2018 年中国肿瘤登记地区前列腺癌死亡情况

Table 5-16b　Mortality of prostate cancer in the registration areas of China,2018

地区 Area	死亡数 No. deaths	粗率 Crude rate/ 100 000^{-1}	构成比 Freq./%	中标率 ASR China/ 100 000^{-1}	世标率 ASR world/ 100 000^{-1}	累积率 Cum. rate 0~74/%	顺位 Rank
合计 All	13 451	5.07	2.30	2.64	2.68	0.19	7
城市地区 Urban areas	7 461	6.30	2.80	3.04	3.09	0.21	7
农村地区 Rural areas	5 990	4.07	1.88	2.27	2.30	0.17	9
东部地区 Eastern areas	7 250	6.65	2.75	3.00	3.07	0.20	7
中部地区 Central areas	2 506	3.78	1.87	2.25	2.25	0.18	10
西部地区 Western areas	3 695	4.10	1.98	2.36	2.37	0.18	8

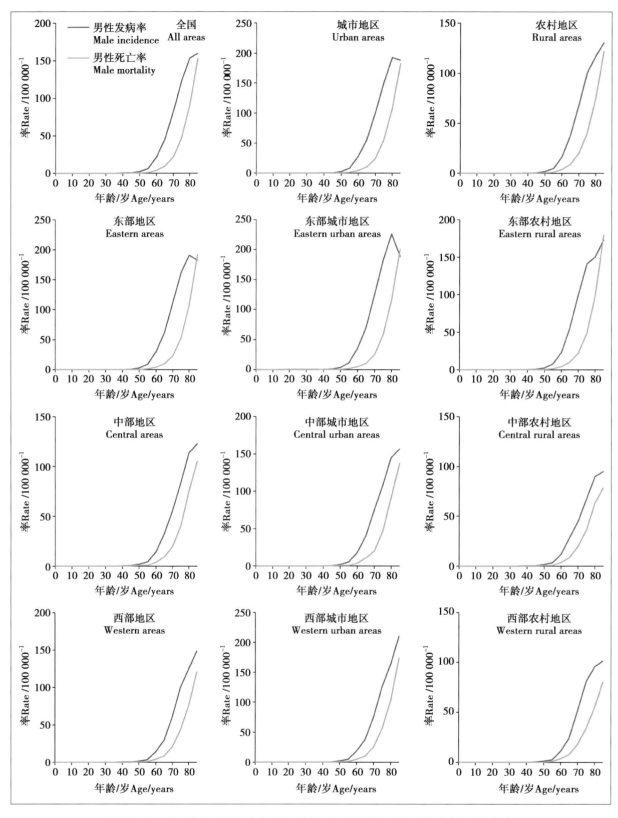

图 5-16a 2018 年中国肿瘤登记地区前列腺癌年龄别发病率和死亡率
Figure 5-16a Age-specific incidence and mortality rates of prostate cancer in the registration areas of China, 2018

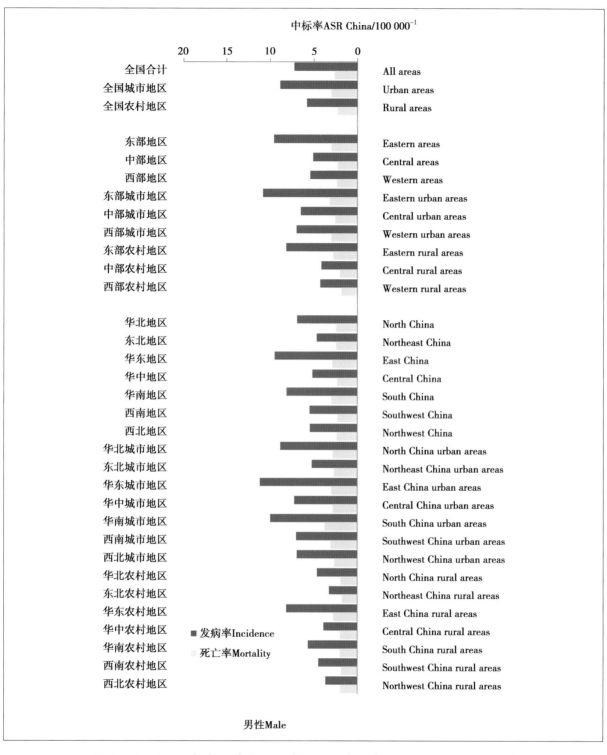

中标率ASR China/100 000⁻¹

全国合计	All areas
全国城市地区	Urban areas
全国农村地区	Rural areas
东部地区	Eastern areas
中部地区	Central areas
西部地区	Western areas
东部城市地区	Eastern urban areas
中部城市地区	Central urban areas
西部城市地区	Western urban areas
东部农村地区	Eastern rural areas
中部农村地区	Central rural areas
西部农村地区	Western rural areas
华北地区	North China
东北地区	Northeast China
华东地区	East China
华中地区	Central China
华南地区	South China
西南地区	Southwest China
西北地区	Northwest China
华北城市地区	North China urban areas
东北城市地区	Northeast China urban areas
华东城市地区	East China urban areas
华中城市地区	Central China urban areas
华南城市地区	South China urban areas
西南城市地区	Southwest China urban areas
西北城市地区	Northwest China urban areas
华北农村地区	North China rural areas
东北农村地区	Northeast China rural areas
华东农村地区	East China rural areas
华中农村地区	Central China rural areas
华南农村地区	South China rural areas
西南农村地区	Southwest China rural areas
西北农村地区	Northwest China rural areas

■ 发病率Incidence
　 死亡率Mortality

男性Male

图 5-16b　2018 年中国肿瘤登记地区不同地区前列腺癌发病率和死亡率
Figure 5-16b　Incidence and mortality rates of prostate cancer in different registration areas of China, 2018

17 肾及泌尿系统不明

2018 年,中国肿瘤登记地区肾及泌尿系统不明癌位居癌症发病谱第 17 位。新发病例数为 27 375 例,占全部癌症发病的 1.75%;其中男性 17 154 例,女性 10 221 例,城市地区 15 766 例,农村地区 11 609 例。发病率为 5.23/10 万,中标发病率为 3.30/10 万,世标发病率 3.27/10 万;男性中标发病率为女性的 1.74 倍,城市中标发病率为农村的 1.53 倍;0~74 岁累积发病率为 0.39%(表 5-17a)。

2018 年,中国肿瘤登记地区肾及泌尿系统不明癌位居癌症死亡谱第 19 位,死亡病例数为 9 900 例,占全部癌症死亡的 1.09%;其中男性 6 384 例,女性 3 516 例,城市地区 5 721 例,农村地区 4 179 例。死亡率为 1.89/10 万,中标死亡率 1.06/10 万,世标死亡率 1.07/10 万;男性中标死亡率为女性的 2.02 倍,城市中标死亡率为农村的 1.46 倍。0~74 岁累积死亡率为 0.12%(表 5-17b)。

按部位划分,肾癌发病率为 4.04/10 万,中标发病率为 2.62/10 万;肾癌死亡率为 1.37/10 万,中标死亡率为 0.78/10 万。肾盂癌的发病率为 0.50/10 万,中标发病率为 0.29/10 万;肾盂癌死亡率为 0.22/10 万,中标死亡率为 0.12/10 万。输尿管癌的发病率为 0.57/10 万,中标发病率为 0.32/10 万;输尿管癌死亡率为 0.25/10 万,中标死亡率为 0.13/10 万(表 5-17c ~ 表 5-17h)。

17 Kidney & unspecified urinary organs

Cancer of the kidney & unspecified urinary organs was the 17th most common cancer in the registration areas of China in 2018. There were 27 375 new cancer cases(17 154 males and 10 221 females,15 766 in urban areas and 11 609 in rural areas),accounting for 1.75% of new cases of all cancers. The crude incidence rate was 5.23 per 100 000, with ASR China 3.30 per 100 000 and ASR world 3.27 per 100 000, respectively. Subgroup analyses showed that the incidence of ASR China was 1.74 times in males as that in females, and it was 1.53 times in urban areas as that in rural areas. The cumulative incidence rate for subjects aged 0 to 74 years was 0.39%(Table 5-17a).

Cancer of the kidney & unspecified urinary organs was the 19th most common cause of cancer deaths in the registration areas of China. A total of 9 900 cases died of cancer of kidney and unspecified urinary organs in 2018(6 384 males and 3 516 females,5 721 in urban areas and 4 179 in rural areas),accounting for 1.09% of all cancer deaths. The crude mortality rate was 1.89 per 100 000,with ASR China 1.06 per 100 000 and ASR world 1.07 per 100 000,respectively. Subgroup analyses showed that the mortality of ASR China was 2.02 times in males as that in females, and it was 1.46 times in urban areas as that in rural areas. The cumulative mortality rate for subjects aged 0 to 74 years was 0.12%(Table 5-17b).

By subsite, the renal cancer incidence was 4.04 per 100 000 with ASR China 2.62 per 100 000;and the mortality was 1.37 per 100 000,with ASR China 0.78 per 100 000. The cancer incidence of renal pelvis was 0.50 per 100 000,with ASR China 0.29 per 100 000;and the mortality was 0.22 per 100 000, with ASR China 0.12 per 100 000. The ureter cancer incidence was 0.57 per 100 000,with ASR China 0.32 per 100 000;and the mortality was 0.25 per 100 000,with ASR China 0.13 per 100 000(Table 5-17c- Table 5-17h).

肾及泌尿系统不明癌年龄别发病率在 20 岁年龄组之前均处于较低水平,自 20~24 岁组开始快速上升,至 75~79 岁组达高峰,80 岁组以后降低;年龄别死亡率从 40~44 岁组开始迅速上升;男性各年龄别发病率和死亡率均明显高于女性(图5-17a)。

城市地区肾及泌尿系统不明癌的发病率和死亡率均高于农村地区。中标发病率和中标死亡率均以东部地区最高,其次是中部地区,西部地区最低。在七大行政区中,东北地区发病率和死亡率最高,西南地区发病率和死亡率最低(表 5-17a,表5-17b,图 5-17b)。

肾(除外肾盂)是肾及泌尿系统不明癌发生的最主要的亚部位,占全部病例的 77.22%,其次为输尿管,占 10.90%;肾盂占 9.64%;其他泌尿器官占 2.25%(图 5-17c)。

全部肾及泌尿系统不明癌病例中有明确组织学类型的病例占 68.03%,其中透明细胞腺癌是最主要的病理类型,占 75.28%;其次是乳头状腺癌,占 3.40%;肾嫌色细胞癌,占 3.22%,肾集合管癌占 0.51%,其他类型癌占 17.59%(图 5-17d)。

The age-specific incidence of cancer of kidney and unspecified urinary organs was low before 20 years old. It increased rapidly from the age group of 20-24 years and peaked at the age group of 75-79 years, and then it decreased at the age group of 80 years. Age-specific mortality rates increased rapidly from the age group of 40-44 years. Age-specific incidence and mortality rates in males were generally higher than those in females (Figure 5-17a).

The incidence and mortality rates of cancer in kidney & unspecified urinary organs were higher in urban areas than in rural areas. Eastern areas had the highest incidence and mortality rates, followed by the central areas and western areas. Among the seven administrative districts, Northeast China had the highest incidence and mortality. Southwest China had the lowest incidence and mortality (Table 5-17a, Table 5-17b, Figure 5-17b).

Kidney (except for the renal pelvis) was the most common subsite of cancer in kidney & unspecified urinary organs, accounting for 77.22% of total cases, followed by ureter (10.90%), renal pelvis (9.64%), and other urinary organs (2.25%) (Figure 5-17c).

About 68.03% cases of cancer in kidney and unspecified urinary organs had morphological verification. Among those, clear cell adenocarcinoma was the most common histological type, accounting for 75.28% of all cases, followed by papillary adenocarcinoma (3.40%), chromophobe renal cell carcinoma (3.22%), collecting duct carcinoma (0.51%), and others (17.59%) (Figure 5-17d).

表 5-17a 2018 年中国肿瘤登记地区肾及泌尿系统不明癌发病情况

Table 5-17a Incidence of cancer of kidney & unspecified urinary organs in the registration areas of China,2018

地区 Area	性别 Sex	病例数 No. cases	粗率 Crude rate/ 100 000^{-1}	构成比 Freq. /%	中标率 ASR China/ 100 000^{-1}	世标率 ASR World/ 100 000^{-1}	累积率 Cum. rate 0~74/%	顺位 Rank
合计 All	合计 Both	27 375	5. 23	1. 75	3. 30	3. 27	0. 39	17
	男性 Male	17 154	6. 46	1. 99	4. 20	4. 16	0. 49	13
	女性 Female	10 221	3. 97	1. 45	2. 42	2. 39	0. 28	16
城市地区 Urban areas	合计 Both	15 766	6. 68	2. 08	4. 06	4. 01	0. 47	16
	男性 Male	9 971	8. 41	2. 45	5. 27	5. 22	0. 62	11
	女性 Female	5 795	4. 93	1. 65	2. 88	2. 83	0. 33	15
农村地区 Rural areas	合计 Both	11 609	4. 04	1. 44	2. 64	2. 62	0. 31	17
	男性 Male	7 183	4. 89	1. 58	3. 29	3. 25	0. 39	15
	女性 Female	4 426	3. 16	1. 26	2. 01	2. 00	0. 23	16
东部地区 Eastern areas	合计 Both	16 507	7. 60	2. 15	4. 43	4. 36	0. 52	16
	男性 Male	10 521	9. 65	2. 57	5. 83	5. 73	0. 68	11
	女性 Female	5 986	5. 54	1. 67	3. 09	3. 05	0. 36	15
中部地区 Central areas	合计 Both	5 478	4. 22	1. 57	2. 89	2. 88	0. 34	17
	男性 Male	3 376	5. 09	1. 76	3. 59	3. 57	0. 43	14
	女性 Female	2 102	3. 31	1. 33	2. 20	2. 19	0. 26	16
西部地区 Western areas	合计 Both	5 390	3. 06	1. 20	2. 04	2. 02	0. 23	20
	男性 Male	3 257	3. 61	1. 25	2. 47	2. 44	0. 28	14
	女性 Female	2 133	2. 48	1. 14	1. 62	1. 59	0. 18	17

表 5-17b 2018 年中国肿瘤登记地区肾及泌尿系统不明癌死亡情况

Table 5-17b Mortality of cancer of kidney & unspecified urinary organs in the registration areas of China,2018

地区 Area	性别 Sex	死亡数 No. deaths	粗率 Crude rate/ 100 000^{-1}	构成比 Freq. /%	中标率 ASR China/ 100 000^{-1}	世标率 ASR World/ 100 000^{-1}	累积率 Cum. rate 0~74/%	顺位 Rank
合计 All	合计 Both	9 900	1. 89	1. 09	1. 06	1. 07	0. 12	18
	男性 Male	6 384	2. 40	1. 09	1. 43	1. 45	0. 16	15
	女性 Female	3 516	1. 36	1. 07	0. 71	0. 71	0. 07	15
城市地区 Urban areas	合计 Both	5 721	2. 42	1. 36	1. 27	1. 28	0. 13	17
	男性 Male	3 687	3. 11	1. 38	1. 74	1. 76	0. 19	14
	女性 Female	2 034	1. 73	1. 32	0. 83	0. 84	0. 08	15
农村地区 Rural areas	合计 Both	4 179	1. 46	0. 85	0. 87	0. 87	0. 10	20
	男性 Male	2 697	1. 83	0. 85	1. 16	1. 16	0. 13	15
	女性 Female	1 482	1. 06	0. 85	0. 59	0. 60	0. 06	17
东部地区 Eastern areas	合计 Both	5 607	2. 58	1. 34	1. 27	1. 27	0. 14	17
	男性 Male	3 641	3. 34	1. 38	1. 77	1. 78	0. 19	13
	女性 Female	1 966	1. 82	1. 27	0. 82	0. 81	0. 08	15
中部地区 Central areas	合计 Both	2 104	1. 62	1. 00	1. 03	1. 03	0. 12	19
	男性 Male	1 349	2. 04	1. 01	1. 36	1. 38	0. 16	15
	女性 Female	755	1. 19	0. 99	0. 70	0. 69	0. 07	15
西部地区 Western areas	合计 Both	2 189	1. 24	0. 77	0. 77	0. 78	0. 09	20
	男性 Male	1 394	1. 55	0. 75	1. 00	1. 01	0. 11	17
	女性 Female	795	0. 92	0. 82	0. 54	0. 56	0. 06	18

表 5-17c　2018 年中国肿瘤登记地区肾癌发病情况

Table 5-17c　Incidence of kidney cancer in the registration areas of China,2018

地区 Area	性别 Sex	病例数 No. cases	粗率 Crude rate/ 100 000^{-1}	构成比 Freq. /%	中标率 ASR China/ 100 000^{-1}	世标率 ASR World/ 100 000^{-1}	累积率 Cum. rate 0~74/%
合计	合计 Both	21 139	4.04	1.35	2.62	2.59	0.30
All	男性 Male	13 585	5.12	1.58	3.39	3.35	0.40
	女性 Female	7 554	2.93	1.07	1.86	1.84	0.21
城市地区	合计 Both	12 105	5.13	1.60	3.21	3.18	0.37
Urban areas	男性 Male	7 924	6.69	1.95	4.28	4.23	0.50
	女性 Female	4 181	3.56	1.19	2.17	2.15	0.25
农村地区	合计 Both	9 034	3.15	1.12	2.10	2.08	0.24
Rural areas	男性 Male	5 661	3.85	1.25	2.63	2.60	0.31
	女性 Female	3 373	2.41	0.96	1.57	1.57	0.18
东部地区	合计 Both	12 840	5.91	1.67	3.57	3.51	0.41
Eastern areas	男性 Male	8 422	7.72	2.06	4.78	4.69	0.56
	女性 Female	4 418	4.09	1.23	2.39	2.37	0.28
中部地区	合计 Both	4 261	3.29	1.22	2.29	2.28	0.27
Central areas	男性 Male	2 670	4.03	1.40	2.87	2.86	0.34
	女性 Female	1 591	2.51	1.01	1.71	1.71	0.20
西部地区	合计 Both	4 038	2.29	0.90	1.57	1.54	0.17
Western areas	男性 Male	2 493	2.77	0.96	1.92	1.90	0.21
	女性 Female	1 545	1.79	0.82	1.21	1.18	0.13

表 5-17d　2018 年中国肿瘤登记地区肾癌死亡情况

Table 5-17d　Mortality of kidney cancer in the registration areas of China,2018

地区 Area	性别 Sex	死亡数 No. deaths	粗率 Crude rate/ 100 000^{-1}	构成比 Freq. /%	中标率 ASR China/ 100 000^{-1}	世标率 ASR world/ 100 000^{-1}	累积率 Cum. rate 0~74/%
合计	合计 Both	7 147	1.37	0.78	0.78	0.79	0.09
All	男性 Male	4 782	1.80	0.82	1.09	1.10	0.12
	女性 Female	2 365	0.92	0.72	0.49	0.50	0.05
城市地区	合计 Both	4 058	1.72	0.97	0.93	0.94	0.10
Urban areas	男性 Male	2 759	2.33	1.04	1.32	1.34	0.15
	女性 Female	1 299	1.11	0.85	0.56	0.56	0.06
农村地区	合计 Both	3 089	1.08	0.63	0.65	0.66	0.08
Rural areas	男性 Male	2 023	1.38	0.64	0.88	0.88	0.10
	女性 Female	1 066	0.76	0.61	0.43	0.44	0.05
东部地区	合计 Both	4 021	1.85	0.96	0.94	0.94	0.10
Eastern areas	男性 Male	2 728	2.50	1.03	1.35	1.36	0.15
	女性 Female	1 293	1.20	0.83	0.56	0.56	0.06
中部地区	合计 Both	1 544	1.19	0.73	0.77	0.77	0.09
Central areas	男性 Male	1 006	1.52	0.75	1.03	1.04	0.12
	女性 Female	538	0.85	0.71	0.51	0.51	0.05
西部地区	合计 Both	1 582	0.90	0.56	0.56	0.58	0.06
Western areas	男性 Male	1 048	1.16	0.56	0.76	0.77	0.09
	女性 Female	534	0.62	0.55	0.37	0.40	0.04

表 5-17e 2018 年中国肿瘤登记地区肾盂癌发病情况

Table 5-17e Incidence of cancer of renal pelvis in the registration areas of China, 2018

地区 Area	性别 Sex	病例数 No. cases	粗率 Crude rate/ 100 000^{-1}	构成比 Freq./%	中标率 ASR China/ 100 000^{-1}	世标率 ASR World/ 100 000^{-1}	累积率 Cum. rate 0~74/%
合计 All	合计 Both	2 638	0.50	0.17	0.29	0.29	0.04
	男性 Male	1 545	0.58	0.18	0.36	0.36	0.04
	女性 Female	1 093	0.42	0.16	0.23	0.23	0.03
城市地区 Urban areas	合计 Both	1 600	0.68	0.21	0.38	0.37	0.04
	男性 Male	906	0.76	0.22	0.45	0.45	0.05
	女性 Female	694	0.59	0.20	0.30	0.30	0.03
农村地区 Rural areas	合计 Both	1 038	0.36	0.13	0.22	0.22	0.03
	男性 Male	639	0.43	0.14	0.28	0.28	0.03
	女性 Female	399	0.28	0.11	0.16	0.17	0.02
东部地区 Eastern areas	合计 Both	1 561	0.72	0.20	0.37	0.37	0.04
	男性 Male	892	0.82	0.22	0.46	0.45	0.05
	女性 Female	669	0.62	0.19	0.30	0.29	0.03
中部地区 Central areas	合计 Both	477	0.37	0.14	0.24	0.24	0.03
	男性 Male	292	0.44	0.15	0.30	0.30	0.03
	女性 Female	185	0.29	0.12	0.18	0.18	0.02
西部地区 Western areas	合计 Both	600	0.34	0.13	0.22	0.21	0.03
	男性 Male	361	0.40	0.14	0.26	0.26	0.03
	女性 Female	239	0.28	0.13	0.17	0.17	0.02

表 5-17f 2018 年中国肿瘤登记地区肾盂癌死亡情况

Table 5-17f Mortality of cancer of renal pelvis in the registration areas of China, 2018

地区 Area	性别 Sex	死亡数 No. deaths	粗率 Crude rate/ 100 000^{-1}	构成比 Freq./%	中标率 ASR China/ 100 000^{-1}	世标率 ASR World/ 100 000^{-1}	累积率 Cum. rate 0~74/%
合计 All	合计 Both	1 149	0.22	0.13	0.12	0.12	0.01
	男性 Male	709	0.27	0.12	0.16	0.16	0.02
	女性 Female	440	0.17	0.13	0.08	0.08	0.01
城市地区 Urban areas	合计 Both	683	0.29	0.16	0.15	0.15	0.02
	男性 Male	399	0.34	0.15	0.19	0.19	0.02
	女性 Female	284	0.24	0.18	0.11	0.11	0.01
农村地区 Rural areas	合计 Both	466	0.16	0.09	0.09	0.09	0.01
	男性 Male	310	0.21	0.10	0.13	0.13	0.01
	女性 Female	156	0.11	0.09	0.06	0.06	0.01
东部地区 Eastern areas	合计 Both	611	0.28	0.15	0.13	0.13	0.01
	男性 Male	372	0.34	0.14	0.17	0.18	0.02
	女性 Female	239	0.22	0.15	0.09	0.09	0.01
中部地区 Central areas	合计 Both	257	0.20	0.12	0.12	0.12	0.01
	男性 Male	162	0.24	0.12	0.16	0.16	0.02
	女性 Female	95	0.15	0.12	0.09	0.08	0.01
西部地区 Western areas	合计 Both	281	0.16	0.10	0.10	0.10	0.01
	男性 Male	175	0.19	0.09	0.12	0.12	0.01
	女性 Female	106	0.12	0.11	0.07	0.07	0.01

表 5-17g　2018 年中国肿瘤登记地区输尿管癌发病情况

Table 5-17g　Incidence of ureter cancer in the registration areas of China,2018

地区 Area	性别 Sex	病例数 No. cases	粗率 Crude rate/ 100 000⁻¹	构成比 Freq./%	中标率 ASR China/ 100 000⁻¹	世标率 ASR World/ 100 000⁻¹	累积率 Cum. rate 0~74/%
合计	合计 Both	2 983	0.57	0.19	0.32	0.32	0.04
All	男性 Male	1 655	0.62	0.19	0.37	0.37	0.05
	女性 Female	1 328	0.52	0.19	0.28	0.27	0.03
城市地区	合计 Both	1 729	0.73	0.23	0.39	0.39	0.05
Urban areas	男性 Male	942	0.79	0.23	0.45	0.45	0.05
	女性 Female	787	0.67	0.22	0.34	0.33	0.04
农村地区	合计 Both	1 254	0.44	0.16	0.26	0.26	0.03
Rural areas	男性 Male	713	0.49	0.16	0.30	0.30	0.04
	女性 Female	541	0.39	0.15	0.22	0.22	0.03
东部地区	合计 Both	1 754	0.81	0.23	0.41	0.40	0.05
Eastern areas	男性 Male	987	0.91	0.24	0.48	0.48	0.06
	女性 Female	767	0.71	0.21	0.34	0.33	0.04
中部地区	合计 Both	622	0.48	0.18	0.30	0.30	0.04
Central areas	男性 Male	342	0.52	0.18	0.34	0.35	0.04
	女性 Female	280	0.44	0.18	0.26	0.26	0.03
西部地区	合计 Both	607	0.34	0.14	0.21	0.21	0.03
Western areas	男性 Male	326	0.36	0.13	0.23	0.23	0.03
	女性 Female	281	0.33	0.15	0.19	0.19	0.02

表 5-17h　2018 年中国肿瘤登记地区输尿管癌死亡情况

Table 5-17h　Mortality of ureter cancer in the registration areas of China,2018

地区 Area	性别 Sex	死亡数 No. deaths	粗率 Crude rate/ 100 000⁻¹	构成比 Freq./%	中标率 ASR China/ 100 000⁻¹	世标率 ASR world/ 100 000⁻¹	累积率 Cum. rate 0~74/%
合计	合计 Both	1 305	0.25	0.14	0.13	0.13	0.01
All	男性 Male	705	0.27	0.12	0.15	0.15	0.01
	女性 Female	600	0.23	0.18	0.11	0.11	0.01
城市地区	合计 Both	801	0.34	0.19	0.16	0.16	0.01
Urban areas	男性 Male	415	0.35	0.16	0.18	0.18	0.02
	女性 Female	386	0.33	0.25	0.14	0.14	0.01
农村地区	合计 Both	504	0.18	0.10	0.10	0.10	0.01
Rural areas	男性 Male	290	0.2	0.09	0.12	0.12	0.01
	女性 Female	214	0.15	0.12	0.08	0.08	0.01
东部地区	合计 Both	796	0.37	0.19	0.16	0.16	0.02
Eastern areas	男性 Male	426	0.39	0.16	0.19	0.19	0.02
	女性 Female	370	0.34	0.24	0.14	0.14	0.01
中部地区	合计 Both	237	0.18	0.11	0.11	0.11	0.01
Central areas	男性 Male	138	0.21	0.10	0.13	0.13	0.01
	女性 Female	99	0.16	0.13	0.09	0.09	0.01
西部地区	合计 Both	272	0.15	0.10	0.09	0.09	0.01
Western areas	男性 Male	141	0.16	0.08	0.10	0.10	0.01
	女性 Female	131	0.15	0.14	0.08	0.08	0.01

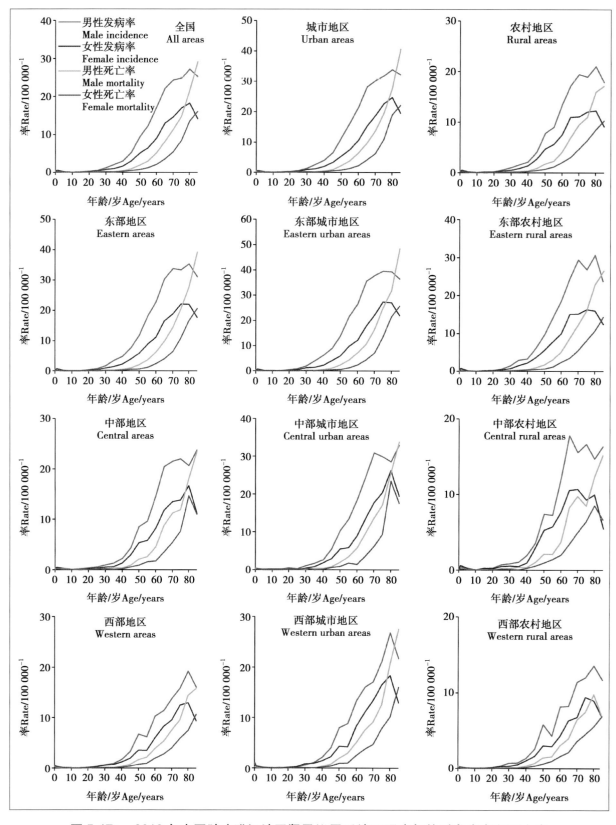

图 5-17a　2018 年中国肿瘤登记地区肾及泌尿系统不明癌年龄别发病率和死亡率

Figure 5-17a　Age-specific incidence and mortality rates of cancer of kidney & unspecified urinary organs in the registration areas of China, 2018

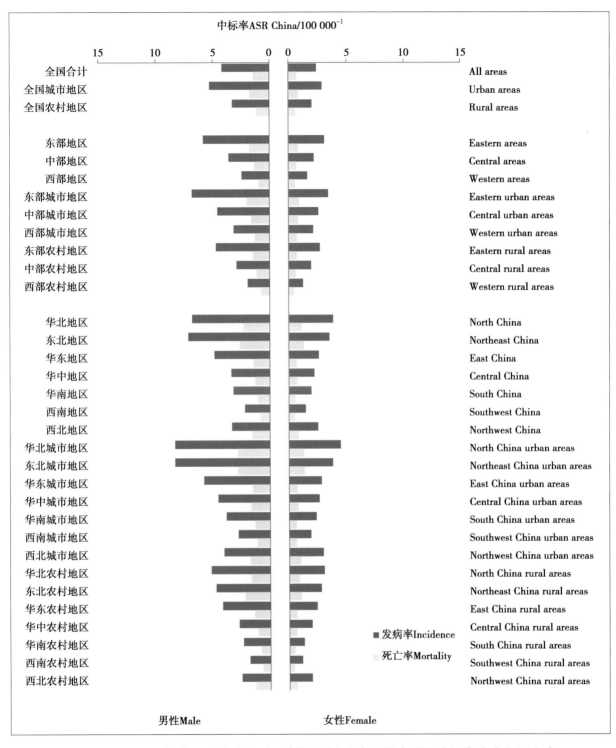

中标率ASR China/100 000^{-1}

图 5-17b　2018 年中国肿瘤登记地区肾及泌尿系统不明癌不同地区发病率和死亡率
Figure 5-17b　Incidence and mortality rates of cancer of kidney & unspecified
urinary organs in different registration areas of China, 2018

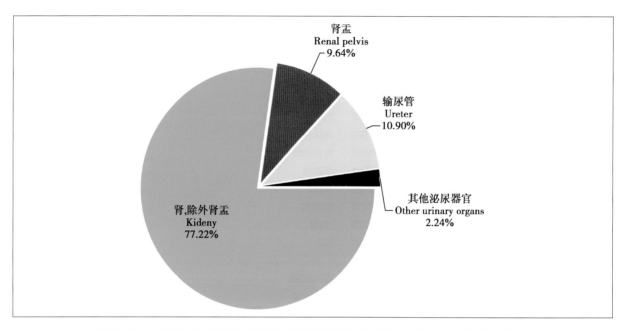

图 5-17c　2018 年中国肿瘤登记地区肾及泌尿系统不明癌亚部位分布情况
Figure 5-17c　Subsite distribution of cancer of kidney & unspecified
urinary organs in the registration areas of China,2018

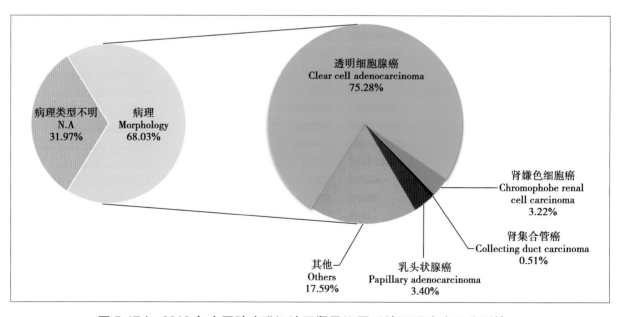

图 5-17d　2018 年中国肿瘤登记地区肾及泌尿系统不明癌病理分型情况
Figure 5-17d　Morphological distribution of cancer of kidney & unspecified
urinary organs in the registration areas of China,2018

18 膀胱

2018 年，中国肿瘤登记地区膀胱癌位居癌症发病谱第 16 位。新发病例数为 30 616 例，占全部癌症发病的 1.96%；其中男性 24 132 例，女性 6 484 例，城市地区 16 041 例，农村地区 14 575 例。发病率为 5.85/10 万，中标发病率为 3.34/10 万，世标发病率为 3.31/10 万；男性中标发病率为女性的 3.96 倍，城市中标发病率为农村的 1.23 倍。0~74 岁累积发病率为 0.38%（表 5-18a）。

2018 年，中国肿瘤登记地区膀胱癌位居癌症死亡谱第 16 位。膀胱癌死亡病例 13 322 例，占全部癌症死亡的 1.46%；其中男性 10 408 例，女性 2 914 例，城市地区 6 927 例，农村地区 6 395 例。膀胱癌死亡率为 2.55/10 万，中标死亡率 1.26/10 万，世标死亡率 1.27/10 万；男性中标死亡率为女性的 4.13 倍，城市中标死亡率为农村的 1.16 倍。0~74 岁累积死亡率为 0.11%（表 5-18b）。

膀胱癌的年龄别发病率和死亡率呈明显的性别差异。男性发病率自 40~45 岁组开始快速上升，至 85 岁及以上年龄组达到高峰。女性发病率自 50~54 岁组缓慢上升，至 80~84 岁达到高峰。男性年龄别峰值发病率是女性的 4.20 倍。男性膀胱癌死亡率自 55~59 岁组开始快速上升，至 85 岁及以上年龄组达到高峰。女性死亡率自 60~64 岁组快速上升，至 85 岁及以上年龄组达到高峰。男性年龄别峰值死亡率是女性的 4.57 倍（图 5-18a）。

18 Bladder

Bladder cancer ranked 16th for cancer incidence in the registration areas of China in 2018. There were 30 616 new cases of bladder cancer（24 132 males and 6 484 females, 16 041 in urban areas and 14 575 in rural areas）, accounting for 1.96% of all new cancer cases. The crude incidence rate was 5.85 per 100 000, with ASR China 3.34 per 100 000 and ASR World 3.31 per 100 000, respectively. The incidence of ASR China was 3.96 times in males as that in females, and it was 1.23 times in urban areas as that in rural areas. The cumulative incidence rate for subjects aged from 0 to 74 years was 0.38%（Table 5-18a）.

Bladder cancer ranked 16th for cancer mortality in the registration areas of China in 2018. A total of 13 322 cases died of bladder cancer（10 408 males and 2 914 females, 6 927 in urban areas and 6 395 in rural areas）, accounting for 1.46% of all cancer deaths. The crude mortality rate was 2.55 per 100 000, with ASR China 1.26 per 100 000 and ASR World 1.27 per 100 000, respectively. The mortality of ASR China was 4.13 times in males as that in females, and it was 1.16 times in urban areas as that in rural areas. The cumulative mortality rate for subjects aged from 0 to 74 years was 0.11%（Table 5-18b）.

Trends of age-specific incidence and mortality rates showed differences between males and females. The incidence rate in males increased rapidly from the age group of 40-45 years and peaked at the age group of 85 + years. The incidence rate in females increased slowly from the age group of 50-54 years and peaked at the age group of 80-84 years. The peak incidence rate in males was 4.20 times as that in females. The mortality rate in males and females increased rapidly from the age group of 55-59 years and 60-64 years, respectively, and peaked at the age group of 85 + years coincidentally. The peak mortality rate in males was 4.57 times as that in females（Figure 5-18a）.

膀胱癌的发病率和死亡率呈现地域差异。东部地区的发病率和死亡率高于中部和西部地区，中部和西部地区发病率和死亡率水平接近。七大行政区中，男性中标发病率和中标死亡率均为东北地区最高，西南地区最低；女性中标发病率和中标死亡率最高的均为东北地区，华南地区最低（表5-18a，表5-18b，图5-18b）。

约20.01%的膀胱癌新发病例具有明确的亚部位信息，其中膀胱侧壁的比例最高，占35.66%，其次是膀胱三角区（18.32%）、膀胱后壁（12.24%）、交搭跨越（8.61%）、膀胱顶（7.15%）、膀胱前壁（6.55%）、输尿管口（5.36%）、膀胱颈（4.82%）和脐尿管（1.29%）（图5-18c）。

全部膀胱癌病例中有明确组织学类型的病例占67.24%，其中移行细胞癌是最主要的病理类型，占77.22%；其次是其他类型（9.60%）、鳞状细胞癌（7.42%）和腺癌（5.76%）（图5-18d）。

The incidence and mortality rates (ASR China) of bladder cancer varied geographically. Eastern areas had the highest incidence and mortality rates, and the incidence and mortality in central areas and western areas were similar. Among seven administrative districts, Northeast China had the highest and Southwest China had the lowest incidence and mortality rate for males. The highest incidence and mortality rates were shown in Northeast China, and the lowest incidence and mortality rates were shown in South China for females (Table 5-18a, Table 5-18b, Figure 5-18b).

About 20.01% of the bladder cancer cases had complete information on subsite. Among them, lateral wall was the most common subsite (35.66%), followed by trigone (18.32%), posterior wall (12.24%), overlapping (8.61%), dome (7.15%), anterior wall (6.55%), ureteric orifice (5.36%), bladder neck (4.82%) and urachus (1.29%) (Figure 5-18c).

About 67.24% of the bladder cancer cases could be morphologically classified. Transitional cell carcinoma was the most common histological type, accounting for 77.22% of all cases, followed by other types (9.60%), squamous cell carcinoma (7.42%) and adenocarcinoma (5.76%) (Figure 5-18d).

表 5-18a 2018 年中国肿瘤登记地区膀胱癌发病情况
Table 5-18a Incidence of bladder cancer in the registration areas of China, 2018

地区 Area	性别 Sex	病例数 No. cases	粗率 Crude rate/ 100 000⁻¹	构成比 Freq./%	中标率 ASR China/ 100 000⁻¹	世标率 ASR World/ 100 000⁻¹	累积率 Cum. rate 0~74/%	顺位 Rank
合计	合计 Both	30 616	5.85	1.96	3.34	3.31	0.38	16
All	男性 Male	24 132	9.09	2.80	5.43	5.40	0.61	7
	女性 Female	6 484	2.52	0.92	1.37	1.35	0.15	17
城市地区	合计 Both	16 041	6.80	2.12	3.71	3.68	0.42	15
Urban areas	男性 Male	12 484	10.54	3.07	6.00	5.97	0.67	8
	女性 Female	3 557	3.03	1.01	1.57	1.55	0.17	17
农村地区	合计 Both	14 575	5.08	1.81	3.02	2.99	0.35	16
Rural areas	男性 Male	11 648	7.92	2.57	4.94	4.89	0.56	7
	女性 Female	2 927	2.09	0.83	1.19	1.17	0.14	19
东部地区	合计 Both	16 133	7.43	2.10	3.81	3.77	0.44	17
Eastern areas	男性 Male	12 756	11.70	3.12	6.31	6.26	0.71	8
	女性 Female	3 377	3.12	0.94	1.51	1.48	0.17	17
中部地区	合计 Both	6 097	4.70	1.74	2.98	2.96	0.34	16
Central areas	男性 Male	4 788	7.22	2.50	4.79	4.78	0.55	7
	女性 Female	1 309	2.06	0.83	1.25	1.22	0.14	18
西部地区	合计 Both	8 386	4.76	1.87	2.93	2.90	0.32	15
Western areas	男性 Male	6 588	7.31	2.53	4.66	4.61	0.51	7
	女性 Female	1 798	2.09	0.96	1.26	1.24	0.14	19

表 5-18b 2018 年中国肿瘤登记地区膀胱癌死亡情况
Table 5-18b Mortality of bladder cancer in the registration areas of China, 2018

地区 Area	性别 Sex	死亡数 No. deaths	粗率 Crude rate/ 100 000⁻¹	构成比 Freq./%	中标率 ASR China/ 100 000⁻¹	世标率 ASR World/ 100 000⁻¹	累积率 Cum. rate 0~74/%	顺位 Rank
合计	合计 Both	13 322	2.55	1.46	1.26	1.27	0.11	16
All	男性 Male	10 408	3.92	1.78	2.11	2.15	0.18	11
	女性 Female	2 914	1.13	0.89	0.51	0.51	0.04	16
城市地区	合计 Both	6 927	2.93	1.65	1.36	1.38	0.11	15
Urban areas	男性 Male	5 342	4.51	2.00	2.26	2.31	0.18	10
	女性 Female	1 585	1.35	1.03	0.56	0.57	0.04	16
农村地区	合计 Both	6 395	2.23	1.30	1.17	1.17	0.11	16
Rural areas	男性 Male	5 066	3.45	1.59	1.97	2.00	0.17	11
	女性 Female	1 329	0.95	0.76	0.46	0.46	0.04	19
东部地区	合计 Both	6 991	3.22	1.67	1.36	1.37	0.11	15
Eastern areas	男性 Male	5 442	4.99	2.06	2.33	2.39	0.19	10
	女性 Female	1 549	1.43	1.00	0.53	0.54	0.04	16
中部地区	合计 Both	2 702	2.08	1.28	1.18	1.18	0.11	16
Central areas	男性 Male	2 071	3.12	1.54	1.89	1.92	0.17	11
	女性 Female	631	0.99	0.83	0.53	0.52	0.05	17
西部地区	合计 Both	3 629	2.06	1.28	1.16	1.16	0.11	17
Western areas	男性 Male	2 895	3.21	1.55	1.91	1.93	0.18	11
	女性 Female	734	0.85	0.76	0.45	0.45	0.04	19

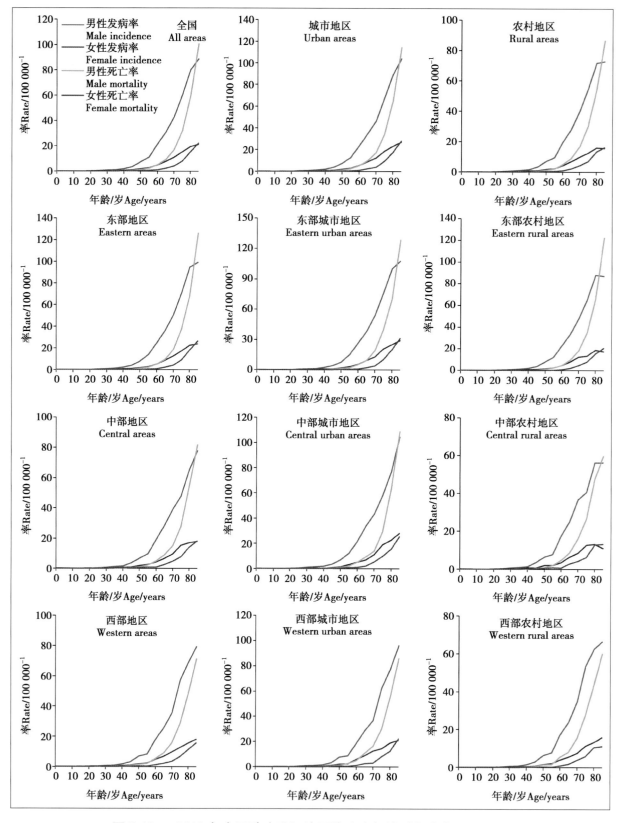

图 5-18a　2018 年中国肿瘤登记地区膀胱癌年龄别发病率和死亡率

Figure 5-18a　Age-specific incidence and mortality rates of bladder cancer
in the registration areas of China, 2018

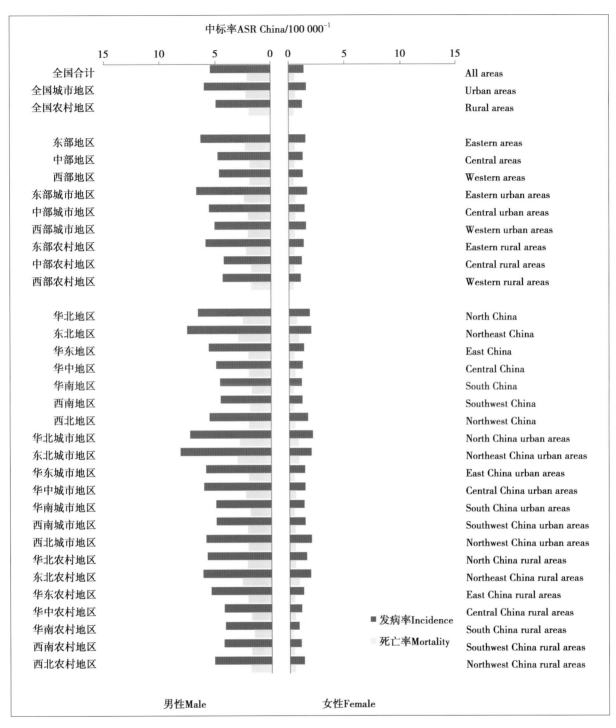

中标率ASR China/100 000^{-1}

全国合计	All areas
全国城市地区	Urban areas
全国农村地区	Rural areas
东部地区	Eastern areas
中部地区	Central areas
西部地区	Western areas
东部城市地区	Eastern urban areas
中部城市地区	Central urban areas
西部城市地区	Western urban areas
东部农村地区	Eastern rural areas
中部农村地区	Central rural areas
西部农村地区	Western rural areas
华北地区	North China
东北地区	Northeast China
华东地区	East China
华中地区	Central China
华南地区	South China
西南地区	Southwest China
西北地区	Northwest China
华北城市地区	North China urban areas
东北城市地区	Northeast China urban areas
华东城市地区	East China urban areas
华中城市地区	Central China urban areas
华南城市地区	South China urban areas
西南城市地区	Southwest China urban areas
西北城市地区	Northwest China urban areas
华北农村地区	North China rural areas
东北农村地区	Northeast China rural areas
华东农村地区	East China rural areas
华中农村地区	Central China rural areas
华南农村地区	South China rural areas
西南农村地区	Southwest China rural areas
西北农村地区	Northwest China rural areas

■ 发病率Incidence
　死亡率Mortality

男性Male　　　女性Female

图 5-18b　2018 年中国肿瘤登记不同地区膀胱癌发病率和死亡率
Figure 5-18b　Incidence and mortality rates of bladder cancer in different registration areas of China,2018

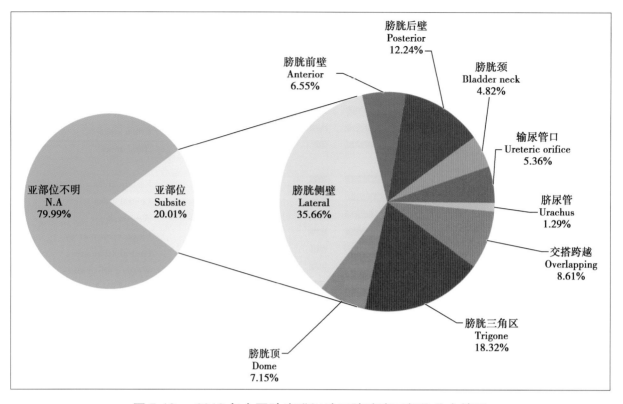

图 5-18c　2018 年中国肿瘤登记地区膀胱癌亚部位分布情况

Figure 5-18c　Subsite distribution of bladder cancer in the registration areas of China,2018

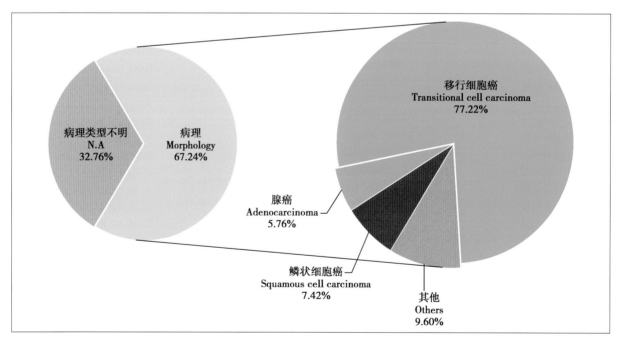

图 5-18d　2018 年中国肿瘤登记地区膀胱癌病理分型情况

Figure 5-18d　Morphological distribution of bladder cancer in the registration areas of China,2018

19 脑

2018年,中国肿瘤登记地区脑瘤位居癌症发病谱的第12位。新发病例数为40 188例,占全部癌症发病的2.57%;其中男性18 668例,女性21 520例,城市地区18 392例,农村地区21 796例。脑瘤发病率为7.68/10万,中标发病率为5.46/10万,世标发病率为5.37/10万;女性中标发病率为男性的1.10倍。0~74岁累积发病率为0.56%(表5-19a)。

2018年,中国肿瘤登记地区脑瘤位居癌症死亡谱的第10位。脑瘤死亡病例为22 124例,占全部癌症死亡的2.42%;其中男性12 224例,女性9 900例,城市地区9 583例,农村地区12 541例。脑瘤死亡率为4.23/10万,中标死亡率2.83/10万,世标死亡率2.82/10万;男性中标死亡率为女性的1.32倍。0~74岁累积死亡率为0.30%(表5-19b)。

脑瘤年龄别发病率20岁前处于较低水平,之后均随年龄增长而升高,在80~84岁组达高峰。脑瘤年龄别死亡率40岁前处于较低水平,之后均随年龄增长而升高,并在85岁及以上年龄组达到高峰(图5-19a)。

脑瘤的中标发病率和死亡率城市地区均高于农村地区。中标发病率以东部地区最高,其次为中部地区,西部地区最低。中标死亡率以中部地区最高,东部地区和西部地区接近。在七大行政区中,华南地区男性和女性的中标发病率最高,东北地区男性和女性的中标发病率最低;华中地区男性和西北地区女性的中标死亡率最高,华南地区男性和女性的中标死亡率最低(表5-19a,表5-19b,图5-19b)。

约37.96%的脑瘤新发病例具有明确的亚部位信息,其中大脑占23.47%,额叶占21.25%,颞叶占13.11%,小脑占11.30%,交搭跨越占9.55%,脑室占6.80%,顶叶占5.74%,脑干占5.67%,枕叶占3.11%(图5-19c)。

19 Brain

Brain tumor ranked 12th for cancer incidence in the registration areas of China in 2018. There were 40 188 new cases of brain tumor(18 668 males and 21 520 females,18 392 in urban areas and 21 796 in rural areas),accounting for 2.57% of all cancer cases. The crude incidence rate of brain tumor was 7.68 per 100 000,with ASR China 5.46 per 100 000 and ASR World 5.37 per 100 000,respectively. The ASR China was 1.10 times in females as that in males. The cumulative incidence rate for subjects aged from 0 to 74 years was 0.56% (Table 5-19a).

Brain tumor was the 10th most common cause of cancer deaths in the registration areas of China in 2018. The number of deaths due to brain tumor was 22 124(12 224 males and 9 900 females,9 583 in urban areas and 12 541 in rural areas),accounting for 2.42% of all cancer deaths. The crude mortality rate of brain tumor was 4.23 per 100 000,with ASR China 2.83 per 100 000 and ASR World 2.82 per 100 000,respectively. The ASR China was 1.32 times in males as that in females. The cumulative mortality rate for subjects aged from 0 to 74 years was 0.30% (Table 5-19b).

The age-specific incidence rate of brain tumor was relatively low before 20 years old and increased with age after that. It reached peak at the age group of 80-84 years. The age-specific mortality rate of brain tumor was relatively low before 40 years old and increased with age after that. It reached peak at the age group of 85+ years(Figure 5-19a).

The incidence and mortality rates(ASR China)of brain tumor were higher in urban areas than in rural areas. The incidence rate(ASR China)was highest in eastern areas,followed by central and western areas. Central areas had the highest mortality rate(ASR China),and the mortality rates in eastern areas and western areas were similar. Among the seven administrative districts,the highest incidence rates(ASR China)were shown in South China for both sexes,while Northeast China had the lowest incidence rates(ASR China)for both sexes. The highest mortality rates(ASR China)were found in Central China and Northwest China for males and females,respectively,while South China had the lowest mortality rates(ASR China)for both sexes(Table 5-19a,Table 5-19b,Figure 5-19b).

About 37.67% of brain tumor cases had specified sub categorical information. Among those,23.47% of cases occurred in cerebrum,followed by frontal lobe of brain(21.25%),temporal lobe(13.11%),cerebellum(11.30%),overlapping(9.55%),cerebral ventricle(6.80%),parietal lobe(5.74%),brain stem(5.67%)and occipital lobe(3.11%)(Figure 5-19c).

表 5-19a 2018 年中国肿瘤登记地区脑瘤发病情况
Table 5-19a Incidence of brain tumor in the registration areas of China,2018

地区 Area	性别 Sex	病例数 No. cases	粗率 Crude rate/ 100 000^{-1}	构成比 Freq./%	中标率 ASR China/ 100 000^{-1}	世标率 ASR World/ 100 000^{-1}	累积率 Cum. rate 0~74/%	顺位 Rank
合计	合计 Both	40 188	7.68	2.57	5.46	5.37	0.56	12
All	男性 Male	18 668	7.03	2.17	5.21	5.11	0.53	11
	女性 Female	21 520	8.35	3.06	5.71	5.62	0.60	10
城市地区	合计 Both	18 392	7.79	2.43	5.35	5.26	0.55	13
Urban areas	男性 Male	8 364	7.06	2.06	5.07	4.98	0.51	13
	女性 Female	10 028	8.53	2.86	5.61	5.53	0.59	10
农村地区	合计 Both	21 796	7.59	2.70	5.55	5.45	0.57	11
Rural areas	男性 Male	10 304	7.01	2.27	5.31	5.21	0.53	9
	女性 Female	11 492	8.20	3.26	5.79	5.69	0.61	10
东部地区	合计 Both	19 666	9.06	2.56	6.00	5.90	0.62	12
Eastern areas	男性 Male	8 801	8.07	2.15	5.62	5.51	0.56	13
	女性 Female	10 865	10.05	3.03	6.37	6.26	0.67	9
中部地区	合计 Both	9 063	6.99	2.59	5.34	5.29	0.55	12
Central areas	男性 Male	4 381	6.61	2.29	5.21	5.15	0.53	8
	女性 Female	4 682	7.38	2.96	5.47	5.44	0.57	11
西部地区	合计 Both	11 459	6.50	2.56	4.83	4.71	0.50	12
Western areas	男性 Male	5 486	6.08	2.11	4.68	4.55	0.47	9
	女性 Female	5 973	6.93	3.19	4.98	4.87	0.52	11

表 5-19b 2018 年中国肿瘤登记地区脑瘤死亡情况
Table 5-19b Mortality of brain tumor in the registration areas of China,2018

地区 Area	性别 Sex	死亡数 No. deaths	粗率 Crude rate/ 100 000^{-1}	构成比 Freq./%	中标率 ASR China/ 100 000^{-1}	世标率 ASR World/ 100 000^{-1}	累积率 Cum. rate 0~74/%	顺位 Rank
合计	合计 Both	22 124	4.23	2.42	2.83	2.82	0.30	10
All	男性 Male	12 224	4.60	2.09	3.22	3.19	0.34	8
	女性 Female	9 900	3.84	3.02	2.44	2.45	0.26	9
城市地区	合计 Both	9 583	4.06	2.28	2.62	2.61	0.27	12
Urban areas	男性 Male	5 320	4.49	2.00	3.03	3.00	0.32	11
	女性 Female	4 263	3.63	2.77	2.22	2.24	0.23	10
农村地区	合计 Both	12 541	4.37	2.55	3.00	3.00	0.32	9
Rural areas	男性 Male	6 904	4.70	2.17	3.37	3.35	0.35	7
	女性 Female	5 637	4.02	3.23	2.63	2.64	0.28	9
东部地区	合计 Both	9 809	4.52	2.34	2.76	2.75	0.28	12
Eastern areas	男性 Male	5 390	4.94	2.04	3.19	3.16	0.33	11
	女性 Female	4 419	4.09	2.85	2.34	2.35	0.24	10
中部地区	合计 Both	5 495	4.24	2.61	3.04	3.04	0.33	9
Central areas	男性 Male	3 062	4.62	2.28	3.44	3.42	0.37	7
	女性 Female	2 433	3.84	3.19	2.64	2.65	0.28	9
西部地区	合计 Both	6 820	3.87	2.41	2.78	2.77	0.29	10
Western areas	男性 Male	3 772	4.18	2.02	3.11	3.07	0.32	7
	女性 Female	3 048	3.54	3.15	2.43	2.46	0.26	9

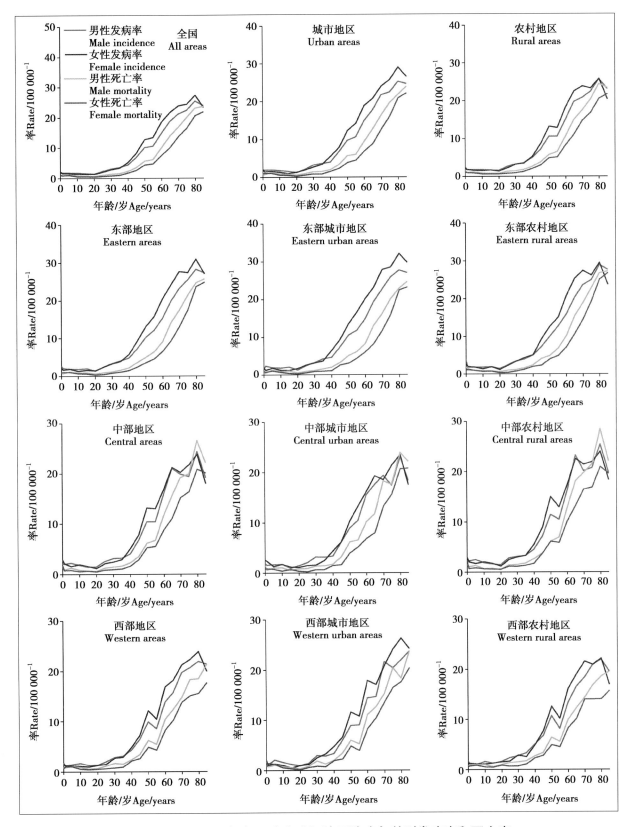

图 5-19a　2018 年中国肿瘤登记地区脑瘤年龄别发病率和死亡率

Figure 5-19a　Age-specific incidence and mortality rates of brain tumor in the registration areas of China, 2018

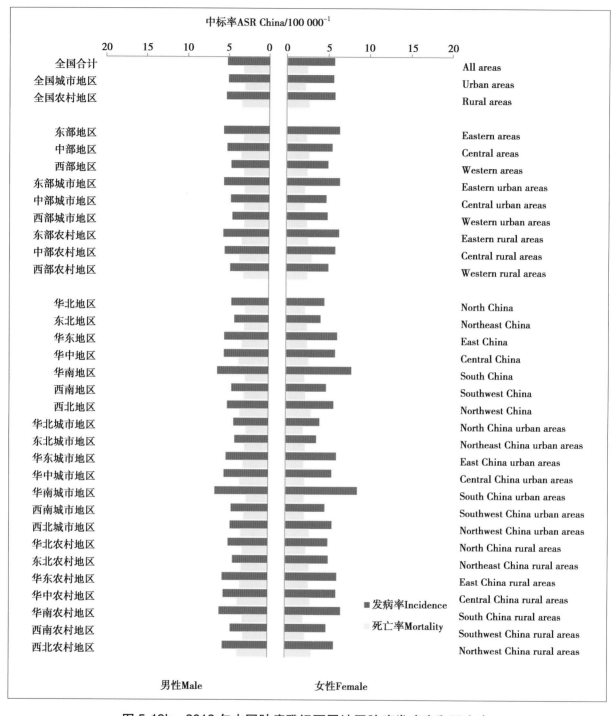

图 5-19b　2018 年中国肿瘤登记不同地区脑瘤发病率和死亡率

Figure 5-19b　Incidence and mortality rates of brain tumor in different registration areas of China,2018

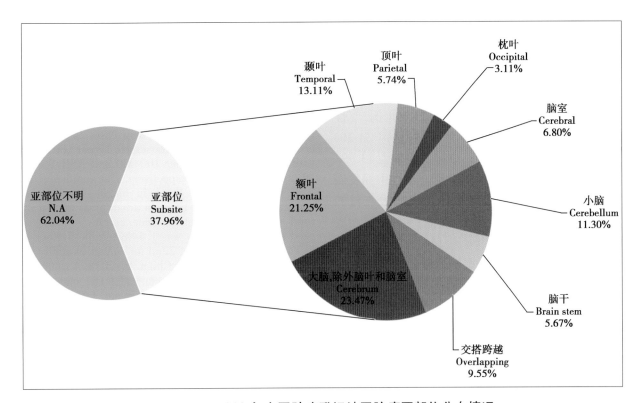

图 5-19c 2018 年中国肿瘤登记地区脑瘤亚部位分布情况

Figure 5-19c Subsite distribution of brain tumor in the registration areas of China, 2018

20 甲状腺

2018 年,中国肿瘤登记地区甲状腺癌位居癌症发病谱第 8 位。新发病例数为 84 593 例,占全部癌症发病的 5.41%;其中男性 21 198 例,女性 63 395 例,城市地区 50 330 例,农村地区 34 263 例。发病率为 16.17/10 万,中标发病率为 13.99/10 万,世标发病率为 12.01/10 万。女性中标发病率为男性的 2.93 倍,城市中标发病率为农村的 1.79 倍。0~74 岁累积发病率为 1.14%(表 5-20a)。

2018 年,中国肿瘤登记地区甲状腺癌位居癌症死亡谱第 22 位。因甲状腺癌死亡病例 3 232 例,占全部癌症死亡的 0.35%;其中男性 1 187 例,女性 2 045 例,城市地区 1 643 例,农村地区 1 589 例。甲状腺癌死亡率为 0.62/10 万,中标死亡率为 0.38/10 万,世标死亡率为 0.37/10 万;女性中标死亡率为男性的 1.69 倍,城市中标死亡率为农村的 1.17 倍。0~74 岁累积死亡率为 0.04%(表 5-20b)。

甲状腺癌年龄别发病率呈明显的性别差异。女性自 15~19 岁组开始快速上升,至 50~54 岁组达高峰;而男性从 20~24 岁组开始呈缓慢上升趋势。女性各年龄别发病率均明显高于男性。甲状腺癌年龄别死亡率从 40~44 岁组开始缓慢上升,至 85 岁及以上组到达高峰(图 5-20a)。

城市地区的甲状腺癌发病率和死亡率均高于农村地区。中标发病率以东部地区最高,其次是中部地区,西部地区最低;中标死亡率以中部地区最高,其次是西部地区,东部地区最低。七大行政区中,东北地区男性和女性中标发病率最高,西北地区男性和女性的中标发病率最低;东北地区男性和女性中标死亡率最高,西南地区男性和华南地区女性的中标发病率最低(表 5-20a、表 5-20b、图 5-20b)。

全部甲状腺癌病例中有明确组织学类型的病例占 87.60%,其中乳头状腺癌是最主要的病理类型,占 93.43%;其次是其他类型、滤泡性腺癌和髓样癌,分别占 5.12%、1.27% 和 0.18%(图 5-20c)。

20 Thyroid

Thyroid cancer was the 8th most common cancer in the registration areas of China in 2018. There were 84 593 new cases of thyroid cancer(21 198 males and 63 395 females,50 330 in urban areas and 34 263 in rural areas),accounting for 5.41% of new cases of all cancers. The crude incidence rate was 16.17 per 100 000, with ASR China 13.99 per 100 000 and ASR World 12.01 per 100 000, respectively. The incidence of ASR China was 2.93 times in females as that in males, and it was 1.79 times in urban areas as that in rural areas. The cumulative incidence rate for subjects aged from 0 to 74 years was 1.14%(Table 5-20a).

Thyroid cancer ranked 22nd for cancer mortality in the registration areas of China in 2018. A total of 3 232 cases died of thyroid cancer(1 187 males and 2 045 females,1 643 in urban areas and 1 589 in rural areas),accounting for 0.35% of all cancer deaths. The crude mortality rate was 0.62 per 100 000, with ASR China 0.38 per 100 000 and ASR World 0.37 per 100 000, respectively. The mortality of ASR China was 1.69 times in females as that in males, and it was 1.17 times in urban areas as that in rural areas. The cumulative mortality rate for subjects aged from 0 to 74 years was 0.04%(Table 5-20b).

The age-specific incidence rate of thyroid cancer showed differences between males and females. The incidence rate in females increased rapidly from the age group of 15-19 years and peaked at the age group of 50-54 years, while the incidence rate in males increased from the age group of 20-24 years with a slower speed. The age-specific incidence rates in females were generally higher than those in males. The age-specific mortality rate of thyroid cancer increased slowly from the age group of 40-44 years, and peaked at the age group of over 85 years(Figure 5-20a).

The incidence and mortality rates of thyroid cancer were higher in urban areas than those in rural areas. Eastern areas had the highest incidence rate(ASR China), followed by central and western areas. Central areas had the highest mortality rate(ASR China), followed by western and eastern areas. Among the seven administrative districts, the highest incidence rates(ASR China) were shown in Northeast China for both sexes, while the lowest incidence rates were shown in Northwest China for both sexes. The highest mortality rates(ASR China) were shown in Northeast China for both sexes, while the lowest mortality rates(ASR China) were shown in Southwest China and South China for males and females, respectively(Table 5-20a, Table 5-20b, Figure 5-20b).

About 87.60% cases of thyroid cancer had morphological verification. Among those, papillary thyroid cancer was the most common histological type, accounting for 93.43% of all cases, followed by other types(5.12%),follicular adenoma(1.27%) and medullary thyroid cancer(0.18%)(Figure 5-20c).

表 5-20a 2018 年中国肿瘤登记地区甲状腺癌发病情况
Table 5-20a Incidence of thyroid cancer in the registration areas of China,2018

地区 Area	性别 Sex	病例数 No. cases	粗率 Crude rate/ 100 000^{-1}	构成比 Freq./%	中标率 ASR China/ 100 000^{-1}	世标率 ASR World/ 100 000^{-1}	累积率 Cum. rate 0~74/%	顺位 Rank
合计	合计 Both	84 593	16. 17	5. 41	13. 99	12. 01	1. 14	8
All	男性 Male	21 198	7. 98	2. 46	7. 16	6. 04	0. 57	9
	女性 Female	63 395	24. 60	9. 01	20. 95	18. 09	1. 72	4
城市地区	合计 Both	50 330	21. 32	6. 65	18. 26	15. 58	1. 46	6
Urban areas	男性 Male	13 183	11. 13	3. 24	9. 89	8. 29	0. 77	7
	女性 Female	37 147	31. 60	10. 59	26. 60	22. 86	2. 16	3
农村地区	合计 Both	34 263	11. 93	4. 25	10. 31	8. 95	0. 86	8
Rural areas	男性 Male	8 015	5. 45	1. 77	4. 86	4. 17	0. 40	12
	女性 Female	26 248	18. 73	7. 44	15. 97	13. 92	1. 33	5
东部地区	合计 Both	55 451	25. 54	7. 23	21. 95	18. 74	1. 75	6
Eastern areas	男性 Male	14 316	13. 13	3. 50	11. 81	9. 89	0. 91	7
	女性 Female	41 135	38. 06	11. 49	32. 07	27. 59	2. 60	3
中部地区	合计 Both	16 241	12. 52	4. 65	10. 78	9. 41	0. 90	8
Central areas	男性 Male	3 778	5. 70	1. 97	5. 05	4. 35	0. 41	12
	女性 Female	12 463	19. 65	7. 88	16. 66	14. 61	1. 39	5
西部地区	合计 Both	12 901	7. 32	2. 88	6. 41	5. 52	0. 52	10
Western areas	男性 Male	3 104	3. 44	1. 19	3. 04	2. 62	0. 25	15
	女性 Female	9 797	11. 37	5. 23	9. 92	8. 56	0. 81	7

表 5-20b 2018 年中国肿瘤登记地区甲状腺癌死亡情况
Table 5-20b Mortality of thyroid cancer in the registration areas of China,2018

地区 Area	性别 Sex	死亡数 No. deaths	粗率 Crude rate/ 100 000^{-1}	构成比 Freq./%	中标率 ASR China/ 100 000^{-1}	世标率 ASR World/ 100 000^{-1}	累积率 Cum. rate 0~74/%	顺位 Rank
合计	合计 Both	3 232	0. 62	0. 35	0. 38	0. 37	0. 04	22
All	男性 Male	1 187	0. 45	0. 20	0. 28	0. 28	0. 03	19
	女性 Female	2 045	0. 79	0. 62	0. 47	0. 45	0. 05	20
城市地区	合计 Both	1 643	0. 70	0. 39	0. 41	0. 39	0. 04	22
Urban areas	男性 Male	627	0. 53	0. 24	0. 32	0. 31	0. 03	19
	女性 Female	1 016	0. 86	0. 66	0. 49	0. 47	0. 05	20
农村地区	合计 Both	1 589	0. 55	0. 32	0. 35	0. 34	0. 04	22
Rural areas	男性 Male	560	0. 38	0. 18	0. 25	0. 25	0. 03	19
	女性 Female	1 029	0. 73	0. 59	0. 46	0. 44	0. 05	20
东部地区	合计 Both	1 539	0. 71	0. 37	0. 38	0. 37	0. 04	22
Eastern areas	男性 Male	576	0. 53	0. 22	0. 30	0. 29	0. 03	19
	女性 Female	963	0. 89	0. 62	0. 46	0. 45	0. 05	20
中部地区	合计 Both	783	0. 60	0. 37	0. 41	0. 40	0. 04	22
Central areas	男性 Male	282	0. 43	0. 21	0. 29	0. 29	0. 03	19
	女性 Female	501	0. 79	0. 66	0. 52	0. 50	0. 05	20
西部地区	合计 Both	910	0. 52	0. 32	0. 35	0. 34	0. 04	22
Western areas	男性 Male	329	0. 36	0. 18	0. 25	0. 25	0. 03	19
	女性 Female	581	0. 67	0. 60	0. 45	0. 42	0. 04	20

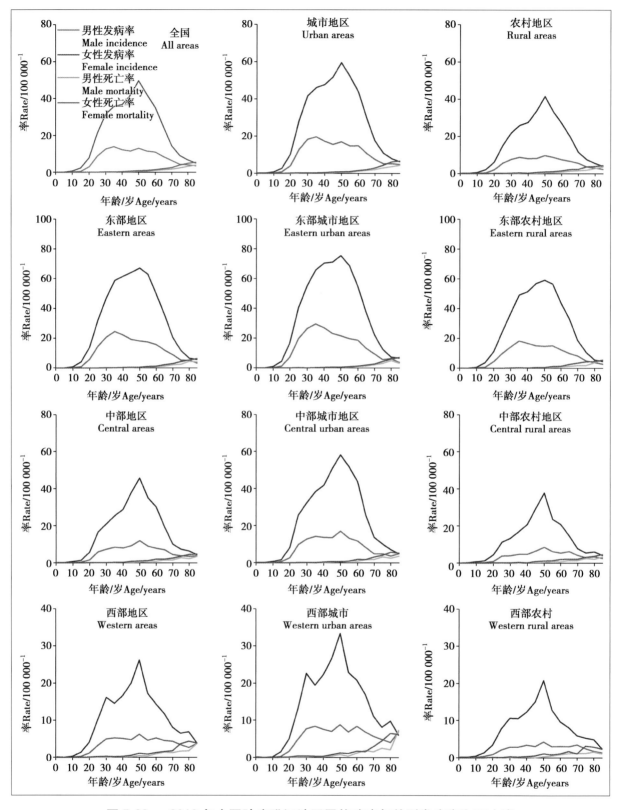

图 5-20a　2018 年中国肿瘤登记地区甲状腺癌年龄别发病率和死亡率

Figure 5-20a　Age-specific incidence and mortality rates of thyroid cancer in the registration areas of China, 2018

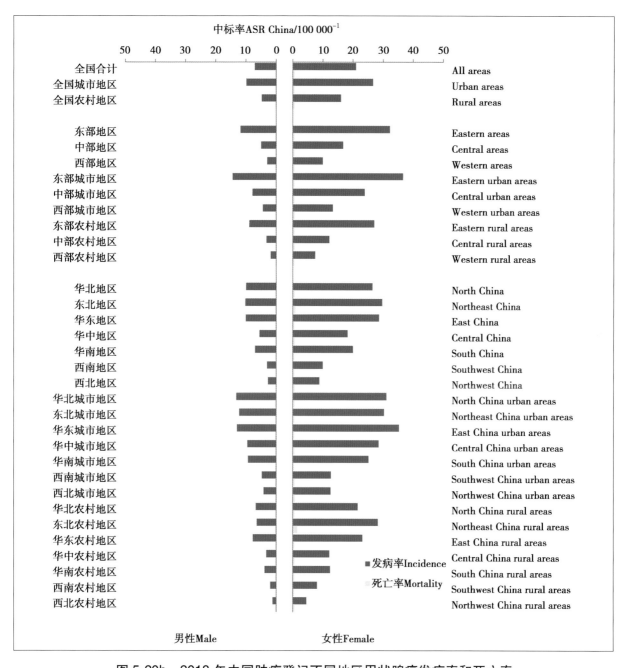

图 5-20b　2018 年中国肿瘤登记不同地区甲状腺癌发病率和死亡率

Figure 5-20b　Incidence and mortality rates of thyroid cancer in different registration areas of China,2018

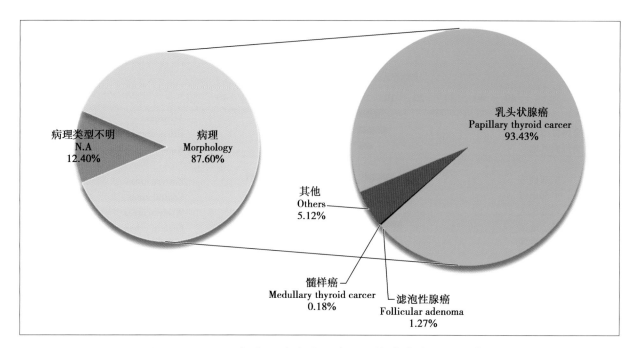

图 5-20c　2018 年中国肿瘤登记地区甲状腺癌病理分型情况

Figure 5-20c　Morphological distribution of thyroid cancer in the
registration areas of China, 2018

21 淋巴瘤

2018 年,中国肿瘤登记地区淋巴瘤位居癌症发病谱第 14 位。新发病例数为 34 440 例,占全部癌症发病的 2.20%;其中男性 19 748 例,女性 14 692 例;城市地区 18 107 例,农村地区 16 333 例。发病率为 6.58/10 万,中标发病率为 4.38/10 万,世标发病率为 4.29/10 万;男性中标发病率是女性的 1.37 倍,城市中标发病率是农村的 1.26 倍。0~74 岁累积发病率为 0.49%(表 5-21a)。

2018 年,中国肿瘤登记地区淋巴瘤位居癌症死亡谱第 12 位。因淋巴瘤死亡病例 19 372 例,占全部癌症死亡的 2.12%;其中男性 11 751 例,女性 7 621 例,城市地区 9 787 例,农村地区 9 585 例。淋巴瘤死亡率为 3.70/10 万,中标死亡率 2.25/10 万,世标死亡率 2.21/10 万;男性中标死亡率为女性的 1.63 倍,城市中标死亡率为农村的 1.20 倍。0~74 岁累积死亡率为 0.25%(表 5-21b)。

淋巴瘤年龄别发病率在 35 岁以前处于较低水平,自 35~39 岁组开始快速上升,男性和女性发病率分别于 80~84 岁组和 75~79 岁组达到高峰。淋巴瘤年龄别死亡率从 40~44 岁组开始快速上升,男性死亡率至 85 岁及以上年龄组达到高峰,女性死亡率至 80~84 岁组达到高峰。总体上,男性年龄别发病率和死亡率均高于女性(图 5-21a)。

城市地区淋巴瘤的发病率和死亡率均高于农村地区。中标发病率和死亡率均为东部地区最高,其次是中部地区,西部地区最低。七大行政区中,华南地区的中标发病率和中标死亡率最高,西北地区的中标发病率和中标死亡率最低(表 5-21a,表 5-21b,图 5-21b)。

全部淋巴瘤病例中,非霍奇金淋巴瘤的其他和未特指类型(ICD-10:C85)是最主要的病理类型,占 40.40%;其次是多发性骨髓瘤和恶性浆细胞性肿瘤(C90),占 24.23%;弥漫性非霍奇金淋巴瘤(C83),占 20.16%;霍奇金淋巴瘤(C81),占 4.70%;周围和皮肤 T 细胞淋巴瘤(C84),占 4.11%;滤泡性非霍奇金淋巴瘤(C82),占 4.11%;其他和未特指的淋巴、造血和有关组织的恶性肿瘤(C96),占 1.15%;以及恶性免疫增生性疾病(C88),占 1.14%(图 5-21c)。

21 Lymphoma

Lymphoma ranked 14th for cancer incidence in the registration areas of China in 2018. There were 34 440 new cases of lymphoma(19 748 males and 14 692 females,18 107 in urban areas and 16 333 in rural areas), accounting for 2.20% of all new cancer cases. The crude incidence rate was 6.58 per 100 000, with ASR China 4.38 per 100 000 and ASR World 4.29 per 100 000, respectively. The incidence of the ASR China was 1.37 times in males as that in females, and it was 1.26 times in urban areas as that in rural areas. The cumulative incidence rate for subjects aged from 0 to 74 years was 0.49%(Table 5-21a).

Lymphoma ranked 12th for cancer mortality in the registration areas of China in 2018. A total of 19 372 cases died of lymphoma(11 751 males and 7 621 females,9 787 in urban areas and 9 585 in rural areas), accounting for 2.12% of all cancer deaths. The crude mortality rate was 3.70 per 100 000, with ASR China 2.25 per 100 000 and ASR World 2.21 per 100 000, respectively. The mortality rate of the ASR China was 1.63 times in males as that in females, and it was 1.20 times in the urban areas as that in rural areas. The cumulative mortality rate for subjects aged from 0 to 74 years was 0.25%(Table 5-21b).

The age-specific incidence rate of lymphoma was relatively low before 35 years old and increased rapidly from the age group of 35-39 years and then peaked at the age group of 80-84 years and 75-79 years for males and females, respectively. The age-specific mortality rate of lymphoma increased rapidly from the age group of 40-44 years, and peaked at the age group of 85 years and above and 80-84 years for males and females, respectively. The age-specific incidence and mortality rates of lymphoma were generally higher in males than those in females(Figure 5-21a).

The incidence and mortality rates of lymphoma were higher in urban areas than those in rural areas. Eastern areas had the highest incidence rate and mortality rate(ASR China), followed by the central areas and western areas. Among the seven administrative districts, the highest incidence and mortality rates(ASR China) were shown in South China, while the lowest incidence and mortality rates(ASR China) rates were shown in Northwest China(Table 5-21a, Table 5-21b, Figure 5-21b).

Among all lymphoma cases, other and unspecified types of non-Hodgkin's(ICD-10:C85) was the most common histological type, accounting for 40.40% of all cases, followed by multiple myeloma & malignant plasma cell neoplasms(C90, 24.23%), diffuse non-Hodgkin's lymphoma(C83, 20.16%), Hodgkin's disease(C81,4.70%), peripheral & cutaneous T-cell lymphoma(C84, 4.11%), follicular non-Hodgkin's lymphoma(C82,4.11%), other and unspecified malignant neoplasms of lymphoid, hematopoietic and related tissue(C96 1.15%), and malignant immunoproliferative disease(C88,1.14%)(Figure 5-21c).

表 5-21a 2018 年中国肿瘤登记地区淋巴瘤发病情况
Table 5-21a Incidence of lymphoma in the registration areas of China,2018

地区 Area	性别 Sex	病例数 No. cases	粗率 Crude rate/ 100 000⁻¹	构成比 Freq./%	中标率 ASR China/ 100 000⁻¹	世标率 ASR World/ 100 000⁻¹	累积率 Cum. rate 0~74/%	顺位 Rank
合计 All	合计 Both	34 440	6.58	2.20	4.38	4.29	0.49	14
	男性 Male	19 748	7.44	2.30	5.07	4.98	0.57	10
	女性 Female	14 692	5.70	2.09	3.70	3.61	0.41	13
城市地区 Urban areas	合计 Both	18 107	7.67	2.39	4.91	4.80	0.54	14
	男性 Male	10 283	8.68	2.53	5.70	5.58	0.63	10
	女性 Female	7 824	6.66	2.23	4.15	4.04	0.46	12
农村地区 Rural areas	合计 Both	16 333	5.69	2.02	3.91	3.84	0.44	15
	男性 Male	9 465	6.44	2.08	4.53	4.46	0.51	10
	女性 Female	6 868	4.90	1.95	3.29	3.22	0.37	14
东部地区 Eastern areas	合计 Both	18 722	8.62	2.44	5.24	5.11	0.58	14
	男性 Male	10 547	9.67	2.58	6.04	5.93	0.67	10
	女性 Female	8 175	7.56	2.28	4.48	4.34	0.50	13
中部地区 Central areas	合计 Both	7 219	5.57	2.07	4.04	3.99	0.45	14
	男性 Male	4 235	6.39	2.21	4.77	4.72	0.54	9
	女性 Female	2 984	4.71	1.89	3.30	3.27	0.37	14
西部地区 Western areas	合计 Both	8 499	4.82	1.90	3.44	3.35	0.38	14
	男性 Male	4 966	5.51	1.91	3.98	3.89	0.44	11
	女性 Female	3 533	4.10	1.89	2.90	2.81	0.32	14

表 5-21b 2018 年中国肿瘤登记地区淋巴瘤死亡情况

Table 5-21b Mortality of lymphoma in the registration areas of China,2018

地区 Area	性别 Sex	死亡数 No. deaths	粗率 Crude rate/ 100 000⁻¹	构成比 Freq./%	中标率 ASR China/ 100 000⁻¹	世标率 ASR World/ 100 000⁻¹	累积率 Cum. rate 0~74/%	顺位 Rank
合计 All	合计 Both	19 372	3.70	2.12	2.25	2.22	0.25	12
	男性 Male	11 751	4.43	2.01	2.81	2.77	0.31	9
	女性 Female	7 621	2.96	2.32	1.72	1.69	0.19	13
城市地区 Urban areas	合计 Both	9 787	4.15	2.33	2.39	2.36	0.26	11
	男性 Male	5 969	5.04	2.24	3.03	2.99	0.33	8
	女性 Female	3 818	3.25	2.48	1.80	1.77	0.20	13
农村地区 Rural areas	合计 Both	9 585	3.34	1.95	2.12	2.09	0.24	12
	男性 Male	5 782	3.93	1.82	2.60	2.57	0.30	10
	女性 Female	3 803	2.71	2.18	1.65	1.62	0.19	13
东部地区 Eastern areas	合计 Both	10 506	4.84	2.51	2.60	2.56	0.29	9
	男性 Male	6 289	5.77	2.38	3.26	3.22	0.36	8
	女性 Female	4 217	3.90	2.72	1.99	1.96	0.22	12
中部地区 Central areas	合计 Both	4 111	3.17	1.95	2.14	2.10	0.25	13
	男性 Male	2 508	3.78	1.87	2.65	2.62	0.30	9
	女性 Female	1 603	2.53	2.10	1.63	1.61	0.19	13
西部地区 Western areas	合计 Both	4 755	2.70	1.68	1.82	1.79	0.20	14
	男性 Male	2 954	3.28	1.58	2.27	2.24	0.25	10
	女性 Female	1 801	2.09	1.86	1.37	1.34	0.16	14

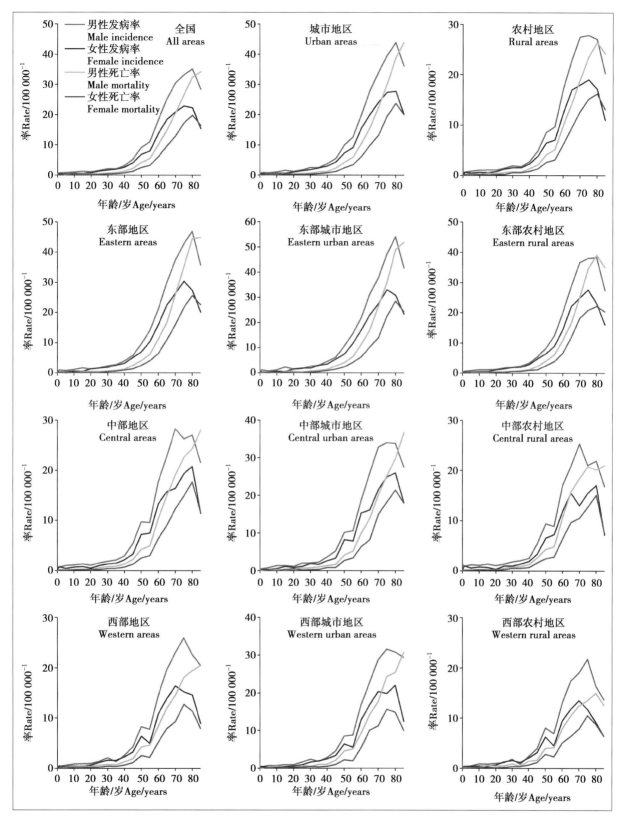

图 5-21a　2018 年中国肿瘤登记地区淋巴瘤年龄别发病率和死亡率

Figure 5-21a　Age-specific incidence and mortality rates of lymphoma in the registration areas of China, 2018

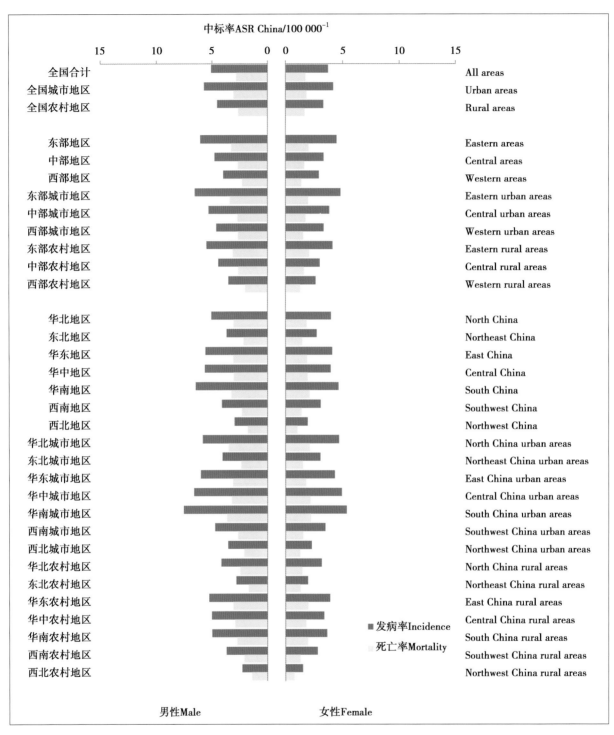

图 5-21b　2018 年中国肿瘤登记不同地区淋巴瘤发病率和死亡率

Figure 5-21b　Incidence and mortality rates of lymphoma in different registration areas of China, 2018

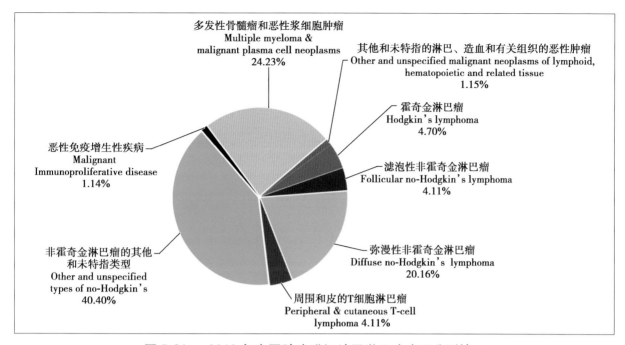

图 5-21c　2018 年中国肿瘤登记地区淋巴瘤病理分型情况

Figure 5-21c　Morphological distribution of lymphoma in the registration areas of China,2018

22 白血病

2018 年,中国肿瘤登记地区白血病位居癌症发病谱第 15 位。新发病例数为 31 788 例,占全部癌症发病的 2.03%;其中男性 18 114 例,女性 13 674 例;城市地区 15 088 例,农村地区 16 700 例。白血病发病率为 6.08/10 万,中标发病率为 4.66/10 万,世标发病率为 4.80/10 万;男性中标发病率为女性的 1.30 倍。0~74 岁累积率为 0.45%(表 5-22a)。

2018 年,中国肿瘤登记地区白血病位居癌症死亡谱第 11 位。因白血病死亡病例为 20 038 例,占全部癌症死亡的 2.20%;其中男性 11 723 例,女性 8 315 例;城市地区 9 397 例,农村地区 10 641 例。白血病死亡率为 3.83/10 万,中标死亡率为 2.68/10 万,世标死亡率为 2.68/10 万;男性中标死亡率为女性的 1.43 倍。0~74 岁累积死亡率为 0.27%(表 5-22b)。

白血病年龄别发病率在 0~4 岁年龄组出现一个小高峰,在 5~39 岁趋于平缓,40 岁后开始快速上升,至 80~84 岁年龄组达到高峰。白血病年龄别死亡率从 40~44 岁组开始快速上升,男性死亡率至 85 岁及以上年龄组达到高峰,女性死亡率至 80~84 岁组达到高峰(图 5-22a)。

22 Leukemia

Leukemia ranked 15th for cancer incidence in the registration areas of China in 2018. There were 31 788 new cases of leukemia(18 114 males and 13 674 females,15 088 in urban areas and 16 700 in rural areas), accounting for 2.03% of all cancer cases. The crude incidence rate was 6.08 per 100 000,with ASR China 4.66 per 100 000 and ASR World 4.80 per 100 000, respectively. The incidence of ASR China was 1.30 times in males as that in females. The cumulative incidence rate for subjects aged from 0 to 74 years was 0.45%(Table 5-22a).

Leukemia ranked 11th for cancer mortality in the registration areas of China in 2018. A total of 20 038 cases died of leukemia(11 723 males and 8 315 females,9 397 in urban areas and 10 641 in rural areas), accounting for 2.20% of all cancer deaths. The crude mortality rate was 3.83 per 100 000,with ASR China 2.68 per 100 000 and ASR World 2.68 per 100 000,respectively. The mortality of ASR China was 1.43 times in males as that in females. The cumulative mortality rate for subjects aged from 0 to 74 years was 0.27%(Table 5-22b).

The first peak of the age-specific incidence rate of leukemia occurred in the age group of 0-4 years. Age-specific incidence and mortality rates were relatively stable at 5-39 years and dramatically increased after the age of 40,and peaked at the age group of 80-84 years. The age-specific mortality rate of leukemia increased rapidly from the age group of 40-44 years, and peaked at the age group of 85 years and above and 80-84 years for males and females, respectively (Figure 5-22a).

城市地区白血病发病率和死亡率与农村地区接近。东部地区的中标发病率最高,其次是中部地区和西部地区。七大行政区中,华南地区中标发病率和中标死亡率最高,西北地区中标发病率和中标死亡率最低(表5-22a,表5-22b,图5-22b)。

全部白血病新发病例中,髓样白血病(ICD-10:C92)是最主要的病理类型,占35.81%;其次是未特指细胞类型的白血病(C95),占33.94%;淋巴样白血病(C91),占22.29%;特指细胞类型的其他白血病(C94),占4.28%;以及单核细胞白血病(C93),占3.68%(图5-22c)。

2018年,中国肿瘤登记地区淋巴样白血病新发病例为6 146例,发病率为1.17/10万(中标率为1.00/10万,世标率为1.15/10万),占全部癌症发病的0.39%。淋巴样白血病死亡病例为3 871例,死亡率为0.74/10万(中标率为0.57/10万,世标率为0.58/10万),占全部癌症死亡的0.42%(表5-22c,表5-22d)。

2018年,中国肿瘤登记地区髓样白血病新发病例为16 279例,发病率为3.11/10万(中标率为2.28/10万,世标率为2.22/10万),占全部癌症发病的1.04%。髓样白血病死亡病例为8 244例,死亡率为1.58/10万(中标率为1.04/10万,世标率为1.02/10万),占全部癌症死亡的0.90%(表5-22e,表5-22f)。

The incidence and mortality rates of leukemia in urban areas were close to those in rural areas. Eastern areas had the highest incidence rate(ASR China), followed by central areas and western areas. Among the seven administrative districts, South China had the highest incidence and mortality rates(ASR China) while Northwest China had the lowest incidence and mortality rates(ASR China)(Table 5-22a, Table 5-22b, Figure 5-22b).

Among all leukemia cases, myeloid leukemia(ICD-10:C92) was the most common histological type, accounting for 35.81% of all cases, followed by leukemia of unspecified cell type(C95, 33.94%), lymphoid leukemia(C91, 22.29%), other leukemias(C94, 4.28%) and monocytic leukemia(C93, 3.68%)(Figure 5-22c).

There were 6 146 new cases diagnosed as lymphoid leukemia in the registration areas of China in 2018, accounting for 0.39% of all cancer cases. The crude incidence rate was 1.17 per 100 000, with ASR China 1.00 per 100 000 and ASR World 1.15 per 100 000, respectively. A total of 3 871 cases died of lymphoid leukemia, accounting for 0.42% of all cancer deaths. The crude mortality rate was 0.74 per 100 000, with ASR China 0.57 per 100 000 and ASR World 0.58 per 100 000, respectively(Table 5-22c, Table 5-22d).

There were 16 279 new cases diagnosed as myeloid leukemia in the registration areas of China in 2018, accounting for 1.04% of all cancer cases. The crude incidence rate was 3.11 per 100 000, with ASR China 2.28 per 100 000 and ASR World 2.22 per 100 000, respectively. A total of 8 244 cases died of myeloid leukemia, accounting for 0.90% of all cancer deaths. The crude mortality rate of myeloid leukemia was 1.58 per 100 000, with ASR China 1.04 per 100 000 and ASR World 1.02 per 100 000, respectively(Table 5-22e, Table 5-22f).

表 5-22a　2018 年中国肿瘤登记地区白血病发病情况

Table 5-22a　Incidence of leukemia in the registration areas of China,2018

地区 Area	性别 Sex	病例数 No. cases	粗率 Crude rate/ 100 000^{-1}	构成比 Freq./%	中标率 ASR China/ 100 000^{-1}	世标率 ASR World/ 100 000^{-1}	累积率 Cum. rate 0~74/%	顺位 Rank
合计	合计 Both	31 788	6. 08	2. 03	4. 66	4. 80	0. 45	15
All	男性 Male	18 114	6. 82	2. 11	5. 27	5. 41	0. 51	12
	女性 Female	13 674	5. 31	1. 94	4. 06	4. 20	0. 39	14
城市地区	合计 Both	15 088	6. 39	1. 99	4. 69	4. 89	0. 45	17
Urban areas	男性 Male	8 710	7. 35	2. 14	5. 43	5. 63	0. 52	12
	女性 Female	6 378	5. 43	1. 82	3. 98	4. 17	0. 38	14
农村地区	合计 Both	16 700	5. 82	2. 07	4. 61	4. 72	0. 44	14
Rural areas	男性 Male	9 404	6. 40	2. 07	5. 12	5. 22	0. 49	11
	女性 Female	7 296	5. 21	2. 07	4. 11	4. 21	0. 39	13
东部地区	合计 Both	16 611	7. 65	2. 17	5. 45	5. 65	0. 52	15
Eastern areas	男性 Male	9 519	8. 73	2. 33	6. 24	6. 45	0. 61	12
	女性 Female	7 092	6. 56	1. 98	4. 70	4. 88	0. 44	14
中部地区	合计 Both	7 041	5. 43	2. 01	4. 48	4. 62	0. 43	15
Central areas	男性 Male	4 019	6. 06	2. 10	5. 04	5. 17	0. 48	11
	女性 Female	3 022	4. 76	1. 91	3. 91	4. 06	0. 37	13
西部地区	合计 Both	8 136	4. 61	1. 82	3. 73	3. 79	0. 35	16
Western areas	男性 Male	4 576	5. 08	1. 76	4. 12	4. 19	0. 39	13
	女性 Female	3 560	4. 13	1. 90	3. 33	3. 39	0. 32	13

表 5-22b　2018 年中国肿瘤登记地区白血病死亡情况

Table 5-22b　Mortality of leukemia in the registration areas of China,2018

地区 Area	性别 Sex	死亡数 No. deaths	粗率 Crude rate/ 100 000^{-1}	构成比 Freq./%	中标率 ASR China/ 100 000^{-1}	世标率 ASR World/ 100 000^{-1}	累积率 Cum. rate 0~74/%	顺位 Rank
合计	合计 Both	20 038	3. 83	2. 20	2. 68	2. 68	0. 27	11
All	男性 Male	11 723	4. 42	2. 01	3. 17	3. 15	0. 31	10
	女性 Female	8 315	3. 23	2. 53	2. 21	2. 22	0. 22	12
城市地区	合计 Both	9 397	3. 98	2. 24	2. 61	2. 62	0. 26	13
Urban areas	男性 Male	5 499	4. 64	2. 06	3. 10	3. 11	0. 31	9
	女性 Female	3 898	3. 32	2. 54	2. 15	2. 17	0. 21	12
农村地区	合计 Both	10 641	3. 71	2. 16	2. 73	2. 72	0. 27	11
Rural areas	男性 Male	6 224	4. 23	1. 96	3. 20	3. 17	0. 31	8
	女性 Female	4 417	3. 15	2. 53	2. 26	2. 27	0. 23	10
东部地区	合计 Both	9 979	4. 60	2. 38	2. 85	2. 84	0. 28	11
Eastern areas	男性 Male	5 804	5. 32	2. 20	3. 38	3. 37	0. 34	9
	女性 Female	4 175	3. 86	2. 69	2. 35	2. 36	0. 23	13
中部地区	合计 Both	4 479	3. 45	2. 13	2. 64	2. 63	0. 26	11
Central areas	男性 Male	2 702	4. 08	2. 01	3. 19	3. 17	0. 31	8
	女性 Female	1 777	2. 80	2. 33	2. 09	2. 08	0. 22	12
西部地区	合计 Both	5 580	3. 16	1. 97	2. 44	2. 45	0. 24	11
Western areas	男性 Male	3 217	3. 57	1. 73	2. 80	2. 79	0. 27	9
	女性 Female	2 363	2. 74	2. 44	2. 09	2. 11	0. 21	11

表 5-22c　2018 年中国肿瘤登记地区淋巴样白血病发病情况
Table 5-22c　Incidence of lymphoid leukemia in the registration areas of China, 2018

地区 Area	性别 Sex	病例数 No. cases	粗率 Crude rate/ 100 000^{-1}	构成比 Freq./%	中标率 ASR China/ 100 000^{-1}	世标率 ASR World/ 100 000^{-1}	累积率 Cum. rate 0~74/%
合计 All	合计 Both	6 146	1.17	0.39	1.00	1.15	0.09
	男性 Male	3 529	1.33	0.41	1.12	1.29	0.10
	女性 Female	2 617	1.02	0.37	0.88	1.02	0.08
城市地区 Urban areas	合计 Both	3 187	1.35	0.42	1.14	1.34	0.10
	男性 Male	1 819	1.54	0.45	1.28	1.49	0.12
	女性 Female	1 368	1.16	0.39	1.01	1.20	0.09
农村地区 Rural areas	合计 Both	2 959	1.03	0.37	0.89	1.00	0.08
	男性 Male	1 710	1.16	0.38	1.00	1.13	0.09
	女性 Female	1 249	0.89	0.35	0.78	0.87	0.07
东部地区 Eastern areas	合计 Both	3 459	1.59	0.45	1.35	1.59	0.12
	男性 Male	1 984	1.82	0.49	1.50	1.77	0.14
	女性 Female	1 475	1.36	0.41	1.19	1.42	0.10
中部地区 Central areas	合计 Both	1 269	0.98	0.36	0.87	0.97	0.08
	男性 Male	732	1.10	0.38	0.98	1.09	0.09
	女性 Female	537	0.85	0.34	0.75	0.85	0.07
西部地区 Western areas	合计 Both	1 418	0.80	0.32	0.68	0.75	0.06
	男性 Male	813	0.90	0.31	0.76	0.83	0.07
	女性 Female	605	0.70	0.32	0.60	0.66	0.05

表 5-22d　2018 年中国肿瘤登记地区淋巴样白血病死亡情况
Table 5-22d　Mortality of lymphoid leukemia in the registration areas of China, 2018

地区 Area	性别 Sex	死亡数 No. deaths	粗率 Crude rate/ 100 000^{-1}	构成比 Freq./%	中标率 ASR China/ 100 000^{-1}	世标率 ASR World/ 100 000^{-1}	累积率 Cum. rate 0~74/%
合计 All	合计 Both	3 871	0.74	0.42	0.57	0.58	0.05
	男性 Male	2 273	0.86	0.39	0.66	0.68	0.06
	女性 Female	1 598	0.62	0.49	0.47	0.48	0.04
城市地区 Urban areas	合计 Both	1 903	0.81	0.45	0.59	0.61	0.05
	男性 Male	1 118	0.94	0.42	0.69	0.71	0.06
	女性 Female	785	0.67	0.51	0.49	0.51	0.05
农村地区 Rural areas	合计 Both	1 968	0.69	0.40	0.54	0.55	0.05
	男性 Male	1 155	0.79	0.36	0.64	0.64	0.06
	女性 Female	813	0.58	0.47	0.45	0.45	0.04
东部地区 Eastern areas	合计 Both	1 890	0.87	0.45	0.63	0.65	0.06
	男性 Male	1 093	1.00	0.41	0.74	0.75	0.07
	女性 Female	797	0.74	0.51	0.53	0.55	0.05
中部地区 Central areas	合计 Both	840	0.65	0.40	0.52	0.52	0.05
	男性 Male	505	0.76	0.38	0.62	0.63	0.06
	女性 Female	335	0.53	0.44	0.42	0.41	0.04
西部地区 Western areas	合计 Both	1 141	0.65	0.40	0.52	0.53	0.05
	男性 Male	675	0.75	0.36	0.61	0.62	0.05
	女性 Female	466	0.54	0.48	0.44	0.44	0.04

表 5-22e　2018 年中国肿瘤登记地区髓样白血病发病情况

Table 5-22e　Incidence of myeloid leukemia in the registration areas of China,2018

地区 Area	性别 Sex	病例数 No. cases	粗率 Crude rate/ 100 000^{-1}	构成比 Freq. /%	中标率 ASR China/ 100 000^{-1}	世标率 ASR World/ 100 000^{-1}	累积率 Cum. rate 0~74/%
合计	合计 Both	16 279	3.11	1.04	2.28	2.22	0.23
All	男性 Male	9 308	3.51	1.08	2.59	2.53	0.26
	女性 Female	6 971	2.71	0.99	1.97	1.92	0.19
城市地区	合计 Both	8 474	3.59	1.12	2.50	2.45	0.25
Urban areas	男性 Male	4 953	4.18	1.22	2.95	2.88	0.29
	女性 Female	3 521	3.00	1.00	2.07	2.03	0.21
农村地区	合计 Both	7 805	2.72	0.97	2.08	2.02	0.21
Rural areas	男性 Male	4 355	2.96	0.96	2.28	2.23	0.23
	女性 Female	3 450	2.46	0.98	1.88	1.81	0.18
东部地区	合计 Both	9 926	4.57	1.29	3.09	3.02	0.31
Eastern areas	男性 Male	5 680	5.21	1.39	3.55	3.47	0.36
	女性 Female	4 246	3.93	1.19	2.66	2.59	0.26
中部地区	合计 Both	2 918	2.25	0.83	1.79	1.76	0.18
Central areas	男性 Male	1 688	2.55	0.88	2.05	2.01	0.20
	女性 Female	1 230	1.94	0.78	1.53	1.51	0.15
西部地区	合计 Both	3 435	1.95	0.77	1.55	1.48	0.15
Western areas	男性 Male	1 940	2.15	0.75	1.72	1.65	0.16
	女性 Female	1 495	1.74	0.80	1.37	1.31	0.13

表 5-22f　2018 年中国肿瘤登记地区髓样白血病死亡情况

Table 5-22f　Mortality of myeloid leukemia in the registration areas of China,2018

地区 Area	性别 Sex	死亡数 No. deaths	粗率 Crude rate/ 100 000^{-1}	构成比 Freq. /%	中标率 ASR China/ 100 000^{-1}	世标率 ASR World/ 100 000^{-1}	累积率 Cum. rate 0~74/%
合计	合计 Both	8 244	1.58	0.90	1.04	1.02	0.11
All	男性 Male	4 833	1.82	0.83	1.23	1.21	0.13
	女性 Female	3 411	1.32	1.04	0.86	0.85	0.09
城市地区	合计 Both	4 389	1.86	1.04	1.15	1.14	0.12
Urban areas	男性 Male	2 593	2.19	0.97	1.38	1.36	0.14
	女性 Female	1 796	1.53	1.17	0.93	0.92	0.10
农村地区	合计 Both	3 855	1.34	0.78	0.94	0.92	0.10
Rural areas	男性 Male	2 240	1.52	0.70	1.09	1.07	0.11
	女性 Female	1 615	1.15	0.93	0.80	0.78	0.08
东部地区	合计 Both	4 850	2.23	1.16	1.31	1.28	0.13
Eastern areas	男性 Male	2 853	2.62	1.08	1.57	1.54	0.16
	女性 Female	1 997	1.85	1.29	1.07	1.05	0.11
中部地区	合计 Both	1 562	1.20	0.74	0.87	0.87	0.09
Central areas	男性 Male	963	1.45	0.72	1.08	1.07	0.11
	女性 Female	599	0.94	0.79	0.67	0.68	0.07
西部地区	合计 Both	1 832	1.04	0.65	0.77	0.76	0.08
Western areas	男性 Male	1 017	1.13	0.55	0.85	0.83	0.09
	女性 Female	815	0.95	0.84	0.70	0.69	0.07

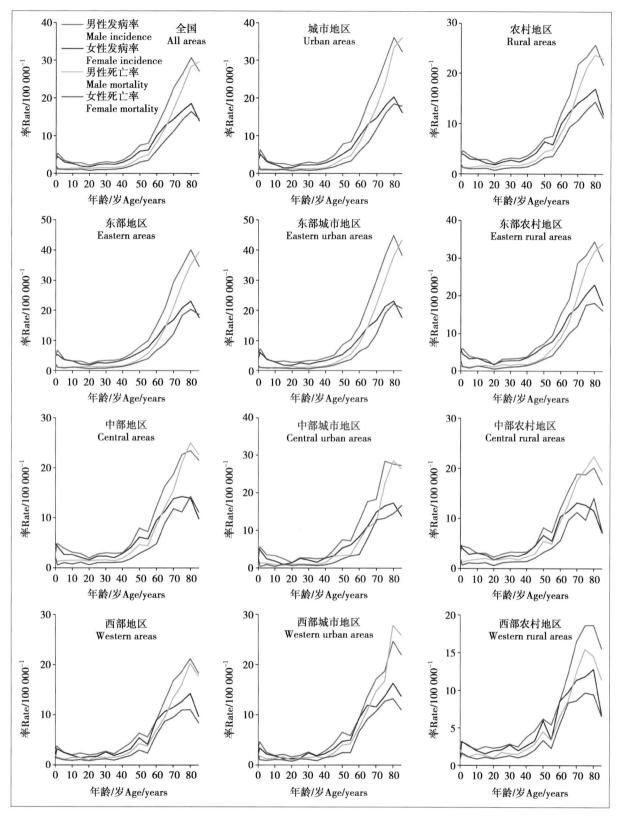

图 5-22a　2018 年中国肿瘤登记地区白血病年龄别发病率和死亡率

Figure 5-22a　Age-specific incidence and mortality rates of leukemia in the registration areas of China, 2018

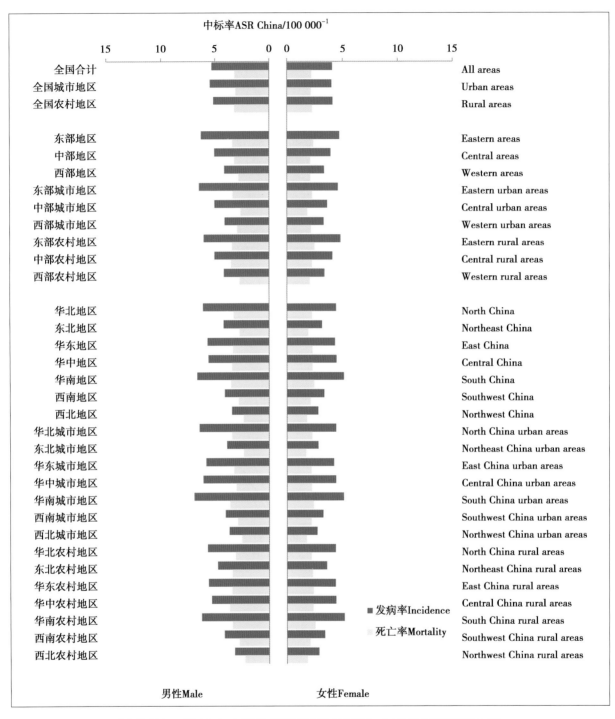

中标率ASR China/100 000⁻¹

全国合计	All areas
全国城市地区	Urban areas
全国农村地区	Rural areas
东部地区	Eastern areas
中部地区	Central areas
西部地区	Western areas
东部城市地区	Eastern urban areas
中部城市地区	Central urban areas
西部城市地区	Western urban areas
东部农村地区	Eastern rural areas
中部农村地区	Central rural areas
西部农村地区	Western rural areas
华北地区	North China
东北地区	Northeast China
华东地区	East China
华中地区	Central China
华南地区	South China
西南地区	Southwest China
西北地区	Northwest China
华北城市地区	North China urban areas
东北城市地区	Northeast China urban areas
华东城市地区	East China urban areas
华中城市地区	Central China urban areas
华南城市地区	South China urban areas
西南城市地区	Southwest China urban areas
西北城市地区	Northwest China urban areas
华北农村地区	North China rural areas
东北农村地区	Northeast China rural areas
华东农村地区	East China rural areas
华中农村地区	Central China rural areas
华南农村地区	South China rural areas
西南农村地区	Southwest China rural areas
西北农村地区	Northwest China rural areas

■ 发病率Incidence
死亡率Mortality

男性Male　　　　女性Female

图 5-22b　2018 年中国肿瘤登记不同地区白血病发病率和死亡率

Figure 5-22b　Incidence and mortality rates of leukemia in different registration areas of China, 2018

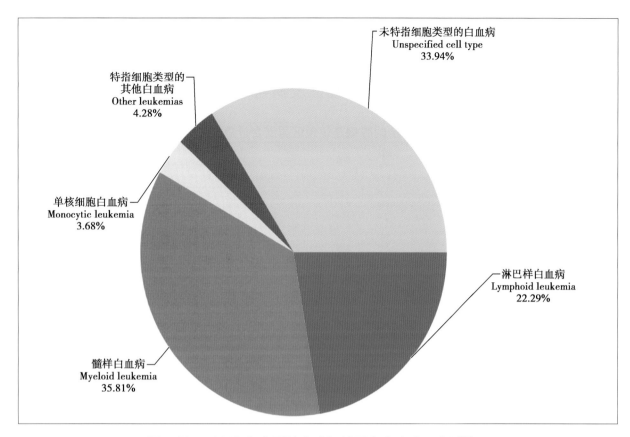

图 5-22c 2018 年中国肿瘤登记地区白血病病理分型情况

Figure 5-22c Morphological distribution of leukemia in the registration
areas of China,2018

附录

附录 1　2018 年全国肿瘤登记地区癌症发病与死亡结果

附表 1-1　2018 年全国肿瘤登记地区男女合计癌症发病主要指标

部位 Site		病例数 No. cases	构成 Freq. /%	年龄组								
				0~	1~4	5~9	10~14	15~19	20~24	25~29	30~34	35~39
唇	Lip	976	0.06	0.02	0.01	0.01	0.02	0.01	0.00	0.02	0.02	0.02
舌	Tongue	4 615	0.30	0.00	0.01	0.02	0.03	0.00	0.05	0.11	0.25	0.37
口	Mouth	5 948	0.38	0.02	0.03	0.03	0.03	0.07	0.06	0.11	0.23	0.25
唾液腺	Salivary glands	3 220	0.21	0.00	0.02	0.02	0.06	0.11	0.15	0.26	0.32	0.35
扁桃腺	Tonsil	907	0.06	0.00	0.02	0.03	0.00	0.01	0.01	0.02	0.02	0.04
其他口咽	Other oropharynx	1 375	0.09	0.00	0.00	0.01	0.01	0.01	0.02	0.01	0.02	0.05
鼻咽	Nasopharynx	19 564	1.25	0.00	0.05	0.04	0.12	0.28	0.42	0.82	1.81	2.69
下咽	Hypopharynx	2 652	0.17	0.02	0.00	0.00	0.00	0.00	0.01	0.01	0.01	0.03
咽,部位不明	Pharynx unspecified	1 354	0.09	0.00	0.01	0.01	0.00	0.00	0.01	0.03	0.02	0.03
食管	Esophagus	93 945	6.01	0.00	0.01	0.00	0.02	0.02	0.05	0.14	0.19	0.43
胃	Stomach	141 415	9.04	0.09	0.01	0.03	0.09	0.18	0.36	1.17	2.26	3.20
小肠	Small intestine	6 443	0.41	0.00	0.02	0.00	0.01	0.01	0.03	0.09	0.16	0.25
结肠	Colon	78 460	5.02	0.00	0.03	0.01	0.07	0.21	0.37	0.95	1.83	2.83
直肠	Rectum	79 281	5.07	0.02	0.02	0.02	0.02	0.09	0.24	0.68	1.51	2.17
肛门	Anus	1 894	0.12	0.00	0.00	0.00	0.00	0.01	0.02	0.06	0.04	0.07
肝脏	Liver	143 438	9.17	1.25	0.44	0.14	0.18	0.29	0.68	1.84	4.26	7.62
胆囊及其他	Gallbladder etc.	21 260	1.36	0.00	0.00	0.00	0.00	0.01	0.03	0.06	0.14	0.31
胰腺	Pancreas	37 617	2.41	0.00	0.02	0.01	0.02	0.06	0.10	0.20	0.38	0.67
鼻、鼻窦及其他	Nose,sinuses etc.	2 269	0.15	0.02	0.04	0.03	0.03	0.05	0.08	0.09	0.10	0.17
喉	Larynx	9 898	0.63	0.02	0.01	0.01	0.01	0.02	0.00	0.03	0.04	0.10
气管、支气管、肺	Trachea,bronchus & lung	340 332	21.76	0.06	0.08	0.04	0.15	0.25	0.69	1.92	3.99	7.43
其他胸腔器官	Other thoracic organs	5 191	0.33	0.30	0.22	0.08	0.09	0.21	0.18	0.29	0.39	0.44
骨	Bone	9 208	0.59	0.13	0.20	0.37	1.03	1.03	0.57	0.60	0.57	0.61
皮肤黑色素瘤	Melanoma of skin	2 860	0.18	0.04	0.05	0.05	0.06	0.04	0.05	0.09	0.11	0.13
皮肤其他	Other skin	14 679	0.94	0.09	0.12	0.11	0.12	0.19	0.17	0.30	0.44	0.58
间皮瘤	Mesothelioma	790	0.05	0.00	0.00	0.00	0.01	0.01	0.01	0.02	0.03	0.03
卡波氏肉瘤	Kaposi sarcoma	175	0.01	0.00	0.00	0.00	0.01	0.01	0.01	0.02	0.01	0.02
结缔组织、软组织	Connective & soft tissue	4 982	0.32	0.50	0.34	0.24	0.25	0.33	0.29	0.39	0.49	0.60
乳腺	Breast	110 863	7.19	0.00	0.07	0.01	0.06	0.39	1.65	6.09	16.40	30.76
外阴	Vulva	1 261	0.08	0.00	0.00	0.01	0.01	0.02	0.03	0.06	0.09	0.15
阴道	Vagina	795	0.05	0.12	0.02	0.01	0.01	0.02	0.01	0.04	0.05	0.09
子宫颈	Cervix uteri	46 626	2.98	0.00	0.05	0.01	0.02	0.07	0.51	3.26	8.21	13.98
子宫体	Corpus uteri	22 856	1.46	0.04	0.00	0.00	0.03	0.02	0.17	0.86	1.71	3.13
子宫,部位不明	Uterus unspecified	4 361	0.28	0.00	0.00	0.00	0.00	0.02	0.00	0.07	0.33	0.49	0.85
卵巢	Ovary	20 193	1.29	0.08	0.09	0.23	0.56	1.16	1.81	2.54	2.90	3.83
其他女性生殖器	Other female genital organs	1 448	0.09	0.00	0.04	0.01	0.00	0.04	0.08	0.10	0.08	0.18
胎盘	Placenta	204	0.01	0.00	0.00	0.00	0.02	0.03	0.11	0.21	0.18	0.15
阴茎	Penis	2 048	0.13	0.00	0.00	0.01	0.00	0.01	0.01	0.07	0.12	0.19
前列腺	Prostate	33 856	2.16	0.04	0.01	0.01	0.02	0.01	0.02	0.04	0.10	0.07
睾丸	Testis	1 256	0.08	0.32	0.32	0.03	0.04	0.15	0.35	0.60	0.85	0.63
其他男性生殖器	Other male genital organs	502	0.03	0.04	0.00	0.01	0.01	0.03	0.02	0.03	0.06	0.04
肾	Kidney	21 139	1.35	0.36	0.48	0.13	0.06	0.11	0.19	0.42	0.92	1.42
肾盂	Renal pelvis	2 638	0.17	0.00	0.00	0.00	0.00	0.00	0.01	0.01	0.03	0.06
输尿管	Ureter	2 983	0.19	0.00	0.00	0.01	0.00	0.00	0.00	0.01	0.01	0.04
膀胱	Bladder	30 616	1.96	0.02	0.03	0.02	0.02	0.04	0.10	0.28	0.51	0.70
其他泌尿器官	Other urinary organs	615	0.04	0.00	0.00	0.01	0.00	0.00	0.00	0.01	0.00	0.02
眼	Eye	856	0.05	0.92	0.44	0.07	0.02	0.02	0.03	0.04	0.05	0.05
脑、神经系统	Brain,nervous system	40 188	2.57	2.17	1.75	1.72	1.61	1.47	1.38	2.21	3.04	3.47
甲状腺	Thyroid	84 593	5.41	0.00	0.03	0.06	0.35	1.36	5.31	14.87	22.03	24.74
肾上腺	Adrenal gland	1 494	0.10	0.52	0.22	0.07	0.02	0.02	0.03	0.06	0.11	0.13
其他内分泌腺	Other endocrine	2 216	0.14	0.02	0.05	0.06	0.17	0.12	0.09	0.21	0.28	0.36
霍奇金淋巴瘤	Hodgkin lymphoma	1 608	0.10	0.04	0.02	0.08	0.09	0.19	0.23	0.30	0.27	0.23
非霍奇金淋巴瘤	Non-Hodgkin lymphoma	24 148	1.54	0.26	0.54	0.51	0.68	0.71	0.73	1.03	1.51	1.60
免疫增生性疾病	Immunoproliferative diseases	391	0.03	0.00	0.01	0.01	0.00	0.01	0.01	0.02	0.01	0.02
多发性骨髓瘤	Multiple myeloma	8 293	0.53	0.02	0.06	0.02	0.04	0.05	0.03	0.09	0.12	0.17
淋巴样白血病	Lymphoid leukemia	6 146	0.39	0.99	2.70	1.54	1.06	0.58	0.40	0.50	0.39	0.37
髓样白血病	Myeloid leukemia	16 279	1.04	1.33	1.33	0.85	0.59	0.81	0.93	1.27	1.64	1.50
白血病,未特指	Leukemia unspecified	9 363	0.60	1.53	1.36	1.09	0.82	0.82	0.62	0.76	0.76	0.75
其他或未指明部位	Other and unspecified	27 828	1.78	1.55	0.93	0.54	0.61	0.62	0.61	0.85	1.17	1.48
所有部位合计	All sites	1 563 923	100.00	12.63	11.51	8.02	9.22	11.48	17.71	40.30	68.10	95.49
所有部位除外 C44	All sites except C44	1 549 244	99.06	12.54	11.39	7.91	9.10	11.29	17.54	40.00	67.66	94.91

Appendix

Appendix 1　Cancer incidence and mortality in registration areas of China,2018

Appendix Table 1-1　Cancer incidence in registration areas of China,both sexes in 2018

Age group										粗率 Crude rate/ 100 000⁻¹	中标率 ASR China/ 100 000⁻¹	世标率 ASR world/ 100 000⁻¹	累积率 Cum. Rate/%		ICD-10
40~44	45~49	50~54	55~59	60~64	65~69	70~74	75~79	80~84	85+				0~64	0~74	
0.05	0.09	0.18	0.26	0.38	0.65	0.83	1.03	1.22	1.49	0.19	0.11	0.11	0.01	0.01	C00
0.50	0.89	1.44	1.58	2.38	2.58	2.78	2.75	3.05	2.73	0.88	0.58	0.56	0.04	0.06	C01-C02
0.46	0.73	1.41	1.80	2.85	3.45	4.80	5.17	5.73	5.94	1.14	0.70	0.69	0.04	0.08	C03-C06
0.47	0.69	0.97	0.94	1.35	1.69	1.70	1.59	1.59	1.70	0.62	0.44	0.42	0.03	0.05	C07-C08
0.09	0.21	0.29	0.39	0.47	0.51	0.51	0.48	0.33	0.59	0.17	0.11	0.11	0.01	0.01	C09
0.10	0.16	0.37	0.50	0.86	0.97	0.90	1.13	0.84	0.67	0.26	0.16	0.16	0.01	0.02	C10
4.26	5.96	7.79	6.82	8.30	8.27	7.62	6.24	5.48	3.85	3.74	2.71	2.53	0.20	0.28	C11
0.11	0.37	0.89	1.12	1.83	1.94	1.82	1.39	1.41	0.87	0.51	0.31	0.32	0.02	0.04	C12-C13
0.10	0.15	0.27	0.43	0.71	0.83	1.18	1.28	1.36	1.05	0.26	0.16	0.16	0.01	0.02	C14
1.54	4.80	14.57	22.37	48.38	73.56	94.53	109.47	114.75	106.61	17.96	10.20	10.29	0.46	1.30	C15
5.99	12.82	26.74	35.84	70.54	101.53	129.40	147.91	161.78	142.54	27.03	15.92	15.84	0.80	1.95	C16
0.46	0.92	1.56	1.83	3.24	4.35	5.00	5.79	5.90	5.15	1.23	0.75	0.74	0.04	0.09	C17
4.72	8.75	15.79	21.33	37.01	50.79	63.07	77.23	94.81	90.02	15.00	8.94	8.83	0.47	1.04	C18
4.74	9.23	17.99	22.00	39.96	55.11	64.91	75.23	82.51	72.62	15.15	9.07	9.00	0.49	1.09	C19-C20
0.13	0.22	0.45	0.50	0.90	1.05	1.43	1.89	2.27	2.22	0.36	0.22	0.22	0.01	0.02	C21
15.54	26.22	43.18	44.89	69.51	83.45	94.73	106.01	117.30	114.52	27.42	17.21	16.90	1.07	1.97	C22
0.74	1.62	3.38	4.73	9.80	13.91	19.46	24.81	31.19	32.20	4.06	2.30	2.30	0.10	0.27	C23-C24
1.49	3.31	6.48	9.33	17.53	24.48	33.38	42.46	50.71	51.81	7.19	4.13	4.12	0.20	0.49	C25
0.25	0.40	0.73	0.61	1.00	1.28	1.38	1.55	1.73	1.70	0.43	0.29	0.28	0.02	0.03	C30-C31
0.29	0.96	2.37	3.91	6.05	7.13	8.12	8.21	8.17	6.17	1.89	1.12	1.14	0.07	0.15	C32
14.82	31.79	68.79	94.35	176.48	241.69	297.44	343.95	375.22	335.31	65.05	38.23	38.20	2.00	4.70	C33-C34
0.53	0.97	1.47	1.71	2.51	2.78	2.79	3.14	2.88	2.73	0.99	0.69	0.68	0.05	0.07	C37-C38
0.84	1.19	1.92	2.11	3.20	4.75	6.71	7.27	8.06	7.29	1.76	1.30	1.27	0.07	0.13	C40-C41
0.25	0.37	0.77	0.75	1.32	1.60	1.94	2.43	2.75	3.32	0.55	0.35	0.34	0.02	0.04	C43
0.79	1.32	2.28	2.94	5.22	7.64	11.61	15.60	23.33	33.90	2.81	1.63	1.62	0.07	0.17	C44
0.04	0.11	0.20	0.29	0.39	0.57	0.53	0.62	0.54	0.55	0.15	0.10	0.09	0.01	0.01	C45
0.02	0.03	0.02	0.04	0.08	0.06	0.10	0.13	0.19	0.16	0.03	0.02	0.02	0.00	0.00	C46
0.68	0.91	1.30	1.30	1.86	2.17	2.35	3.15	3.20	2.95	0.95	0.72	0.70	0.05	0.07	C47,C49
54.47	84.60	92.21	82.09	96.17	81.08	67.32	57.79	50.71	39.91	43.02	30.35	28.39	2.32	3.07	C50
0.30	0.41	0.59	0.63	1.01	1.56	1.92	1.95	2.56	2.04	0.49	0.30	0.29	0.02	0.03	C51
0.15	0.40	0.42	0.50	0.81	0.88	1.11	1.09	0.94	0.62	0.31	0.20	0.19	0.01	0.02	C52
23.30	33.12	45.14	35.08	35.37	31.41	26.94	24.99	19.50	13.68	18.10	12.95	12.00	0.99	1.28	C53
6.85	14.60	26.50	22.62	21.28	18.30	14.21	10.87	8.73	5.51	8.87	5.93	5.76	0.49	0.65	C54
1.81	2.74	4.10	3.39	3.21	3.43	3.08	3.14	3.14	3.35	1.69	1.15	1.09	0.08	0.12	C55
6.73	11.82	16.66	14.16	17.41	17.40	16.99	14.42	13.66	9.33	7.84	5.54	5.27	0.40	0.57	C56
0.39	0.74	1.21	1.08	1.60	1.49	1.31	1.14	0.85	0.95	0.56	0.37	0.37	0.03	0.04	C57
0.12	0.14	0.05	0.02	0.02	0.02	0.01	0.00	0.00	0.03	0.08	0.09	0.07	0.01	0.01	C58
0.28	0.67	0.96	1.13	2.09	2.48	3.44	3.24	4.25	5.09	0.77	0.49	0.48	0.03	0.06	C60
0.26	0.55	2.28	6.35	21.70	45.80	82.96	123.25	153.97	160.29	12.75	7.24	7.14	0.16	0.80	C61
0.59	0.50	0.56	0.34	0.46	0.53	0.62	0.74	1.04	1.11	0.47	0.44	0.40	0.03	0.03	C62
0.03	0.07	0.13	0.21	0.44	0.63	0.85	1.37	1.48	1.33	0.19	0.12	0.12	0.01	0.01	C63
2.13	3.67	6.40	8.09	10.30	13.18	13.34	12.93	13.23	11.14	4.04	2.62	2.59	0.17	0.30	C64
0.11	0.21	0.46	0.66	1.16	1.86	2.44	3.10	3.28	3.16	0.50	0.29	0.29	0.01	0.04	C66
0.04	0.18	0.31	0.58	1.44	2.10	3.10	3.96	4.78	3.42	0.57	0.32	0.32	0.01	0.04	C66
1.23	2.24	4.55	6.84	13.26	19.32	26.81	36.85	46.75	48.43	5.85	3.34	3.31	0.15	0.38	C67
0.03	0.05	0.06	0.12	0.29	0.43	0.53	0.74	1.00	0.82	0.12	0.07	0.07	0.00	0.01	C68
0.08	0.10	0.16	0.21	0.26	0.38	0.39	0.55	0.60	0.69	0.16	0.12	0.15	0.01	0.01	C69
4.88	7.57	11.52	12.06	16.80	20.26	22.61	23.47	26.54	23.58	7.68	5.46	5.37	0.35	0.56	C70-C72,D32-D33, D42-D43
24.33	26.59	31.03	26.73	23.01	16.65	10.44	6.85	5.49	4.38	16.17	13.99	12.01	1.00	1.14	C73
0.15	0.26	0.40	0.49	0.60	0.73	0.78	0.99	1.10	0.90	0.29	0.20	0.21	0.01	0.02	C74
0.38	0.47	0.62	0.77	0.92	0.94	0.84	0.76	0.83	0.67	0.42	0.33	0.31	0.02	0.03	C75
0.19	0.22	0.36	0.35	0.49	0.67	0.74	0.98	0.94	0.68	0.31	0.26	0.24	0.02	0.02	C81
2.23	3.39	5.76	6.57	11.08	14.46	17.30	19.02	19.61	15.13	4.62	3.11	3.04	0.18	0.34	C82-C86,C96
0.03	0.05	0.05	0.10	0.20	0.26	0.34	0.32	0.40	0.21	0.07	0.05	0.05	0.00	0.01	C88
0.43	0.93	1.87	2.52	4.40	6.40	7.24	7.49	7.17	4.40	1.59	0.97	0.97	0.05	0.12	C90
0.50	0.71	1.08	1.17	1.99	2.56	2.56	2.98	2.82	1.17	1.17	1.00	1.15	0.06	0.09	C91
1.80	2.49	3.76	4.07	6.25	8.31	10.03	11.12	12.90	9.42	3.11	2.28	2.22	0.13	0.23	C92-C94,D45-D47
0.96	1.28	1.84	1.85	3.04	4.16	5.68	6.72	7.85	6.95	1.79	1.38	1.43	0.08	0.13	C95
2.29	3.65	6.34	7.01	11.47	15.60	18.96	23.67	30.00	37.06	5.32	3.40	3.40	0.19	0.36	O&U
149.08	244.07	394.65	448.56	722.19	930.79	1 117.21	1 283.80	1 422.68	1 318.34	298.94	190.16	185.49	11.10	21.34	C00-C97,D32-D33, D42-D43,D45-D47
148.29	242.75	392.38	445.61	716.97	923.15	1 105.60	1 268.21	1 399.35	1 284.43	296.13	188.53	183.87	11.03	21.17	C00-C97,D32-D33, D42-D43,D45-D47 exc. C44

附表 1-2　2018 年全国肿瘤登记地区男性癌症发病主要指标

部位	Site	病例数 No. cases	构成 Freq. /%	0~	1~4	5~9	10~14	15~19	20~24	25~29	30~34	35~39
唇	Lip	570	0.07	0.04	0.01	0.00	0.02	0.01	0.01	0.02	0.02	0.04
舌	Tongue	3 028	0.35	0.00	0.02	0.02	0.04	0.00	0.05	0.12	0.33	0.48
口	Mouth	3 865	0.45	0.04	0.03	0.04	0.03	0.07	0.05	0.12	0.23	0.32
唾液腺	Salivary glands	1 792	0.21	0.00	0.02	0.02	0.06	0.08	0.14	0.21	0.33	0.28
扁桃腺	Tonsil	661	0.08	0.00	0.03	0.03	0.00	0.01	0.02	0.03	0.04	0.08
其他口咽	Other oropharynx	1 171	0.14	0.00	0.00	0.01	0.01	0.01	0.03	0.02	0.03	0.08
鼻咽	Nasopharynx	13 912	1.62	0.00	0.06	0.05	0.18	0.38	0.47	1.05	2.36	3.78
下咽	Hypopharynx	2 469	0.29	0.04	0.01	0.01	0.01	0.00	0.01	0.02	0.02	0.05
咽,部位不明	Pharynx unspecified	1 051	0.12	0.00	0.02	0.01	0.00	0.00	0.00	0.03	0.02	0.04
食管	Esophagus	69 821	8.11	0.00	0.02	0.01	0.01	0.02	0.06	0.12	0.21	0.49
胃	Stomach	98 542	11.45	0.14	0.02	0.03	0.09	0.19	0.35	0.91	1.86	3.26
小肠	Small intestine	3 729	0.43	0.00	0.02	0.00	0.01	0.01	0.03	0.12	0.18	0.29
结肠	Colon	44 282	5.15	0.00	0.03	0.03	0.07	0.27	0.32	1.05	1.98	3.05
直肠	Rectum	48 406	5.63	0.04	0.02	0.02	0.03	0.10	0.23	0.75	1.56	2.31
肛门	Anus	1 077	0.13	0.00	0.00	0.00	0.01	0.01	0.02	0.06	0.04	0.06
肝脏	Liver	106 248	12.35	1.62	0.53	0.14	0.23	0.37	0.88	2.77	6.96	12.78
胆囊及其他	Gallbladder etc.	10 293	1.20	0.00	0.00	0.01	0.00	0.01	0.03	0.07	0.18	0.31
胰腺	Pancreas	21 565	2.51	0.00	0.02	0.00	0.01	0.05	0.08	0.17	0.38	0.84
鼻、鼻窦及其他	Nose, sinuses etc.	1 436	0.17	0.00	0.02	0.01	0.01	0.08	0.09	0.11	0.15	0.19
喉	Larynx	8 994	1.05	0.04	0.00	0.02	0.01	0.01	0.02	0.04	0.02	0.14
气管、支气管、肺	Trachea, bronchus & lung	221 553	25.75	0.04	0.05	0.06	0.22	0.26	0.76	1.81	3.43	6.63
其他胸腔器官	Other thoracic organs	3 152	0.37	0.25	0.24	0.07	0.13	0.32	0.23	0.38	0.46	0.48
骨	Bone	5 381	0.63	0.14	0.18	0.40	1.15	1.29	0.65	0.66	0.69	0.77
皮肤黑色素瘤	Melanoma of skin	1 465	0.17	0.04	0.04	0.07	0.05	0.03	0.06	0.07	0.08	0.13
皮肤其他	Other skin	7 338	0.85	0.07	0.07	0.15	0.15	0.16	0.15	0.32	0.44	0.59
间皮瘤	Mesothelioma	429	0.05	0.00	0.00	0.00	0.00	0.01	0.02	0.01	0.03	0.03
卡波氏肉瘤	Kaposi sarcoma	123	0.01	0.00	0.00	0.01	0.01	0.00	0.04	0.02	0.02
结缔组织、软组织	Connective & soft tissue	2 701	0.31	0.49	0.42	0.26	0.27	0.30	0.34	0.37	0.51	0.65
乳腺	Breast	1 512	0.18	0.04	0.00	0.01	0.01	0.01	0.02	0.09	0.15	0.18
外阴	Vulva	—	—	—	—	—	—	—	—	—	—	—
阴道	Vagina	—	—	—	—	—	—	—	—	—	—	—
子宫颈	Cervix uteri	—	—	—	—	—	—	—	—	—	—	—
子宫体	Corpus uteri	—	—	—	—	—	—	—	—	—	—	—
子宫,部位不明	Uterus unspecified	—	—	—	—	—	—	—	—	—	—	—
卵巢	Ovary	—	—	—	—	—	—	—	—	—	—	—
其他女性生殖器	Other female genital organs	—	—	—	—	—	—	—	—	—	—	—
胎盘	Placenta	—	—	—	—	—	—	—	—	—	—	—
阴茎	Penis	2 048	0.24	0.00	0.00	0.01	0.00	0.01	0.01	0.07	0.12	0.19
前列腺	Prostate	33 856	3.93	0.04	0.01	0.01	0.02	0.01	0.02	0.04	0.10	0.07
睾丸	Testis	1 256	0.15	0.32	0.32	0.03	0.04	0.15	0.35	0.60	0.85	0.63
其他男性生殖器	Other male genital organs	502	0.06	0.00	0.00	0.01	0.00	0.03	0.02	0.03	0.06	0.04
肾	Kidney	13 585	1.58	0.46	0.46	0.13	0.05	0.12	0.21	0.53	1.13	1.93
肾盂	Renal pelvis	1 545	0.18	0.00	0.00	0.01	0.00	0.01	0.02	0.01	0.05	0.09
输尿管	Ureter	1 655	0.19	0.00	0.02	0.00	0.00	0.00	0.01	0.02	0.01	0.03
膀胱	Bladder	24 132	2.80	0.04	0.03	0.03	0.02	0.05	0.12	0.38	0.77	1.08
其他泌尿器官	Other urinary organs	369	0.04	0.00	0.00	0.02	0.01	0.00	0.00	0.01	0.01	0.02
眼	Eye	463	0.05	0.85	0.51	0.07	0.01	0.02	0.03	0.02	0.04	0.06
脑、神经系统	Brain, nervous system	18 668	2.17	2.22	1.85	1.86	1.79	1.58	1.41	2.35	3.18	3.58
甲状腺	Thyroid	21 198	2.46	0.00	0.02	0.02	0.17	0.56	2.92	8.78	12.67	13.94
肾上腺	Adrenal gland	827	0.10	0.42	0.26	0.09	0.03	0.02	0.05	0.09	0.09	0.12
其他内分泌腺	Other endocrine	1 050	0.12	0.04	0.06	0.08	0.23	0.14	0.08	0.15	0.22	0.23
霍奇金淋巴瘤	Hodgkin lymphoma	987	0.11	0.00	0.03	0.10	0.12	0.25	0.24	0.28	0.30	0.19
非霍奇金淋巴瘤	Non-Hodgkin lymphoma	13 857	1.61	0.39	0.64	0.66	0.84	0.95	0.85	1.13	1.71	1.67
免疫增生性疾病	Immunoproliferative diseases	259	0.03	0.00	0.00	0.01	0.03	0.01	0.01	0.04	0.01	0.02
多发性骨髓瘤	Multiple myeloma	4 645	0.54	0.00	0.04	0.03	0.04	0.07	0.02	0.10	0.13	0.19
淋巴样白血病	Lymphoid leukemia	3 529	0.41	0.95	2.91	1.65	1.06	0.73	0.50	0.54	0.43	0.40
髓样白血病	Myeloid leukemia	9 308	1.08	1.38	0.47	0.60	0.85	1.10	0.89	1.33	1.79	1.65
白血病,未特指	Leukemia unspecified	5 277	0.61	1.55	1.43	1.18	0.85	0.93	0.68	0.87	0.85	0.83
其他或未指明部位	Other and unspecified	14 835	1.72	1.38	0.99	0.57	0.69	0.65	0.65	0.88	1.05	1.34
所有部位合计	All sites	860 417	100.00	13.07	12.41	8.63	9.67	11.45	14.21	29.77	48.25	66.65
所有部位除外 C44	All sites except C44	853 079	99.15	12.99	12.34	8.48	9.52	11.29	14.06	29.45	47.81	66.06

Appendix Table 1-2　Cancer incidence in registration areas of China, male in 2018

Age group										粗率 Crude rate/ 100 000⁻¹	中标率 ASR China/ 100 000⁻¹	世标率 ASR world/ 100 000⁻¹	累积率 Cum. Rate/%		ICD-10
40~44	45~49	50~54	55~59	60~64	65~69	70~74	75~79	80~84	85+				0~64	0~74	
0.05	0.10	0.23	0.36	0.47	0.85	0.86	1.37	1.13	1.81	0.21	0.13	0.13	0.01	0.02	C00
0.67	1.16	2.11	2.26	3.34	3.36	3.59	3.40	3.32	2.79	1.14	0.77	0.75	0.05	0.09	C01-C02
0.60	1.04	2.00	2.68	3.99	4.53	5.98	6.53	7.05	7.70	1.46	0.93	0.92	0.06	0.11	C03-C06
0.41	0.67	1.01	1.07	1.76	2.02	2.15	1.99	2.28	2.43	0.67	0.48	0.46	0.03	0.05	C07-C08
0.13	0.29	0.43	0.60	0.73	0.75	0.79	0.67	0.44	0.80	0.25	0.17	0.17	0.01	0.02	C09
0.16	0.26	0.65	0.91	1.52	1.63	1.57	1.85	1.56	1.20	0.44	0.28	0.28	0.02	0.03	C10
5.98	8.45	11.08	9.89	12.24	12.25	10.79	8.62	7.82	4.91	5.24	3.82	3.59	0.28	0.39	C11
0.20	0.68	1.63	2.14	3.48	3.65	3.35	2.55	2.83	1.90	0.93	0.58	0.59	0.04	0.08	C12-C13
0.14	0.25	0.46	0.76	1.21	1.33	1.96	1.88	1.87	1.42	0.40	0.25	0.25	0.01	0.03	C14
2.32	7.81	24.39	37.71	78.74	113.62	139.88	157.53	161.55	152.32	26.30	15.67	15.90	0.76	2.03	C15
6.57	15.62	36.01	51.92	105.68	151.82	192.87	216.24	229.79	198.71	37.12	22.55	22.60	1.11	2.84	C16
0.53	1.04	1.85	2.07	3.72	5.23	6.08	7.02	6.92	6.64	1.40	0.89	0.88	0.05	0.11	C17
5.03	9.56	17.47	25.13	44.24	60.26	73.80	89.47	108.25	110.53	16.68	10.33	10.24	0.54	1.21	C18
5.12	10.49	21.09	28.41	51.94	71.01	82.37	94.60	103.07	93.62	18.23	11.26	11.24	0.61	1.38	C19-C20
0.14	0.24	0.50	0.57	1.12	1.29	1.74	2.16	2.47	2.97	0.41	0.25	0.25	0.01	0.03	C21
25.89	43.71	69.69	71.71	106.97	121.34	131.54	143.40	154.58	152.72	40.02	26.22	25.68	1.71	2.98	C22
0.75	1.55	3.22	4.94	10.19	14.41	19.44	24.30	29.20	33.91	3.88	2.31	2.32	0.11	0.28	C23-C24
1.86	4.24	8.29	11.86	21.70	28.95	38.52	47.24	56.14	60.29	8.12	4.91	4.92	0.25	0.58	C25
0.30	0.52	0.90	0.85	1.31	1.83	1.62	2.02	2.25	1.95	0.54	0.37	0.36	0.02	0.04	C30-C31
0.50	1.73	4.32	7.29	11.39	13.27	15.04	15.28	14.96	12.08	3.39	2.06	2.10	0.13	0.27	C32
14.24	34.90	82.25	122.37	240.62	336.75	415.90	485.12	522.28	479.22	83.45	50.48	50.72	2.54	6.30	C33-C34
0.59	1.16	1.52	2.12	3.14	3.75	3.37	3.89	3.90	3.90	1.19	0.84	0.83	0.05	0.09	C37-C38
0.97	1.34	2.20	2.39	3.68	5.80	8.34	9.06	9.28	9.65	2.03	1.53	1.49	0.08	0.15	C40-C41
0.27	0.32	0.72	0.79	1.38	1.80	1.96	2.60	3.13	4.43	0.55	0.36	0.36	0.02	0.04	C43
0.91	1.38	2.40	3.19	5.73	8.28	12.14	16.24	24.42	31.25	2.76	1.72	1.70	0.08	0.18	C44
0.04	0.10	0.18	0.30	0.48	0.71	0.53	0.77	0.80	0.66	0.16	0.10	0.10	0.01	0.01	C45
0.02	0.03	0.03	0.05	0.12	0.11	0.16	0.18	0.30	0.35	0.05	0.03	0.03	0.00	0.00	C46
0.61	0.96	1.38	1.41	2.04	2.55	2.65	3.68	3.92	3.63	1.02	0.77	0.76	0.05	0.07	C47,C49
0.35	0.59	0.84	0.91	1.38	1.72	1.98	2.64	2.14	3.10	0.57	0.38	0.37	0.02	0.04	C50
—	—	—	—	—	—	—	—	—	—	—	—	—	—	—	C51
—	—	—	—	—	—	—	—	—	—	—	—	—	—	—	C52
—	—	—	—	—	—	—	—	—	—	—	—	—	—	—	C53
—	—	—	—	—	—	—	—	—	—	—	—	—	—	—	C54
—	—	—	—	—	—	—	—	—	—	—	—	—	—	—	C55
—	—	—	—	—	—	—	—	—	—	—	—	—	—	—	C56
—	—	—	—	—	—	—	—	—	—	—	—	—	—	—	C57
—	—	—	—	—	—	—	—	—	—	—	—	—	—	—	C58
0.28	0.67	0.96	1.13	2.09	2.48	3.44	3.24	4.25	5.09	0.77	0.49	0.48	0.03	0.06	C60
0.26	0.55	2.28	6.35	21.70	45.80	82.96	123.25	153.97	160.29	12.75	7.24	7.14	0.16	0.80	C61
0.59	0.50	0.56	0.34	0.46	0.53	0.62	0.74	1.04	1.11	0.47	0.44	0.40	0.03	0.03	C62
0.03	0.07	0.13	0.21	0.44	0.63	0.85	1.37	1.48	1.33	0.19	0.12	0.12	0.01	0.01	C63
2.73	4.73	8.33	10.53	13.68	17.13	17.40	16.47	17.23	15.89	5.12	3.39	3.35	0.22	0.40	C64
0.17	0.25	0.67	0.94	1.43	2.15	2.73	3.43	3.70	3.59	0.58	0.36	0.36	0.02	0.04	C65
0.05	0.20	0.33	0.77	1.83	2.42	3.50	4.07	5.10	4.25	0.62	0.37	0.37	0.02	0.05	C66
1.78	3.53	7.23	11.05	21.58	31.09	43.09	60.73	80.26	89.11	9.09	5.43	5.40	0.24	0.61	C67
0.03	0.04	0.09	0.14	0.34	0.52	0.71	0.88	1.21	1.46	0.14	0.08	0.08	0.00	0.01	C68
0.09	0.12	0.17	0.29	0.28	0.43	0.45	0.39	0.74	0.71	0.17	0.13	0.17	0.01	0.01	C69
4.47	6.90	10.24	10.65	15.01	18.82	21.27	22.44	25.52	23.90	7.03	5.21	5.11	0.32	0.53	C70-C72,D32-D33, D42-D43
12.17	11.54	12.98	11.55	11.01	8.52	6.46	4.40	4.09	3.54	7.98	7.16	6.04	0.49	0.57	C73
0.13	0.26	0.33	0.61	0.75	0.86	0.86	1.27	1.26	1.15	0.31	0.22	0.23	0.01	0.02	C74
0.35	0.37	0.54	0.66	0.98	1.02	0.94	0.92	1.07	0.80	0.40	0.31	0.30	0.02	0.03	C75
0.23	0.29	0.47	0.48	0.67	0.84	0.97	1.25	1.15	1.20	0.37	0.30	0.29	0.02	0.03	C81
2.44	3.78	6.62	7.63	12.78	16.72	20.36	22.61	24.15	20.41	5.22	3.61	3.54	0.21	0.39	C82-C86,C96
0.01	0.06	0.06	0.13	0.25	0.37	0.57	0.44	0.66	0.40	0.10	0.06	0.06	0.00	0.01	C88
0.48	1.02	2.04	2.78	4.70	7.25	8.59	8.91	9.17	6.29	1.75	1.10	1.09	0.06	0.14	C90
0.51	0.72	1.21	1.35	2.21	2.81	3.65	4.68	4.39	4.34	1.33	1.12	1.29	0.07	0.10	C91
1.97	2.79	4.21	4.55	7.06	9.73	12.15	13.73	16.68	13.81	3.51	2.59	2.53	0.15	0.26	C92-C94,D45-D47
1.04	1.43	2.02	2.08	3.26	4.75	7.01	8.08	9.63	8.94	1.99	1.55	1.60	0.09	0.15	C95
2.10	3.45	6.50	7.86	12.79	18.02	21.86	26.17	34.38	44.18	5.59	3.66	3.69	0.20	0.40	O&U
107.27	193.49	366.82	478.73	859.61	1 167.76	1 441.38	1 681.77	1 868.79	1 798.64	324.09	205.39	203.62	11.04	24.08	C00-C97,D32-D33, D42-D43,D45-D47
106.37	192.11	364.42	475.54	853.88	1 159.48	1 429.23	1 665.53	1 844.36	1 767.39	321.32	203.68	201.92	10.96	23.90	C00-C97,D32-D33, D42-D43,D45-D47 exc. C44

部位	Site	病例数 No. cases	构成 Freq. /%	0~	1~4	5~9	10~14	15~19	20~24	25~29	30~34	35~39
唇	Lip	406	0.06	0.00	0.01	0.01	0.01	0.00	0.00	0.02	0.03	0.00
舌	Tongue	1 587	0.23	0.00	0.00	0.01	0.02	0.01	0.05	0.10	0.17	0.26
口	Mouth	2 083	0.30	0.00	0.03	0.02	0.02	0.07	0.07	0.09	0.22	0.18
唾液腺	Salivary glands	1 428	0.20	0.00	0.02	0.02	0.06	0.14	0.16	0.31	0.30	0.41
扁桃腺	Tonsil	246	0.03	0.00	0.01	0.02	0.01	0.02	0.01	0.02	0.01	0.03
其他口咽	Other oropharynx	204	0.03	0.00	0.00	0.00	0.01	0.01	0.01	0.01	0.02	0.02
鼻咽	Nasopharynx	5 652	0.80	0.00	0.03	0.03	0.06	0.18	0.37	0.57	1.26	1.58
下咽	Hypopharynx	183	0.03	0.00	0.00	0.00	0.00	0.00	0.01	0.01	0.00	0.01
咽,部位不明	Pharynx unspecified	303	0.04	0.00	0.01	0.01	0.01	0.01	0.02	0.03	0.02	0.03
食管	Esophagus	24 124	3.43	0.00	0.00	0.00	0.02	0.02	0.05	0.16	0.17	0.37
胃	Stomach	42 873	6.09	0.04	0.00	0.02	0.10	0.17	0.37	1.44	2.67	3.14
小肠	Small intestine	2 714	0.39	0.00	0.02	0.01	0.01	0.00	0.03	0.06	0.14	0.20
结肠	Colon	34 178	4.86	0.00	0.02	0.00	0.07	0.14	0.42	0.84	1.67	2.61
直肠	Rectum	30 875	4.39	0.00	0.02	0.01	0.01	0.07	0.25	0.60	1.47	2.04
肛门	Anus	817	0.12	0.00	0.00	0.01	0.00	0.02	0.02	0.05	0.05	0.09
肝脏	Liver	37 190	5.29	0.83	0.34	0.13	0.11	0.20	0.48	0.87	1.52	2.37
胆囊及其他	Gallbladder etc.	10 967	1.56	0.00	0.00	0.00	0.01	0.01	0.03	0.05	0.11	0.30
胰腺	Pancreas	16 052	2.28	0.00	0.01	0.01	0.04	0.07	0.13	0.24	0.38	0.50
鼻、鼻窦及其他	Nose,sinuses etc.	833	0.12	0.04	0.05	0.04	0.05	0.02	0.06	0.07	0.05	0.15
喉	Larynx	904	0.13	0.00	0.02	0.00	0.02	0.00	0.03	0.01	0.06	0.05
气管、支气管、肺	Trachea,bronchus & lung	118 779	16.88	0.08	0.12	0.04	0.06	0.24	0.62	2.02	4.56	8.25
其他胸腔器官	Other thoracic organs	2 039	0.29	0.36	0.21	0.08	0.06	0.08	0.12	0.19	0.31	0.40
骨	Bone	3 827	0.54	0.12	0.22	0.35	0.90	0.74	0.48	0.54	0.45	0.45
皮肤黑色素瘤	Melanoma of skin	1 395	0.20	0.04	0.06	0.02	0.06	0.05	0.04	0.10	0.13	0.13
皮肤其他	Other skin	7 341	1.04	0.12	0.17	0.07	0.09	0.22	0.18	0.27	0.44	0.58
间皮瘤	Mesothelioma	361	0.05	0.00	0.00	0.02	0.00	0.01	0.01	0.04	0.03	0.03
卡波氏肉瘤	Kaposi sarcoma	52	0.01	0.00	0.00	0.00	0.01	0.02	0.00	0.01	0.00	0.02
结缔组织、软组织	Connective & soft tissue	2 281	0.32	0.52	0.26	0.22	0.23	0.37	0.24	0.42	0.48	0.55
乳腺	Breast	110 863	15.76	0.00	0.07	0.01	0.06	0.39	1.65	6.09	16.40	30.76
外阴	Vulva	1 261	0.18	0.00	0.00	0.01	0.01	0.02	0.03	0.06	0.09	0.15
阴道	Vagina	795	0.11	0.12	0.02	0.01	0.01	0.02	0.01	0.04	0.05	0.09
子宫颈	Cervix uteri	46 626	6.63	0.00	0.05	0.01	0.02	0.07	0.51	3.26	8.21	13.98
子宫体	Corpus uteri	22 856	3.25	0.04	0.00	0.00	0.03	0.00	0.17	0.86	1.71	3.13
子宫,部位不明	Uterus unspecified	4 361	0.62	0.00	0.00	0.00	0.00	0.02	0.10	0.33	0.49	0.85
卵巢	Ovary	20 193	2.87	0.08	0.09	0.23	0.56	1.16	1.81	2.54	2.90	3.83
其他女性生殖器	Other female genital organs	1 448	0.21	0.00	0.04	0.01	0.03	0.04	0.08	0.10	0.08	0.18
胎盘	Placenta	204	0.03	0.00	0.00	0.00	0.02	0.03	0.11	0.21	0.18	0.15
阴茎	Penis	—	—	—	—	—	—	—	—	—	—	—
前列腺	Prostate	—	—	—	—	—	—	—	—	—	—	—
睾丸	Testis	—	—	—	—	—	—	—	—	—	—	—
其他男性生殖器	Other male genital organs	—	—	—	—	—	—	—	—	—	—	—
肾	Kidney	7 554	1.07	0.24	0.50	0.13	0.07	0.10	0.17	0.32	0.71	0.91
肾盂	Renal pelvis	1 093	0.16	0.00	0.01	0.01	0.00	0.00	0.01	0.00	0.02	0.03
输尿管	Ureter	1 328	0.19	0.00	0.00	0.00	0.00	0.01	0.01	0.01	0.01	0.05
膀胱	Bladder	6 484	0.92	0.00	0.02	0.01	0.01	0.02	0.08	0.18	0.26	0.31
其他泌尿器官	Other urinary organs	246	0.03	0.00	0.00	0.00	0.00	0.00	0.00	0.01	0.00	0.01
眼	Eye	393	0.06	0.99	0.36	0.07	0.03	0.02	0.02	0.05	0.06	0.03
脑、神经系统	Brain,nervous system	21 520	3.06	2.10	1.63	1.56	1.40	1.34	1.34	2.07	2.90	3.37
甲状腺	Thyroid	63 395	9.01	0.00	0.04	0.10	0.56	2.26	7.83	21.15	31.51	35.73
肾上腺	Adrenal gland	667	0.09	0.63	0.18	0.05	0.02	0.02	0.02	0.03	0.13	0.14
其他内分泌腺	Other endocrine	1 166	0.17	0.00	0.04	0.04	0.10	0.11	0.10	0.28	0.34	0.49
霍奇金淋巴瘤	Hodgkin lymphoma	621	0.09	0.08	0.01	0.04	0.06	0.12	0.23	0.32	0.23	0.27
非霍奇金淋巴瘤	Non-Hodgkin lymphoma	10 291	1.46	0.12	0.42	0.33	0.49	0.44	0.60	0.93	1.31	1.53
免疫增生性疾病	Immunoproliferative diseases	132	0.02	0.00	0.02	0.01	0.00	0.01	0.01	0.00	0.01	0.02
多发性骨髓瘤	Multiple myeloma	3 648	0.52	0.04	0.09	0.01	0.04	0.02	0.03	0.08	0.11	0.15
淋巴样白血病	Lymphoid leukemia	2 617	0.37	1.03	2.45	1.41	1.05	0.42	0.29	0.45	0.35	0.34
髓样白血病	Myeloid leukemia	6 971	0.99	1.27	0.71	0.58	0.76	0.74	0.87	1.21	1.48	1.34
白血病,未特指	Leukemia unspecified	4 086	0.58	1.51	1.28	1.00	0.78	0.71	0.55	0.64	0.66	0.66
其他或未指明部位	Other and unspecified	12 993	1.85	1.75	0.86	0.52	0.52	0.59	0.57	0.82	1.30	1.62
所有部位合计	All sites	703 506	100.00	12.14	10.48	7.33	8.70	11.51	21.40	51.17	88.22	124.85
所有部位除外 C44	All sites except C44	696 165	98.96	12.02	10.31	7.26	8.61	11.29	21.21	50.91	87.78	124.27

Appendix Table 1-3　Cancer incidence in registration areas of China, female in 2018

Age group										粗率 Crude rate/ 100 000⁻¹	中标率 ASR China/ 100 000⁻¹	世标率 ASR world/ 100 000⁻¹	累积率 Cum. Rate/%		ICD-10
40~44	45~49	50~54	55~59	60~64	65~69	70~74	75~79	80~84	85+				0~64	0~74	
0.04	0.08	0.13	0.16	0.29	0.45	0.80	0.71	1.30	1.27	0.16	0.09	0.09	0.00	0.01	C00
0.33	0.61	0.75	0.89	1.41	1.82	2.00	2.16	2.83	2.69	0.62	0.39	0.37	0.02	0.04	C01-C02
0.32	0.41	0.81	0.92	1.70	2.39	3.66	3.95	4.64	4.77	0.81	0.48	0.47	0.02	0.05	C03-C06
0.53	0.70	0.92	0.81	0.94	1.36	1.26	1.24	1.03	1.21	0.55	0.41	0.38	0.03	0.04	C07-C08
0.05	0.13	0.14	0.17	0.22	0.28	0.23	0.30	0.25	0.44	0.10	0.06	0.06	0.00	0.01	C09
0.04	0.06	0.07	0.08	0.19	0.32	0.26	0.49	0.25	0.33	0.08	0.05	0.05	0.00	0.01	C10
2.51	3.42	4.39	3.71	4.32	4.35	4.55	4.09	3.57	3.14	2.19	1.58	1.46	0.11	0.16	C11
0.02	0.05	0.12	0.09	0.16	0.25	0.34	0.35	0.25	0.18	0.07	0.04	0.04	0.00	0.01	C12-C13
0.06	0.06	0.07	0.10	0.20	0.32	0.43	0.73	0.94	0.80	0.12	0.07	0.07	0.00	0.01	C14
0.74	1.73	4.45	6.80	17.71	34.04	50.61	66.14	76.49	76.03	9.36	4.89	4.86	0.16	0.58	C15
5.39	9.97	17.20	19.51	35.04	51.91	67.94	86.30	106.17	104.96	16.64	9.54	9.32	0.48	1.07	C16
0.38	0.80	1.26	1.59	2.75	3.47	3.95	4.68	5.07	4.15	1.05	0.62	0.61	0.04	0.07	C17
4.39	7.92	14.05	17.47	29.71	41.44	52.67	66.18	83.82	76.30	13.26	7.61	7.47	0.40	0.87	C18
4.35	7.95	14.81	15.48	27.85	39.43	48.00	57.77	65.70	58.57	11.98	6.96	6.84	0.37	0.81	C19-C20
0.12	0.20	0.39	0.42	0.69	0.81	1.12	1.63	2.11	1.72	0.32	0.19	0.18	0.01	0.02	C21
4.94	8.43	15.90	17.66	31.66	46.08	59.09	72.29	86.83	88.97	14.43	8.25	8.17	0.42	0.95	C22
0.73	1.69	3.55	4.52	9.40	13.43	19.48	25.26	32.83	31.06	4.26	2.29	2.28	0.10	0.27	C23-C24
1.11	2.36	4.62	6.77	13.32	20.07	28.39	38.15	46.27	46.13	6.23	3.38	3.35	0.15	0.39	C25
0.20	0.28	0.55	0.37	0.69	0.73	1.16	1.13	1.30	1.54	0.32	0.21	0.21	0.01	0.02	C30-C31
0.07	0.18	0.37	0.49	0.66	1.07	1.42	1.42	2.63	2.22	0.35	0.20	0.20	0.01	0.02	C32
15.41	28.62	54.94	65.91	111.67	147.92	182.74	216.66	254.97	239.06	46.10	26.54	26.25	1.46	3.12	C33-C34
0.47	0.76	1.41	1.30	1.88	1.83	2.22	2.46	2.04	1.95	0.79	0.54	0.53	0.04	0.06	C37-C38
0.71	1.03	1.63	1.82	2.70	3.72	5.14	5.65	7.07	5.71	1.49	1.07	1.04	0.06	0.10	C40-C41
0.23	0.41	0.82	0.71	1.26	1.40	1.93	2.27	2.45	2.58	0.54	0.34	0.33	0.02	0.04	C43
0.67	1.27	2.15	2.69	4.70	7.01	11.09	15.01	22.44	35.68	2.85	1.55	1.54	0.07	0.16	C44
0.05	0.12	0.23	0.29	0.29	0.44	0.54	0.48	0.34	0.47	0.14	0.09	0.09	0.01	0.01	C45
0.01	0.03	0.01	0.03	0.04	0.06	0.05	0.08	0.09	0.03	0.02	0.01	0.01	0.00	0.00	C46
0.74	0.86	1.21	1.18	1.69	1.79	2.06	2.67	2.60	2.49	0.89	0.66	0.65	0.04	0.06	C47,C49
54.47	84.60	92.21	82.09	96.17	81.08	67.32	57.79	50.71	39.91	43.02	30.35	28.39	2.32	3.07	C50
0.30	0.41	0.59	0.63	1.01	1.56	1.92	1.95	2.56	2.04	0.49	0.30	0.29	0.02	0.03	C51
0.15	0.40	0.42	0.50	0.81	0.88	1.11	1.09	0.94	0.62	0.31	0.20	0.19	0.01	0.02	C52
23.30	33.12	45.14	35.08	35.37	31.41	26.94	24.99	19.50	13.68	18.10	12.95	12.00	0.99	1.28	C53
6.85	14.60	26.50	22.62	21.28	18.30	14.21	10.87	8.73	5.51	8.87	5.93	5.76	0.49	0.65	C54
1.81	2.74	4.10	3.39	3.21	3.43	3.08	3.14	3.77	3.35	1.69	1.15	1.09	0.08	0.12	C55
6.73	11.82	16.66	14.16	17.41	17.40	16.99	14.42	13.66	9.33	7.84	5.54	5.27	0.40	0.57	C56
0.39	0.74	1.21	1.08	1.60	1.49	1.31	1.14	0.85	0.95	0.56	0.37	0.37	0.03	0.04	C57
0.12	0.14	0.05	0.02	0.02	0.02	0.01	0.00	0.00	0.03	0.08	0.09	0.07	0.01	—	C58
—	—	—	—	—	—	—	—	—	—	—	—	—	—	—	C60
—	—	—	—	—	—	—	—	—	—	—	—	—	—	—	C61
—	—	—	—	—	—	—	—	—	—	—	—	—	—	—	C62
—	—	—	—	—	—	—	—	—	—	—	—	—	—	—	C63
1.51	2.60	4.42	5.60	6.88	9.29	9.42	9.74	9.96	7.96	2.93	1.86	1.84	0.12	0.21	C64
0.05	0.16	0.25	0.38	0.88	1.57	2.15	2.81	2.94	2.87	0.42	0.23	0.23	0.01	0.03	C65
0.03	0.15	0.28	0.39	1.04	1.78	2.70	3.86	4.51	2.87	0.52	0.28	0.27	0.01	0.03	C66
0.68	0.92	1.78	2.56	4.85	7.71	11.06	15.31	19.34	21.23	2.52	1.37	1.35	0.06	0.15	C67
0.03	0.05	0.04	0.10	0.23	0.34	0.36	0.62	0.83	0.38	0.10	0.05	0.05	0.00	0.01	C68
0.07	0.08	0.15	0.13	0.25	0.33	0.34	0.70	0.49	0.68	0.15	0.11	0.14	0.01	0.01	C69
5.29	8.25	12.84	13.50	18.62	21.68	23.91	24.40	27.37	23.36	8.35	5.71	5.62	0.37	0.60	C70-C72,D32-D33, D42-D43
36.78	41.90	49.61	42.14	35.14	24.67	14.30	9.06	6.64	4.94	24.60	20.95	18.09	1.52	1.72	C73
0.16	0.26	0.47	0.37	0.44	0.59	0.71	0.75	0.96	0.74	0.26	0.18	0.19	0.01	0.02	C74
0.42	0.58	0.71	0.88	0.87	0.87	0.75	0.62	0.63	0.59	0.45	0.35	0.33	0.02	0.03	C75
0.15	0.15	0.24	0.22	0.31	0.50	0.51	0.73	0.63	0.50	0.24	0.21	0.19	0.01	0.02	C81
2.02	2.99	4.87	5.49	9.37	12.23	14.33	15.77	15.91	11.61	3.99	2.62	2.54	0.15	0.29	C82-C86,C96
0.05	0.05	0.05	0.08	0.15	0.15	0.13	0.21	0.18	0.09	0.05	0.03	0.03	0.00	0.00	C88
0.38	0.85	1.70	2.24	4.10	5.57	5.93	6.22	5.54	3.14	1.42	0.84	0.85	0.05	0.11	C90
0.49	0.69	0.94	0.99	1.77	2.31	2.14	2.41	2.40	1.81	1.02	0.88	1.02	0.06	0.08	C91
1.63	2.19	3.30	3.58	5.44	6.90	7.98	8.77	9.80	6.48	2.71	1.97	1.92	0.12	0.19	C92-C94,D45-D47
0.87	1.13	1.65	1.62	2.82	3.58	4.39	5.49	6.39	5.41	1.59	1.21	1.26	0.07	0.11	C95
2.48	3.85	6.17	6.15	10.15	13.22	16.16	21.42	26.41	32.30	5.04	3.15	3.13	0.18	0.33	O&U
191.87	295.54	423.30	417.92	583.35	697.00	803.31	924.98	1 057.93	997.07	273.02	176.98	169.40	11.18	18.68	C00-C97,D32-D33, D42-D43,D45-D47
191.20	294.27	421.15	415.23	578.64	690.00	792.22	909.97	1 035.49	961.39	270.18	175.42	167.86	11.11	18.52	C00-C97,D32-D33, D42-D43,D45-D47 exc. C44

部位 Site		病例数 No. cases	构成 Freq. /%	年龄组								
				0~	1~4	5~9	10~14	15~19	20~24	25~29	30~34	35~39
唇	Lip	378	0.05	0.00	0.00	0.00	0.00	0.00	0.00	0.01	0.01	0.02
舌	Tongue	2 475	0.33	0.00	0.00	0.01	0.02	0.00	0.06	0.14	0.25	0.31
口	Mouth	2 899	0.38	0.00	0.00	0.02	0.02	0.02	0.05	0.09	0.22	0.22
唾液腺	Salivary glands	1 525	0.20	0.00	0.00	0.02	0.06	0.18	0.16	0.31	0.34	0.36
扁桃腺	Tonsil	480	0.06	0.00	0.01	0.01	0.00	0.03	0.01	0.01	0.02	0.04
其他口咽	Other oropharynx	691	0.09	0.00	0.00	0.00	0.01	0.00	0.01	0.02	0.03	0.04
鼻咽	Nasopharynx	9 104	1.20	0.00	0.02	0.05	0.12	0.26	0.35	1.02	1.92	2.84
下咽	Hypopharynx	1 452	0.19	0.04	0.00	0.00	0.00	0.00	0.01	0.01	0.02	0.04
咽,部位不明	Pharynx unspecified	622	0.08	0.00	0.01	0.01	0.00	0.00	0.01	0.01	0.02	0.03
食管	Esophagus	33 601	4.44	0.00	0.00	0.00	0.02	0.03	0.05	0.10	0.11	0.38
胃	Stomach	59 979	7.92	0.17	0.01	0.01	0.12	0.15	0.38	1.17	2.18	3.12
小肠	Small intestine	3 455	0.46	0.00	0.01	0.00	0.01	0.00	0.03	0.10	0.15	0.27
结肠	Colon	45 051	5.95	0.00	0.01	0.02	0.07	0.13	0.42	1.01	1.82	3.05
直肠	Rectum	39 053	5.16	0.00	0.00	0.01	0.01	0.08	0.25	0.67	1.39	2.29
肛门	Anus	863	0.11	0.00	0.00	0.01	0.00	0.02	0.01	0.02	0.03	0.07
肝脏	Liver	62 003	8.19	1.33	0.47	0.12	0.15	0.24	0.50	1.62	3.55	6.35
胆囊及其他	Gallbladder etc.	10 363	1.37	0.00	0.00	0.00	0.00	0.01	0.04	0.06	0.14	0.32
胰腺	Pancreas	18 932	2.50	0.00	0.00	0.02	0.03	0.04	0.13	0.17	0.37	0.62
鼻、鼻窦及其他	Nose, sinuses etc.	1 065	0.14	0.04	0.03	0.02	0.06	0.05	0.08	0.06	0.10	0.18
喉	Larynx	5 117	0.68	0.04	0.04	0.00	0.00	0.00	0.02	0.02	0.03	0.08
气管、支气管、肺	Trachea, bronchus & lung	161 972	21.39	0.08	0.07	0.05	0.14	0.19	0.66	1.84	4.00	7.89
其他胸腔器官	Other thoracic organs	2 656	0.35	0.33	0.23	0.04	0.10	0.23	0.20	0.30	0.43	0.50
骨	Bone	3 598	0.48	0.12	0.10	0.35	0.89	0.91	0.55	0.52	0.44	0.52
皮肤黑色素瘤	Melanoma of skin	1 460	0.19	0.00	0.05	0.05	0.04	0.06	0.05	0.10	0.09	0.16
皮肤其他	Other skin	7 209	0.95	0.08	0.09	0.05	0.08	0.16	0.16	0.31	0.50	0.64
间皮瘤	Mesothelioma	429	0.06	0.00	0.00	0.01	0.00	0.01	0.02	0.01	0.02	0.01
卡波氏肉瘤	Kaposi sarcoma	114	0.02	0.00	0.00	0.00	0.01	0.02	0.01	0.03	0.00	0.04
结缔组织、软组织	Connective & soft tissue	2 601	0.34	0.58	0.43	0.28	0.27	0.38	0.28	0.38	0.53	0.66
乳腺	Breast	60 395	8.08	0.00	0.02	0.00	0.02	0.22	1.23	6.07	17.38	34.08
外阴	Vulva	638	0.08	0.00	0.00	0.00	0.00	0.04	0.01	0.07	0.06	0.16
阴道	Vagina	360	0.05	0.18	0.04	0.00	0.00	0.04	0.00	0.03	0.05	0.11
子宫颈	Cervix uteri	20 109	2.66	0.00	0.00	0.02	0.00	0.06	0.45	2.93	7.52	13.22
子宫体	Corpus uteri	11 697	1.54	0.00	0.00	0.00	0.02	0.04	0.25	0.98	1.73	3.43
子宫,部位不明	Uterus unspecified	1 671	0.22	0.00	0.00	0.00	0.02	0.00	0.04	0.21	0.40	0.64
卵巢	Ovary	10 381	1.37	0.09	0.12	0.26	0.53	1.33	1.93	2.90	3.21	4.02
其他女性生殖器	Other female genital organs	769	0.10	0.00	0.06	0.02	0.02	0.04	0.04	0.06	0.10	0.20
胎盘	Placenta	91	0.01	0.00	0.00	0.00	0.00	0.04	0.11	0.20	0.22	0.13
阴茎	Penis	887	0.12	0.00	0.00	0.02	0.00	0.02	0.00	0.09	0.11	0.19
前列腺	Prostate	19 448	2.57	0.08	0.00	0.00	0.00	0.02	0.04	0.05	0.09	0.11
睾丸	Testis	634	0.08	0.32	0.31	0.05	0.02	0.22	0.45	0.83	1.01	0.70
其他男性生殖器	Other male genital organs	286	0.04	0.00	0.00	0.00	0.00	0.02	0.01	0.02	0.05	0.05
肾	Kidney	12 105	1.60	0.42	0.53	0.12	0.10	0.09	0.22	0.42	1.12	1.73
肾盂	Renal pelvis	1 600	0.21	0.00	0.00	0.01	0.00	0.01	0.01	0.00	0.04	0.08
输尿管	Ureter	1 729	0.23	0.00	0.00	0.00	0.00	0.00	0.01	0.00	0.01	0.05
膀胱	Bladder	16 041	2.12	0.00	0.02	0.02	0.03	0.04	0.10	0.33	0.55	0.75
其他泌尿器官	Other urinary organs	332	0.04	0.00	0.00	0.01	0.00	0.00	0.00	0.02	0.00	0.02
眼	Eye	350	0.05	0.95	0.40	0.04	0.01	0.02	0.04	0.04	0.04	0.04
脑、神经系统	Brain, nervous system	18 392	2.43	1.87	1.68	1.78	1.53	1.24	1.26	2.00	2.92	3.45
甲状腺	Thyroid	50 330	6.65	0.00	0.04	0.04	0.34	1.63	7.09	20.75	30.14	32.98
肾上腺	Adrenal gland	671	0.09	0.75	0.30	0.07	0.00	0.02	0.03	0.06	0.08	0.13
其他内分泌腺	Other endocrine	969	0.13	0.04	0.09	0.08	0.19	0.17	0.10	0.20	0.25	0.34
霍奇金淋巴瘤	Hodgkin lymphoma	745	0.10	0.08	0.04	0.06	0.09	0.22	0.29	0.33	0.30	0.25
非霍奇金淋巴瘤	Non-Hodgkin lymphoma	12 716	1.68	0.17	0.54	0.46	0.62	0.83	0.77	1.09	1.71	1.96
免疫增生性疾病	Immunoproliferative diseases	245	0.03	0.00	0.02	0.01	0.04	0.03	0.01	0.04	0.01	0.04
多发性骨髓瘤	Multiple myeloma	4 401	0.58	0.04	0.06	0.03	0.06	0.04	0.03	0.08	0.09	0.21
淋巴样白血病	Lymphoid leukemia	3 187	0.42	1.00	3.58	1.80	1.26	0.63	0.42	0.49	0.39	0.40
髓样白血病	Myeloid leukemia	8 474	1.12	1.70	0.99	0.65	0.67	0.81	0.89	1.34	1.75	1.61
白血病,未特指	Leukemia unspecified	3 427	0.45	1.08	1.09	0.70	0.55	0.62	0.49	0.56	0.47	0.49
其他或未指明部位	Other and unspecified	14 307	1.89	1.99	1.06	0.58	0.54	0.56	0.50	0.88	1.14	1.56
所有部位合计	All sites	757 307	100.00	13.29	12.24	7.80	8.53	11.12	19.04	46.01	75.97	106.01
所有部位除外 C44	All sites except C44	750 098	99.05	13.20	12.15	7.75	8.44	10.96	18.88	45.70	75.47	105.37

Age group										粗率 Crude rate/ 100 000⁻¹	中标率 ASR China/ 100 000⁻¹	世标率 ASR world/ 100 000⁻¹	累积率 Cum. Rate/%		ICD-10
40~44	45~49	50~54	55~59	60~64	65~69	70~74	75~79	80~84	85+				0~64	0~74	
0.05	0.06	0.16	0.27	0.31	0.43	0.69	0.92	1.18	1.17	0.16	0.09	0.09	0.00	0.01	C00
0.52	1.03	1.63	2.00	2.70	3.00	3.30	3.05	3.74	3.70	1.05	0.65	0.64	0.04	0.07	C01-C02
0.43	0.79	1.38	2.12	3.10	3.55	4.79	5.47	6.02	6.80	1.23	0.72	0.71	0.04	0.08	C03-C06
0.51	0.68	0.95	0.87	1.37	1.61	1.69	1.86	1.64	2.21	0.65	0.46	0.43	0.03	0.05	C07-C08
0.11	0.25	0.31	0.51	0.54	0.68	0.49	0.51	0.33	0.71	0.20	0.13	0.13	0.01	0.01	C09
0.11	0.20	0.40	0.61	0.97	0.94	0.98	1.01	1.02	0.64	0.29	0.18	0.18	0.01	0.02	C10
4.40	6.07	7.72	6.91	8.18	7.91	7.77	6.03	5.63	3.91	3.86	2.75	2.56	0.20	0.28	C11
0.14	0.44	1.11	1.36	2.19	2.29	1.98	1.41	1.66	0.96	0.62	0.36	0.37	0.03	0.05	C12-C13
0.07	0.13	0.31	0.53	0.73	0.79	1.13	1.14	1.36	1.03	0.26	0.15	0.15	0.01	0.02	C14
1.30	4.12	12.58	19.36	37.52	53.80	69.26	79.14	85.05	83.13	14.23	7.81	7.91	0.38	0.99	C15
5.77	11.62	23.76	33.40	62.70	89.65	114.47	134.04	152.77	140.43	25.41	14.42	14.33	0.72	1.74	C16
0.44	0.96	1.71	2.06	3.79	4.97	5.80	7.25	7.22	6.44	1.46	0.86	0.85	0.05	0.10	C17
5.25	9.62	18.43	26.75	44.98	61.68	78.04	99.47	123.60	118.15	19.09	10.84	10.73	0.56	1.26	C18
4.66	9.18	18.68	24.04	43.30	58.15	67.37	78.70	88.92	78.90	16.54	9.52	9.48	0.52	1.15	C19-C20
0.17	0.22	0.45	0.55	0.89	1.00	1.24	2.04	2.07	1.92	0.37	0.21	0.21	0.01	0.02	C21
13.90	23.55	39.19	43.42	64.52	76.83	86.63	101.13	113.71	116.27	26.27	15.84	15.61	0.99	1.81	C22
0.74	1.56	3.33	5.12	9.76	13.79	19.26	26.59	35.21	37.01	4.39	2.36	2.36	0.11	0.27	C23-C24
1.53	3.33	6.76	10.51	18.52	25.32	35.39	46.98	56.24	59.89	8.02	4.41	4.40	0.21	0.51	C25
0.21	0.41	0.66	0.63	1.10	1.29	1.44	1.75	1.61	1.74	0.45	0.29	0.28	0.02	0.03	C30-C31
0.31	0.99	2.62	4.57	6.89	8.15	8.96	8.46	8.40	7.05	2.17	1.24	1.26	0.08	0.16	C32
15.07	31.50	68.37	99.88	181.81	242.24	296.29	350.05	388.85	353.57	68.62	38.83	38.84	2.06	4.75	C33-C34
0.51	1.01	1.60	2.00	2.76	2.99	3.26	3.50	3.30	3.35	1.13	0.76	0.74	0.05	0.08	C37-C38
0.71	1.02	1.52	1.77	2.74	3.89	5.06	6.48	7.79	6.90	1.52	1.10	1.07	0.06	0.10	C40-C41
0.26	0.40	0.80	0.76	1.43	1.83	2.28	2.78	2.87	4.02	0.62	0.38	0.37	0.02	0.04	C43
0.80	1.37	2.14	3.32	5.80	8.07	11.91	16.60	24.07	34.56	3.05	1.70	1.69	0.08	0.18	C44
0.05	0.08	0.21	0.34	0.44	0.79	0.60	0.78	0.85	0.75	0.18	0.11	0.11	0.01	0.01	C45
0.03	0.04	0.04	0.06	0.12	0.11	0.14	0.16	0.26	0.21	0.05	0.03	0.03	0.00	0.00	C46
0.72	0.85	1.44	1.44	2.13	2.63	2.69	3.75	4.35	3.88	1.10	0.80	0.79	0.05	0.08	C47,C49
61.22	94.09	101.40	98.68	117.97	100.40	85.89	78.93	68.30	52.33	51.38	34.95	32.87	2.66	3.59	C50
0.30	0.31	0.52	0.62	1.14	1.79	2.19	2.18	3.22	2.73	0.54	0.31	0.30	0.02	0.04	C51
0.16	0.32	0.36	0.52	0.84	0.79	1.16	0.82	0.98	0.85	0.31	0.19	0.19	0.01	0.02	C52
22.31	30.43	41.74	34.79	32.98	27.61	23.53	22.00	16.74	11.87	17.11	12.02	11.15	0.93	1.19	C53
7.40	15.01	28.29	26.18	23.47	20.99	16.07	13.53	10.16	5.57	9.95	6.49	6.32	0.53	0.72	C54
1.34	2.08	3.24	3.07	2.76	3.21	2.24	2.52	3.31	3.51	1.42	0.93	0.88	0.07	0.10	C55
7.50	13.02	17.42	15.88	19.47	18.58	18.95	17.04	17.11	12.23	8.83	6.09	5.80	0.44	0.63	C56
0.41	0.92	1.24	1.46	1.74	1.62	1.59	1.53	0.89	1.09	0.65	0.42	0.41	0.03	0.05	C57
0.12	0.11	0.02	0.04	0.00	0.00	0.03	0.00	0.00	0.06	0.08	0.08	0.07	0.00	0.01	C58
0.23	0.58	0.97	0.95	1.87	2.31	3.06	3.23	4.49	5.26	0.75	0.46	0.45	0.03	0.05	C60
0.32	0.58	2.80	8.06	27.88	55.51	100.79	150.05	193.16	188.29	16.41	8.87	8.74	0.20	0.98	C61
0.67	0.47	0.64	0.33	0.42	0.54	0.58	0.77	1.02	1.38	0.54	0.50	0.45	0.03	0.04	C62
0.03	0.10	0.12	0.32	0.58	0.79	0.96	1.69	1.93	1.81	0.24	0.14	0.14	0.01	0.02	C63
2.79	4.44	7.50	10.12	12.63	16.30	16.91	16.29	16.57	14.24	5.13	3.21	3.18	0.21	0.37	C64
0.10	0.25	0.53	0.84	1.37	2.46	3.13	4.49	4.51	4.45	0.68	0.38	0.37	0.02	0.04	C65
0.04	0.20	0.32	0.72	1.75	2.32	3.69	5.30	6.56	4.84	0.73	0.39	0.39	0.02	0.05	C66
1.33	2.38	4.69	7.81	14.58	21.53	29.04	41.75	52.99	59.11	6.80	3.71	3.68	0.16	0.42	C67
0.03	0.05	0.06	0.13	0.32	0.48	0.60	0.90	1.20	1.14	0.14	0.08	0.08	0.00	0.01	C68
0.06	0.08	0.13	0.18	0.19	0.40	0.31	0.49	0.59	0.75	0.15	0.11	0.14	0.01	0.01	C69
4.70	7.26	11.03	12.46	16.88	19.28	22.90	24.18	27.35	25.73	7.79	5.35	5.26	0.34	0.55	C70-C72,D32-D33, D42-D43
32.48	33.55	38.03	33.30	29.46	20.40	12.61	8.21	6.68	5.59	21.32	18.26	15.58	1.30	1.46	C73
0.12	0.20	0.41	0.44	0.61	0.72	0.69	0.94	1.15	0.96	0.28	0.19	0.21	0.01	0.02	C74
0.36	0.48	0.51	0.81	0.87	0.77	0.80	0.67	0.79	0.57	0.41	0.32	0.31	0.02	0.03	C75
0.25	0.21	0.31	0.31	0.49	0.59	0.66	0.94	0.90	0.78	0.32	0.27	0.25	0.02	0.02	C81
2.56	3.69	6.31	7.61	12.12	15.74	19.47	22.79	24.79	19.61	5.39	3.49	3.39	0.20	0.38	C82-C86,C96
0.05	0.06	0.07	0.15	0.24	0.32	0.48	0.49	0.38	0.25	0.10	0.07	0.07	0.00	0.01	C88
0.51	0.91	1.98	2.80	4.96	7.24	8.46	8.93	8.91	5.91	1.86	1.09	1.09	0.06	0.14	C90
0.47	0.78	1.11	1.31	2.14	3.07	3.42	4.06	4.15	3.24	1.35	1.14	1.34	0.07	0.10	C91
1.98	2.56	3.99	4.71	6.98	9.60	11.50	13.87	15.80	11.99	3.59	2.50	2.45	0.15	0.25	C92-C94,D45-D47
0.67	0.94	1.39	1.53	2.35	3.45	4.41	5.86	7.50	7.54	1.44	1.05	1.09	0.06	0.10	C95
2.54	3.81	6.78	8.02	12.45	16.89	19.61	26.96	36.47	45.52	6.06	3.68	3.70	0.20	0.39	O&U
161.05	252.38	402.22	484.11	748.53	938.93	1 121.71	1 326.21	1 504.91	1 427.22	320.83	198.15	192.91	11.68	21.98	C00-C97,D32-D33, D42-D43,D45-D47
160.26	251.01	400.08	480.78	742.72	930.86	1 109.79	1 309.61	1 480.84	1 392.66	317.77	196.45	191.23	11.60	21.80	C00-C97,D32-D33, D42-D43,D45-D47 exc. C44

部位 Site		病例数 No. cases	构成 Freq. /%	年龄组								
				0~	1~4	5~9	10~14	15~19	20~24	25~29	30~34	35~39
唇	Lip	209	0.05	0.00	0.00	0.00	0.00	0.00	0.00	0.01	0.00	0.04
舌	Tongue	1 610	0.40	0.00	0.00	0.02	0.02	0.00	0.07	0.15	0.31	0.43
口	Mouth	1 850	0.46	0.00	0.00	0.03	0.00	0.02	0.03	0.08	0.19	0.25
唾液腺	Salivary glands	831	0.20	0.00	0.00	0.03	0.03	0.12	0.16	0.27	0.34	0.24
扁桃腺	Tonsil	358	0.09	0.00	0.02	0.00	0.00	0.02	0.02	0.01	0.02	0.05
其他口咽	Other oropharynx	600	0.15	0.00	0.00	0.00	0.00	0.00	0.01	0.02	0.04	0.05
鼻咽	Nasopharynx	6 478	1.59	0.00	0.04	0.06	0.21	0.35	0.37	1.41	2.49	4.03
下咽	Hypopharynx	1 380	0.34	0.08	0.00	0.00	0.00	0.00	0.01	0.01	0.03	0.06
咽,部位不明	Pharynx unspecified	486	0.12	0.00	0.02	0.00	0.00	0.00	0.00	0.00	0.02	0.02
食管	Esophagus	25 809	6.35	0.00	0.00	0.00	0.00	0.03	0.04	0.08	0.09	0.40
胃	Stomach	41 142	10.12	0.32	0.02	0.02	0.10	0.17	0.31	0.91	1.72	3.01
小肠	Small intestine	1 994	0.49	0.00	0.02	0.00	0.00	0.00	0.04	0.12	0.16	0.34
结肠	Colon	25 384	6.25	0.00	0.02	0.05	0.07	0.15	0.39	1.17	1.78	3.16
直肠	Rectum	24 028	5.91	0.00	0.00	0.00	0.02	0.12	0.27	0.74	1.40	2.40
肛门	Anus	478	0.12	0.00	0.00	0.00	0.00	0.00	0.00	0.01	0.02	0.07
肝脏	Liver	45 830	11.28	1.97	0.59	0.09	0.17	0.29	0.68	2.44	5.82	10.74
胆囊及其他	Gallbladder etc.	5 084	1.25	0.00	0.00	0.00	0.00	0.00	0.03	0.04	0.16	0.34
胰腺	Pancreas	10 711	2.64	0.00	0.00	0.00	0.02	0.03	0.04	0.14	0.40	0.77
鼻、鼻窦及其他	Nose, sinuses etc.	690	0.17	0.00	0.02	0.02	0.03	0.07	0.12	0.09	0.16	0.19
喉	Larynx	4 662	1.15	0.08	0.00	0.00	0.00	0.00	0.00	0.04	0.04	0.15
气管、支气管、肺	Trachea, bronchus & lung	103 359	25.43	0.08	0.04	0.05	0.21	0.19	0.71	1.68	3.09	6.50
其他胸腔器官	Other thoracic organs	1 616	0.40	0.24	0.23	0.02	0.14	0.32	0.25	0.40	0.51	0.53
骨	Bone	2 099	0.52	0.16	0.09	0.31	1.01	1.23	0.59	0.61	0.53	0.73
皮肤黑色素瘤	Melanoma of skin	742	0.18	0.00	0.02	0.06	0.02	0.03	0.08	0.09	0.04	0.15
皮肤其他	Other skin	3 676	0.90	0.08	0.04	0.06	0.09	0.13	0.13	0.37	0.53	0.58
间皮瘤	Mesothelioma	250	0.06	0.00	0.00	0.00	0.00	0.00	0.03	0.01	0.03	0.01
卡波氏肉瘤	Kaposi sarcoma	74	0.02	0.00	0.00	0.00	0.02	0.00	0.03	0.06	0.00	0.05
结缔组织、软组织	Connective & soft tissue	1 401	0.34	0.63	0.45	0.31	0.26	0.34	0.32	0.36	0.56	0.74
乳腺	Breast	773	0.19	0.08	0.00	0.02	0.00	0.00	0.03	0.11	0.15	0.24
外阴	Vulva	—	—	—	—	—	—	—	—	—	—	—
阴道	Vagina	—	—	—	—	—	—	—	—	—	—	—
子宫颈	Cervix uteri	—	—	—	—	—	—	—	—	—	—	—
子宫体	Corpus uteri	—	—	—	—	—	—	—	—	—	—	—
子宫,部位不明	Uterus unspecified	—	—	—	—	—	—	—	—	—	—	—
卵巢	Ovary	—	—	—	—	—	—	—	—	—	—	—
其他女性生殖器	Other female genital organs	—	—	—	—	—	—	—	—	—	—	—
胎盘	Placenta	—	—	—	—	—	—	—	—	—	—	—
阴茎	Penis	887	0.22	0.00	0.00	0.02	0.00	0.02	0.00	0.09	0.11	0.19
前列腺	Prostate	19 448	4.78	0.08	0.00	0.02	0.00	0.02	0.04	0.05	0.09	0.11
睾丸	Testis	634	0.16	0.32	0.31	0.05	0.02	0.22	0.45	0.83	1.01	0.70
其他男性生殖器	Other male genital organs	286	0.07	0.00	0.00	0.00	0.02	0.00	0.01	0.02	0.05	0.05
肾	Kidney	7 924	1.95	0.47	0.56	0.13	0.09	0.12	0.27	0.56	1.31	2.43
肾盂	Renal pelvis	906	0.22	0.00	0.00	0.02	0.00	0.02	0.01	0.00	0.05	0.12
输尿管	Ureter	942	0.23	0.00	0.00	0.00	0.00	0.00	0.01	0.00	0.02	0.02
膀胱	Bladder	12 484	3.07	0.00	0.04	0.02	0.03	0.07	0.11	0.41	0.82	1.16
其他泌尿器官	Other urinary organs	199	0.05	0.00	0.00	0.02	0.00	0.00	0.00	0.02	0.00	0.03
眼	Eye	177	0.04	0.71	0.43	0.03	0.00	0.02	0.04	0.01	0.03	0.07
脑、神经系统	Brain, nervous system	8 364	2.06	1.74	1.91	1.99	1.77	1.53	1.21	2.08	3.19	3.58
甲状腺	Thyroid	13 183	3.24	0.00	0.04	0.00	0.12	0.73	4.13	12.91	18.31	19.68
肾上腺	Adrenal gland	369	0.09	0.55	0.36	0.11	0.00	0.00	0.05	0.08	0.07	0.12
其他内分泌腺	Other endocrine	466	0.11	0.08	0.09	0.13	0.29	0.19	0.09	0.14	0.20	0.23
霍奇金淋巴瘤	Hodgkin lymphoma	463	0.11	0.00	0.07	0.08	0.12	0.30	0.27	0.35	0.30	0.20
非霍奇金淋巴瘤	Non-Hodgkin lymphoma	7 200	1.77	0.16	0.72	0.64	0.80	1.16	0.88	1.19	2.00	1.99
免疫增生性疾病	Immunoproliferative diseases	162	0.04	0.00	0.00	0.00	0.07	0.03	0.01	0.08	0.01	0.04
多发性骨髓瘤	Multiple myeloma	2 458	0.60	0.00	0.04	0.05	0.03	0.07	0.03	0.07	0.12	0.24
淋巴样白血病	Lymphoid leukemia	1 819	0.45	0.79	3.82	1.87	1.27	0.79	0.56	0.46	0.45	0.46
髓样白血病	Myeloid leukemia	4 953	1.22	1.74	1.13	0.64	0.82	1.05	0.96	1.44	2.07	1.78
白血病,未特指	Leukemia unspecified	1 938	0.48	1.26	1.40	0.74	0.57	0.78	0.52	0.68	0.46	0.47
其他或未指明部位	Other and unspecified	7 581	1.87	1.74	1.12	0.64	0.61	0.62	0.49	0.89	0.91	1.42
所有部位合计	All sites	406 447	100.00	13.35	13.51	8.32	9.02	11.35	14.89	33.79	52.24	71.39
所有部位除外 C44	All sites except C44	402 771	99.10	13.27	13.47	8.25	8.93	11.21	14.75	33.42	51.71	70.81

Appendix Table 1-5　Cancer incidence in urban registration areas of China, male in 2018

Age group										粗率 Crude rate/ 100 000⁻¹	中标率 ASR China/ 100 000⁻¹	世标率 ASR world/ 100 000⁻¹	累积率 Cum. Rate/%		ICD-10
40~44	45~49	50~54	55~59	60~64	65~69	70~74	75~79	80~84	85+				0~64	0~74	
0.04	0.06	0.20	0.34	0.35	0.52	0.66	1.15	1.08	1.73	0.18	0.10	0.10	0.01	0.01	C00
0.71	1.33	2.41	2.94	3.88	3.77	4.31	3.65	4.15	3.45	1.36	0.87	0.85	0.06	0.10	C01-C02
0.59	1.20	1.98	3.22	4.51	4.53	5.64	6.80	6.42	8.20	1.56	0.95	0.95	0.06	0.11	C03-C06
0.44	0.65	0.98	1.02	1.82	1.95	1.97	2.15	2.56	2.93	0.70	0.48	0.46	0.03	0.05	C07-C08
0.15	0.34	0.47	0.83	0.84	1.04	0.82	0.73	0.40	1.12	0.30	0.19	0.19	0.01	0.02	C09
0.19	0.35	0.71	1.14	1.74	1.63	1.81	1.77	1.93	1.04	0.51	0.31	0.31	0.02	0.04	C10
6.18	8.49	11.18	10.11	12.29	11.97	11.35	8.23	7.90	4.83	5.47	3.92	3.66	0.29	0.40	C11
0.25	0.84	2.12	2.62	4.28	4.42	3.72	2.73	3.47	2.16	1.16	0.70	0.72	0.05	0.09	C12-C13
0.09	0.22	0.55	0.97	1.30	1.22	1.86	1.65	1.82	1.29	0.41	0.24	0.25	0.02	0.03	C14
2.00	6.85	21.94	34.25	64.39	87.54	105.66	115.77	122.92	118.65	21.78	12.50	12.72	0.65	1.62	C15
6.04	13.72	31.21	47.36	94.88	134.12	170.23	194.75	216.46	193.99	34.72	20.23	20.28	1.00	2.52	C16
0.47	1.11	2.00	2.33	4.47	6.21	6.97	8.99	8.18	7.94	1.68	1.02	1.01	0.06	0.12	C17
5.43	10.65	20.44	31.86	54.37	74.50	92.42	114.65	141.16	144.80	21.42	12.60	12.54	0.65	1.48	C18
5.20	10.49	22.31	31.55	57.70	76.58	87.84	97.43	111.27	100.44	20.28	12.01	12.03	0.66	1.48	C19-C20
0.15	0.25	0.54	0.57	1.14	1.27	1.52	2.34	2.16	2.07	0.40	0.24	0.24	0.01	0.03	C21
23.42	39.84	63.92	70.64	101.71	114.07	120.46	134.68	147.93	149.55	38.68	24.33	23.95	1.60	2.78	C22
0.73	1.57	3.41	5.52	10.23	14.95	19.89	26.21	33.64	38.23	4.29	2.43	2.44	0.11	0.28	C23-C24
2.06	4.10	8.93	13.51	23.00	30.07	40.68	50.39	60.47	69.72	9.04	5.22	5.24	0.27	0.62	C25
0.24	0.52	0.89	0.96	1.42	1.95	1.75	2.38	2.05	1.90	0.58	0.38	0.37	0.02	0.04	C30-C31
0.55	1.75	4.85	8.59	13.08	15.33	16.56	15.95	14.95	14.32	3.93	2.30	2.36	0.15	0.30	C32
13.10	32.64	78.93	126.78	246.96	337.17	414.33	489.36	529.02	498.69	87.23	50.53	50.89	2.55	6.31	C33-C34
0.57	1.32	1.73	2.55	3.50	3.90	4.04	4.42	4.26	4.83	1.36	0.93	0.91	0.06	0.10	C37-C38
0.84	1.18	1.81	1.97	3.28	4.88	5.66	8.15	9.04	9.41	1.77	1.31	1.27	0.07	0.12	C40-C41
0.25	0.34	0.80	0.81	1.38	2.04	2.26	2.96	3.64	5.70	0.63	0.38	0.38	0.02	0.04	C43
0.89	1.65	2.24	3.74	6.46	8.93	12.07	18.22	26.88	32.88	3.10	1.83	1.80	0.08	0.19	C44
0.04	0.07	0.20	0.39	0.59	0.95	0.64	1.04	1.14	1.29	0.21	0.12	0.13	0.01	0.01	C45
0.02	0.04	0.06	0.08	0.16	0.14	0.21	0.19	0.34	0.43	0.06	0.04	0.04	0.00	0.00	C46
0.64	0.87	1.60	1.63	2.37	3.18	2.77	4.15	5.29	4.83	1.18	0.86	0.85	0.05	0.08	C47,C49
0.39	0.59	0.91	1.02	1.65	1.72	2.05	3.07	2.56	3.71	0.65	0.41	0.40	0.03	0.04	C50
—	—	—	—	—	—	—	—	—	—	—	—	—	—	—	C51
—	—	—	—	—	—	—	—	—	—	—	—	—	—	—	C52
—	—	—	—	—	—	—	—	—	—	—	—	—	—	—	C53
—	—	—	—	—	—	—	—	—	—	—	—	—	—	—	C54
—	—	—	—	—	—	—	—	—	—	—	—	—	—	—	C55
—	—	—	—	—	—	—	—	—	—	—	—	—	—	—	C56
—	—	—	—	—	—	—	—	—	—	—	—	—	—	—	C57
—	—	—	—	—	—	—	—	—	—	—	—	—	—	—	C58
0.23	0.58	0.97	0.95	1.87	2.31	3.06	3.23	4.49	5.26	0.75	0.46	0.45	0.03	0.05	C60
0.32	0.58	2.80	8.06	27.88	55.51	100.79	150.05	193.16	188.29	16.41	8.87	8.74	0.20	0.98	C61
0.67	0.47	0.64	0.33	0.43	0.54	0.58	0.77	1.02	1.38	0.54	0.50	0.45	0.03	0.04	C62
0.03	0.10	0.12	0.32	0.58	0.79	0.96	1.69	1.93	1.81	0.24	0.14	0.14	0.01	0.02	C63
3.80	6.04	10.14	13.78	17.27	21.75	21.91	21.02	21.37	19.50	6.69	4.28	4.23	0.28	0.50	C64
0.15	0.27	0.80	1.25	1.68	2.86	3.56	4.69	4.49	4.75	0.76	0.45	0.45	0.02	0.05	C65
0.04	0.24	0.39	1.02	2.20	2.86	4.01	4.96	6.76	6.04	0.79	0.45	0.45	0.02	0.05	C66
2.00	3.74	7.46	12.70	23.69	34.74	46.55	67.99	89.34	104.50	10.54	6.00	5.97	0.26	0.67	C67
0.01	0.03	0.07	0.15	0.42	0.66	0.74	1.19	1.25	1.90	0.17	0.10	0.10	0.00	0.01	C68
0.08	0.11	0.19	0.21	0.18	0.41	0.29	0.27	0.57	0.86	0.15	0.11	0.14	0.01	0.01	C69
3.94	6.71	9.75	10.72	14.89	17.74	21.75	22.45	25.29	24.68	7.06	5.07	4.98	0.32	0.51	C70-C72,D32-D33, D42-D43
17.18	15.54	16.96	14.75	14.88	10.66	7.52	5.27	5.23	4.75	11.13	9.89	8.29	0.68	0.77	C73
0.11	0.18	0.34	0.53	0.78	0.91	0.85	1.08	1.36	1.12	0.31	0.21	0.23	0.01	0.02	C74
0.28	0.39	0.45	0.70	0.96	0.79	0.96	1.00	0.91	0.86	0.39	0.31	0.30	0.02	0.03	C75
0.35	0.26	0.42	0.45	0.76	0.84	0.93	1.08	1.19	1.12	0.39	0.32	0.30	0.02	0.03	C81
2.79	4.10	7.31	8.78	13.66	18.32	22.47	27.21	30.52	25.97	6.08	4.04	3.95	0.23	0.43	C82-C86,C96
0.03	0.06	0.08	0.20	0.31	0.47	0.74	0.65	0.63	0.52	0.14	0.09	0.09	0.00	0.01	C88
0.59	1.02	2.16	3.16	5.23	8.26	9.97	10.65	11.48	8.37	2.07	1.24	1.24	0.06	0.16	C90
0.47	0.82	1.40	1.44	2.32	3.36	4.20	5.53	5.80	5.09	1.54	1.28	1.49	0.08	0.12	C91
2.12	2.91	4.76	5.32	7.95	11.75	14.17	17.80	21.31	17.34	4.18	2.95	2.88	0.17	0.29	C92-C94,D45-D47
0.78	1.03	1.61	1.71	2.65	4.01	5.58	6.88	8.98	9.84	1.64	1.20	1.26	0.07	0.11	C95
2.26	3.69	7.11	8.99	14.25	20.05	22.41	29.17	40.58	53.42	6.40	3.98	4.03	0.22	0.43	O&U
109.87	191.92	365.24	504.83	878.63	1 170.13	1 434.17	1 708.61	1 950.71	1 917.51	343.02	209.37	207.52	11.32	24.35	C00-C97,D32-D33, D42-D43,D45-D47
108.98	190.27	363.00	501.09	872.17	1 161.20	1 422.10	1 690.39	1 923.83	1 884.63	339.91	207.54	205.72	11.24	24.16	C00-C97,D32-D33, D42-D43,D45-D47 exc. C44

部位 Site		病例数 No. cases	构成 Freq./%	年龄组								
				0~	1~4	5~9	10~14	15~19	20~24	25~29	30~34	35~39
唇	Lip	169	0.05	0.00	0.00	0.00	0.00	0.00	0.00	0.01	0.02	0.00
舌	Tongue	863	0.25	0.00	0.00	0.00	0.02	0.00	0.06	0.13	0.19	0.20
口	Mouth	1 049	0.30	0.00	0.00	0.00	0.04	0.02	0.07	0.09	0.26	0.20
唾液腺	Salivary glands	694	0.20	0.00	0.00	0.00	0.08	0.24	0.15	0.35	0.33	0.48
扁桃腺	Tonsil	122	0.03	0.00	0.00	0.02	0.00	0.04	0.00	0.00	0.01	0.03
其他口咽	Other oropharynx	91	0.03	0.00	0.00	0.00	0.02	0.00	0.01	0.01	0.02	0.02
鼻咽	Nasopharynx	2 626	0.75	0.00	0.00	0.04	0.02	0.17	0.32	0.63	1.37	1.68
下咽	Hypopharynx	72	0.02	0.00	0.00	0.00	0.00	0.00	0.01	0.00	0.00	0.01
咽,部位不明	Pharynx unspecified	136	0.04	0.00	0.00	0.02	0.00	0.00	0.00	0.02	0.01	0.03
食管	Esophagus	7 792	2.22	0.00	0.00	0.00	0.04	0.02	0.07	0.12	0.13	0.36
胃	Stomach	18 837	5.37	0.00	0.00	0.00	0.14	0.13	0.46	1.43	2.62	3.22
小肠	Small intestine	1 461	0.42	0.00	0.00	0.00	0.02	0.00	0.03	0.08	0.13	0.20
结肠	Colon	19 667	5.61	0.00	0.00	0.00	0.08	0.11	0.46	0.86	1.86	2.94
直肠	Rectum	15 025	4.28	0.00	0.00	0.02	0.00	0.04	0.24	0.60	1.39	2.17
肛门	Anus	385	0.11	0.00	0.00	0.02	0.00	0.04	0.03	0.02	0.04	0.07
肝脏	Liver	16 173	4.61	0.61	0.34	0.14	0.12	0.18	0.31	0.80	1.35	2.04
胆囊及其他	Gallbladder etc.	5 279	1.50	0.00	0.00	0.00	0.00	0.02	0.06	0.08	0.12	0.31
胰腺	Pancreas	8 221	2.34	0.00	0.00	0.04	0.04	0.04	0.22	0.20	0.35	0.48
鼻、鼻窦及其他	Nose,sinuses etc.	375	0.11	0.09	0.04	0.00	0.08	0.00	0.04	0.02	0.03	0.02
喉	Larynx	455	0.13	0.00	0.00	0.00	0.00	0.00	0.03	0.00	0.02	0.02
气管、支气管、肺	Trachea,bronchus & lung	58 613	16.71	0.09	0.10	0.05	0.06	0.20	0.61	2.00	4.88	9.26
其他胸腔器官	Other thoracic organs	1 040	0.30	0.44	0.22	0.07	0.06	0.13	0.15	0.21	0.36	0.47
骨	Bone	1 499	0.43	0.09	0.12	0.39	0.76	0.55	0.50	0.43	0.36	0.32
皮肤黑色素瘤	Melanoma of skin	718	0.20	0.00	0.08	0.04	0.06	0.09	0.01	0.12	0.13	0.17
皮肤其他	Other skin	3 533	1.01	0.09	0.16	0.04	0.08	0.18	0.20	0.26	0.47	0.69
间皮瘤	Mesothelioma	179	0.05	0.00	0.00	0.00	0.02	0.00	0.02	0.01	0.00	0.01
卡波氏肉瘤	Kaposi sarcoma	40	0.01	0.00	0.00	0.00	0.00	0.04	0.00	0.00	0.00	0.03
结缔组织、软组织	Connective & soft tissue	1 200	0.34	0.53	0.40	0.25	0.27	0.42	0.24	0.41	0.49	0.59
乳腺	Breast	60 395	17.21	0.00	0.02	0.00	0.02	0.22	1.23	6.07	17.38	34.08
外阴	Vulva	638	0.18	0.00	0.00	0.00	0.00	0.04	0.01	0.07	0.06	0.16
阴道	Vagina	360	0.10	0.18	0.04	0.00	0.00	0.04	0.00	0.03	0.05	0.11
子宫颈	Cervix uteri	20 109	5.73	0.00	0.00	0.00	0.00	0.06	0.45	2.93	7.52	13.22
子宫体	Corpus uteri	11 697	3.33	0.00	0.00	0.00	0.02	0.04	0.25	0.98	1.73	3.43
子宫,部位不明	Uterus unspecified	1 671	0.48	0.00	0.00	0.00	0.02	0.00	0.04	0.21	0.40	0.62
卵巢	Ovary	10 381	2.96	0.09	0.12	0.26	0.53	1.33	1.93	2.90	3.21	4.02
其他女性生殖器	Other female genital organs	769	0.22	0.00	0.06	0.02	0.02	0.04	0.04	0.06	0.10	0.20
胎盘	Placenta	91	0.03	0.00	0.00	0.00	0.00	0.04	0.11	0.20	0.22	0.13
阴茎	Penis	—	—	—	—	—	—	—	—	—	—	—
前列腺	Prostate	—	—	—	—	—	—	—	—	—	—	—
睾丸	Testis	—	—	—	—	—	—	—	—	—	—	—
其他男性生殖器	Other male genital organs	—	—	—	—	—	—	—	—	—	—	—
肾	Kidney	4 181	1.19	0.35	0.50	0.12	0.12	0.06	0.17	0.28	0.93	1.04
肾盂	Renal pelvis	694	0.20	0.00	0.00	0.00	0.00	0.00	0.01	0.00	0.03	0.04
输尿管	Ureter	787	0.22	0.00	0.00	0.00	0.00	0.00	0.00	0.00	0.00	0.07
膀胱	Bladder	3 557	1.01	0.00	0.00	0.02	0.02	0.02	0.08	0.24	0.29	0.34
其他泌尿器官	Other urinary organs	133	0.04	0.00	0.00	0.00	0.00	0.00	0.00	0.01	0.00	0.00
眼	Eye	173	0.05	1.23	0.36	0.05	0.02	0.02	0.04	0.07	0.05	0.01
脑、神经系统	Brain,nervous system	10 028	2.86	2.01	1.42	1.54	1.27	0.92	1.31	1.92	2.67	3.33
甲状腺	Thyroid	37 147	10.59	0.00	0.04	0.09	0.58	2.62	10.19	28.54	41.63	46.03
肾上腺	Adrenal gland	302	0.09	0.96	0.24	0.04	0.00	0.04	0.01	0.03	0.10	0.14
其他内分泌腺	Other endocrine	503	0.14	0.00	0.08	0.00	0.08	0.15	0.11	0.26	0.31	0.46
霍奇金淋巴瘤	Hodgkin lymphoma	282	0.08	0.18	0.00	0.00	0.06	0.13	0.32	0.31	0.30	0.29
非霍奇金淋巴瘤	Non-Hodgkin lymphoma	5 516	1.57	0.18	0.34	0.25	0.43	0.46	0.66	1.00	1.43	1.92
免疫增生性疾病	Immunoproliferative diseases	83	0.02	0.00	0.04	0.02	0.00	0.02	0.01	0.00	0.01	0.03
多发性骨髓瘤	Multiple myeloma	1 943	0.55	0.09	0.08	0.02	0.08	0.02	0.03	0.09	0.06	0.18
淋巴样白血病	Lymphoid leukemia	1 368	0.39	1.23	3.32	1.72	1.25	0.44	0.28	0.52	0.33	0.33
髓样白血病	Myeloid leukemia	3 521	1.00	1.66	0.82	0.65	0.51	0.55	0.81	1.24	1.44	1.45
白血病,未特指	Leukemia unspecified	1 489	0.42	0.88	0.88	0.67	0.53	0.44	0.46	0.45	0.47	0.51
其他或未指明部位	Other and unspecified	6 726	1.92	2.28	1.00	0.51	0.47	0.50	0.52	0.87	1.37	1.70
所有部位合计	All sites	350 860	100.00	13.22	10.83	7.21	7.97	10.87	23.40	58.17	99.04	140.01
所有部位除外 C44	All sites except C44	347 327	98.99	13.13	10.67	7.18	7.89	10.68	23.20	57.91	98.57	139.32

Appendix Table 1-6　Cancer incidence in urban registration areas of China,female in 2018

40~44	45~49	50~54	55~59	60~64	65~69	70~74	75~79	80~84	85+	粗率 Crude rate/ 100 000⁻¹	中标率 ASR China/ 100 000⁻¹	世标率 ASR world/ 100 000⁻¹	累积率 Cum. Rate/% 0~64	0~74	ICD-10
0.05	0.06	0.11	0.20	0.27	0.34	0.71	0.71	1.26	0.79	0.14	0.08	0.08	0.00	0.01	C00
0.33	0.74	0.83	1.06	1.53	2.26	2.34	2.52	3.40	3.88	0.74	0.44	0.42	0.03	0.05	C01-C02
0.28	0.37	0.76	1.01	1.70	2.60	3.98	4.28	5.69	5.81	0.89	0.51	0.49	0.02	0.06	C03-C06
0.58	0.72	0.92	0.71	0.92	1.28	1.44	1.60	0.89	1.70	0.59	0.44	0.40	0.03	0.04	C07-C08
0.07	0.15	0.14	0.18	0.18	0.24	0.33	0.18	0.31	0.42	0.10	0.07	0.06	0.00	0.01	C09
0.02	0.06	0.09	0.08	0.21	0.28	0.20	0.34	0.28	0.36	0.08	0.05	0.05	0.00	0.01	C10
2.62	3.63	4.17	3.69	4.12	4.00	4.38	4.08	3.78	3.27	2.23	1.59	1.46	0.11	0.15	C11
0.03	0.03	0.09	0.10	0.11	0.24	0.33	0.24	0.19	0.12	0.06	0.04	0.04	0.00	0.00	C12-C13
0.05	0.04	0.07	0.09	0.17	0.38	0.43	0.68	0.98	0.85	0.12	0.06	0.06	0.00	0.01	C14
0.61	1.37	3.01	4.36	10.92	21.27	34.77	46.72	53.99	58.20	6.63	3.33	3.29	0.11	0.39	C15
5.49	9.51	16.14	19.33	30.84	46.78	61.62	80.32	100.52	102.84	16.02	8.92	8.70	0.45	0.99	C16
0.41	0.81	1.41	1.80	3.12	3.78	4.69	5.71	6.43	5.39	1.24	0.70	0.69	0.04	0.08	C17
5.08	8.59	16.37	21.60	35.69	49.31	64.42	86.04	109.19	99.45	16.73	9.17	9.01	0.47	1.04	C18
4.12	7.86	14.97	16.48	29.04	40.38	47.97	62.13	70.58	63.78	12.78	7.15	7.04	0.38	0.83	C19-C20
0.18	0.20	0.37	0.52	0.66	0.74	0.98	1.77	2.00	1.82	0.33	0.19	0.18	0.01	0.02	C21
4.42	7.13	13.93	16.01	27.71	40.93	54.57	71.45	85.64	92.91	13.76	7.53	7.44	0.37	0.85	C22
0.75	1.55	3.24	4.71	9.30	12.66	18.67	26.93	36.50	36.16	4.49	2.30	2.28	0.10	0.26	C23-C24
1.00	2.55	4.53	7.49	14.08	20.73	30.38	43.97	52.78	53.00	6.99	3.63	3.59	0.16	0.41	C25
0.18	0.31	0.43	0.31	0.78	0.66	1.13	1.19	1.26	1.41	0.32	0.20	0.20	0.01	0.02	C30-C31
0.06	0.22	0.34	0.52	0.76	1.22	1.76	1.84	3.03	1.94	0.39	0.21	0.21	0.01	0.02	C32
17.03	30.36	57.57	72.79	117.31	150.72	184.44	226.79	273.85	251.71	49.86	27.86	27.53	1.56	3.24	C33-C34
0.46	0.71	1.46	1.45	2.02	2.10	2.52	2.69	2.52	2.30	0.88	0.59	0.58	0.04	0.06	C37-C38
0.58	0.87	1.22	1.57	2.19	2.93	4.48	5.00	6.76	5.15	1.28	0.89	0.87	0.05	0.09	C40-C41
0.27	0.46	0.79	0.71	1.47	1.62	2.29	2.62	2.24	2.85	0.61	0.37	0.37	0.02	0.04	C43
0.71	1.09	2.05	2.90	5.15	7.24	11.77	15.17	21.77	35.73	3.01	1.58	1.57	0.07	0.16	C44
0.06	0.10	0.22	0.29	0.29	0.64	0.55	0.54	0.61	0.36	0.15	0.09	0.09	0.01	0.01	C45
0.03	0.04	0.02	0.04	0.08	0.09	0.08	0.14	0.19	0.06	0.03	0.02	0.02	0.00	0.00	C46
0.80	0.83	1.28	1.25	1.90	2.09	2.62	3.40	3.59	3.21	1.02	0.74	0.73	0.05	0.07	C47,C49
61.22	94.09	101.40	98.68	117.97	100.40	85.89	78.93	68.30	52.33	51.38	34.95	32.87	2.66	3.59	C50
0.30	0.31	0.52	0.62	1.14	1.79	2.19	2.18	3.22	2.73	0.54	0.31	0.30	0.02	0.04	C51
0.16	0.32	0.36	0.52	0.84	0.79	1.16	0.82	0.98	0.85	0.31	0.19	0.19	0.01	0.02	C52
22.31	30.43	41.74	34.79	32.98	27.61	23.53	22.00	16.74	11.87	17.11	12.02	11.15	0.93	1.19	C53
7.40	15.01	28.29	26.18	23.47	20.99	16.07	13.53	10.16	5.57	9.95	6.49	6.32	0.53	0.72	C54
1.34	2.08	3.24	3.07	2.76	3.21	2.24	2.24	2.52	3.31	1.42	0.93	0.88	0.07	0.10	C55
7.50	13.02	17.42	15.88	19.47	18.58	18.95	17.04	17.11	12.23	8.83	6.09	5.80	0.44	0.63	C56
0.41	0.92	1.24	1.46	1.74	1.62	1.59	1.53	0.89	1.09	0.65	0.42	0.41	0.03	0.05	C57
0.12	0.11	0.02	0.04	0.00	0.00	0.03	0.00	0.00	0.06	0.08	0.08	0.07	0.00	0.01	C58
—	—	—	—	—	—	—	—	—	—	—	—	—	—	—	C60
—	—	—	—	—	—	—	—	—	—	—	—	—	—	—	C61
—	—	—	—	—	—	—	—	—	—	—	—	—	—	—	C62
—	—	—	—	—	—	—	—	—	—	—	—	—	—	—	C63
1.80	2.84	4.81	6.43	8.03	11.04	12.17	12.11	12.63	10.54	3.56	2.17	2.15	0.14	0.25	C64
0.04	0.22	0.26	0.43	1.07	2.07	2.72	4.32	4.52	4.24	0.59	0.30	0.30	0.01	0.03	C65
0.04	0.16	0.25	0.42	1.31	1.79	3.38	5.61	6.39	4.00	0.67	0.34	0.33	0.01	0.04	C66
0.66	1.00	1.85	2.89	5.57	8.80	12.45	18.53	23.17	27.25	3.03	1.57	1.55	0.06	0.17	C67
0.04	0.07	0.06	0.11	0.23	0.31	0.45	0.65	1.17	0.61	0.11	0.06	0.06	0.00	0.01	C68
0.05	0.04	0.06	0.15	0.20	0.40	0.33	0.68	0.61	0.67	0.15	0.11	0.14	0.01	0.01	C69
5.45	7.82	12.34	14.22	18.85	20.77	23.98	25.71	29.05	26.47	8.53	5.61	5.53	0.37	0.59	C70-C72,D32-D33, D42-D43
47.72	51.70	59.57	51.99	43.89	29.79	17.43	10.81	7.88	6.18	31.60	26.60	22.86	1.92	2.16	C73
0.13	0.22	0.48	0.36	0.43	0.53	0.53	0.82	0.98	0.85	0.26	0.17	0.19	0.01	0.02	C74
0.44	0.56	0.56	0.92	0.79	0.76	0.66	0.37	0.70	0.36	0.43	0.33	0.31	0.02	0.03	C75
0.14	0.17	0.21	0.17	0.23	0.34	0.40	0.82	0.65	0.55	0.24	0.21	0.19	0.01	0.02	C81
2.34	3.27	5.28	6.43	10.60	13.26	16.63	18.87	20.09	15.14	4.69	2.95	2.85	0.17	0.32	C82-C86,C96
0.07	0.06	0.07	0.09	0.17	0.19	0.23	0.34	0.19	0.06	0.07	0.05	0.05	0.00	0.01	C88
0.43	0.80	1.80	2.44	4.70	6.26	7.03	7.41	6.81	4.18	1.65	0.94	0.95	0.05	0.12	C90
0.46	0.74	0.83	1.18	1.97	2.79	2.67	2.75	2.80	1.94	1.16	1.01	1.20	0.06	0.09	C91
1.83	2.21	3.20	4.10	6.02	7.52	8.97	10.41	11.28	8.24	3.00	2.07	2.03	0.12	0.21	C92-C94,D45-D47
0.57	0.84	1.17	1.35	2.05	2.91	3.30	4.96	6.29	4.18	1.27	0.90	0.93	0.05	0.08	C95
2.81	3.92	6.44	7.05	10.66	13.85	16.96	24.99	33.10	39.97	5.72	3.41	3.39	0.19	0.34	O&U
212.06	313.28	440.01	463.22	619.72	715.99	825.62	987.88	1 139.19	1 083.10	298.46	189.02	180.46	12.03	19.74	C00-C97,D32-D33, D42-D43,D45-D47
211.35	312.20	437.97	460.32	614.57	708.75	813.85	972.71	1 117.42	1 047.37	295.46	187.44	178.89	11.96	19.57	C00-C97,D32-D33, D42-D43,D45-D47 exc. C44

附表 1-7 2018 年全国农村肿瘤登记地区男女合计癌症发病主要指标

部位	Site	病例数 No. cases	构成 Freq. /%	0~	1~4	5~9	10~14	15~19	20~24	25~29	30~34	35~39
唇	Lip	598	0.07	0.03	0.01	0.01	0.03	0.01	0.01	0.02	0.03	0.02
舌	Tongue	2 140	0.27	0.00	0.01	0.02	0.04	0.01	0.05	0.08	0.25	0.42
口	Mouth	3 049	0.38	0.03	0.05	0.04	0.03	0.10	0.07	0.13	0.23	0.27
唾液腺	Salivary glands	1 695	0.21	0.00	0.03	0.02	0.07	0.07	0.15	0.22	0.30	0.34
扁桃腺	Tonsil	427	0.05	0.00	0.03	0.04	0.01	0.01	0.01	0.02	0.03	0.04
其他口咽	Other oropharynx	684	0.08	0.00	0.00	0.01	0.01	0.01	0.03	0.01	0.01	0.06
鼻咽	Nasopharynx	10 460	1.30	0.00	0.07	0.03	0.13	0.29	0.48	0.65	1.71	2.54
下咽	Hypopharynx	1 200	0.15	0.00	0.01	0.01	0.01	0.00	0.00	0.02	0.03	0.03
咽,部位不明	Pharynx unspecified	732	0.09	0.00	0.01	0.01	0.01	0.01	0.02	0.04	0.02	0.04
食管	Esophagus	60 344	7.48	0.00	0.01	0.01	0.01	0.01	0.05	0.18	0.27	0.48
胃	Stomach	81 436	10.10	0.03	0.01	0.04	0.08	0.20	0.35	1.17	2.34	3.28
小肠	Small intestine	2 988	0.37	0.00	0.02	0.01	0.01	0.01	0.03	0.09	0.17	0.23
结肠	Colon	33 409	4.14	0.00	0.04	0.01	0.07	0.27	0.33	0.90	1.83	2.64
直肠	Rectum	40 228	4.99	0.03	0.03	0.02	0.03	0.09	0.23	0.69	1.62	2.07
肛门	Anus	1 031	0.13	0.00	0.00	0.00	0.01	0.01	0.02	0.09	0.05	0.07
肝脏	Liver	81 435	10.10	1.19	0.41	0.15	0.20	0.32	0.82	2.01	4.90	8.79
胆囊及其他	Gallbladder etc.	10 897	1.35	0.00	0.00	0.01	0.01	0.01	0.02	0.06	0.15	0.29
胰腺	Pancreas	18 685	2.32	0.00	0.03	0.00	0.02	0.07	0.09	0.23	0.39	0.72
鼻,鼻窦及其他	Nose, sinuses etc.	1 204	0.15	0.00	0.04	0.03	0.01	0.04	0.07	0.12	0.10	0.16
喉	Larynx	4 781	0.59	0.00	0.01	0.02	0.03	0.01	0.03	0.02	0.05	0.11
气管、支气管、肺	Trachea, bronchus & lung	178 360	22.11	0.03	0.09	0.05	0.15	0.29	0.71	1.98	3.99	7.01
其他胸腔器官	Other thoracic organs	2 535	0.31	0.27	0.22	0.10	0.09	0.19	0.16	0.28	0.34	0.39
骨	Bone	5 610	0.70	0.14	0.28	0.39	1.13	1.11	0.58	0.67	0.68	0.70
皮肤黑色素瘤	Melanoma of skin	1 400	0.17	0.07	0.05	0.04	0.07	0.02	0.05	0.07	0.12	0.11
皮肤其他	Other skin	7 470	0.93	0.10	0.13	0.16	0.15	0.21	0.17	0.28	0.39	0.53
间皮瘤	Mesothelioma	361	0.04	0.00	0.00	0.01	0.00	0.01	0.01	0.03	0.04	0.05
卡波氏肉瘤	Kaposi sarcoma	61	0.01	0.00	0.00	0.01	0.01	0.00	0.01	0.01	0.02	0.00
结缔组织、软组织	Connective & soft tissue	2 381	0.30	0.44	0.28	0.21	0.24	0.30	0.30	0.40	0.47	0.54
乳腺	Breast	50 468	6.35	0.00	0.11	0.03	0.10	0.51	1.97	6.11	15.46	27.59
外阴	Vulva	623	0.08	0.00	0.00	0.01	0.01	0.00	0.04	0.05	0.12	0.15
阴道	Vagina	435	0.05	0.07	0.00	0.01	0.01	0.01	0.00	0.05	0.05	0.06
子宫颈	Cervix uteri	26 517	3.29	0.00	0.10	0.01	0.03	0.08	0.55	3.55	8.88	14.70
子宫体	Corpus uteri	11 159	1.38	0.07	0.04	0.00	0.00	0.04	0.01	0.10	0.77	1.70	2.84
子宫,部位不明	Uterus unspecified	2 690	0.33	0.00	0.00	0.01	0.00	0.01	0.00	0.42	0.59	1.05
卵巢	Ovary	9 812	1.22	0.07	0.06	0.20	0.59	1.05	1.73	2.24	2.60	3.65
其他女性生殖器	Other female genital organs	679	0.08	0.00	0.02	0.00	0.04	0.04	0.10	0.13	0.07	0.17
胎盘	Placenta	113	0.01	0.00	0.00	0.00	0.03	0.03	0.11	0.21	0.13	0.16
阴茎	Penis	1 161	0.14	0.00	0.00	0.01	0.00	0.01	0.02	0.05	0.13	0.19
前列腺	Prostate	14 408	1.79	0.00	0.01	0.01	0.04	0.01	0.01	0.03	0.11	0.04
睾丸	Testis	622	0.08	0.32	0.33	0.02	0.05	0.10	0.27	0.43	0.70	0.56
其他男性生殖器	Other male genital organs	216	0.03	0.06	0.00	0.00	0.02	0.03	0.03	0.03	0.07	0.03
肾	Kidney	9 034	1.12	0.31	0.43	0.13	0.03	0.12	0.17	0.42	0.75	1.14
肾盂	Renal pelvis	1 038	0.13	0.00	0.01	0.01	0.00	0.00	0.01	0.01	0.02	0.04
输尿管	Ureter	1 254	0.16	0.00	0.01	0.00	0.00	0.01	0.01	0.02	0.01	0.03
膀胱	Bladder	14 575	1.81	0.03	0.03	0.02	0.01	0.03	0.11	0.25	0.48	0.66
其他泌尿器官	Other urinary organs	283	0.04	0.00	0.00	0.01	0.01	0.00	0.00	0.00	0.00	0.01
眼	Eye	506	0.06	0.88	0.47	0.09	0.03	0.02	0.02	0.03	0.06	0.05
脑、神经系统	Brain, nervous system	21 796	2.70	2.41	1.80	1.68	1.66	1.63	1.46	2.38	3.15	3.49
甲状腺	Thyroid	34 263	4.25	0.00	0.03	0.07	0.36	1.18	4.00	10.16	14.61	17.15
肾上腺	Adrenal gland	823	0.10	0.34	0.16	0.07	0.03	0.02	0.03	0.06	0.13	0.13
其他内分泌腺	Other endocrine	1 247	0.15	0.00	0.03	0.05	0.15	0.09	0.08	0.22	0.30	0.38
霍奇金淋巴瘤	Hodgkin lymphoma	863	0.11	0.00	0.01	0.09	0.10	0.16	0.19	0.27	0.24	0.22
非霍奇金淋巴瘤	Non-Hodgkin lymphoma	11 432	1.42	0.34	0.54	0.54	0.71	0.63	0.70	0.98	1.32	1.26
免疫增生性疾病	Immunoproliferative diseases	146	0.02	0.00	0.00	0.01	0.00	0.00	0.00	0.00	0.00	0.00
多发性骨髓瘤	Multiple myeloma	3 892	0.48	0.00	0.07	0.02	0.03	0.05	0.03	0.10	0.15	0.13
淋巴样白血病	Lymphoid leukemia	2 959	0.37	0.99	1.99	1.35	0.92	0.56	0.38	0.50	0.40	0.35
髓样白血病	Myeloid leukemia	7 805	0.97	1.02	0.74	0.55	0.90	1.01	0.88	1.21	1.54	1.39
白血病,未特指	Leukemia unspecified	5 936	0.74	1.90	1.57	1.37	1.01	0.97	0.72	0.91	1.02	0.99
其他或未指明部位	Other and unspecified	13 521	1.68	1.19	0.82	0.52	0.66	0.67	0.68	0.83	1.20	1.40
所有部位合计	All sites	806 616	100.00	12.10	10.93	8.18	9.70	11.73	16.73	35.72	60.90	85.81
所有部位除外 C44	All sites except C44	799 146	99.07	11.99	10.80	8.02	9.55	11.52	16.56	35.44	60.51	85.27

Appendix Table 1-7　Cancer incidence in rural registration areas of China, both sexes in 2018

| Age group | | | | | | | | | | 粗率 Crude rate/ 100 000⁻¹ | 中标率 ASR China/ 100 000⁻¹ | 世标率 ASR world/ 100 000⁻¹ | 累积率 Cum. Rate/% | | ICD-10 |
40~44	45~49	50~54	55~59	60~64	65~69	70~74	75~79	80~84	85+				0~64	0~74	
0.04	0.11	0.19	0.25	0.44	0.84	0.95	1.12	1.26	1.80	0.21	0.13	0.13	0.01	0.01	C00
0.49	0.77	1.29	1.20	2.10	2.22	2.34	2.48	2.41	1.77	0.75	0.51	0.49	0.03	0.06	C01-C02
0.49	0.68	1.44	1.52	2.63	3.37	4.82	4.92	5.46	5.09	1.06	0.69	0.67	0.04	0.08	C03-C06
0.44	0.69	0.98	1.00	1.34	1.76	1.70	1.37	1.55	1.20	0.59	0.43	0.41	0.03	0.05	C07-C08
0.08	0.17	0.27	0.28	0.42	0.37	0.52	0.45	0.33	0.46	0.15	0.10	0.10	0.01	0.01	C09
0.10	0.12	0.34	0.40	0.76	0.99	0.84	1.24	0.67	0.71	0.24	0.15	0.15	0.01	0.02	C10
4.16	5.86	7.84	6.75	8.41	8.59	7.49	6.43	5.34	3.79	3.64	2.67	2.51	0.19	0.27	C11
0.09	0.31	0.70	0.91	1.51	1.63	1.68	1.38	1.17	0.78	0.42	0.26	0.27	0.02	0.03	C12-C13
0.13	0.18	0.24	0.35	0.69	0.86	1.23	1.40	1.36	1.06	0.25	0.16	0.16	0.01	0.02	C14
1.74	5.35	16.18	25.02	58.16	90.75	116.01	135.57	142.38	129.95	21.02	12.28	12.39	0.54	1.57	C15
6.17	13.81	29.17	37.99	77.60	111.86	142.09	159.85	170.17	144.63	28.36	17.22	17.14	0.86	2.13	C16
0.47	0.89	1.44	1.63	2.74	3.81	4.32	4.53	4.67	3.86	1.04	0.66	0.65	0.04	0.08	C17
4.27	8.02	13.64	16.55	29.83	41.31	50.33	58.09	68.03	62.05	11.64	7.28	7.15	0.39	0.85	C18
4.81	9.27	17.43	20.20	36.95	52.47	62.82	72.25	76.54	66.37	14.01	8.67	8.58	0.47	1.04	C19-C20
0.10	0.22	0.44	0.46	0.91	1.09	1.58	1.75	2.45	2.51	0.36	0.22	0.22	0.01	0.03	C21
16.89	28.43	46.43	46.17	74.01	89.22	101.62	110.20	120.65	112.79	28.36	18.39	18.00	1.15	2.10	C22
0.74	1.67	3.43	4.40	9.83	14.02	19.63	23.27	27.45	27.42	3.80	2.24	2.24	0.10	0.27	C23-C24
1.46	3.29	6.25	8.30	16.64	23.75	31.66	38.56	45.56	43.76	6.51	3.89	3.88	0.19	0.46	C25
0.29	0.38	0.78	0.60	0.91	1.27	1.34	1.38	1.83	1.66	0.42	0.29	0.28	0.02	0.03	C30-C31
0.27	0.93	2.17	3.33	5.30	6.24	7.40	7.99	7.96	5.31	1.67	1.02	1.03	0.06	0.13	C32
14.61	32.03	69.13	89.48	171.67	241.22	298.42	338.70	362.54	317.17	62.12	37.68	37.62	1.96	4.65	C33-C34
0.54	0.93	1.36	1.46	2.29	2.61	2.39	2.83	2.48	2.12	0.88	0.63	0.62	0.04	0.07	C37-C38
0.96	1.32	2.25	2.40	3.61	5.50	8.12	7.95	8.32	7.68	1.95	1.47	1.43	0.08	0.15	C40-C41
0.25	0.34	0.75	0.74	1.23	1.41	1.66	2.13	2.65	2.62	0.49	0.32	0.32	0.02	0.03	C43
0.78	1.28	2.39	2.61	4.69	7.26	11.35	14.73	22.64	33.26	2.60	1.57	1.56	0.07	0.16	C44
0.04	0.14	0.19	0.25	0.33	0.38	0.48	0.48	0.26	0.35	0.13	0.09	0.08	0.01	0.01	C45
0.01	0.02	0.00	0.02	0.05	0.05	0.07	0.09	0.12	0.11	0.02	0.02	0.02	0.00	0.00	C46
0.64	0.95	1.19	1.17	1.62	1.77	2.06	2.62	2.12	2.02	0.83	0.65	0.63	0.04	0.06	C47,C49
48.74	76.69	84.67	67.39	76.16	63.90	51.22	39.30	34.39	28.04	36.02	26.30	24.44	2.03	2.60	C50
0.31	0.49	0.64	0.63	0.88	1.35	1.68	1.76	1.95	1.39	0.44	0.29	0.28	0.02	0.03	C51
0.15	0.46	0.48	0.47	0.79	0.95	1.07	1.34	0.91	0.41	0.31	0.20	0.20	0.01	0.02	C52
24.15	35.37	47.92	35.33	37.56	34.78	29.90	27.61	22.06	15.41	18.92	13.76	12.75	1.04	1.36	C53
6.39	14.25	25.04	19.46	19.27	15.90	12.60	8.54	7.40	5.45	7.96	5.44	5.27	0.45	0.59	C54
2.20	3.29	4.80	3.67	3.63	3.63	3.80	3.69	4.21	3.19	1.92	1.34	1.26	0.10	0.14	C55
6.07	10.81	16.04	12.64	15.52	16.36	15.29	12.14	10.47	6.55	7.00	5.06	4.81	0.37	0.52	C56
0.37	0.59	1.18	0.75	1.47	1.36	1.07	0.80	0.82	0.81	0.48	0.33	0.33	0.02	0.04	C57
0.12	0.17	0.07	0.01	0.04	0.03	0.00	0.00	0.00	0.00	0.08	0.09	0.07	0.01	0.01	C58
0.32	0.75	0.95	1.29	2.28	2.62	3.77	3.25	4.03	4.91	0.79	0.52	0.51	0.03	0.06	C60
0.21	0.52	1.87	4.85	16.24	37.53	68.10	100.61	117.38	130.79	9.80	5.81	5.73	0.12	0.65	C61
0.53	0.53	0.50	0.34	0.48	0.53	0.64	0.71	1.06	0.82	0.42	0.39	0.35	0.02	0.03	C62
0.03	0.05	0.14	0.12	0.32	0.50	0.75	1.10	1.06	0.82	0.15	0.10	0.10	0.00	0.01	C63
1.58	3.04	5.51	6.30	8.19	10.47	10.32	10.04	10.13	8.07	3.15	2.10	2.08	0.14	0.24	C64
0.12	0.17	0.41	0.50	0.97	1.33	1.85	1.91	2.14	1.88	0.36	0.22	0.22	0.01	0.03	C65
0.04	0.16	0.29	0.46	1.15	1.90	2.60	2.79	3.12	2.02	0.44	0.26	0.26	0.01	0.03	C66
1.16	2.12	4.43	5.98	12.06	17.40	24.92	32.63	40.94	37.82	5.08	3.02	2.99	0.14	0.35	C67
0.04	0.04	0.06	0.11	0.25	0.38	0.48	0.61	0.81	0.50	0.10	0.06	0.06	0.00	0.01	C68
0.09	0.13	0.19	0.23	0.33	0.36	0.46	0.61	0.62	0.64	0.18	0.13	0.17	0.01	0.01	C69
5.03	7.82	11.91	11.71	16.73	21.11	22.37	22.87	25.78	21.44	7.59	5.55	5.45	0.35	0.57	C70-C72,D32-D33, D42-D43
17.59	20.84	25.33	20.94	17.21	13.38	8.60	5.68	4.38	3.18	11.93	10.31	8.95	0.75	0.86	C73
0.17	0.31	0.38	0.52	0.59	0.73	0.87	1.04	1.05	0.85	0.29	0.21	0.21	0.01	0.02	C74
0.40	0.47	0.72	0.74	0.97	1.09	0.88	0.84	0.86	0.78	0.43	0.34	0.32	0.02	0.03	C75
0.15	0.22	0.40	0.38	0.49	0.73	0.80	1.01	0.83	0.78	0.30	0.25	0.23	0.01	0.02	C81
1.96	3.15	5.31	5.65	10.14	13.34	15.45	15.77	14.80	10.68	3.98	2.77	2.72	0.16	0.31	C82-C86,C96
0.02	0.05	0.04	0.07	0.16	0.20	0.23	0.17	0.41	0.18	0.05	0.03	0.03	0.00	0.00	C88
0.37	0.95	1.78	2.26	3.89	5.67	6.20	6.26	5.55	2.90	1.36	0.86	0.86	0.05	0.11	C90
0.53	0.64	1.05	1.05	1.85	2.11	2.43	3.00	2.50	2.41	1.03	0.89	1.00	0.06	0.08	C91
1.66	2.44	3.58	3.50	5.60	7.18	8.79	8.76	10.20	6.86	2.72	2.08	2.02	0.13	0.21	C92-C94,D45-D47
1.20	1.57	2.20	2.14	3.67	4.78	6.75	7.45	8.17	6.37	2.07	1.65	1.70	0.10	0.15	C95
2.08	3.52	5.98	6.13	10.60	14.48	18.41	20.85	23.97	28.66	4.71	3.15	3.13	0.18	0.34	O&U
139.17	237.21	388.49	417.26	698.47	923.70	1 113.38	1 247.31	1 346.17	1210.09	280.94	183.13	178.95	10.60	20.79	C00-C97,D32-D33, D42-D43,D45-D47
138.39	235.93	386.10	414.65	693.78	916.44	1 102.03	1 232.58	1 323.53	1 176.83	278.34	181.56	177.39	10.53	20.63	C00-C97,D32-D33, D42-D43,D45-D47 exc. C44

附表 1-8　2018 年全国农村肿瘤登记地区男性癌症发病主要指标

部位 Site		病例数 No. cases	构成 Freq./%	年龄组								
				0~	1~4	5~9	10~14	15~19	20~24	25~29	30~34	35~39
唇	Lip	361	0.08	0.06	0.01	0.00	0.04	0.02	0.01	0.02	0.03	0.05
舌	Tongue	1 418	0.31	0.00	0.03	0.02	0.06	0.00	0.04	0.09	0.35	0.52
口	Mouth	2 015	0.44	0.06	0.06	0.04	0.05	0.10	0.07	0.15	0.27	0.38
唾液腺	Salivary glands	961	0.21	0.00	0.03	0.01	0.08	0.06	0.13	0.17	0.32	0.32
扁桃腺	Tonsil	303	0.07	0.00	0.04	0.06	0.00	0.01	0.03	0.04	0.06	0.05
其他口咽	Other oropharynx	571	0.13	0.00	0.00	0.02	0.01	0.01	0.04	0.02	0.01	0.10
鼻咽	Nasopharynx	7 434	1.64	0.00	0.08	0.03	0.17	0.39	0.55	0.77	2.24	3.55
下咽	Hypopharynx	1 089	0.24	0.00	0.01	0.01	0.01	0.00	0.00	0.03	0.00	0.05
咽,部位不明	Pharynx unspecified	565	0.12	0.00	0.01	0.01	0.00	0.00	0.00	0.05	0.02	0.06
食管	Esophagus	44 012	9.69	0.00	0.03	0.01	0.01	0.01	0.07	0.15	0.32	0.56
胃	Stomach	57 400	12.64	0.00	0.03	0.04	0.08	0.21	0.38	0.90	1.99	3.49
小肠	Small intestine	1 735	0.38	0.00	0.01	0.00	0.01	0.02	0.03	0.13	0.19	0.24
结肠	Colon	18 898	4.16	0.00	0.04	0.01	0.07	0.36	0.27	0.96	2.15	2.95
直肠	Rectum	24 378	5.37	0.06	0.03	0.03	0.04	0.09	0.20	0.77	1.70	2.22
肛门	Anus	599	0.13	0.00	0.00	0.00	0.01	0.01	0.03	0.10	0.06	0.05
肝脏	Liver	60 418	13.31	1.34	0.47	0.18	0.27	0.43	1.02	3.03	7.96	14.59
胆囊及其他	Gallbladder etc.	5 209	1.15	0.00	0.00	0.01	0.00	0.00	0.03	0.09	0.19	0.28
胰腺	Pancreas	10 854	2.39	0.00	0.04	0.00	0.00	0.00	0.06	0.11	0.37	0.90
鼻、鼻窦及其他	Nose, sinuses etc.	746	0.16	0.00	0.03	0.01	0.00	0.08	0.07	0.13	0.14	0.20
喉	Larynx	4 332	0.95	0.00	0.00	0.03	0.01	0.01	0.03	0.04	0.04	0.14
气管、支气管、肺	Trachea, bronchus & lung	118 194	26.04	0.00	0.06	0.07	0.23	0.31	0.79	1.92	3.73	6.74
其他胸腔器官	Other thoracic organs	1 536	0.34	0.26	0.24	0.11	0.12	0.31	0.21	0.37	0.41	0.44
骨	Bone	3 282	0.72	0.13	0.25	0.46	1.24	1.33	0.70	0.71	0.83	0.81
皮肤黑色素瘤	Melanoma of skin	723	0.16	0.06	0.06	0.07	0.07	0.02	0.04	0.05	0.12	0.12
皮肤其他	Other skin	3 662	0.81	0.06	0.10	0.21	0.19	0.18	0.17	0.28	0.37	0.60
间皮瘤	Mesothelioma	179	0.04	0.00	0.00	0.00	0.00	0.01	0.01	0.00	0.02	0.06
卡波氏肉瘤	Kaposi sarcoma	49	0.01	0.00	0.00	0.01	0.01	0.00	0.02	0.02	0.04	0.02
结缔组织、软组织	Connective & soft tissue	1 300	0.29	0.38	0.39	0.22	0.27	0.28	0.35	0.37	0.46	0.57
乳腺	Breast	739	0.16	0.00	0.00	0.00	0.01	0.02	0.01	0.07	0.15	0.13
外阴	Vulva	—	—	—	—	—	—	—	—	—	—	—
阴道	Vagina	—	—	—	—	—	—	—	—	—	—	—
子宫颈	Cervix uteri	—	—	—	—	—	—	—	—	—	—	—
子宫体	Corpus uteri	—	—	—	—	—	—	—	—	—	—	—
子宫,部位不明	Uterus unspecified	—	—	—	—	—	—	—	—	—	—	—
卵巢	Ovary	—	—	—	—	—	—	—	—	—	—	—
其他女性生殖器	Other female genital organs	—	—	—	—	—	—	—	—	—	—	—
胎盘	Placenta	—	—	—	—	—	—	—	—	—	—	—
阴茎	Penis	1 161	0.26	0.00	0.00	0.01	0.00	0.01	0.02	0.05	0.13	0.19
前列腺	Prostate	14 408	3.17	0.00	0.01	0.01	0.04	0.01	0.01	0.03	0.11	0.04
睾丸	Testis	622	0.14	0.32	0.33	0.02	0.05	0.10	0.27	0.43	0.70	0.56
其他男性生殖器	Other male genital organs	216	0.05	0.06	0.00	0.02	0.02	0.03	0.03	0.03	0.07	0.03
肾	Kidney	5 661	1.25	0.45	0.38	0.13	0.02	0.12	0.17	0.50	0.97	1.47
肾盂	Renal pelvis	639	0.14	0.00	0.00	0.00	0.00	0.00	0.02	0.02	0.05	0.07
输尿管	Ureter	713	0.16	0.00	0.03	0.00	0.00	0.00	0.00	0.04	0.00	0.05
膀胱	Bladder	11 648	2.57	0.06	0.03	0.03	0.01	0.05	0.14	0.36	0.71	1.01
其他泌尿器官	Other urinary organs	170	0.04	0.00	0.00	0.02	0.01	0.00	0.00	0.00	0.01	0.01
眼	Eye	286	0.06	0.96	0.57	0.09	0.02	0.02	0.03	0.03	0.05	0.06
脑、神经系统	Brain, nervous system	10 304	2.27	2.62	1.80	1.76	1.80	1.62	1.56	2.56	3.18	3.57
甲状腺	Thyroid	8 015	1.77	0.00	0.01	0.03	0.20	0.44	2.03	5.58	7.72	8.83
肾上腺	Adrenal gland	458	0.10	0.32	0.18	0.07	0.05	0.03	0.04	0.09	0.12	0.13
其他内分泌腺	Other endocrine	584	0.13	0.00	0.04	0.04	0.19	0.10	0.07	0.15	0.24	0.23
霍奇金淋巴瘤	Hodgkin lymphoma	524	0.12	0.00	0.00	0.12	0.12	0.21	0.23	0.22	0.31	0.19
非霍奇金淋巴瘤	Non-Hodgkin lymphoma	6 657	1.47	0.57	0.59	0.67	0.87	0.81	0.83	1.08	1.45	1.38
免疫增生性疾病	Immunoproliferative diseases	97	0.02	0.00	0.00	0.01	0.00	0.00	0.00	0.00	0.00	0.00
多发性骨髓瘤	Multiple myeloma	2 187	0.48	0.00	0.04	0.02	0.05	0.07	0.02	0.13	0.14	0.15
淋巴样白血病	Lymphoid leukemia	1 710	0.38	1.09	2.22	1.49	0.92	0.69	0.45	0.61	0.41	0.35
髓样白血病	Myeloid leukemia	4 355	0.96	1.09	0.85	0.56	0.88	1.13	0.84	1.24	1.55	1.53
白血病,未特指	Leukemia unspecified	3 339	0.74	1.79	1.55	1.49	1.04	1.03	0.80	1.02	1.15	1.15
其他或未指明部位	Other and unspecified	7 254	1.60	1.09	0.89	0.52	0.75	0.67	0.76	0.88	1.17	1.28
所有部位合计	All sites	453 970	100.00	12.84	11.56	8.86	10.11	11.52	13.72	26.66	44.75	62.44
所有部位除外 C44	All sites except C44	450 308	99.19	12.77	11.47	8.64	9.92	11.33	13.55	26.38	44.38	61.84

Appendix Table 1-8　Cancer incidence in rural registration areas of China，male in 2018

| Age group | | | | | | | | | | 粗率 Crude rate/ 100 000⁻¹ | 中标率 ASR China/ 100 000⁻¹ | 世标率 ASR world/ 100 000⁻¹ | 累积率 Cum. Rate/% | | ICD-10 |
40~44	45~49	50~54	55~59	60~64	65~69	70~74	75~79	80~84	85+	$100\,000^{-1}$	$100\,000^{-1}$	$100\,000^{-1}$	0~64	0~74	
0.05	0.13	0.25	0.38	0.57	1.13	1.02	1.56	1.17	1.91	0.25	0.16	0.16	0.01	0.02	C00
0.64	1.03	1.88	1.66	2.87	3.00	2.99	3.18	2.55	2.09	0.96	0.68	0.65	0.05	0.08	C01-C02
0.61	0.90	2.01	2.20	3.53	4.54	6.27	6.30	7.64	7.18	1.37	0.91	0.90	0.05	0.11	C03-C06
0.39	0.69	1.04	1.10	1.71	2.07	2.30	1.85	2.02	1.91	0.65	0.47	0.45	0.03	0.05	C07-C08
0.11	0.24	0.39	0.40	0.63	0.60	0.75	0.62	0.48	0.45	0.21	0.14	0.15	0.01	0.02	C09
0.14	0.19	0.61	0.72	1.33	1.63	1.37	1.92	1.22	1.36	0.39	0.25	0.26	0.02	0.03	C10
5.81	8.42	11.00	9.70	12.19	12.49	10.32	8.96	7.75	5.00	5.06	3.74	3.53	0.27	0.39	C11
0.16	0.54	1.23	1.72	2.77	2.99	3.03	2.40	2.23	1.64	0.74	0.47	0.49	0.03	0.06	C12-C13
0.18	0.27	0.39	0.57	1.13	1.43	2.04	2.08	1.91	1.55	0.38	0.25	0.25	0.01	0.03	C14
2.59	8.59	26.37	40.73	91.42	135.83	168.39	192.80	197.61	187.78	29.94	18.41	18.65	0.85	2.38	C15
6.99	17.18	39.89	55.92	115.22	166.90	211.73	234.39	242.24	203.68	39.05	24.53	24.57	1.21	3.10	C16
0.58	0.99	1.73	1.85	3.06	4.40	5.34	5.36	5.73	5.27	1.18	0.78	0.77	0.04	0.09	C17
4.71	8.67	15.07	19.24	35.29	48.14	58.29	68.21	77.53	74.44	12.86	8.37	8.24	0.45	0.98	C18
5.06	10.50	20.10	25.68	46.86	66.27	77.80	92.20	95.41	86.43	16.58	10.61	10.55	0.57	1.29	C19-C20
0.13	0.24	0.47	0.57	1.10	1.31	1.93	2.01	2.76	3.91	0.41	0.26	0.26	0.01	0.03	C21
27.89	46.88	74.36	72.65	111.63	127.54	140.77	150.76	160.78	156.06	41.10	27.80	27.14	1.81	3.15	C22
0.77	1.53	3.07	4.43	10.15	13.94	19.07	22.69	25.05	29.36	3.54	2.20	2.21	0.10	0.27	C23-C24
1.71	4.35	7.77	10.42	20.55	27.99	36.72	44.57	52.11	50.35	7.38	4.64	4.63	0.23	0.56	C25
0.36	0.51	0.91	0.76	1.21	1.74	1.51	1.72	2.44	2.00	0.51	0.35	0.34	0.02	0.04	C30-C31
0.46	1.71	3.89	6.14	9.90	11.52	13.78	14.71	14.96	9.73	2.95	1.85	1.88	0.11	0.24	C32
15.16	36.75	84.93	118.51	235.02	336.40	417.21	481.54	515.99	458.71	80.41	50.40	50.53	2.52	6.29	C33-C34
0.61	1.04	1.35	1.75	2.82	3.63	2.81	3.44	3.56	2.91	1.04	0.77	0.76	0.05	0.08	C37-C38
1.08	1.48	2.52	2.75	4.04	6.58	10.56	9.84	9.50	9.91	2.23	1.72	1.67	0.09	0.18	C40-C41
0.29	0.31	0.66	0.77	1.39	1.60	1.71	2.30	2.65	3.09	0.49	0.33	0.33	0.02	0.04	C43
0.92	1.16	2.53	2.71	5.09	7.73	12.20	14.58	22.13	29.54	2.49	1.62	1.60	0.07	0.17	C44
0.03	0.13	0.15	0.22	0.38	0.50	0.44	0.55	0.48	0.00	0.12	0.08	0.08	0.01	0.01	C45
0.02	0.03	0.01	0.02	0.08	0.08	0.11	0.16	0.27	0.27	0.03	0.03	0.02	0.00	0.00	C46
0.59	1.02	1.21	1.22	1.74	2.01	2.55	3.28	2.65	2.36	0.88	0.70	0.68	0.04	0.07	C47,C49
0.31	0.59	0.77	0.82	1.15	1.72	1.93	2.27	1.75	2.45	0.50	0.34	0.33	0.02	0.04	C50
—	—	—	—	—	—	—	—	—	—	—	—	—	—	—	C51
—	—	—	—	—	—	—	—	—	—	—	—	—	—	—	C52
—	—	—	—	—	—	—	—	—	—	—	—	—	—	—	C53
—	—	—	—	—	—	—	—	—	—	—	—	—	—	—	C54
—	—	—	—	—	—	—	—	—	—	—	—	—	—	—	C55
—	—	—	—	—	—	—	—	—	—	—	—	—	—	—	C56
—	—	—	—	—	—	—	—	—	—	—	—	—	—	—	C57
—	—	—	—	—	—	—	—	—	—	—	—	—	—	—	C58
0.32	0.75	0.95	1.29	2.28	2.62	3.77	3.25	4.03	4.91	0.79	0.52	0.51	0.03	0.06	C60
0.21	0.52	1.87	4.85	16.24	37.53	68.10	100.61	117.38	130.79	9.80	5.81	5.73	0.12	0.65	C61
0.53	0.53	0.50	0.34	0.48	0.52	0.64	0.71	1.06	0.82	0.42	0.39	0.35	0.02	0.03	C62
0.03	0.05	0.14	0.12	0.32	0.50	0.75	1.10	1.06	0.82	0.15	0.10	0.10	0.00	0.01	C63
1.87	3.65	6.87	7.70	10.50	13.20	13.64	12.63	13.37	12.09	3.85	2.63	2.60	0.17	0.31	C64
0.18	0.23	0.56	0.66	1.22	1.54	2.04	2.37	2.97	2.36	0.43	0.28	0.28	0.02	0.03	C65
0.05	0.17	0.27	0.55	1.50	2.04	3.08	3.31	3.56	2.36	0.49	0.30	0.30	0.01	0.04	C66
1.60	3.36	7.05	9.61	19.72	27.98	40.20	54.60	71.80	72.89	7.92	4.94	4.89	0.22	0.56	C67
0.04	0.05	0.10	0.12	0.27	0.40	0.69	0.62	1.17	1.00	0.12	0.07	0.07	0.00	0.01	C68
0.10	0.13	0.15	0.35	0.37	0.44	0.58	0.49	0.90	0.55	0.19	0.15	0.19	0.01	0.02	C69
4.90	7.05	10.63	10.60	15.11	19.73	20.86	22.43	25.74	23.09	7.01	5.31	5.21	0.33	0.53	C70-C72,D32-D33, D42-D43
8.12	8.28	9.77	8.75	7.59	6.69	5.58	3.67	3.02	2.27	5.45	4.86	4.17	0.34	0.40	C73
0.15	0.33	0.32	0.67	0.72	0.82	0.86	1.43	1.17	1.18	0.31	0.23	0.23	0.01	0.03	C74
0.40	0.36	0.61	0.63	0.99	1.22	0.93	0.84	1.22	0.73	0.40	0.31	0.30	0.02	0.03	C75
0.14	0.31	0.52	0.50	0.60	0.84	1.00	1.40	1.11	1.27	0.36	0.29	0.27	0.02	0.03	C81
2.17	3.53	6.06	6.62	11.99	15.36	18.60	18.73	18.20	14.54	4.53	3.23	3.18	0.19	0.36	C82-C86,C96
0.00	0.06	0.04	0.07	0.19	0.29	0.42	0.26	0.69	0.27	0.07	0.04	0.04	0.00	0.01	C88
0.40	1.01	1.94	2.45	4.23	6.38	7.44	7.43	7.00	4.09	1.49	0.97	0.96	0.05	0.12	C90
0.55	0.64	1.07	1.27	2.10	2.35	3.19	3.96	3.08	3.54	1.16	1.00	1.13	0.06	0.09	C91
1.84	2.69	3.76	3.87	6.28	8.01	10.48	10.29	12.36	10.09	2.96	2.28	2.23	0.14	0.23	C92-C94,D45-D47
1.26	1.75	2.35	2.41	3.80	5.38	8.19	9.09	10.24	8.19	2.27	1.84	1.87	0.10	0.17	C95
1.97	3.26	6.01	6.88	11.50	16.29	21.39	23.63	28.60	34.45	4.93	3.39	3.39	0.18	0.37	O&U
105.17	194.77	368.10	455.92	842.80	1 165.74	1 447.38	1 659.11	1 792.29	1 673.43	308.83	201.84	200.10	10.78	23.85	C00-C97,D32-D33, D42-D43,D45-D47
104.25	193.61	365.56	453.21	837.71	1 158.02	1 435.18	1 644.53	1 770.16	1 643.90	306.34	200.22	198.50	10.71	23.68	C00-C97,D32-D33, D42-D43,D45-D47 exc. C44

部位 Site		病例数 No. cases	构成 Freq. /%	年龄组								
				0~	1~4	5~9	10~14	15~19	20~24	25~29	30~34	35~39
唇	Lip	237	0.07	0.00	0.02	0.03	0.01	0.00	0.00	0.02	0.03	0.00
舌	Tongue	722	0.20	0.00	0.00	0.03	0.03	0.01	0.05	0.08	0.15	0.33
口	Mouth	1 034	0.29	0.00	0.05	0.04	0.01	0.10	0.06	0.10	0.18	0.16
唾液腺	Salivary glands	734	0.21	0.00	0.03	0.04	0.06	0.08	0.17	0.28	0.27	0.36
扁桃腺	Tonsil	124	0.04	0.00	0.02	0.03	0.01	0.00	0.01	0.03	0.00	0.03
其他口咽	Other oropharynx	113	0.03	0.00	0.00	0.00	0.00	0.01	0.01	0.00	0.01	0.03
鼻咽	Nasopharynx	3 026	0.86	0.00	0.05	0.03	0.08	0.18	0.40	0.53	1.15	1.48
下咽	Hypopharynx	111	0.03	0.00	0.00	0.00	0.00	0.00	0.00	0.01	0.00	0.01
咽,部位不明	Pharynx unspecified	167	0.05	0.00	0.02	0.00	0.01	0.01	0.03	0.03	0.03	0.02
食管	Esophagus	16 332	4.63	0.00	0.00	0.00	0.01	0.01	0.03	0.20	0.21	0.38
胃	Stomach	24 036	6.82	0.07	0.00	0.04	0.07	0.19	0.31	1.46	2.72	3.07
小肠	Small intestine	1 253	0.36	0.00	0.03	0.01	0.00	0.00	0.03	0.05	0.14	0.21
结肠	Colon	14 511	4.11	0.00	0.03	0.00	0.07	0.17	0.38	0.83	1.49	2.30
直肠	Rectum	15 850	4.49	0.00	0.03	0.01	0.01	0.09	0.26	0.60	1.55	1.91
肛门	Anus	432	0.12	0.00	0.00	0.00	0.00	0.00	0.01	0.08	0.05	0.10
肝脏	Liver	21 017	5.96	1.02	0.34	0.11	0.11	0.21	0.60	0.93	1.68	2.69
胆囊及其他	Gallbladder etc.	5 688	1.61	0.00	0.00	0.00	0.01	0.00	0.01	0.03	0.10	0.30
胰腺	Pancreas	7 831	2.22	0.00	0.02	0.00	0.04	0.09	0.06	0.27	0.41	0.52
鼻、鼻窦及其他	Nose, sinuses etc.	458	0.13	0.00	0.06	0.05	0.03	0.00	0.07	0.11	0.06	0.13
喉	Larynx	449	0.13	0.00	0.03	0.00	0.04	0.00	0.03	0.01	0.10	0.07
气管、支气管、肺	Trachea, bronchus & lung	60 166	17.06	0.07	0.13	0.04	0.07	0.26	0.62	2.04	4.26	7.28
其他胸腔器官	Other thoracic organs	999	0.28	0.29	0.19	0.09	0.06	0.05	0.10	0.18	0.26	0.34
骨	Bone	2 328	0.66	0.15	0.31	0.32	1.01	0.87	0.47	0.63	0.53	0.58
皮肤黑色素瘤	Melanoma of skin	677	0.19	0.07	0.05	0.01	0.07	0.00	0.05	0.09	0.13	0.10
皮肤其他	Other skin	3 808	1.08	0.15	0.18	0.10	0.10	0.25	0.18	0.28	0.41	0.46
间皮瘤	Mesothelioma	182	0.05	0.00	0.00	0.03	0.00	0.00	0.01	0.06	0.06	0.05
卡波氏肉瘤	Kaposi sarcoma	12	0.00	0.00	0.00	0.00	0.01	0.00	0.00	0.01	0.00	0.01
结缔组织、软组织	Connective & soft tissue	1 081	0.31	0.51	0.15	0.20	0.21	0.32	0.25	0.43	0.47	0.51
乳腺	Breast	50 468	14.31	0.00	0.11	0.03	0.10	0.51	1.97	6.11	15.46	27.59
外阴	Vulva	623	0.18	0.00	0.00	0.01	0.01	0.00	0.04	0.05	0.12	0.15
阴道	Vagina	435	0.12	0.07	0.00	0.01	0.01	0.00	0.01	0.05	0.05	0.06
子宫颈	Cervix uteri	26 517	7.52	0.00	0.10	0.01	0.03	0.08	0.55	3.55	8.88	14.70
子宫体	Corpus uteri	11 159	3.16	0.07	0.00	0.00	0.04	0.01	0.10	0.77	1.70	2.84
子宫,部位不明	Uterus unspecified	2 690	0.76	0.00	0.00	0.00	0.01	0.00	0.03	0.42	0.59	1.05
卵巢	Ovary	9 812	2.78	0.07	0.06	0.20	0.59	1.05	1.73	2.24	2.60	3.65
其他女性生殖器	Other female genital organs	679	0.19	0.00	0.02	0.00	0.04	0.04	0.10	0.13	0.07	0.17
胎盘	Placenta	113	0.03	0.00	0.00	0.00	0.00	0.03	0.03	0.11	0.21	0.13	0.16
阴茎	Penis	—	—	—	—	—	—	—	—	—	—	—
前列腺	Prostate	—	—	—	—	—	—	—	—	—	—	—
睾丸	Testis	—	—	—	—	—	—	—	—	—	—	—
其他男性生殖器	Other male genital organs	—	—	—	—	—	—	—	—	—	—	—
肾	Kidney	3 373	0.96	0.15	0.50	0.13	0.04	0.13	0.17	0.35	0.51	0.79
肾盂	Renal pelvis	399	0.11	0.00	0.02	0.01	0.00	0.00	0.00	0.00	0.00	0.02
输尿管	Ureter	541	0.15	0.00	0.00	0.00	0.00	0.01	0.01	0.01	0.02	0.02
膀胱	Bladder	2 927	0.83	0.00	0.03	0.00	0.00	0.01	0.08	0.13	0.23	0.29
其他泌尿器官	Other urinary organs	113	0.03	0.00	0.00	0.00	0.00	0.00	0.00	0.01	0.00	0.02
眼	Eye	220	0.06	0.80	0.35	0.09	0.04	0.03	0.00	0.04	0.07	0.04
脑、神经系统	Brain, nervous system	11 492	3.26	2.18	1.80	1.58	1.49	1.63	1.36	2.20	3.12	3.40
甲状腺	Thyroid	26 248	7.44	0.00	0.05	0.10	0.55	2.01	6.08	15.02	21.87	25.90
肾上腺	Adrenal gland	365	0.10	0.36	0.13	0.06	0.00	0.01	0.02	0.02	0.15	0.13
其他内分泌腺	Other endocrine	663	0.19	0.00	0.02	0.05	0.11	0.08	0.09	0.30	0.37	0.52
霍奇金淋巴瘤	Hodgkin lymphoma	339	0.10	0.00	0.02	0.05	0.07	0.12	0.16	0.32	0.17	0.26
非霍奇金淋巴瘤	Non-Hodgkin lymphoma	4 775	1.35	0.07	0.48	0.39	0.54	0.43	0.56	0.88	1.19	1.14
免疫增生性疾病	Immunoproliferative diseases	49	0.01	0.00	0.00	0.00	0.00	0.00	0.00	0.00	0.01	0.01
多发性骨髓瘤	Multiple myeloma	1 705	0.48	0.00	0.10	0.01	0.01	0.03	0.03	0.08	0.16	0.12
淋巴样白血病	Lymphoid leukemia	1 249	0.35	0.87	1.74	1.18	0.91	0.40	0.30	0.40	0.38	0.36
髓样白血病	Myeloid leukemia	3 450	0.98	0.94	0.61	0.53	0.94	0.87	0.92	1.19	1.52	1.24
白血病,未特指	Leukemia unspecified	2 597	0.74	2.03	1.60	1.23	0.96	0.89	0.62	0.80	0.84	0.81
其他或未指明部位	Other and unspecified	6 267	1.78	1.31	0.74	0.52	0.55	0.66	0.60	0.77	1.23	1.54
所有部位合计	All sites	352 646	100.00	11.25	10.20	7.41	9.22	11.97	19.91	45.37	77.92	110.39
所有部位除外 C44	All sites except C44	348 838	98.92	11.11	10.02	7.31	9.12	11.72	19.74	45.09	77.51	109.92

Appendix Table 1-9　Cancer incidence in rural registration areas of China, female in 2018

Age group										粗率 Crude rate/ 100 000⁻¹	中标率 ASR China/ 100 000⁻¹	世标率 ASR world/ 100 000⁻¹	累积率 Cum. Rate/%		ICD-10
40~44	45~49	50~54	55~59	60~64	65~69	70~74	75~79	80~84	85+				0~64	0~74	
0.04	0.10	0.14	0.12	0.31	0.55	0.87	0.71	1.34	1.74	0.17	0.10	0.10	0.00	0.01	C00
0.33	0.51	0.68	0.73	1.30	1.43	1.70	1.84	2.29	1.56	0.52	0.34	0.33	0.02	0.04	C01-C02
0.36	0.45	0.85	0.84	1.70	2.19	3.39	3.66	3.68	3.77	0.74	0.46	0.45	0.02	0.05	C03-C06
0.49	0.68	0.92	0.89	0.96	1.44	1.11	0.92	1.17	0.75	0.52	0.39	0.37	0.03	0.04	C07-C08
0.04	0.10	0.14	0.16	0.20	0.23	0.28	0.30	0.22	0.46	0.09	0.06	0.06	0.00	0.01	C09
0.06	0.06	0.06	0.08	0.17	0.35	0.31	0.62	0.22	0.29	0.08	0.05	0.05	0.00	0.01	C10
2.42	3.25	4.57	3.73	4.51	4.66	4.70	4.11	3.37	3.01	2.16	1.57	1.47	0.11	0.16	C11
0.02	0.06	0.15	0.08	0.21	0.26	0.35	0.45	0.30	0.23	0.08	0.05	0.05	0.00	0.01	C12-C13
0.07	0.08	0.08	0.11	0.23	0.28	0.44	0.77	0.91	0.75	0.12	0.07	0.07	0.00	0.01	C14
0.84	2.03	5.64	8.97	23.94	45.39	64.35	83.12	97.36	93.09	11.66	6.29	6.26	0.21	0.76	C15
5.30	10.35	18.06	19.67	38.89	56.48	73.42	91.54	111.42	106.99	17.15	10.08	9.87	0.50	1.15	C16
0.35	0.80	1.14	1.40	2.41	3.20	3.32	3.78	3.81	2.95	0.89	0.55	0.54	0.03	0.07	C17
3.81	7.35	12.15	13.81	24.22	34.44	42.49	48.82	60.29	54.16	10.36	6.21	6.09	0.33	0.72	C18
4.55	8.02	14.68	14.60	26.76	38.58	48.03	53.97	61.16	53.58	11.31	6.78	6.66	0.37	0.80	C19-C20
0.06	0.21	0.41	0.34	0.71	0.87	1.25	1.52	2.21	1.62	0.31	0.19	0.18	0.01	0.02	C21
5.38	9.51	17.51	19.12	35.29	50.65	63.02	73.03	87.93	85.21	15.00	8.89	8.80	0.47	1.04	C22
0.71	1.81	3.80	4.36	9.50	14.11	20.18	23.80	29.41	26.18	4.06	2.28	2.27	0.10	0.27	C23-C24
1.21	2.20	4.69	6.13	12.62	19.49	26.67	33.05	40.23	39.56	5.59	3.16	3.13	0.14	0.37	C25
0.22	0.25	0.65	0.43	0.61	0.80	1.18	1.07	1.34	1.45	0.33	0.22	0.21	0.01	0.02	C30-C31
0.07	0.14	0.39	0.46	0.57	0.94	1.11	1.84	2.25	2.49	0.32	0.19	0.19	0.01	0.02	C32
14.04	27.18	52.77	59.81	106.49	145.43	181.26	207.80	237.46	226.96	42.94	25.36	25.11	1.37	3.01	C33-C34
0.48	0.81	1.37	1.16	1.74	1.58	1.97	2.26	1.60	1.62	0.71	0.50	0.49	0.03	0.05	C37-C38
0.83	1.16	1.97	2.04	3.17	4.42	5.70	6.22	7.35	6.26	1.66	1.22	1.19	0.07	0.12	C40-C41
0.20	0.37	0.84	0.71	1.07	1.21	1.62	1.96	2.64	2.32	0.48	0.31	0.30	0.02	0.03	C43
0.63	1.42	2.23	2.51	4.29	6.79	10.51	14.87	23.05	35.63	2.72	1.52	1.51	0.07	0.15	C44
0.04	0.14	0.24	0.28	0.28	0.26	0.52	0.42	0.09	0.58	0.13	0.09	0.09	0.01	0.01	C45
0.00	0.02	0.00	0.02	0.01	0.03	0.02	0.03	0.00	0.00	0.01	0.01	0.01	0.00	0.00	C46
0.69	0.88	1.16	1.13	1.50	1.53	1.57	2.02	1.69	1.80	0.77	0.60	0.58	0.04	0.06	C47、C49
48.74	76.69	84.67	67.39	76.16	63.90	51.22	39.30	34.39	28.04	36.02	26.30	24.44	2.03	2.60	C50
0.31	0.49	0.64	0.63	0.88	1.35	1.68	1.76	1.95	1.39	0.44	0.29	0.28	0.02	0.03	C51
0.15	0.46	0.48	0.47	0.79	0.95	1.07	1.34	0.91	0.41	0.31	0.20	0.20	0.01	0.02	C52
24.15	35.37	47.92	35.33	37.56	34.78	29.90	27.61	22.06	15.41	18.92	13.76	12.75	1.04	1.36	C53
6.39	14.25	25.04	19.46	19.27	15.90	12.60	8.54	7.40	5.45	7.96	5.44	5.27	0.45	0.59	C54
2.20	3.29	4.80	3.67	3.63	3.63	3.30	3.69	4.24	3.19	1.92	1.34	1.26	0.10	0.14	C55
6.07	10.81	16.04	12.64	15.52	16.36	15.29	12.14	10.47	6.55	7.00	5.06	4.81	0.37	0.52	C56
0.37	0.59	1.18	0.75	1.47	1.36	1.07	0.80	0.82	0.81	0.48	0.33	0.33	0.02	0.04	C57
0.12	0.17	0.07	0.01	0.04	0.03	0.00	0.00	0.00	0.00	0.08	0.09	0.07	0.01	0.01	C58
—	—	—	—	—	—	—	—	—	—	—	—	—	—	—	C60
—	—	—	—	—	—	—	—	—	—	—	—	—	—	—	C61
—	—	—	—	—	—	—	—	—	—	—	—	—	—	—	C62
—	—	—	—	—	—	—	—	—	—	—	—	—	—	—	C63
1.27	2.40	4.11	4.87	5.82	7.73	7.03	7.68	7.48	5.50	2.41	1.57	1.57	0.11	0.18	C64
0.06	0.11	0.25	0.34	0.71	1.12	1.66	1.49	1.47	1.56	0.28	0.16	0.17	0.01	0.02	C65
0.02	0.14	0.31	0.36	0.79	1.76	2.12	2.32	2.77	1.80	0.39	0.22	0.22	0.01	0.03	C66
0.69	0.84	1.73	2.27	4.19	6.75	9.85	12.49	15.79	15.47	2.09	1.19	1.17	0.05	0.14	C67
0.03	0.04	0.03	0.09	0.23	0.37	0.28	0.59	0.52	0.17	0.08	0.05	0.05	0.00	0.01	C68
0.08	0.12	0.23	0.10	0.29	0.28	0.35	0.71	0.39	0.70	0.16	0.12	0.14	0.01	0.01	C69
5.16	8.60	13.24	12.85	18.41	22.50	23.85	23.26	25.82	20.39	8.20	5.79	5.69	0.37	0.61	C70-C72,D32-D33, D42-D43
27.51	33.73	41.44	33.40	27.11	20.12	11.58	7.53	5.49	3.77	18.73	15.97	13.92	1.17	1.33	C73
0.19	0.29	0.45	0.37	0.45	0.64	0.87	0.68	0.95	0.64	0.26	0.18	0.19	0.01	0.02	C74
0.41	0.59	0.83	0.85	0.95	0.97	0.83	0.83	0.56	0.81	0.47	0.37	0.34	0.03	0.03	C75
0.15	0.13	0.27	0.26	0.38	0.63	0.61	0.65	0.61	0.46	0.24	0.20	0.19	0.01	0.02	C81
1.74	2.76	4.53	4.65	8.23	11.30	12.34	13.06	12.02	8.23	3.41	2.31	2.26	0.14	0.26	C82-C86,C96
0.04	0.04	0.04	0.07	0.12	0.11	0.04	0.09	0.17	0.12	0.03	0.02	0.02	0.00	0.00	C88
0.34	0.88	1.62	2.07	3.55	4.95	4.98	5.18	4.37	2.14	1.22	0.75	0.75	0.04	0.09	C90
0.51	0.65	1.03	0.82	1.60	1.87	1.68	2.11	2.03	1.68	0.89	0.78	0.87	0.05	0.07	C91
1.47	2.18	3.38	3.12	4.90	6.35	7.12	7.35	8.43	4.81	2.46	1.88	1.81	0.11	0.18	C92-C94,D45-D47
1.13	1.38	2.05	1.86	3.54	4.17	5.15	5.95	6.49	5.33	1.85	1.46	1.52	0.09	0.14	C95
2.19	3.78	5.96	5.35	9.67	12.65	15.47	18.30	20.20	24.97	4.47	2.92	2.89	0.17	0.31	O&U
174.74	280.75	409.59	377.75	549.94	680.12	783.98	869.96	982.54	914.78	251.68	166.28	159.60	10.43	17.75	C00-C97,D32-D33, D42-D43,D45-D47
174.10	279.34	407.36	375.24	545.66	673.33	773.47	855.08	959.48	879.16	248.96	164.76	158.09	10.36	17.60	C00-C97,D32-D33, D42-D43,D45-D47 exc. C44

附表 1-10　2018 年全国肿瘤登记地区男女合计癌症死亡主要指标

部位 Site		死亡数 No. deaths	构成 Freq./%	年龄组								
				0~	1~4	5~9	10~14	15~19	20~24	25~29	30~34	35~39
唇	Lip	309	0.03	0.00	0.00	0.00	0.00	0.00	0.00	0.00	0.00	0.00
舌	Tongue	2 312	0.25	0.02	0.00	0.00	0.00	0.00	0.01	0.03	0.06	0.10
口	Mouth	3 092	0.34	0.00	0.00	0.00	0.00	0.01	0.01	0.01	0.04	0.05
唾液腺	Salivary glands	992	0.11	0.00	0.00	0.00	0.00	0.00	0.01	0.02	0.03	0.05
扁桃腺	Tonsil	384	0.04	0.00	0.00	0.00	0.00	0.00	0.00	0.00	0.00	0.01
其他口咽	Other oropharynx	850	0.09	0.00	0.00	0.00	0.00	0.00	0.01	0.01	0.01	0.04
鼻咽	Nasopharynx	10 099	1.11	0.00	0.01	0.00	0.02	0.05	0.06	0.16	0.34	0.66
下咽	Hypopharynx	1 426	0.16	0.00	0.00	0.00	0.00	0.00	0.00	0.01	0.00	0.02
咽,部位不明	Pharynx unspecified	1 024	0.11	0.00	0.00	0.01	0.00	0.01	0.00	0.01	0.01	0.02
食管	Esophagus	74 902	8.21	0.17	0.00	0.00	0.00	0.00	0.03	0.05	0.10	0.19
胃	Stomach	103 378	11.33	0.11	0.00	0.01	0.02	0.06	0.21	0.54	1.18	1.62
小肠	Small intestine	3 635	0.40	0.00	0.01	0.00	0.01	0.00	0.01	0.03	0.04	0.08
结肠	Colon	34 571	3.79	0.02	0.00	0.01	0.02	0.08	0.13	0.29	0.52	0.71
直肠	Rectum	40 124	4.40	0.00	0.00	0.01	0.01	0.04	0.10	0.24	0.48	0.78
肛门	Anus	1 268	0.14	0.00	0.00	0.00	0.00	0.00	0.01	0.01	0.02	0.05
肝脏	Liver	126 122	13.82	0.45	0.18	0.08	0.13	0.26	0.45	1.23	3.13	5.78
胆囊及其他	Gallbladder etc.	16 140	1.77	0.00	0.00	0.00	0.00	0.00	0.01	0.02	0.08	0.15
胰腺	Pancreas	33 455	3.67	0.02	0.00	0.00	0.01	0.02	0.02	0.10	0.25	0.41
鼻、鼻窦及其他	Nose, sinuses etc.	1 149	0.13	0.02	0.02	0.01	0.00	0.02	0.02	0.02	0.04	0.06
喉	Larynx	5 652	0.62	0.00	0.00	0.00	0.00	0.00	0.01	0.01	0.02	0.05
气管、支气管、肺	Trachea, bronchus & lung	253 701	27.81	0.00	0.03	0.02	0.08	0.07	0.28	0.61	1.43	2.76
其他胸腔器官	Other thoracic organs	2 590	0.28	0.06	0.02	0.02	0.03	0.06	0.09	0.12	0.10	0.13
骨	Bone	6 593	0.72	0.04	0.03	0.09	0.26	0.45	0.29	0.21	0.23	0.23
皮肤黑色素瘤	Melanoma of skin	1 459	0.16	0.00	0.00	0.00	0.00	0.00	0.01	0.04	0.04	0.06
皮肤其他	Other skin	4 314	0.47	0.02	0.00	0.01	0.02	0.01	0.02	0.03	0.05	0.08
间皮瘤	Mesothelioma	560	0.06	0.00	0.00	0.00	0.00	0.00	0.01	0.00	0.01	0.03
卡波氏肉瘤	Kaposi sarcoma	147	0.02	0.00	0.00	0.00	0.01	0.01	0.01	0.01	0.01	0.00
结缔组织、软组织	Connective & soft tissue	1 710	0.19	0.04	0.11	0.09	0.05	0.08	0.07	0.08	0.09	0.12
乳腺	Breast	24 883	2.79	0.00	0.00	0.00	0.01	0.03	0.08	0.53	1.87	3.71
外阴	Vulva	534	0.06	0.00	0.00	0.00	0.00	0.00	0.01	0.02	0.02	0.04
阴道	Vagina	267	0.03	0.00	0.00	0.01	0.01	0.00	0.00	0.01	0.02	0.02
子宫颈	Cervix uteri	14 737	1.62	0.00	0.01	0.00	0.00	0.00	0.12	0.47	1.13	2.03
子宫体	Corpus uteri	4 760	0.52	0.00	0.00	0.00	0.00	0.01	0.02	0.08	0.24	0.29
子宫,部位不明	Uterus unspecified	2 036	0.22	0.00	0.00	0.00	0.00	0.00	0.00	0.07	0.09	0.19
卵巢	Ovary	9 404	1.03	0.00	0.01	0.00	0.01	0.17	0.15	0.34	0.48	0.67
其他女性生殖器	Other female genital organs	503	0.06	0.00	0.00	0.00	0.01	0.00	0.01	0.00	0.04	0.03
胎盘	Placenta	26	0.00	0.00	0.00	0.00	0.00	0.00	0.01	0.02	0.04	0.01
阴茎	Penis	675	0.07	0.00	0.00	0.00	0.00	0.00	0.01	0.01	0.03	0.06
前列腺	Prostate	13 451	1.47	0.00	0.02	0.00	0.01	0.03	0.01	0.02	0.05	0.04
睾丸	Testis	285	0.03	0.00	0.03	0.01	0.01	0.03	0.04	0.07	0.08	0.07
其他男性生殖器	Other male genital organs	171	0.02	0.00	0.00	0.00	0.00	0.01	0.02	0.01	0.01	0.01
肾	Kidney	7 147	0.78	0.22	0.15	0.05	0.02	0.03	0.03	0.08	0.14	0.14
肾盂	Renal pelvis	1 149	0.13	0.00	0.00	0.00	0.00	0.00	0.00	0.01	0.01	0.01
输尿管	Ureter	1 305	0.14	0.00	0.00	0.00	0.00	0.00	0.00	0.00	0.00	0.01
膀胱	Bladder	13 322	1.46	0.00	0.01	0.00	0.01	0.01	0.01	0.03	0.02	0.06
其他泌尿器官	Other urinary organs	299	0.03	0.00	0.00	0.00	0.00	0.00	0.00	0.00	0.00	0.00
眼	Eye	324	0.04	0.02	0.12	0.03	0.01	0.00	0.01	0.01	0.01	0.01
脑、神经系统	Brain, nervous system	22 124	2.42	1.10	0.92	1.08	0.76	0.65	0.56	0.89	1.14	1.33
甲状腺	Thyroid	3 232	0.35	0.00	0.00	0.00	0.01	0.01	0.05	0.11	0.13	0.19
肾上腺	Adrenal gland	950	0.10	0.11	0.07	0.07	0.01	0.00	0.01	0.01	0.04	0.04
其他内分泌腺	Other endocrine	602	0.07	0.00	0.01	0.02	0.04	0.03	0.01	0.03	0.03	0.03
霍奇金淋巴瘤	Hodgkin lymphoma	825	0.09	0.04	0.00	0.01	0.02	0.03	0.04	0.04	0.04	0.07
非霍奇金淋巴瘤	Non-Hodgkin lymphoma	13 474	1.48	0.02	0.15	0.12	0.20	0.27	0.26	0.29	0.49	0.51
免疫增生性疾病	Immunoproliferative diseases	97	0.01	0.00	0.01	0.00	0.00	0.00	0.00	0.00	0.00	0.00
多发性骨髓瘤	Multiple myeloma	4 976	0.55	0.04	0.02	0.03	0.04	0.05	0.03	0.05	0.05	0.09
淋巴样白血病	Lymphoid leukemia	3 871	0.42	0.50	0.37	0.40	0.42	0.44	0.25	0.36	0.28	0.24
髓样白血病	Myeloid leukemia	8 244	0.90	0.32	0.32	0.23	0.25	0.26	0.30	0.38	0.45	0.53
白血病,未特指	Leukemia unspecified	7 923	0.87	1.07	0.51	0.47	0.52	0.56	0.41	0.53	0.54	0.52
其他或未指明部位	Other and unspecified	18 282	2.00	0.36	0.28	0.25	0.26	0.26	0.27	0.34	0.46	0.59
所有部位合计	All sites	912 425	100.00	4.75	3.38	3.15	3.29	4.01	4.33	7.84	14.16	22.15
所有部位除外 C44	All sites except C44	908 111	99.53	4.73	3.38	3.14	3.27	3.99	4.31	7.80	14.11	22.07

Appendix Table 1-10　Cancer mortality in　registration areas of China, both sexes in 2018

Age group										粗率 Crude rate/ 100 000^(-1)	中标率 ASR China/ 100 000^(-1)	世标率 ASR world/ 100 000^(-1)	累积率 Cum. Rate/%		ICD-10
40~44	45~49	50~54	55~59	60~64	65~69	70~74	75~79	80~84	85+				0~64	0~74	
0.01	0.01	0.03	0.05	0.08	0.16	0.27	0.43	0.58	1.10	0.06	0.03	0.03	0.00	0.00	C00
0.19	0.26	0.57	0.69	1.04	1.41	1.47	2.00	2.67	3.51	0.44	0.26	0.26	0.01	0.03	C01-C02
0.11	0.27	0.59	0.67	1.23	1.72	2.56	3.55	4.76	6.55	0.59	0.33	0.33	0.01	0.04	C03-C06
0.05	0.11	0.21	0.28	0.37	0.54	0.92	0.88	1.23	1.67	0.19	0.11	0.11	0.01	0.01	C07-C08
0.02	0.07	0.11	0.11	0.22	0.21	0.26	0.30	0.30	0.53	0.07	0.04	0.04	0.00	0.01	C09
0.03	0.07	0.25	0.25	0.22	0.39	0.59	0.69	0.88	0.88	0.16	0.10	0.10	0.01	0.01	C10
1.18	2.06	3.30	3.35	4.87	6.18	6.29	6.72	6.09	6.09	1.93	1.24	1.21	0.08	0.14	C11
0.05	0.17	0.44	0.62	0.83	0.96	1.05	1.02	1.09	0.90	0.27	0.16	0.17	0.01	0.02	C12-C13
0.03	0.08	0.19	0.20	0.46	0.57	1.00	1.23	1.42	1.77	0.20	0.11	0.11	0.01	0.01	C14
0.93	2.80	8.94	14.37	31.91	51.73	76.61	101.89	121.87	125.52	14.32	7.87	7.89	0.30	0.94	C15
3.18	6.49	13.72	19.13	40.64	67.24	99.05	135.40	172.31	173.19	19.76	11.09	10.98	0.43	1.27	C16
0.17	0.37	0.53	0.81	1.57	2.29	3.11	4.15	5.37	6.01	0.69	0.40	0.40	0.02	0.05	C17
1.16	2.37	4.31	6.14	11.80	18.40	27.15	43.05	68.27	90.48	6.61	3.60	3.58	0.14	0.37	C18
1.61	3.11	5.74	7.50	14.74	23.14	33.37	50.23	72.32	85.55	7.67	4.26	4.22	0.17	0.45	C19-C20
0.07	0.12	0.20	0.25	0.45	0.72	0.99	1.66	1.94	2.59	0.24	0.14	0.14	0.01	0.01	C21
11.99	20.66	34.22	37.08	57.85	74.04	88.80	104.04	125.09	133.45	24.11	14.77	14.54	0.87	1.68	C22
0.40	0.93	1.98	3.03	6.40	10.26	14.22	21.40	28.79	32.48	3.09	1.69	1.69	0.07	0.19	C23-C24
1.06	2.42	5.01	7.74	14.20	21.68	30.18	40.48	51.96	55.12	6.39	3.59	3.58	0.16	0.42	C25
0.08	0.13	0.30	0.28	0.43	0.61	0.86	1.20	1.28	1.77	0.22	0.13	0.13	0.01	0.01	C30-C31
0.10	0.34	0.88	1.58	2.59	3.68	5.11	6.66	8.94	7.91	1.08	0.61	0.61	0.03	0.07	C32
6.55	15.58	37.10	54.08	111.55	171.25	238.57	316.79	389.23	397.84	48.49	27.18	27.16	1.15	3.20	C33-C34
0.19	0.31	0.58	0.68	1.22	1.46	1.89	2.25	2.44	3.21	0.50	0.31	0.31	0.02	0.03	C37-C38
0.41	0.68	1.12	1.36	2.51	3.90	5.08	7.46	8.25	8.18	1.26	0.81	0.80	0.04	0.08	C40-C41
0.10	0.16	0.23	0.37	0.55	0.80	1.06	1.51	2.09	3.02	0.28	0.16	0.16	0.01	0.02	C43
0.14	0.22	0.44	0.52	0.91	1.50	2.77	4.75	9.43	22.48	0.82	0.41	0.43	0.01	0.03	C44
0.02	0.06	0.12	0.14	0.33	0.42	0.39	0.56	0.51	0.57	0.11	0.06	0.06	0.00	0.01	C45
0.00	0.02	0.02	0.04	0.05	0.07	0.08	0.13	0.25	0.18	0.03	0.02	0.02	0.00	0.00	C46
0.13	0.22	0.36	0.35	0.64	0.85	0.97	1.37	2.18	2.71	0.33	0.22	0.22	0.01	0.02	C47,C49
6.77	11.85	17.18	17.36	22.41	22.63	23.25	28.80	37.45	46.87	9.66	5.98	5.81	0.41	0.64	C50
0.07	0.09	0.19	0.23	0.39	0.42	0.84	1.32	1.44	2.28	0.21	0.11	0.11	0.01	0.01	C51
0.02	0.08	0.15	0.12	0.20	0.30	0.44	0.46	0.72	0.62	0.10	0.06	0.06	0.00	0.01	C52
4.19	7.01	11.99	10.07	11.32	14.49	15.92	18.44	20.40	16.49	5.72	3.62	3.49	0.24	0.39	C53
0.68	1.41	3.15	3.41	4.71	5.33	6.24	7.16	8.17	7.55	1.85	1.09	1.08	0.07	0.13	C54
0.39	0.72	1.28	1.18	1.60	2.20	2.74	3.33	3.59	4.56	0.79	0.47	0.46	0.03	0.05	C55
1.63	3.57	6.32	6.83	9.41	10.84	12.17	12.49	12.56	10.60	3.65	2.24	2.21	0.15	0.26	C56
0.06	0.13	0.26	0.39	0.44	0.64	0.80	0.75	0.81	0.83	0.20	0.12	0.11	0.01	0.01	C57
0.03	0.02	0.00	0.00	0.00	0.00	0.01	0.00	0.00	0.00	0.01	0.01	0.01	0.00	0.00	C58
0.07	0.16	0.22	0.15	0.55	0.71	0.98	1.41	3.02	4.12	0.25	0.15	0.15	0.01	0.01	C60
0.08	0.20	0.50	1.13	4.13	9.48	21.85	46.97	90.86	153.82	5.07	2.64	2.68	0.03	0.19	C61
0.09	0.08	0.08	0.09	0.15	0.24	0.27	0.51	0.69	1.20	0.11	0.08	0.08	0.00	0.01	C62
0.02	0.02	0.03	0.05	0.10	0.18	0.28	0.49	0.66	1.11	0.06	0.04	0.04	0.00	0.00	C63
0.26	0.58	1.10	1.69	2.78	4.29	6.13	7.74	10.95	13.75	1.37	0.78	0.79	0.04	0.09	C64
0.03	0.08	0.13	0.20	0.37	0.71	0.95	1.38	2.30	2.95	0.22	0.12	0.12	0.00	0.01	C65
0.02	0.03	0.09	0.19	0.41	0.70	1.06	1.98	3.16	3.67	0.25	0.13	0.13	0.00	0.01	C66
0.17	0.36	0.77	1.34	3.01	5.69	10.38	19.39	34.97	53.83	2.55	1.26	1.27	0.03	0.11	C67
0.00	0.01	0.02	0.03	0.10	0.14	0.21	0.44	0.75	1.05	0.06	0.03	0.03	0.00	0.00	C68
0.02	0.03	0.05	0.04	0.07	0.13	0.18	0.30	0.60	0.85	0.06	0.04	0.05	0.00	0.00	C69
2.06	3.12	5.04	5.50	8.84	11.98	15.35	18.17	21.84	22.67	4.23	2.83	2.82	0.16	0.30	C70-C72, D32-D33, D42-D43
0.26	0.45	0.67	0.83	1.25	1.76	2.18	3.22	4.15	4.86	0.62	0.38	0.37	0.02	0.04	C73
0.05	0.09	0.20	0.26	0.37	0.53	0.62	0.94	1.25	1.35	0.18	0.11	0.12	0.01	0.01	C74
0.06	0.04	0.10	0.15	0.22	0.33	0.44	0.58	0.72	0.94	0.12	0.08	0.07	0.00	0.01	C75
0.08	0.07	0.15	0.21	0.26	0.46	0.71	0.89	0.91	0.82	0.16	0.10	0.10	0.01	0.01	C81
0.78	1.28	2.42	2.90	5.54	7.91	11.16	14.81	18.32	18.17	2.58	1.57	1.55	0.08	0.17	C82-C86,C96
0.00	0.01	0.00	0.00	0.03	0.07	0.12	0.16	0.21	0.11	0.02	0.01	0.01	0.00	0.00	C88
0.17	0.37	0.77	1.21	2.35	3.82	4.75	5.78	6.05	4.49	0.95	0.56	0.56	0.03	0.07	C90
0.32	0.48	0.65	0.74	1.29	1.84	2.32	3.04	3.72	3.57	0.74	0.57	0.58	0.03	0.05	C91
0.63	0.93	1.49	1.83	3.07	4.66	6.10	8.18	9.62	9.39	1.58	1.04	1.02	0.05	0.11	C92-C94,D45-D47
0.63	0.90	1.43	1.55	2.81	4.03	5.78	7.04	8.46	7.84	1.51	1.08	1.08	0.06	0.11	C95
0.98	1.79	3.02	4.01	6.97	10.44	14.15	19.63	26.42	34.76	3.49	2.08	2.07	0.10	0.22	O&U
43.50	83.35	160.08	204.86	377.41	560.11	770.99	1 037.95	1 336.25	1 479.18	174.41	100.82	100.15	4.66	11.31	C00-C97, D32-D33, D42-D43, D45-D47
43.36	83.13	159.64	204.34	376.50	558.60	768.22	1 033.20	1 326.82	1 456.70	173.58	100.40	99.72	4.65	11.28	C00-C97, D32-D33, D42-D43, D45-D47 exc. C44

附表 1-11　2018 年全国肿瘤登记地区男性癌症死亡主要指标

部位	Site	死亡数 No. deaths	构成 Freq./%	年龄组								
				0~	1~4	5~9	10~14	15~19	20~24	25~29	30~34	35~39
唇	Lip	190	0.03	0.00	0.00	0.00	0.00	0.00	0.00	0.00	0.00	0.00
舌	Tongue	1 575	0.27	0.00	0.00	0.00	0.00	0.00	0.01	0.01	0.07	0.15
口	Mouth	2 044	0.35	0.00	0.00	0.01	0.00	0.00	0.00	0.02	0.05	0.08
唾液腺	Salivary glands	630	0.11	0.00	0.00	0.00	0.00	0.00	0.01	0.03	0.03	0.07
扁桃腺	Tonsil	298	0.05	0.00	0.00	0.00	0.00	0.00	0.00	0.00	0.01	0.00
其他口咽	Other oropharynx	703	0.12	0.00	0.00	0.01	0.01	0.00	0.02	0.01	0.01	0.05
鼻咽	Nasopharynx	7 492	1.28	0.00	0.01	0.01	0.02	0.09	0.07	0.23	0.46	0.99
下咽	Hypopharynx	1 324	0.23	0.00	0.00	0.00	0.00	0.01	0.01	0.01	0.01	0.03
咽,部位不明	Pharynx unspecified	774	0.13	0.00	0.01	0.01	0.00	0.00	0.00	0.01	0.02	0.02
食管	Esophagus	55 649	9.52	0.00	0.00	0.01	0.00	0.01	0.04	0.04	0.15	0.25
胃	Stomach	72 156	12.35	0.00	0.00	0.01	0.02	0.05	0.19	0.48	1.07	1.61
小肠	Small intestine	2 204	0.38	0.00	0.01	0.00	0.01	0.01	0.01	0.05	0.05	0.12
结肠	Colon	19 393	3.32	0.00	0.01	0.01	0.03	0.08	0.17	0.34	0.49	0.84
直肠	Rectum	24 861	4.25	0.00	0.01	0.01	0.01	0.05	0.10	0.28	0.58	0.89
肛门	Anus	737	0.13	0.00	0.00	0.00	0.00	0.00	0.01	0.03	0.02	0.06
肝脏	Liver	92 906	15.90	0.39	0.20	0.07	0.16	0.33	0.61	1.89	5.17	9.83
胆囊及其他	Gallbladder etc.	7 601	1.30	0.00	0.00	0.01	0.00	0.00	0.01	0.02	0.09	0.18
胰腺	Pancreas	19 409	3.32	0.00	0.01	0.00	0.01	0.01	0.02	0.11	0.26	0.52
鼻、鼻窦及其他	Nose, sinuses etc.	764	0.13	0.00	0.02	0.01	0.00	0.01	0.03	0.02	0.03	0.05
喉	Larynx	4 993	0.85	0.00	0.01	0.00	0.00	0.00	0.01	0.01	0.02	0.07
气管、支气管、肺	Trachea, bronchus & lung	178 041	30.47	0.00	0.04	0.03	0.10	0.10	0.32	0.78	1.77	3.32
其他胸腔器官	Other thoracic organs	1 679	0.29	0.04	0.04	0.03	0.05	0.11	0.13	0.16	0.13	0.16
骨	Bone	3 983	0.68	0.00	0.03	0.09	0.26	0.62	0.38	0.28	0.31	0.28
皮肤黑色素瘤	Melanoma of skin	792	0.14	0.00	0.00	0.01	0.00	0.01	0.02	0.03	0.04	0.08
皮肤其他	Other skin	2 350	0.40	0.00	0.01	0.00	0.04	0.01	0.03	0.03	0.07	0.07
间皮瘤	Mesothelioma	331	0.06	0.00	0.00	0.00	0.00	0.00	0.01	0.00	0.03	0.02
卡波氏肉瘤	Kaposi sarcoma	86	0.01	0.00	0.00	0.00	0.01	0.00	0.01	0.02	0.02	0.00
结缔组织、软组织	Connective & soft tissue	1 003	0.17	0.00	0.14	0.09	0.06	0.08	0.11	0.09	0.11	0.15
乳腺	Breast	589	0.10	0.00	0.00	0.00	0.01	0.00	0.00	0.02	0.02	0.05
外阴	Vulva	—	—	—	—	—	—	—	—	—	—	—
阴道	Vagina	—	—	—	—	—	—	—	—	—	—	—
子宫颈	Cervix uteri	—	—	—	—	—	—	—	—	—	—	—
子宫体	Corpus uteri	—	—	—	—	—	—	—	—	—	—	—
子宫,部位不明	Uterus unspecified	—	—	—	—	—	—	—	—	—	—	—
卵巢	Ovary	—	—	—	—	—	—	—	—	—	—	—
其他女性生殖器	Other female genital organs	—	—	—	—	—	—	—	—	—	—	—
胎盘	Placenta	—	—	—	—	—	—	—	—	—	—	—
阴茎	Penis	675	0.12	0.00	0.00	0.00	0.00	0.01	0.00	0.01	0.03	0.06
前列腺	Prostate	13 451	2.30	0.00	0.02	0.00	0.01	0.03	0.01	0.02	0.05	0.04
睾丸	Testis	285	0.05	0.00	0.03	0.01	0.00	0.03	0.04	0.07	0.08	0.07
其他男性生殖器	Other male genital organs	171	0.03	0.00	0.00	0.00	0.01	0.01	0.00	0.01	0.01	0.00
肾	Kidney	4 782	0.82	0.18	0.15	0.05	0.04	0.05	0.03	0.10	0.17	0.20
肾盂	Renal pelvis	709	0.12	0.00	0.00	0.01	0.00	0.00	0.00	0.01	0.01	0.01
输尿管	Ureter	705	0.12	0.00	0.00	0.00	0.00	0.00	0.00	0.00	0.01	0.00
膀胱	Bladder	10 408	1.78	0.00	0.01	0.01	0.01	0.01	0.01	0.04	0.02	0.09
其他泌尿器官	Other urinary organs	188	0.03	0.00	0.00	0.00	0.00	0.00	0.00	0.00	0.01	0.00
眼	Eye	160	0.03	0.04	0.13	0.03	0.01	0.00	0.02	0.00	0.01	0.00
脑、神经系统	Brain, nervous system	12 224	2.09	1.13	0.87	1.18	0.90	0.75	0.66	1.13	1.41	1.62
甲状腺	Thyroid	1 187	0.20	0.00	0.00	0.00	0.00	0.01	0.03	0.08	0.05	0.12
肾上腺	Adrenal gland	597	0.10	0.11	0.08	0.07	0.01	0.00	0.01	0.02	0.04	0.03
其他内分泌腺	Other endocrine	331	0.06	0.00	0.02	0.03	0.05	0.04	0.02	0.03	0.03	0.00
霍奇金淋巴瘤	Hodgkin lymphoma	535	0.09	0.00	0.00	0.01	0.02	0.03	0.05	0.07	0.04	0.08
非霍奇金淋巴瘤	Non-Hodgkin lymphoma	8 247	1.41	0.00	0.16	0.16	0.23	0.35	0.34	0.39	0.60	0.62
免疫增生性疾病	Immunoproliferative diseases	74	0.01	0.00	0.02	0.00	0.00	0.00	0.00	0.01	0.01	0.00
多发性骨髓瘤	Multiple myeloma	2 895	0.50	0.04	0.02	0.06	0.04	0.05	0.02	0.07	0.06	0.12
淋巴样白血病	Lymphoid leukemia	2 273	0.39	0.53	0.43	0.44	0.43	0.54	0.32	0.40	0.38	0.26
髓样白血病	Myeloid leukemia	4 833	0.83	0.28	0.33	0.21	0.29	0.23	0.35	0.44	0.48	0.65
白血病,未特指	Leukemia unspecified	4 617	0.79	1.02	0.53	0.55	0.61	0.66	0.53	0.68	0.63	0.59
其他或未指明部位	Other and unspecified	10 493	1.80	0.32	0.31	0.30	0.31	0.25	0.34	0.42	0.52	0.59
所有部位合计	All sites	584 397	100.00	4.06	3.61	3.49	3.78	4.60	5.09	8.93	15.68	25.19
所有部位除外 C44	All sites except C44	582 047	99.60	4.06	3.61	3.49	3.75	4.59	5.06	8.91	15.62	25.11

Appendix Table 1-11　Cancer mortality in registration areas of China, male in 2018

Age group										粗率 Crude rate/ 100 000⁻¹	中标率 ASR China/ 100 000⁻¹	世标率 ASR world/ 100 000⁻¹	累积率 Cum. Rate/%		ICD-10
40~44	45~49	50~54	55~59	60~64	65~69	70~74	75~79	80~84	85+				0~64	0~74	
0.01	0.02	0.04	0.07	0.13	0.26	0.31	0.49	0.71	1.37	0.07	0.04	0.04	0.00	0.00	C00
0.26	0.37	0.90	1.01	1.61	2.11	1.95	2.53	3.18	4.60	0.59	0.37	0.37	0.02	0.04	C01-C02
0.15	0.41	0.90	1.04	1.93	2.37	3.52	4.33	5.93	8.23	0.77	0.46	0.46	0.02	0.05	C03-C06
0.05	0.17	0.26	0.41	0.49	0.71	1.18	1.36	1.65	1.55	0.24	0.15	0.14	0.01	0.02	C07-C08
0.04	0.11	0.20	0.19	0.39	0.32	0.43	0.40	0.44	0.66	0.11	0.07	0.07	0.00	0.01	C09
0.05	0.12	0.42	0.41	0.72	1.02	1.14	1.48	1.34	1.15	0.26	0.16	0.16	0.01	0.02	C10
1.66	3.23	5.03	5.17	7.49	9.46	9.29	9.49	8.59	8.59	2.82	1.86	1.82	0.12	0.22	C11
0.09	0.33	0.85	1.19	1.58	1.81	1.88	1.92	2.03	1.73	0.50	0.31	0.31	0.02	0.04	C12-C13
0.06	0.15	0.31	0.34	0.79	0.95	1.51	1.78	1.78	2.88	0.29	0.18	0.18	0.01	0.02	C14
1.48	4.78	15.29	25.00	53.93	82.78	116.52	148.10	171.07	176.31	20.96	12.27	12.36	0.50	1.50	C15
3.67	8.18	18.92	27.88	61.35	101.72	149.21	200.79	246.97	244.17	27.18	16.05	15.95	0.62	1.87	C16
0.22	0.47	0.68	1.07	2.02	2.86	3.83	5.24	6.06	8.06	0.83	0.50	0.50	0.02	0.06	C17
1.28	2.58	4.91	7.16	14.35	22.29	32.74	50.76	79.80	109.51	7.30	4.26	4.25	0.16	0.44	C18
1.78	3.75	6.82	9.94	19.89	31.05	43.22	66.14	92.34	114.34	9.36	5.51	5.48	0.22	0.59	C19-C20
0.08	0.12	0.24	0.34	0.61	0.88	1.17	2.02	2.33	2.79	0.28	0.17	0.17	0.01	0.02	C21
20.54	34.84	56.00	59.91	89.86	109.57	123.68	138.89	163.90	176.57	34.99	22.54	22.15	1.40	2.56	C22
0.44	0.85	1.76	3.08	6.66	10.75	13.69	20.52	26.23	33.95	2.86	1.67	1.68	0.07	0.19	C23-C24
1.36	3.18	6.68	10.05	18.09	26.17	35.59	46.14	58.45	63.43	7.31	4.35	4.36	0.20	0.51	C25
0.10	0.20	0.38	0.42	0.65	0.85	1.21	1.69	1.89	2.21	0.29	0.18	0.18	0.01	0.02	C30-C31
0.19	0.62	1.55	2.96	4.87	6.88	9.27	11.55	16.41	15.45	1.88	1.11	1.11	0.05	0.13	C32
7.92	20.23	51.92	80.65	168.14	259.08	352.24	462.82	552.55	566.24	67.06	39.61	39.69	1.68	4.73	C33-C34
0.22	0.40	0.68	0.90	1.66	2.10	2.49	2.87	3.32	4.52	0.63	0.42	0.42	0.02	0.05	C37-C38
0.50	0.85	1.41	1.71	3.16	4.90	6.09	9.66	9.88	9.61	1.50	1.01	0.99	0.05	0.10	C40-C41
0.10	0.17	0.27	0.38	0.64	0.81	1.17	1.76	2.69	3.54	0.30	0.18	0.18	0.01	0.02	C43
0.18	0.24	0.58	0.70	1.15	2.13	3.47	5.77	11.14	22.80	0.89	0.50	0.51	0.02	0.04	C44
0.03	0.07	0.12	0.17	0.41	0.51	0.43	0.63	0.66	0.93	0.12	0.08	0.08	0.00	0.01	C45
0.01	0.01	0.02	0.06	0.08	0.08	0.13	0.18	0.27	0.27	0.03	0.02	0.02	0.00	0.00	C46
0.16	0.23	0.43	0.39	0.73	1.08	1.12	1.87	2.96	3.01	0.38	0.26	0.26	0.01	0.02	C47,C49
0.07	0.16	0.18	0.37	0.50	0.67	0.82	1.32	1.51	2.70	0.22	0.14	0.13	0.01	0.01	C50
—	—	—	—	—	—	—	—	—	—	—	—	—	—	—	C51
—	—	—	—	—	—	—	—	—	—	—	—	—	—	—	C52
—	—	—	—	—	—	—	—	—	—	—	—	—	—	—	C53
—	—	—	—	—	—	—	—	—	—	—	—	—	—	—	C54
—	—	—	—	—	—	—	—	—	—	—	—	—	—	—	C55
—	—	—	—	—	—	—	—	—	—	—	—	—	—	—	C56
—	—	—	—	—	—	—	—	—	—	—	—	—	—	—	C57
—	—	—	—	—	—	—	—	—	—	—	—	—	—	—	C58
0.07	0.16	0.22	0.15	0.55	0.71	0.98	1.41	3.02	4.12	0.25	0.15	0.15	0.01	0.01	C60
0.08	0.20	0.50	1.13	4.13	9.48	21.85	46.97	90.86	153.82	5.07	2.64	2.68	0.03	0.19	C61
0.09	0.08	0.08	0.09	0.15	0.25	0.27	0.51	0.69	1.20	0.11	0.08	0.08	0.00	0.01	C62
0.02	0.02	0.03	0.05	0.10	0.18	0.28	0.49	0.66	1.11	0.06	0.04	0.04	0.00	0.00	C63
0.33	0.75	1.58	2.41	4.05	6.28	8.59	10.58	14.27	19.48	1.80	1.09	1.10	0.05	0.12	C64
0.05	0.12	0.20	0.28	0.51	0.94	1.29	1.74	2.55	3.72	0.27	0.16	0.16	0.01	0.02	C65
0.03	0.03	0.13	0.25	0.50	0.81	1.21	1.97	3.73	4.25	0.27	0.15	0.15	0.00	0.01	C66
0.24	0.54	1.21	2.17	5.08	9.24	16.89	32.05	59.14	101.19	3.92	2.11	2.15	0.05	0.18	C67
0.00	0.01	0.02	0.05	0.11	0.14	0.30	0.56	1.02	1.86	0.07	0.04	0.04	0.00	0.00	C68
0.01	0.04	0.05	0.04	0.07	0.16	0.22	0.28	0.63	0.75	0.06	0.04	0.05	0.00	0.00	C69
2.33	3.58	5.68	6.24	10.10	13.95	16.96	20.05	23.22	23.73	4.60	3.22	3.19	0.18	0.34	C70-C72,D32-D33, D42-D43
0.19	0.26	0.46	0.62	1.04	1.47	1.80	2.38	3.18	3.98	0.45	0.28	0.28	0.01	0.03	C73
0.04	0.11	0.27	0.38	0.50	0.69	0.80	1.28	1.48	1.95	0.22	0.14	0.15	0.01	0.03	C74
0.04	0.03	0.11	0.14	0.25	0.36	0.56	0.70	0.99	1.20	0.12	0.08	0.08	0.00	0.01	C75
0.09	0.10	0.19	0.30	0.38	0.60	0.88	1.18	1.34	1.20	0.20	0.14	0.13	0.01	0.01	C81
0.99	1.63	3.10	3.68	7.10	9.86	14.00	18.16	22.50	25.72	3.11	1.99	1.96	0.10	0.22	C82-C86,C96
0.00	0.01	0.01	0.00	0.03	0.10	0.19	0.26	0.38	0.18	0.03	0.02	0.02	0.00	0.00	C88
0.19	0.44	0.85	1.44	2.69	4.33	5.52	6.93	8.18	7.22	1.09	0.67	0.67	0.03	0.08	C90
0.34	0.56	0.72	0.86	1.45	2.18	2.91	3.84	4.69	5.31	0.86	0.66	0.68	0.04	0.06	C91
0.70	1.06	1.75	2.15	3.56	5.53	7.48	9.80	12.79	14.12	1.82	1.23	1.21	0.06	0.13	C92-C94,D45-D47
0.75	1.04	1.66	1.79	3.43	4.47	6.79	8.99	10.92	11.22	1.74	1.27	1.27	0.07	0.12	C95
1.05	1.96	3.34	4.83	8.77	12.87	17.43	23.90	30.65	41.12	3.95	2.46	2.47	0.11	0.27	O&U
50.31	99.59	199.89	272.03	518.23	770.77	1 046.52	1 396.54	1 772.99	2 018.59	220.12	133.06	132.70	6.05	15.14	C00-C97,D32-D33, D42-D43,D45-D47
50.14	99.35	199.30	271.34	517.08	768.64	1 043.05	1 390.77	1 761.85	1 995.80	219.24	132.56	132.19	6.04	15.10	C00-C97,D32-D33, D42-D43,D45-D47 exc. C44

部位 Site		死亡数 No. deaths	构成 Freq./%	年龄组								
				0~	1~4	5~9	10~14	15~19	20~24	25~29	30~34	35~39
唇	Lip	119	0.04	0.00	0.00	0.00	0.00	0.00	0.00	0.00	0.01	0.00
舌	Tongue	737	0.22	0.04	0.00	0.00	0.00	0.00	0.02	0.05	0.05	0.06
口	Mouth	1 048	0.32	0.00	0.01	0.00	0.01	0.02	0.01	0.01	0.02	0.02
唾液腺	Salivary glands	362	0.11	0.00	0.00	0.00	0.00	0.01	0.01	0.01	0.03	0.04
扁桃腺	Tonsil	86	0.03	0.00	0.00	0.00	0.00	0.02	0.00	0.01	0.00	0.02
其他口咽	Other oropharynx	147	0.04	0.00	0.00	0.00	0.00	0.00	0.00	0.01	0.00	0.02
鼻咽	Nasopharynx	2 607	0.79	0.00	0.02	0.00	0.01	0.02	0.05	0.08	0.21	0.31
下咽	Hypopharynx	102	0.03	0.00	0.00	0.00	0.00	0.00	0.00	0.01	0.00	0.01
咽,部位不明	Pharynx unspecified	250	0.08	0.00	0.00	0.00	0.00	0.02	0.01	0.00	0.01	0.01
食管	Esophagus	19 253	5.87	0.36	0.00	0.00	0.01	0.00	0.02	0.06	0.05	0.13
胃	Stomach	31 222	9.52	0.24	0.00	0.01	0.02	0.08	0.22	0.59	1.30	1.64
小肠	Small intestine	1 431	0.44	0.00	0.01	0.01	0.00	0.00	0.01	0.02	0.03	0.04
结肠	Colon	15 178	4.63	0.04	0.00	0.00	0.02	0.07	0.08	0.24	0.55	0.58
直肠	Rectum	15 263	4.65	0.00	0.00	0.01	0.01	0.02	0.09	0.19	0.39	0.66
肛门	Anus	531	0.16	0.00	0.00	0.00	0.00	0.01	0.01	0.00	0.03	0.04
肝脏	Liver	33 216	10.13	0.52	0.16	0.10	0.10	0.18	0.27	0.55	1.06	1.65
胆囊及其他	Gallbladder etc.	8 539	2.60	0.00	0.00	0.00	0.00	0.00	0.01	0.01	0.07	0.13
胰腺	Pancreas	14 046	4.28	0.04	0.00	0.01	0.00	0.03	0.02	0.09	0.23	0.29
鼻、鼻窦及其他	Nose,sinuses etc.	385	0.12	0.04	0.02	0.02	0.01	0.03	0.01	0.01	0.04	0.07
喉	Larynx	659	0.20	0.00	0.00	0.01	0.00	0.00	0.01	0.01	0.02	0.02
气管、支气管、肺	Trachea,bronchus & lung	75 660	23.07	0.00	0.02	0.05	0.02	0.05	0.23	0.44	1.08	2.18
其他胸腔器官	Other thoracic organs	911	0.28	0.08	0.00	0.01	0.01	0.02	0.04	0.09	0.06	0.10
骨	Bone	2 610	0.80	0.08	0.02	0.10	0.26	0.27	0.20	0.15	0.14	0.18
皮肤黑色素瘤	Melanoma of skin	667	0.20	0.00	0.01	0.00	0.02	0.00	0.01	0.05	0.04	0.05
皮肤其他	Other skin	1 964	0.60	0.04	0.01	0.01	0.00	0.02	0.02	0.04	0.03	0.08
间皮瘤	Mesothelioma	229	0.07	0.00	0.00	0.00	0.00	0.00	0.01	0.01	0.00	0.03
卡波氏肉瘤	Kaposi sarcoma	61	0.02	0.00	0.00	0.00	0.02	0.03	0.00	0.01	0.01	0.01
结缔组织、软组织	Connective & soft tissue	707	0.22	0.08	0.07	0.09	0.05	0.08	0.04	0.07	0.08	0.08
乳腺	Breast	24 883	7.59	0.00	0.00	0.00	0.01	0.03	0.08	0.53	1.87	3.71
外阴	Vulva	534	0.16	0.00	0.00	0.00	0.00	0.00	0.01	0.02	0.02	0.04
阴道	Vagina	267	0.08	0.00	0.00	0.01	0.01	0.00	0.00	0.01	0.02	0.02
子宫颈	Cervix uteri	14 737	4.49	0.00	0.01	0.00	0.00	0.00	0.12	0.47	1.13	2.03
子宫体	Corpus uteri	4 760	1.45	0.00	0.00	0.00	0.00	0.01	0.02	0.08	0.24	0.29
子宫,部位不明	Uterus unspecified	2 036	0.62	0.00	0.00	0.00	0.00	0.00	0.00	0.07	0.09	0.19
卵巢	Ovary	9 404	2.87	0.00	0.01	0.00	0.01	0.01	0.17	0.15	0.34	0.48	0.67
其他女性生殖器	Other female genital organs	503	0.15	0.00	0.00	0.00	0.01	0.00	0.01	0.00	0.04	0.03
胎盘	Placenta	26	0.01	0.00	0.00	0.00	0.00	0.00	0.01	0.02	0.04	0.01
阴茎	Penis	—	—	—	—	—	—	—	—	—	—	—
前列腺	Prostate	—	—	—	—	—	—	—	—	—	—	—
睾丸	Testis	—	—	—	—	—	—	—	—	—	—	—
其他男性生殖器	Other male genital organs	—	—	—	—	—	—	—	—	—	—	—
肾	Kidney	2 365	0.72	0.28	0.14	0.05	0.01	0.01	0.04	0.06	0.12	0.08
肾盂	Renal pelvis	440	0.13	0.00	0.01	0.00	0.01	0.00	0.01	0.01	0.01	0.01
输尿管	Ureter	600	0.18	0.00	0.00	0.00	0.00	0.00	0.00	0.00	0.00	0.00
膀胱	Bladder	2 914	0.89	0.00	0.01	0.00	0.00	0.01	0.01	0.02	0.02	0.03
其他泌尿器官	Other urinary organs	111	0.03	0.00	0.00	0.00	0.00	0.00	0.00	0.00	0.00	0.00
眼	Eye	164	0.05	0.00	0.11	0.02	0.02	0.01	0.01	0.01	0.02	0.02
脑、神经系统	Brain,nervous system	9 900	3.02	1.07	0.96	0.97	0.60	0.55	0.47	0.64	0.86	1.04
甲状腺	Thyroid	2 045	0.62	0.00	0.00	0.00	0.00	0.02	0.02	0.07	0.14	0.21	0.26
肾上腺	Adrenal gland	353	0.11	0.12	0.05	0.06	0.01	0.00	0.00	0.01	0.04	0.04
其他内分泌腺	Other endocrine	271	0.08	0.00	0.00	0.01	0.02	0.02	0.00	0.02	0.03	0.05
霍奇金淋巴瘤	Hodgkin lymphoma	290	0.09	0.08	0.00	0.01	0.01	0.02	0.03	0.02	0.05	0.05
非霍奇金淋巴瘤	Non-Hodgkin lymphoma	5 227	1.59	0.04	0.13	0.08	0.17	0.18	0.17	0.18	0.37	0.40
免疫增生性疾病	Immunoproliferative diseases	23	0.01	0.00	0.00	0.00	0.00	0.00	0.00	0.00	0.00	0.00
多发性骨髓瘤	Multiple myeloma	2 081	0.63	0.04	0.02	0.00	0.00	0.03	0.05	0.04	0.03	0.07
淋巴样白血病	Lymphoid leukemia	1 598	0.49	0.48	0.29	0.36	0.41	0.33	0.18	0.32	0.18	0.23
髓样白血病	Myeloid leukemia	3 411	1.04	0.36	0.30	0.24	0.20	0.30	0.24	0.33	0.42	0.40
白血病,未特指	Leukemia unspecified	3 306	1.01	1.11	0.48	0.39	0.40	0.45	0.29	0.36	0.44	0.44
其他或未指明部位	Other and unspecified	7 789	2.37	0.40	0.25	0.18	0.20	0.27	0.20	0.26	0.39	0.59
所有部位合计	All sites	328 028	100.00	5.52	3.12	2.76	2.73	3.35	3.53	6.71	12.62	19.06
所有部位除外 C44	All sites except C44	326 064	99.40	5.48	3.12	2.76	2.73	3.33	3.51	6.67	12.58	18.98

Appendix Table 1-12　Cancer mortality in registration areas of China, female in 2018

Age group										粗率 Crude rate/ 100 000⁻¹	中标率 ASR China/ 100 000⁻¹	世标率 ASR world/ 100 000⁻¹	累积率 Cum. Rate/%		ICD-10
40~44	45~49	50~54	55~59	60~64	65~69	70~74	75~79	80~84	85+				0~64	0~74	
0.00	0.00	0.02	0.02	0.03	0.07	0.23	0.36	0.47	0.92	0.05	0.02	0.02	0.00	0.00	C00
0.12	0.15	0.23	0.37	0.47	0.71	1.02	1.52	2.24	2.78	0.29	0.16	0.16	0.01	0.02	C01-C02
0.06	0.13	0.28	0.29	0.52	1.09	1.64	2.86	3.81	5.42	0.41	0.21	0.20	0.01	0.02	C03-C06
0.06	0.05	0.17	0.14	0.25	0.37	0.66	0.44	0.90	1.75	0.14	0.08	0.08	0.00	0.01	C07-C08
0.00	0.03	0.02	0.02	0.05	0.11	0.09	0.21	0.18	0.44	0.03	0.02	0.02	0.00	0.00	C09
0.01	0.01	0.06	0.03	0.06	0.17	0.26	0.35	0.49	0.51	0.06	0.03	0.03	0.00	0.00	C10
0.69	0.87	1.51	1.50	2.22	2.94	3.38	4.22	4.04	4.41	1.01	0.62	0.60	0.04	0.07	C11
0.00	0.01	0.03	0.04	0.07	0.12	0.23	0.21	0.31	0.36	0.04	0.02	0.02	0.00	0.00	C12-C13
0.01	0.01	0.06	0.07	0.12	0.19	0.50	0.73	1.12	1.04	0.10	0.05	0.05	0.00	0.01	C14
0.36	0.79	2.39	3.57	9.66	21.11	37.97	60.23	81.65	91.55	7.47	3.65	3.60	0.09	0.38	C15
2.69	4.77	8.36	10.25	19.71	33.23	50.48	76.44	111.27	125.72	12.12	6.40	6.28	0.25	0.67	C16
0.12	0.26	0.37	0.54	1.12	1.73	2.42	3.16	4.80	4.65	0.56	0.30	0.29	0.01	0.03	C17
1.04	2.15	3.69	5.09	9.21	14.56	21.74	36.10	58.85	77.75	5.89	2.99	2.97	0.11	0.30	C18
1.43	2.46	4.63	5.03	9.53	15.33	23.83	35.89	55.96	66.29	5.92	3.09	3.04	0.12	0.32	C19-C20
0.06	0.12	0.17	0.15	0.28	0.57	0.81	1.33	1.62	2.46	0.21	0.11	0.11	0.00	0.01	C21
3.24	6.23	11.80	13.90	25.50	39.00	55.03	72.61	93.36	104.61	12.89	7.08	7.01	0.32	0.79	C22
0.36	1.02	2.22	2.99	6.14	9.78	14.73	22.20	30.87	31.50	3.31	1.71	1.69	0.06	0.19	C23-C24
0.77	1.64	3.30	5.39	10.28	17.25	24.94	35.37	46.65	49.56	5.45	2.85	2.83	0.11	0.32	C25
0.06	0.07	0.21	0.14	0.22	0.38	0.51	0.76	0.79	1.48	0.15	0.09	0.09	0.00	0.01	C30-C31
0.02	0.04	0.19	0.17	0.29	0.52	1.08	2.25	2.83	2.87	0.26	0.13	0.12	0.00	0.01	C32
5.15	10.84	21.85	27.10	54.38	84.59	128.50	185.13	255.69	285.19	29.36	15.35	15.24	0.62	1.68	C33-C34
0.16	0.21	0.48	0.45	0.78	0.84	1.31	1.70	1.73	2.34	0.35	0.21	0.21	0.01	0.02	C37-C38
0.31	0.50	0.81	1.01	1.86	2.91	4.11	5.47	6.91	7.22	1.01	0.62	0.61	0.03	0.06	C40-C41
0.10	0.14	0.18	0.35	0.45	0.79	0.95	1.29	1.59	2.66	0.26	0.15	0.14	0.01	0.02	C43
0.10	0.20	0.30	0.35	0.67	0.88	2.09	3.82	8.03	22.27	0.76	0.33	0.35	0.01	0.02	C44
0.01	0.06	0.12	0.10	0.24	0.32	0.35	0.49	0.38	0.33	0.09	0.05	0.05	0.00	0.01	C45
0.00	0.03	0.03	0.02	0.03	0.05	0.04	0.10	0.22	0.12	0.02	0.02	0.02	0.00	0.00	C46
0.09	0.21	0.28	0.31	0.56	0.63	0.82	0.92	1.55	2.52	0.27	0.18	0.18	0.01	0.02	C47,C49
6.77	11.85	17.18	17.36	22.41	22.63	23.25	28.80	37.45	46.87	9.66	5.98	5.81	0.41	0.64	C50
0.07	0.09	0.19	0.23	0.39	0.42	0.84	1.32	1.44	2.28	0.21	0.11	0.11	0.01	0.01	C51
0.02	0.08	0.15	0.12	0.20	0.30	0.44	0.46	0.72	0.62	0.10	0.06	0.06	0.00	0.01	C52
4.19	7.01	11.99	10.07	11.32	14.49	15.92	18.44	20.40	16.49	5.72	3.62	3.49	0.24	0.39	C53
0.68	1.41	3.15	3.41	4.71	5.33	6.24	7.16	8.17	7.55	1.85	1.09	1.08	0.07	0.13	C54
0.39	0.72	1.28	1.18	1.60	2.20	2.74	3.33	3.59	4.56	0.79	0.47	0.46	0.03	0.05	C55
1.63	3.57	6.32	6.83	9.41	10.84	12.17	12.49	12.56	10.60	3.65	2.24	2.21	0.15	0.26	C56
0.06	0.13	0.26	0.39	0.44	0.64	0.80	0.75	0.81	0.83	0.20	0.12	0.11	0.01	0.01	C57
0.03	0.02	0.00	0.00	0.00	0.00	0.01	0.00	0.00	0.00	0.01	0.01	0.01	0.00	0.00	C58
—	—	—	—	—	—	—	—	—	—	—	—	—	—	—	C60
—	—	—	—	—	—	—	—	—	—	—	—	—	—	—	C61
—	—	—	—	—	—	—	—	—	—	—	—	—	—	—	C62
—	—	—	—	—	—	—	—	—	—	—	—	—	—	—	C63
0.20	0.40	0.60	0.96	1.49	2.32	3.74	5.17	8.23	9.92	0.92	0.49	0.50	0.02	0.05	C64
0.01	0.03	0.07	0.13	0.22	0.48	0.62	1.05	2.09	2.43	0.17	0.08	0.08	0.00	0.01	C65
0.01	0.03	0.06	0.13	0.33	0.59	0.92	1.98	2.69	3.29	0.23	0.11	0.11	0.00	0.01	C66
0.10	0.18	0.32	0.50	0.92	2.18	4.07	7.98	15.21	22.15	1.13	0.51	0.51	0.01	0.04	C67
0.00	0.01	0.01	0.01	0.09	0.14	0.13	0.33	0.54	0.50	0.04	0.02	0.02	0.00	0.00	C68
0.02	0.02	0.05	0.04	0.06	0.10	0.15	0.32	0.58	0.92	0.06	0.04	0.04	0.00	0.00	C69
1.79	2.65	4.39	4.75	7.57	10.04	13.79	16.47	20.71	21.97	3.84	2.44	2.45	0.14	0.26	C70-C72,D32-D33, D42-D43
0.33	0.64	0.88	1.05	1.46	2.04	2.54	3.98	4.94	5.45	0.79	0.47	0.45	0.03	0.05	C73
0.05	0.07	0.14	0.14	0.23	0.37	0.44	0.63	1.05	0.95	0.14	0.08	0.09	0.00	0.01	C74
0.07	0.06	0.10	0.16	0.19	0.30	0.33	0.48	0.49	0.77	0.11	0.07	0.06	0.00	0.01	C75
0.06	0.04	0.11	0.12	0.15	0.32	0.55	0.63	0.56	0.56	0.11	0.07	0.07	0.00	0.01	C81
0.57	0.92	1.73	2.12	3.97	5.98	8.41	11.79	14.90	13.12	2.03	1.18	1.15	0.05	0.13	C82-C86,C96
0.00	0.00	0.00	0.01	0.02	0.04	0.06	0.06	0.07	0.06	0.01	0.00	0.00	0.00	0.00	C88
0.16	0.30	0.68	0.96	2.00	3.33	4.00	4.74	4.31	2.66	0.81	0.46	0.46	0.02	0.06	C90
0.30	0.40	0.58	0.62	1.13	1.50	1.75	2.32	2.92	2.40	0.62	0.47	0.48	0.03	0.04	C91
0.55	0.79	1.23	1.50	2.58	3.81	4.77	6.71	7.02	6.22	1.32	0.86	0.85	0.05	0.09	C92-C94,D45-D47
0.51	0.77	1.19	1.32	2.38	3.60	5.28	6.44	5.39	5.22	1.28	0.88	0.90	0.05	0.09	C95
0.90	1.62	2.70	3.17	5.14	8.05	10.96	15.79	22.95	30.50	3.02	1.70	1.70	0.08	0.17	O&U
36.53	66.83	119.11	136.67	235.14	352.28	504.18	714.64	979.15	1 118.37	127.30	70.17	69.29	3.24	7.53	C00-C97,D32-D33, D42-D43,D45-D47
36.43	66.63	118.82	136.32	234.47	351.39	502.09	710.81	971.12	1 096.11	126.54	69.84	68.94	3.23	7.50	C00-C97,D32-D33, D42-D43,D45-D47 exc. C44

部位	Site	死亡数 No. deaths	构成 Freq. /%	年龄组								
				0~	1~4	5~9	10~14	15~19	20~24	25~29	30~34	35~39
唇	Lip	110	0.03	0.00	0.00	0.00	0.00	0.00	0.00	0.00	0.00	0.00
舌	Tongue	1 298	0.31	0.00	0.00	0.00	0.00	0.00	0.01	0.03	0.06	0.09
口	Mouth	1 562	0.37	0.00	0.00	0.01	0.00	0.00	0.01	0.01	0.04	0.05
唾液腺	Salivary glands	489	0.12	0.00	0.00	0.00	0.00	0.00	0.01	0.01	0.04	0.05
扁桃腺	Tonsil	196	0.05	0.00	0.00	0.00	0.00	0.00	0.01	0.00	0.00	0.02
其他口咽	Other oropharynx	442	0.11	0.00	0.00	0.00	0.00	0.00	0.01	0.01	0.00	0.02
鼻咽	Nasopharynx	4 726	1.12	0.00	0.01	0.00	0.01	0.04	0.03	0.19	0.35	0.64
下咽	Hypopharynx	821	0.20	0.00	0.00	0.00	0.00	0.00	0.00	0.01	0.01	0.02
咽,部位不明	Pharynx unspecified	457	0.11	0.00	0.00	0.01	0.00	0.00	0.00	0.00	0.01	0.02
食管	Esophagus	27 069	6.44	0.00	0.00	0.01	0.01	0.01	0.04	0.03	0.06	0.17
胃	Stomach	42 711	10.16	0.00	0.00	0.00	0.03	0.06	0.19	0.46	1.24	1.60
小肠	Small intestine	1 997	0.48	0.00	0.01	0.00	0.00	0.01	0.01	0.04	0.03	0.11
结肠	Colon	20 288	4.83	0.00	0.01	0.01	0.03	0.04	0.14	0.27	0.58	0.71
直肠	Rectum	19 364	4.61	0.00	0.00	0.00	0.01	0.03	0.09	0.21	0.45	0.71
肛门	Anus	542	0.13	0.00	0.00	0.00	0.00	0.01	0.01	0.01	0.03	0.02
肝脏	Liver	53 793	12.80	0.37	0.25	0.08	0.12	0.18	0.35	1.02	2.51	4.68
胆囊及其他	Gallbladder etc.	8 142	1.94	0.00	0.00	0.00	0.00	0.00	0.01	0.03	0.10	0.18
胰腺	Pancreas	17 165	4.08	0.04	0.00	0.00	0.03	0.02	0.03	0.10	0.22	0.42
鼻、鼻窦及其他	Nose,sinuses etc.	514	0.12	0.04	0.01	0.01	0.01	0.02	0.02	0.01	0.04	0.06
喉	Larynx	2 811	0.67	0.00	0.00	0.00	0.00	0.01	0.01	0.02	0.02	0.05
气管、支气管、肺	Trachea,bronchus & lung	117 482	27.96	0.00	0.02	0.02	0.07	0.06	0.23	0.48	1.22	2.42
其他胸腔器官	Other thoracic organs	1 411	0.34	0.04	0.02	0.00	0.04	0.03	0.10	0.16	0.10	0.15
骨	Bone	2 696	0.64	0.04	0.03	0.07	0.28	0.48	0.23	0.17	0.20	0.15
皮肤黑色素瘤	Melanoma of skin	699	0.17	0.00	0.01	0.00	0.02	0.01	0.01	0.04	0.02	0.06
皮肤其他	Other skin	1 798	0.43	0.00	0.01	0.00	0.02	0.00	0.01	0.05	0.04	0.06
间皮瘤	Mesothelioma	352	0.08	0.00	0.00	0.00	0.00	0.00	0.01	0.00	0.02	0.02
卡波氏肉瘤	Kaposi sarcoma	90	0.02	0.00	0.00	0.00	0.01	0.04	0.01	0.01	0.01	0.01
结缔组织、软组织	Connective & soft tissue	908	0.22	0.04	0.16	0.08	0.06	0.11	0.08	0.11	0.10	0.12
乳腺	Breast	13 055	3.18	0.00	0.00	0.00	0.00	0.04	0.04	0.52	1.69	3.79
外阴	Vulva	284	0.07	0.00	0.00	0.00	0.00	0.01	0.02	0.02	0.04
阴道	Vagina	138	0.03	0.00	0.00	0.00	0.00	0.00	0.00	0.00	0.01	0.01
子宫颈	Cervix uteri	6 318	1.50	0.00	0.00	0.00	0.00	0.00	0.11	0.41	1.05	2.23
子宫体	Corpus uteri	2 263	0.54	0.00	0.00	0.00	0.00	0.00	0.03	0.12	0.29	0.33
子宫,部位不明	Uterus unspecified	824	0.20	0.00	0.00	0.00	0.00	0.00	0.00	0.01	0.07	0.17
卵巢	Ovary	5 100	1.21	0.00	0.02	0.00	0.00	0.00	0.15	0.14	0.38	0.51	0.68
其他女性生殖器	Other female genital organs	273	0.06	0.00	0.00	0.00	0.00	0.00	0.01	0.00	0.01	0.04
胎盘	Placenta	8	0.00	0.00	0.00	0.00	0.00	0.00	0.00	0.02	0.03	0.00
阴茎	Penis	281	0.07	0.00	0.00	0.00	0.00	0.02	0.00	0.00	0.02	0.03
前列腺	Prostate	7 461	1.78	0.00	0.02	0.00	0.00	0.05	0.01	0.02	0.04	0.05
睾丸	Testis	116	0.03	0.00	0.04	0.00	0.00	0.00	0.05	0.07	0.10	0.04
其他男性生殖器	Other male genital organs	90	0.02	0.00	0.00	0.00	0.00	0.00	0.03	0.01	0.01	0.00
肾	Kidney	4 058	0.97	0.33	0.15	0.03	0.03	0.04	0.05	0.06	0.16	0.10
肾盂	Renal pelvis	683	0.16	0.00	0.00	0.01	0.00	0.00	0.00	0.00	0.01	0.02
输尿管	Ureter	801	0.19	0.00	0.00	0.00	0.00	0.00	0.00	0.00	0.01	0.00
膀胱	Bladder	6 927	1.65	0.00	0.00	0.01	0.02	0.01	0.01	0.03	0.02	0.06
其他泌尿器官	Other urinary organs	179	0.04	0.00	0.00	0.00	0.00	0.00	0.00	0.00	0.00	0.01
眼	Eye	140	0.03	0.04	0.11	0.02	0.02	0.00	0.01	0.01	0.01	0.01
脑、神经系统	Brain,nervous system	9 583	2.28	0.83	0.82	1.13	0.75	0.62	0.40	0.72	1.13	1.16
甲状腺	Thyroid	1 643	0.39	0.00	0.00	0.00	0.01	0.01	0.04	0.16	0.15	0.19
肾上腺	Adrenal gland	469	0.11	0.12	0.08	0.07	0.01	0.00	0.01	0.02	0.03	0.03
其他内分泌腺	Other endocrine	280	0.07	0.00	0.01	0.01	0.02	0.05	0.01	0.05	0.04	0.02
霍奇金淋巴瘤	Hodgkin lymphoma	361	0.09	0.08	0.00	0.00	0.03	0.02	0.02	0.06	0.03	0.05
非霍奇金淋巴瘤	Non-Hodgkin lymphoma	6 714	1.60	0.04	0.15	0.11	0.20	0.30	0.30	0.27	0.42	0.57
免疫增生性疾病	Immunoproliferative diseases	50	0.01	0.00	0.00	0.00	0.00	0.00	0.00	0.01	0.01	0.00
多发性骨髓瘤	Multiple myeloma	2 662	0.63	0.08	0.02	0.03	0.04	0.07	0.03	0.05	0.05	0.11
淋巴样白血病	Lymphoid leukemia	1 903	0.45	0.46	0.46	0.49	0.39	0.45	0.26	0.34	0.23	0.25
髓样白血病	Myeloid leukemia	4 389	1.04	0.50	0.27	0.23	0.20	0.27	0.33	0.35	0.42	0.51
白血病,未特指	Leukemia unspecified	3 105	0.74	0.87	0.37	0.33	0.38	0.39	0.34	0.39	0.39	0.35
其他或未指明部位	Other and unspecified	9 813	2.34	0.42	0.31	0.24	0.25	0.26	0.26	0.32	0.42	0.58
所有部位合计	All sites	420 199	100.00	4.36	3.33	3.01	3.07	3.76	3.97	7.11	12.97	20.38
所有部位除外 C44	All sites except C44	418 401	99.57	4.36	3.32	3.01	3.06	3.76	3.96	7.07	12.93	20.32

Age group										粗率 Crude rate/ $100\ 000^{-1}$	中标率 ASR China/ $100\ 000^{-1}$	世标率 ASR world/ $100\ 000^{-1}$	累积率 Cum. Rate/%		ICD-10
40~44	45~49	50~54	55~59	60~64	65~69	70~74	75~79	80~84	85+				0~64	0~74	
0.01	0.01	0.02	0.03	0.03	0.12	0.25	0.34	0.41	0.93	0.05	0.02	0.02	0.00	0.00	C00
0.22	0.30	0.68	0.78	1.18	1.75	1.60	2.54	3.79	4.56	0.55	0.31	0.31	0.02	0.03	C01-C02
0.07	0.28	0.58	0.91	1.36	1.77	2.47	3.81	5.20	7.65	0.66	0.35	0.35	0.02	0.04	C03-C06
0.04	0.14	0.26	0.29	0.28	0.51	1.02	1.03	1.31	1.89	0.21	0.12	0.12	0.01	0.01	C07-C08
0.02	0.07	0.15	0.12	0.22	0.25	0.26	0.29	0.20	0.75	0.09	0.05	0.05	0.00	0.01	C09
0.04	0.10	0.30	0.30	0.47	0.60	0.72	0.87	0.95	1.00	0.19	0.11	0.11	0.01	0.01	C10
1.17	1.97	3.26	3.45	4.99	6.29	6.60	6.19	6.68	6.12	2.00	1.25	1.22	0.08	0.15	C11
0.07	0.21	0.64	0.87	0.98	1.10	1.14	1.26	1.31	0.96	0.35	0.20	0.21	0.01	0.03	C12-C13
0.02	0.08	0.18	0.20	0.44	0.55	0.88	1.05	1.41	1.99	0.19	0.10	0.11	0.00	0.01	C14
0.78	2.59	8.30	13.28	26.10	37.93	55.34	72.80	90.79	96.44	11.47	6.08	6.12	0.26	0.72	C15
3.22	5.55	12.03	17.15	34.98	56.72	83.09	118.74	156.56	167.01	18.09	9.72	9.61	0.38	1.08	C16
0.17	0.37	0.52	0.99	1.68	2.70	3.87	5.07	6.63	7.37	0.85	0.46	0.46	0.02	0.05	C17
1.16	2.69	4.91	7.62	14.27	22.42	33.76	54.33	89.56	118.33	8.59	4.42	4.40	0.16	0.44	C18
1.51	3.02	5.78	8.15	15.25	22.94	32.96	50.38	77.47	93.49	8.20	4.32	4.30	0.18	0.46	C19-C20
0.06	0.11	0.19	0.25	0.37	0.61	0.79	1.61	1.92	2.56	0.23	0.12	0.12	0.01	0.01	C21
10.56	17.81	30.30	34.56	52.22	67.16	81.03	96.69	121.98	136.41	22.79	13.35	13.19	0.77	1.51	C22
0.39	0.95	1.98	3.15	6.58	10.47	14.48	23.65	32.99	38.33	3.45	1.79	1.78	0.07	0.19	C23-C24
1.15	2.60	5.39	8.59	15.20	22.02	32.05	46.21	59.14	65.38	7.27	3.89	3.89	0.17	0.44	C25
0.06	0.10	0.24	0.20	0.44	0.66	0.69	1.41	1.36	1.89	0.22	0.13	0.12	0.01	0.01	C30-C31
0.14	0.37	0.85	1.77	2.84	3.64	4.99	7.14	9.68	9.40	1.19	0.64	0.64	0.03	0.07	C32
5.80	14.01	34.28	54.49	107.82	165.19	227.84	318.85	404.88	429.55	49.77	26.54	26.56	1.10	3.07	C33-C34
0.19	0.37	0.67	0.82	1.36	1.75	2.20	2.81	2.87	4.06	0.60	0.36	0.36	0.02	0.04	C37-C38
0.31	0.57	0.82	1.22	2.21	3.14	4.10	7.18	8.27	8.15	1.14	0.71	0.69	0.03	0.07	C40-C41
0.09	0.17	0.22	0.37	0.50	0.90	1.10	1.48	2.46	2.88	0.30	0.17	0.16	0.01	0.02	C43
0.14	0.18	0.43	0.46	0.86	1.21	2.69	4.29	8.14	18.65	0.76	0.36	0.37	0.01	0.03	C44
0.03	0.05	0.16	0.17	0.42	0.55	0.57	0.78	0.87	0.89	0.15	0.08	0.08	0.00	0.01	C45
0.00	0.02	0.03	0.08	0.05	0.11	0.12	0.20	0.36	0.14	0.04	0.02	0.02	0.00	0.00	C46
0.15	0.25	0.33	0.44	0.81	0.90	1.03	1.59	2.48	3.31	0.38	0.25	0.25	0.01	0.02	C47,C49
7.14	12.41	17.96	19.71	24.74	24.35	26.68	36.22	47.18	60.93	11.11	6.56	6.39	0.44	0.70	C50
0.07	0.09	0.21	0.20	0.51	0.47	0.73	1.50	1.63	3.15	0.24	0.12	0.12	0.01	0.01	C51
0.01	0.11	0.14	0.14	0.16	0.33	0.58	0.44	0.93	0.85	0.12	0.06	0.06	0.00	0.01	C52
4.04	6.63	11.71	9.83	10.22	12.09	13.08	16.66	18.18	14.17	5.37	3.36	3.22	0.23	0.36	C53
0.58	1.45	2.95	3.49	4.86	5.09	5.84	7.96	9.04	8.30	1.93	1.10	1.09	0.07	0.13	C54
0.27	0.68	1.13	1.11	1.49	1.81	2.29	2.48	3.31	4.12	0.70	0.40	0.39	0.02	0.05	C55
1.93	3.92	6.79	8.28	10.54	11.92	14.13	16.05	16.74	13.93	4.34	2.56	2.53	0.17	0.30	C56
0.06	0.16	0.22	0.55	0.54	0.67	0.93	0.92	1.07	0.97	0.23	0.13	0.13	0.01	0.02	C57
0.01	0.02	0.00	0.00	0.00	0.00	0.00	0.00	0.00	0.00	0.01	0.01	0.01	0.00	0.00	C58
0.01	0.11	0.12	0.19	0.61	0.64	0.77	1.11	2.73	4.23	0.24	0.13	0.13	0.01	0.01	C60
0.08	0.22	0.59	1.29	4.45	10.23	24.14	55.08	107.58	183.46	6.30	3.04	3.09	0.03	0.21	C61
0.13	0.06	0.09	0.11	0.12	0.18	0.19	0.46	0.45	0.86	0.10	0.07	0.07	0.00	0.01	C62
0.02	0.02	0.07	0.06	0.11	0.16	0.27	0.58	0.85	1.21	0.08	0.04	0.04	0.00	0.00	C63
0.27	0.62	1.25	2.09	3.21	5.04	7.19	9.82	14.21	18.47	1.72	0.93	0.94	0.04	0.10	C64
0.03	0.07	0.12	0.20	0.46	0.87	1.32	1.79	3.05	4.27	0.29	0.15	0.15	0.00	0.02	C65
0.02	0.04	0.10	0.22	0.52	0.75	1.06	2.72	4.74	5.59	0.34	0.16	0.16	0.00	0.01	C66
0.18	0.40	0.84	1.43	3.09	5.92	10.35	21.07	38.67	64.06	2.93	1.36	1.38	0.03	0.11	C67
0.01	0.01	0.01	0.03	0.11	0.18	0.27	0.58	0.87	1.57	0.08	0.04	0.04	0.00	0.00	C68
0.01	0.04	0.04	0.04	0.07	0.11	0.16	0.25	0.46	0.75	0.06	0.04	0.04	0.00	0.00	C69
1.73	2.83	4.73	5.22	8.09	10.74	14.44	17.75	21.33	22.92	4.06	2.62	2.61	0.15	0.27	C70-C72,D32-D33, D42-D43
0.31	0.46	0.69	0.80	1.30	1.72	2.44	3.72	5.07	5.66	0.70	0.41	0.39	0.02	0.04	C73
0.05	0.10	0.20	0.31	0.42	0.54	0.60	0.94	1.41	1.49	0.20	0.12	0.12	0.01	0.01	C74
0.05	0.04	0.09	0.18	0.25	0.30	0.50	0.51	0.72	0.78	0.12	0.08	0.07	0.00	0.01	C75
0.06	0.10	0.14	0.22	0.25	0.37	0.63	0.90	0.95	0.78	0.15	0.10	0.09	0.00	0.01	C81
0.75	1.23	2.45	3.11	5.45	8.02	11.59	16.56	21.82	22.78	2.84	1.65	1.62	0.08	0.17	C82-C86,C96
0.00	0.01	0.00	0.01	0.02	0.07	0.17	0.18	0.20	0.11	0.02	0.01	0.01	0.00	0.00	C88
0.18	0.40	0.74	1.26	2.64	4.23	5.51	6.89	7.58	6.19	1.13	0.64	0.64	0.03	0.08	C90
0.31	0.48	0.68	0.72	1.28	2.02	2.63	3.54	4.53	4.23	0.81	0.59	0.61	0.03	0.05	C91
0.65	0.95	1.43	2.09	3.44	5.38	7.24	9.94	12.52	12.63	1.86	1.15	1.14	0.06	0.12	C92-C94,D45-D47
0.43	0.73	1.11	1.24	2.41	3.25	4.25	6.48	8.20	8.51	1.32	0.87	0.88	0.04	0.09	C95
1.03	1.83	3.31	4.75	7.91	11.35	15.60	23.40	33.01	43.92	4.16	2.32	2.33	0.11	0.24	O&U
40.82	78.29	152.28	207.19	364.39	529.55	730.13	1 030.83	1 383.93	1 596.98	178.01	98.01	97.55	4.50	10.80	C00-C97,D32-D33, D42-D43,D45-D47
40.68	78.11	151.85	206.74	363.53	528.34	727.44	1 026.54	1 375.78	1 578.33	177.25	97.65	97.18	4.49	10.77	C00-C97,D32-D33, D42-D43,D45-D47 exc. C44

部位	Site	死亡数 No. deaths	构成 Freq. /%	年龄组								
				0~	1~4	5~9	10~14	15~19	20~24	25~29	30~34	35~39
唇	Lip	66	0.02	0.00	0.00	0.00	0.00	0.00	0.00	0.00	0.00	0.00
舌	Tongue	869	0.33	0.00	0.00	0.00	0.00	0.00	0.01	0.02	0.09	0.15
口	Mouth	1 018	0.38	0.00	0.00	0.02	0.00	0.00	0.00	0.00	0.05	0.07
唾液腺	Salivary glands	308	0.12	0.00	0.00	0.00	0.00	0.00	0.01	0.01	0.05	0.05
扁桃腺	Tonsil	153	0.06	0.00	0.00	0.00	0.00	0.00	0.00	0.00	0.00	0.01
其他口咽	Other oropharynx	372	0.14	0.00	0.00	0.00	0.00	0.00	0.03	0.00	0.00	0.02
鼻咽	Nasopharynx	3 502	1.31	0.00	0.00	0.00	0.02	0.08	0.04	0.29	0.48	0.93
下咽	Hypopharynx	772	0.29	0.00	0.00	0.00	0.00	0.00	0.00	0.01	0.01	0.04
咽,部位不明	Pharynx unspecified	339	0.13	0.00	0.00	0.02	0.00	0.00	0.00	0.00	0.01	0.03
食管	Esophagus	20 894	7.84	0.00	0.00	0.02	0.00	0.02	0.03	0.01	0.08	0.22
胃	Stomach	29 507	11.07	0.00	0.00	0.00	0.02	0.02	0.13	0.50	1.10	1.58
小肠	Small intestine	1 186	0.45	0.00	0.02	0.00	0.00	0.02	0.01	0.06	0.04	0.18
结肠	Colon	11 487	4.31	0.00	0.02	0.02	0.03	0.05	0.21	0.30	0.47	0.86
直肠	Rectum	12 073	4.53	0.00	0.00	0.00	0.02	0.03	0.09	0.25	0.47	0.83
肛门	Anus	317	0.12	0.00	0.00	0.00	0.00	0.00	0.00	0.02	0.02	0.04
肝脏	Liver	39 457	14.81	0.63	0.32	0.09	0.12	0.29	0.53	1.66	4.23	8.09
胆囊及其他	Gallbladder etc.	3 919	1.47	0.00	0.00	0.00	0.00	0.00	0.00	0.04	0.10	0.17
胰腺	Pancreas	9 817	3.68	0.00	0.00	0.00	0.00	0.00	0.05	0.11	0.25	0.58
鼻、鼻窦及其他	Nose,sinuses etc.	348	0.13	0.00	0.02	0.02	0.00	0.00	0.03	0.01	0.03	0.02
喉	Larynx	2 494	0.94	0.00	0.00	0.00	0.00	0.02	0.01	0.01	0.03	0.08
气管、支气管、肺	Trachea,bronchus & lung	82 183	30.84	0.00	0.00	0.02	0.12	0.05	0.27	0.54	1.44	2.80
其他胸腔器官	Other thoracic organs	927	0.35	0.08	0.04	0.00	0.07	0.05	0.15	0.20	0.14	0.21
骨	Bone	1 606	0.60	0.00	0.04	0.05	0.28	0.74	0.29	0.21	0.26	0.19
皮肤黑色素瘤	Melanoma of skin	367	0.14	0.00	0.00	0.00	0.00	0.02	0.02	0.03	0.02	0.06
皮肤其他	Other skin	1 018	0.38	0.00	0.00	0.00	0.03	0.00	0.03	0.04	0.08	0.05
间皮瘤	Mesothelioma	207	0.08	0.00	0.00	0.00	0.00	0.00	0.01	0.00	0.04	0.01
卡波氏肉瘤	Kaposi sarcoma	49	0.02	0.00	0.00	0.00	0.02	0.00	0.00	0.01	0.00	0.00
结缔组织、软组织	Connective & soft tissue	514	0.19	0.00	0.18	0.03	0.07	0.10	0.11	0.13	0.12	0.15
乳腺	Breast	295	0.11	0.00	0.00	0.00	0.00	0.00	0.00	0.01	0.02	0.07
外阴	Vulva	—	—	—	—	—	—	—	—	—	—	—
阴道	Vagina	—	—	—	—	—	—	—	—	—	—	—
子宫颈	Cervix uteri	—	—	—	—	—	—	—	—	—	—	—
子宫体	Corpus uteri	—	—	—	—	—	—	—	—	—	—	—
子宫,部位不明	Uterus unspecified	—	—	—	—	—	—	—	—	—	—	—
卵巢	Ovary	—	—	—	—	—	—	—	—	—	—	—
其他女性生殖器	Other female genital organs	—	—	—	—	—	—	—	—	—	—	—
胎盘	Placenta	—	—	—	—	—	—	—	—	—	—	—
阴茎	Penis	281	0.11	0.00	0.00	0.00	0.00	0.02	0.00	0.00	0.02	0.03
前列腺	Prostate	7 461	2.80	0.00	0.02	0.00	0.00	0.05	0.01	0.02	0.04	0.05
睾丸	Testis	116	0.04	0.00	0.04	0.00	0.00	0.00	0.05	0.07	0.10	0.04
其他男性生殖器	Other male genital organs	90	0.03	0.00	0.00	0.00	0.00	0.00	0.03	0.01	0.01	0.00
肾	Kidney	2 759	1.04	0.24	0.14	0.05	0.05	0.05	0.03	0.08	0.15	0.16
肾盂	Renal pelvis	399	0.15	0.00	0.00	0.02	0.00	0.00	0.00	0.00	0.01	0.02
输尿管	Ureter	415	0.16	0.00	0.00	0.00	0.00	0.00	0.00	0.00	0.01	0.00
膀胱	Bladder	5 342	2.00	0.00	0.00	0.02	0.02	0.02	0.01	0.05	0.02	0.09
其他泌尿器官	Other urinary organs	114	0.04	0.00	0.00	0.00	0.00	0.00	0.00	0.00	0.00	0.01
眼	Eye	64	0.02	0.08	0.13	0.03	0.02	0.00	0.01	0.00	0.00	0.01
脑、神经系统	Brain,nervous system	5 320	2.00	0.79	0.65	1.21	0.92	0.76	0.55	0.92	1.43	1.47
甲状腺	Thyroid	627	0.24	0.00	0.00	0.00	0.00	0.00	0.01	0.07	0.08	0.18
肾上腺	Adrenal gland	295	0.11	0.16	0.13	0.06	0.00	0.00	0.01	0.02	0.03	0.01
其他内分泌腺	Other endocrine	145	0.05	0.00	0.02	0.02	0.02	0.05	0.03	0.05	0.02	0.06
霍奇金淋巴瘤	Hodgkin lymphoma	240	0.09	0.00	0.00	0.00	0.03	0.00	0.01	0.09	0.02	0.06
非霍奇金淋巴瘤	Non-Hodgkin lymphoma	4 120	1.55	0.00	0.16	0.14	0.26	0.37	0.41	0.37	0.57	0.75
免疫增生性疾病	Immunoproliferative diseases	40	0.02	0.00	0.00	0.00	0.00	0.00	0.00	0.01	0.01	0.00
多发性骨髓瘤	Multiple myeloma	1 569	0.59	0.08	0.02	0.06	0.03	0.05	0.01	0.06	0.07	0.17
淋巴样白血病	Lymphoid leukemia	1 118	0.42	0.39	0.56	0.53	0.35	0.51	0.35	0.34	0.33	0.28
髓样白血病	Myeloid leukemia	2 593	0.97	0.24	0.31	0.24	0.23	0.24	0.44	0.37	0.47	0.66
白血病,未特指	Leukemia unspecified	1 788	0.67	0.95	0.43	0.39	0.43	0.46	0.36	0.50	0.45	0.35
其他或未指明部位	Other and unspecified	5 538	2.08	0.39	0.36	0.25	0.29	0.24	0.25	0.39	0.44	0.65
所有部位合计	All sites	266 498	100.00	4.03	3.58	3.28	3.50	4.28	4.68	7.89	13.96	22.53
所有部位除外 C44	All sites except C44	265 480	99.62	4.03	3.58	3.28	3.47	4.28	4.65	7.86	13.89	22.48

| Age group | | | | | | | | | | 粗率 Crude rate/ 100 000^{-1} | 中标率 ASR China/ 100 000^{-1} | 世标率 ASR world/ 100 000^{-1} | 累积率 Cum. Rate/% | | ICD-10 |
40~44	45~49	50~54	55~59	60~64	65~69	70~74	75~79	80~84	85+				0~64	0~74	
0.01	0.02	0.03	0.04	0.05	0.21	0.27	0.31	0.45	1.29	0.06	0.03	0.03	0.00	0.00	C00
0.31	0.42	1.08	1.12	1.89	2.58	2.13	3.04	4.38	5.70	0.73	0.44	0.44	0.03	0.05	C01-C02
0.10	0.46	0.92	1.50	2.28	2.34	3.43	4.38	5.68	8.97	0.86	0.49	0.50	0.03	0.06	C03-C06
0.03	0.22	0.32	0.43	0.35	0.68	1.25	1.58	2.05	1.73	0.26	0.16	0.15	0.01	0.02	C07-C08
0.04	0.11	0.27	0.20	0.38	0.43	0.40	0.35	0.45	1.04	0.13	0.08	0.08	0.01	0.01	C09
0.08	0.20	0.56	0.56	0.87	1.06	1.25	1.58	1.31	1.04	0.31	0.19	0.19	0.01	0.02	C10
1.69	3.16	4.86	5.27	7.83	9.87	9.70	8.84	9.83	8.37	2.96	1.88	1.85	0.12	0.22	C11
0.14	0.41	1.25	1.71	1.91	2.13	2.07	2.50	2.39	1.64	0.65	0.39	0.39	0.03	0.05	C12-C13
0.03	0.15	0.29	0.34	0.84	0.95	1.25	1.35	1.48	3.37	0.29	0.16	0.17	0.01	0.02	C14
1.32	4.66	14.83	24.28	46.47	63.95	88.43	108.85	129.68	134.10	17.63	9.93	10.05	0.46	1.22	C15
3.74	6.66	16.22	25.05	52.85	85.84	126.42	177.38	223.22	234.63	24.90	14.02	13.93	0.54	1.60	C16
0.21	0.49	0.69	1.24	2.11	3.36	4.76	6.19	7.39	9.66	1.00	0.58	0.58	0.03	0.07	C17
1.33	2.98	5.73	9.34	17.80	27.96	42.14	64.15	103.37	144.45	9.69	5.31	5.33	0.20	0.55	C18
1.59	3.66	7.04	11.32	21.34	31.25	44.13	65.30	98.48	124.78	10.19	5.66	5.67	0.23	0.61	C19-C20
0.06	0.13	0.21	0.32	0.50	0.75	1.06	1.96	2.56	2.59	0.27	0.15	0.15	0.01	0.02	C21
18.25	30.51	50.11	56.28	83.41	101.91	113.84	126.38	156.22	177.16	33.30	20.54	20.29	1.27	2.35	C22
0.43	0.91	1.90	3.49	6.85	11.59	14.94	22.45	30.52	40.73	3.31	1.82	1.84	0.07	0.20	C23-C24
1.49	3.39	7.16	11.39	19.57	27.14	36.74	51.31	65.52	73.87	8.28	4.70	4.71	0.22	0.54	C25
0.10	0.17	0.35	0.34	0.64	0.97	1.04	2.08	1.82	2.33	0.29	0.17	0.17	0.01	0.02	C30-C31
0.27	0.67	1.54	3.35	5.46	6.94	9.15	12.41	17.28	18.90	2.10	1.18	1.19	0.06	0.14	C32
7.03	17.83	48.47	82.28	165.95	256.06	342.12	463.19	559.88	603.27	69.36	38.97	39.15	1.63	4.62	C33-C34
0.21	0.49	0.86	1.15	1.76	2.54	3.03	3.84	3.64	5.78	0.78	0.49	0.49	0.03	0.05	C37-C38
0.42	0.60	1.04	1.54	2.97	4.02	4.52	9.26	9.89	9.75	1.36	0.88	0.86	0.04	0.09	C40-C41
0.09	0.22	0.21	0.34	0.51	0.86	1.33	1.81	3.13	3.28	0.31	0.18	0.18	0.01	0.02	C43
0.15	0.22	0.57	0.66	1.05	1.84	3.51	5.19	10.12	20.11	0.86	0.46	0.46	0.01	0.04	C44
0.03	0.04	0.16	0.21	0.53	0.70	0.72	0.85	1.08	1.47	0.17	0.10	0.10	0.01	0.01	C45
0.00	0.01	0.02	0.10	0.07	0.14	0.21	0.23	0.34	0.17	0.04	0.03	0.03	0.00	0.00	C46
0.21	0.23	0.42	0.53	0.93	1.06	1.17	2.00	3.35	3.62	0.43	0.29	0.29	0.02	0.03	C47, C49
0.05	0.18	0.15	0.35	0.50	0.75	0.88	1.54	1.59	3.45	0.25	0.14	0.14	0.01	0.01	C50
—	—	—	—	—	—	—	—	—	—	—	—	—	—	—	C51
—	—	—	—	—	—	—	—	—	—	—	—	—	—	—	C52
—	—	—	—	—	—	—	—	—	—	—	—	—	—	—	C53
—	—	—	—	—	—	—	—	—	—	—	—	—	—	—	C54
—	—	—	—	—	—	—	—	—	—	—	—	—	—	—	C55
—	—	—	—	—	—	—	—	—	—	—	—	—	—	—	C56
—	—	—	—	—	—	—	—	—	—	—	—	—	—	—	C57
—	—	—	—	—	—	—	—	—	—	—	—	—	—	—	C58
0.01	0.11	0.12	0.19	0.61	0.64	0.77	1.11	2.73	4.23	0.24	0.13	0.13	0.01	0.01	C60
0.08	0.22	0.59	1.29	4.45	10.23	24.14	55.08	107.58	183.46	6.30	3.04	3.09	0.03	0.21	C61
0.13	0.06	0.09	0.11	0.12	0.18	0.19	0.46	0.45	0.86	0.10	0.07	0.07	0.00	0.01	C62
0.02	0.02	0.07	0.06	0.11	0.16	0.27	0.58	0.85	1.21	0.08	0.04	0.04	0.00	0.00	C63
0.38	0.82	1.83	3.11	5.03	7.51	10.32	13.91	18.24	26.49	2.33	1.32	1.34	0.06	0.15	C64
0.03	0.11	0.18	0.30	0.61	1.11	1.75	2.31	2.67	5.18	0.34	0.19	0.19	0.01	0.02	C65
0.03	0.02	0.15	0.30	0.61	0.88	1.20	2.50	5.29	6.47	0.35	0.18	0.18	0.01	0.02	C66
0.34	0.57	1.31	2.29	5.20	9.70	17.15	34.32	64.73	114.77	4.51	2.26	2.31	0.05	0.18	C67
0.00	0.02	0.01	0.03	0.15	0.14	0.40	0.69	1.42	2.68	0.10	0.05	0.05	0.00	0.00	C68
0.00	0.05	0.05	0.05	0.11	0.14	0.16	0.08	0.34	0.69	0.05	0.04	0.05	0.00	0.00	C69
1.97	3.35	5.63	5.99	9.41	12.74	16.35	19.68	21.88	23.99	4.49	3.03	3.00	0.17	0.32	C70-C72, D32-D33, D42-D43
0.18	0.30	0.60	0.62	1.15	1.61	2.05	2.96	3.75	4.31	0.53	0.32	0.31	0.02	0.03	C73
0.03	0.10	0.33	0.45	0.54	0.77	0.77	1.15	1.70	1.98	0.25	0.15	0.16	0.01	0.02	C74
0.03	0.03	0.07	0.14	0.36	0.25	0.56	0.58	0.97	1.21	0.12	0.08	0.08	0.00	0.01	C75
0.06	0.14	0.18	0.33	0.38	0.52	0.80	1.27	1.36	1.21	0.20	0.13	0.12	0.01	0.01	C81
0.94	1.58	3.22	3.89	7.19	9.91	15.02	20.10	26.94	32.96	3.48	2.11	2.08	0.10	0.22	C82-C86, C96
0.00	0.02	0.00	0.00	0.04	0.11	0.27	0.31	0.40	0.17	0.03	0.02	0.02	0.00	0.00	C88
0.19	0.52	0.80	1.58	2.96	5.10	6.57	8.46	10.12	9.66	1.32	0.77	0.77	0.03	0.09	C90
0.30	0.63	0.77	0.76	1.53	2.38	3.14	4.61	5.97	6.47	0.94	0.69	0.71	0.04	0.06	C91
0.72	1.06	1.76	2.52	4.05	6.85	8.77	11.84	16.65	18.29	2.19	1.38	1.36	0.07	0.14	C92-C94, D45-D47
0.46	0.86	1.28	1.48	2.70	3.81	6.01	7.92	10.80	11.30	1.51	1.03	1.04	0.05	0.10	C95
1.02	2.05	3.52	5.56	10.06	14.06	19.43	28.75	37.51	49.96	4.67	2.74	2.75	0.13	0.32	O&U
46.36	91.84	189.78	275.78	505.02	738.67	997.96	1 368.92	1 799.43	2 154.82	224.91	129.19	129.26	5.86	14.55	C00-C97, D32-D33, D42-D43, D45-D47
46.21	91.62	189.21	275.13	503.97	736.83	994.45	1 363.73	1 789.32	2 134.71	224.05	128.74	128.79	5.85	14.50	C00-C97, D32-D33, D42-D43, D45-D47 exc. C44

部位	Site	死亡数 No. deaths	构成 Freq./%	0~	1~4	5~9	10~14	15~19	20~24	25~29	30~34	35~39
唇	Lip	44	0.03	0.00	0.00	0.00	0.00	0.00	0.00	0.00	0.00	0.00
舌	Tongue	429	0.28	0.00	0.00	0.00	0.00	0.00	0.01	0.03	0.03	0.04
口	Mouth	544	0.35	0.00	0.00	0.00	0.00	0.00	0.01	0.01	0.02	0.03
唾液腺	Salivary glands	181	0.12	0.00	0.00	0.00	0.00	0.00	0.01	0.01	0.03	0.04
扁桃腺	Tonsil	43	0.03	0.00	0.00	0.00	0.00	0.00	0.02	0.00	0.00	0.03
其他口咽	Other oropharynx	70	0.05	0.00	0.00	0.00	0.00	0.00	0.00	0.00	0.01	0.01
鼻咽	Nasopharynx	1 224	0.80	0.00	0.02	0.00	0.00	0.00	0.03	0.09	0.22	0.35
下咽	Hypopharynx	49	0.03	0.00	0.00	0.00	0.00	0.00	0.00	0.01	0.00	0.00
咽,部位不明	Pharynx unspecified	118	0.08	0.00	0.00	0.00	0.00	0.00	0.00	0.00	0.00	0.01
食管	Esophagus	6 175	4.02	0.00	0.00	0.00	0.02	0.00	0.06	0.05	0.04	0.11
胃	Stomach	13 204	8.59	0.00	0.00	0.00	0.04	0.11	0.25	0.42	1.38	1.62
小肠	Small intestine	811	0.53	0.00	0.00	0.00	0.00	0.00	0.01	0.02	0.01	0.04
结肠	Colon	8 801	5.73	0.00	0.00	0.00	0.00	0.04	0.07	0.24	0.69	0.56
直肠	Rectum	7 291	4.74	0.00	0.00	0.00	0.00	0.02	0.08	0.17	0.43	0.60
肛门	Anus	225	0.15	0.00	0.00	0.00	0.00	0.02	0.01	0.00	0.03	0.00
肝脏	Liver	14 336	9.33	0.09	0.16	0.07	0.12	0.07	0.15	0.39	0.83	1.33
胆囊及其他	Gallbladder etc.	4 223	2.75	0.00	0.00	0.00	0.00	0.00	0.01	0.02	0.11	0.20
胰腺	Pancreas	7 348	4.78	0.09	0.00	0.00	0.04	0.04	0.01	0.09	0.19	0.26
鼻、鼻窦及其他	Nose, sinuses etc.	166	0.11	0.09	0.00	0.00	0.02	0.00	0.04	0.00	0.04	0.10
喉	Larynx	317	0.21	0.00	0.00	0.00	0.00	0.00	0.00	0.01	0.02	0.00
气管、支气管、肺	Trachea, bronchus & lung	35 299	22.97	0.00	0.04	0.02	0.02	0.07	0.18	0.42	1.00	2.05
其他胸腔器官	Other thoracic organs	484	0.31	0.00	0.00	0.00	0.00	0.00	0.04	0.13	0.06	0.08
骨	Bone	1 090	0.71	0.00	0.02	0.11	0.29	0.20	0.17	0.14	0.14	0.10
皮肤黑色素瘤	Melanoma of skin	332	0.22	0.00	0.02	0.00	0.00	0.00	0.00	0.06	0.02	0.05
皮肤其他	Other skin	780	0.51	0.00	0.02	0.00	0.00	0.00	0.00	0.06	0.01	0.07
间皮瘤	Mesothelioma	145	0.09	0.00	0.00	0.00	0.00	0.00	0.00	0.00	0.00	0.02
卡波氏肉瘤	Kaposi sarcoma	41	0.03	0.00	0.00	0.00	0.00	0.07	0.01	0.01	0.01	0.00
结缔组织、软组织	Connective & soft tissue	394	0.26	0.09	0.14	0.14	0.06	0.11	0.06	0.09	0.07	0.09
乳腺	Breast	13 055	8.49	0.00	0.00	0.00	0.00	0.04	0.04	0.52	1.69	3.79
外阴	Vulva	284	0.18	0.00	0.00	0.00	0.00	0.00	0.01	0.02	0.02	0.04
阴道	Vagina	138	0.09	0.00	0.00	0.00	0.00	0.00	0.00	0.00	0.01	0.01
子宫颈	Cervix uteri	6 318	4.11	0.00	0.00	0.00	0.00	0.00	0.11	0.41	1.05	2.23
子宫体	Corpus uteri	2 263	1.47	0.00	0.00	0.00	0.00	0.00	0.03	0.12	0.29	0.33
子宫,部位不明	Uterus unspecified	824	0.54	0.00	0.00	0.00	0.00	0.00	0.00	0.01	0.07	0.17
卵巢	Ovary	5 100	3.32	0.00	0.02	0.00	0.00	0.15	0.14	0.38	0.51	0.68
其他女性生殖器	Other female genital organs	273	0.18	0.00	0.00	0.00	0.00	0.00	0.01	0.00	0.01	0.04
胎盘	Placenta	8	0.01	0.00	0.00	0.00	0.00	0.00	0.00	0.02	0.03	0.00
阴茎	Penis	—	—	—	—	—	—	—	—	—	—	—
前列腺	Prostate	—	—	—	—	—	—	—	—	—	—	—
睾丸	Testis	—	—	—	—	—	—	—	—	—	—	—
其他男性生殖器	Other male genital organs	—	—	—	—	—	—	—	—	—	—	—
肾	Kidney	1 299	0.85	0.44	0.16	0.02	0.00	0.02	0.07	0.05	0.17	0.05
肾盂	Renal pelvis	284	0.18	0.00	0.00	0.00	0.00	0.00	0.00	0.00	0.00	0.01
输尿管	Ureter	386	0.25	0.00	0.00	0.00	0.00	0.00	0.00	0.00	0.00	0.00
膀胱	Bladder	1 585	1.03	0.00	0.00	0.00	0.02	0.00	0.00	0.01	0.02	0.02
其他泌尿器官	Other urinary organs	65	0.04	0.00	0.00	0.00	0.00	0.00	0.00	0.00	0.00	0.00
眼	Eye	76	0.05	0.00	0.10	0.02	0.00	0.00	0.01	0.02	0.02	0.01
脑、神经系统	Brain, nervous system	4 263	2.77	0.88	1.00	1.05	0.57	0.46	0.25	0.51	0.84	0.85
甲状腺	Thyroid	1 016	0.66	0.00	0.00	0.00	0.02	0.07	0.24	0.21	0.21	
肾上腺	Adrenal gland	174	0.11	0.09	0.02	0.09	0.00	0.00	0.01	0.02	0.04	
其他内分泌腺	Other endocrine	135	0.09	0.00	0.00	0.00	0.02	0.06	0.00	0.05	0.05	0.03
霍奇金淋巴瘤	Hodgkin lymphoma	121	0.08	0.18	0.00	0.00	0.02	0.04	0.03	0.02	0.03	0.03
非霍奇金淋巴瘤	Non-Hodgkin lymphoma	2 594	1.69	0.09	0.14	0.07	0.14	0.22	0.18	0.17	0.28	0.40
免疫增生性疾病	Immunoproliferative diseases	10	0.01	0.00	0.00	0.00	0.00	0.00	0.00	0.00	0.00	0.00
多发性骨髓瘤	Multiple myeloma	1 093	0.71	0.09	0.02	0.00	0.00	0.04	0.09	0.06	0.03	0.05
淋巴样白血病	Lymphoid leukemia	785	0.51	0.53	0.36	0.44	0.43	0.39	0.17	0.35	0.13	0.21
髓样白血病	Myeloid leukemia	1 796	1.17	0.79	0.24	0.23	0.18	0.31	0.22	0.33	0.37	0.36
白血病,未特指	Leukemia unspecified	1 317	0.86	0.79	0.30	0.26	0.31	0.31	0.32	0.28	0.33	0.36
其他或未指明部位	Other and unspecified	4 275	2.78	0.44	0.26	0.19	0.19	0.28	0.27	0.26	0.41	0.52
所有部位合计	All sites	153 701	100.00	4.73	3.04	2.70	2.59	3.19	3.23	6.34	12.01	18.28
所有部位除外 C44	All sites except C44	152 921	99.49	4.73	3.02	2.70	2.59	3.19	3.23	6.28	12.00	18.20

Appendix Table 1-15　Cancer mortality in urban registration areas of China, female in 2018

Age group										粗率 Crude rate/ 100 000⁻¹	中标率 ASR China/ 100 000⁻¹	世标率 ASR world/ 100 000⁻¹	累积率 Cum. Rate/%		ICD-10
40~44	45~49	50~54	55~59	60~64	65~69	70~74	75~79	80~84	85+				0~64	0~74	
0.00	0.00	0.00	0.03	0.01	0.03	0.23	0.37	0.37	0.67	0.04	0.02	0.02	0.00	0.00	C00
0.14	0.18	0.26	0.43	0.47	0.95	1.11	2.11	3.31	3.76	0.36	0.19	0.18	0.01	0.02	C01-C02
0.04	0.11	0.23	0.31	0.45	1.22	1.56	3.30	4.80	6.72	0.46	0.22	0.21	0.01	0.02	C03-C06
0.05	0.07	0.20	0.14	0.21	0.34	0.81	0.54	0.70	2.00	0.15	0.08	0.08	0.00	0.01	C07-C08
0.00	0.03	0.03	0.04	0.07	0.07	0.13	0.24	0.00	0.55	0.04	0.02	0.02	0.00	0.00	C09
0.01	0.01	0.02	0.04	0.08	0.16	0.23	0.65	0.90	0.91	0.06	0.03	0.03	0.00	0.00	C10
0.64	0.77	1.63	1.62	2.18	2.83	3.65	3.84	4.10	4.54	1.04	0.62	0.60	0.04	0.07	C11
0.00	0.02	0.01	0.03	0.07	0.10	0.25	0.17	0.42	0.48	0.04	0.02	0.02	0.00	0.00	C12-C13
0.01	0.01	0.07	0.06	0.05	0.17	0.53	0.78	1.35	1.03	0.10	0.05	0.05	0.00	0.00	C14
0.24	0.50	1.62	2.20	5.94	12.85	23.98	40.91	58.88	70.01	5.25	2.42	2.39	0.05	0.24	C15
2.69	4.43	7.75	9.18	17.29	28.63	42.02	66.86	101.87	119.56	11.23	5.72	5.60	0.23	0.58	C16
0.12	0.25	0.36	0.74	1.26	2.05	3.02	4.08	6.01	5.75	0.69	0.35	0.35	0.01	0.04	C17
0.99	2.41	4.07	5.90	10.77	17.08	25.82	45.64	78.23	99.99	7.49	3.59	3.56	0.13	0.34	C18
1.43	2.37	4.50	4.95	9.22	14.94	22.37	37.17	60.23	71.53	6.20	3.07	3.03	0.12	0.31	C19-C20
0.05	0.10	0.16	0.19	0.24	0.47	0.53	1.29	1.40	2.54	0.19	0.10	0.10	0.00	0.01	C21
2.91	5.03	10.05	12.67	21.34	33.65	49.93	70.43	93.90	107.81	12.20	6.34	6.28	0.28	0.69	C22
0.34	0.98	2.07	2.80	6.32	9.38	14.03	24.72	35.01	36.64	3.59	1.75	1.74	0.06	0.18	C23-C24
0.80	1.79	3.59	5.78	10.87	17.09	27.61	41.69	53.89	59.42	6.25	3.12	3.09	0.12	0.34	C25
0.02	0.04	0.14	0.06	0.24	0.36	0.35	0.82	0.98	1.57	0.14	0.08	0.08	0.00	0.01	C30-C31
0.01	0.06	0.15	0.18	0.25	0.45	1.06	2.48	3.45	2.73	0.27	0.13	0.12	0.00	0.01	C32
4.59	10.16	19.79	26.49	50.27	77.57	119.54	191.15	277.72	307.61	30.03	14.89	14.75	0.58	1.56	C33-C34
0.16	0.24	0.47	0.50	0.96	0.98	1.41	1.90	2.24	2.85	0.41	0.24	0.23	0.01	0.03	C37-C38
0.19	0.54	0.61	0.90	1.45	2.29	3.70	5.34	6.95	7.03	0.93	0.54	0.53	0.02	0.05	C40-C41
0.09	0.12	0.23	0.39	0.50	0.95	0.88	1.19	1.91	2.60	0.28	0.15	0.15	0.01	0.02	C43
0.13	0.14	0.28	0.25	0.67	0.60	1.91	3.50	6.53	17.62	0.66	0.28	0.29	0.01	0.02	C44
0.02	0.07	0.17	0.13	0.32	0.41	0.43	0.71	0.70	0.48	0.12	0.07	0.07	0.00	0.01	C45
0.00	0.04	0.03	0.05	0.04	0.07	0.03	0.17	0.37	0.12	0.03	0.02	0.02	0.00	0.00	C46
0.09	0.28	0.24	0.36	0.68	0.74	0.91	1.22	1.77	3.09	0.34	0.21	0.22	0.01	0.02	C47, C49
7.14	12.41	17.96	19.71	24.74	24.35	26.68	36.22	47.18	60.93	11.11	6.56	6.39	0.44	0.70	C50
0.07	0.09	0.21	0.20	0.51	0.47	0.73	1.50	1.63	3.15	0.24	0.12	0.12	0.01	0.01	C51
0.01	0.11	0.14	0.14	0.16	0.33	0.58	0.44	0.93	0.85	0.12	0.06	0.06	0.00	0.01	C52
4.04	6.63	11.71	9.83	10.22	12.09	13.08	16.66	18.18	14.17	5.37	3.36	3.22	0.23	0.36	C53
0.58	1.45	2.95	3.49	4.86	5.09	5.84	7.96	9.04	8.30	1.93	1.10	1.09	0.07	0.13	C54
0.27	0.68	1.13	1.11	1.49	1.81	2.29	2.48	3.31	4.12	0.70	0.40	0.39	0.02	0.05	C55
1.93	3.92	6.79	8.28	10.54	11.92	14.13	16.05	16.74	13.93	4.34	2.56	2.53	0.17	0.30	C56
0.06	0.16	0.22	0.55	0.54	0.67	0.93	0.92	1.07	0.97	0.23	0.13	0.13	0.01	0.02	C57
0.01	0.02	0.00	0.00	0.00	0.00	0.00	0.00	0.00	0.00	0.01	0.01	0.01	0.00	—	C58
—	—	—	—	—	—	—	—	—	—	—	—	—	—	—	C60
—	—	—	—	—	—	—	—	—	—	—	—	—	—	—	C61
—	—	—	—	—	—	—	—	—	—	—	—	—	—	—	C62
—	—	—	—	—	—	—	—	—	—	—	—	—	—	—	C63
0.17	0.41	0.64	1.07	1.41	2.66	4.23	6.19	10.91	12.84	1.11	0.56	0.56	0.02	0.06	C64
0.02	0.02	0.06	0.09	0.31	0.64	0.91	1.33	3.36	3.63	0.24	0.11	0.11	0.00	0.01	C65
0.01	0.06	0.05	0.13	0.43	0.62	0.93	2.92	4.29	4.97	0.33	0.14	0.14	0.00	0.01	C66
0.01	0.23	0.36	0.57	1.00	2.28	3.91	9.35	17.30	28.47	1.35	0.56	0.57	0.01	0.04	C67
0.01	0.01	0.01	0.03	0.08	0.21	0.15	0.48	0.42	0.79	0.06	0.03	0.03	0.00	0.00	C68
0.02	0.04	0.03	0.04	0.04	0.09	0.15	0.41	0.56	0.79	0.06	0.04	0.04	0.00	0.00	C69
1.49	2.31	3.81	4.44	6.78	8.81	12.62	16.05	20.89	22.17	3.63	2.22	2.24	0.12	0.23	C70-C72, D32-D33, D42-D43
0.43	0.62	0.79	0.98	1.46	1.83	2.82	4.39	6.15	6.60	0.86	0.49	0.47	0.03	0.05	C73
0.06	0.10	0.08	0.17	0.29	0.33	0.43	0.75	1.17	1.15	0.15	0.08	0.09	0.00	0.01	C74
0.07	0.06	0.10	0.22	0.13	0.34	0.45	0.44	0.51	0.48	0.11	0.08	0.07	0.00	0.01	C75
0.05	0.06	0.09	0.10	0.12	0.22	0.48	0.58	0.61	0.48	0.10	0.07	0.06	0.00	0.01	C81
0.57	0.88	1.66	2.32	3.72	6.19	8.34	13.43	17.62	15.63	2.21	1.21	1.19	0.05	0.13	C82-C86, C96
0.00	0.00	0.00	0.01	0.00	0.03	0.08	0.07	0.05	0.06	0.01	0.00	0.00	0.00	0.00	C88
0.16	0.28	0.68	0.94	2.31	3.40	4.51	5.51	5.50	3.76	0.93	0.51	0.51	0.02	0.06	C90
0.31	0.32	0.59	0.67	1.04	1.67	2.14	2.58	3.36	2.66	0.67	0.49	0.51	0.03	0.05	C91
0.58	0.84	1.10	1.66	2.84	3.97	5.79	8.26	9.14	8.66	1.53	0.93	0.92	0.05	0.10	C92-C94, D45-D47
0.40	0.60	0.98	0.99	2.11	2.71	4.11	5.20	6.06	6.54	1.12	0.73	0.73	0.04	0.07	C95
1.05	1.61	3.09	3.93	5.79	8.73	11.97	18.67	29.32	39.67	3.64	1.93	1.93	0.09	0.19	O&U
35.30	64.64	113.95	138.09	225.16	327.91	476.34	731.71	1 043.06	1 205.45	130.75	68.81	67.93	3.14	7.17	C00-C97, D32-D33, D42-D43, D45-D47
35.17	64.50	113.68	137.83	224.49	327.30	474.42	728.21	1 036.53	1 187.82	130.08	68.53	67.64	3.14	7.14	C00-C97, D32-D33, D42-D43, D45-D47 exc. C44

部位 Site		死亡数 No. deaths	构成 Freq. /%	年龄组								
				0~	1~4	5~9	10~14	15~19	20~24	25~29	30~34	35~39
唇	Lip	199	0.04	0.00	0.00	0.00	0.00	0.00	0.00	0.00	0.00	0.00
舌	Tongue	1 014	0.21	0.03	0.00	0.00	0.00	0.00	0.01	0.03	0.06	0.11
口	Mouth	1 530	0.31	0.00	0.01	0.00	0.01	0.01	0.01	0.01	0.03	0.05
唾液腺	Salivary glands	503	0.10	0.00	0.00	0.00	0.00	0.01	0.01	0.02	0.01	0.06
扁桃腺	Tonsil	188	0.04	0.00	0.00	0.00	0.00	0.00	0.01	0.00	0.00	0.00
其他口咽	Other oropharynx	408	0.08	0.00	0.00	0.00	0.01	0.01	0.00	0.01	0.01	0.05
鼻咽	Nasopharynx	5 373	1.09	0.00	0.01	0.01	0.02	0.06	0.09	0.13	0.33	0.67
下咽	Hypopharynx	605	0.12	0.00	0.00	0.00	0.00	0.01	0.01	0.00	0.01	0.01
咽,部位不明	Pharynx unspecified	567	0.12	0.00	0.00	0.00	0.00	0.01	0.01	0.01	0.02	0.01
食管	Esophagus	47 833	9.72	0.31	0.00	0.00	0.00	0.00	0.03	0.07	0.14	0.22
胃	Stomach	60 667	12.33	0.20	0.00	0.01	0.01	0.07	0.22	0.60	1.13	1.64
小肠	Small intestine	1 638	0.33	0.00	0.01	0.01	0.01	0.00	0.00	0.02	0.04	0.05
结肠	Colon	14 283	2.90	0.03	0.00	0.01	0.02	0.10	0.12	0.30	0.47	0.71
直肠	Rectum	20 760	4.22	0.00	0.01	0.01	0.01	0.05	0.10	0.26	0.51	0.83
肛门	Anus	726	0.15	0.00	0.00	0.00	0.00	0.00	0.01	0.01	0.01	0.07
肝脏	Liver	72 329	14.69	0.51	0.13	0.08	0.14	0.31	0.52	1.40	3.70	6.79
胆囊及其他	Gallbladder etc.	7 998	1.62	0.00	0.00	0.01	0.00	0.00	0.01	0.00	0.06	0.13
胰腺	Pancreas	16 290	3.31	0.00	0.01	0.01	0.00	0.02	0.01	0.10	0.27	0.39
鼻、鼻窦及其他	Nose, sinuses etc.	635	0.13	0.00	0.02	0.02	0.00	0.02	0.00	0.02	0.03	0.06
喉	Larynx	2 841	0.58	0.00	0.01	0.01	0.00	0.00	0.01	0.00	0.02	0.05
气管、支气管、肺	Trachea, bronchus & lung	136 219	27.67	0.00	0.04	0.03	0.08	0.08	0.31	0.72	1.61	3.07
其他胸部器官	Other thoracic organs	1 179	0.24	0.07	0.02	0.03	0.03	0.09	0.08	0.09	0.09	0.12
骨	Bone	3 897	0.79	0.03	0.02	0.10	0.24	0.43	0.33	0.25	0.25	0.31
皮肤黑色素瘤	Melanoma of skin	760	0.15	0.00	0.00	0.00	0.01	0.00	0.02	0.04	0.05	0.07
皮肤其他	Other skin	2 516	0.51	0.03	0.00	0.01	0.02	0.02	0.03	0.02	0.05	0.09
间皮瘤	Mesothelioma	208	0.04	0.00	0.00	0.00	0.00	0.00	0.01	0.00	0.00	0.03
卡波氏肉瘤	Kaposi sarcoma	57	0.01	0.00	0.00	0.00	0.01	0.00	0.01	0.01	0.02	0.00
结缔组织、软组织	Connective & soft tissue	802	0.16	0.03	0.07	0.10	0.04	0.07	0.07	0.05	0.09	0.11
乳腺	Breast	11 828	2.46	0.00	0.00	0.00	0.01	0.03	0.11	0.54	2.04	3.64
外阴	Vulva	250	0.05	0.00	0.00	0.00	0.00	0.00	0.00	0.01	0.01	0.03
阴道	Vagina	129	0.03	0.00	0.00	0.01	0.01	0.00	0.00	0.01	0.02	0.02
子宫颈	Cervix uteri	8 419	1.71	0.00	0.02	0.00	0.00	0.00	0.12	0.52	1.21	1.84
子宫体	Corpus uteri	2 497	0.51	0.00	0.00	0.00	0.00	0.01	0.01	0.06	0.19	0.26
子宫,部位不明	Uterus unspecified	1 212	0.25	0.00	0.00	0.00	0.00	0.00	0.00	0.12	0.10	0.21
卵巢	Ovary	4 304	0.87	0.00	0.00	0.00	0.01	0.18	0.17	0.30	0.46	0.65
其他女性生殖器	Other female genital organs	230	0.05	0.00	0.00	0.00	0.00	0.00	0.01	0.00	0.06	0.02
胎盘	Placenta	18	0.00	0.00	0.00	0.00	0.00	0.00	0.01	0.02	0.04	0.02
阴茎	Penis	394	0.08	0.00	0.00	0.00	0.00	0.00	0.00	0.01	0.03	0.08
前列腺	Prostate	5 990	1.22	0.00	0.01	0.00	0.01	0.01	0.01	0.01	0.05	0.03
睾丸	Testis	169	0.03	0.00	0.03	0.01	0.01	0.05	0.03	0.06	0.07	0.09
其他男性生殖器	Other male genital organs	81	0.02	0.00	0.00	0.00	0.00	0.01	0.00	0.01	0.01	0.01
肾	Kidney	3 089	0.63	0.14	0.14	0.07	0.02	0.02	0.03	0.09	0.13	0.17
肾盂	Renal pelvis	466	0.09	0.00	0.01	0.00	0.01	0.00	0.01	0.01	0.01	0.00
输尿管	Ureter	504	0.10	0.00	0.00	0.00	0.00	0.00	0.00	0.00	0.00	0.00
膀胱	Bladder	6 395	1.30	0.00	0.01	0.00	0.00	0.01	0.01	0.03	0.01	0.06
其他泌尿器官	Other urinary organs	120	0.02	0.00	0.00	0.00	0.00	0.00	0.00	0.00	0.00	0.00
眼	Eye	184	0.04	0.00	0.12	0.03	0.01	0.01	0.01	0.00	0.01	0.01
脑、神经系统	Brain, nervous system	12 541	2.55	1.33	0.99	1.04	0.76	0.68	0.68	1.03	1.14	1.50
甲状腺	Thyroid	1 589	0.32	0.00	0.00	0.00	0.01	0.01	0.06	0.07	0.11	0.19
肾上腺	Adrenal gland	481	0.10	0.10	0.06	0.06	0.01	0.00	0.01	0.01	0.05	0.05
其他内分泌腺	Other endocrine	322	0.07	0.00	0.01	0.02	0.05	0.02	0.01	0.01	0.02	0.03
霍奇金淋巴瘤	Hodgkin lymphoma	464	0.09	0.00	0.00	0.01	0.01	0.03	0.05	0.03	0.05	0.08
非霍奇金淋巴瘤	Non-Hodgkin lymphoma	6 760	1.37	0.00	0.15	0.13	0.20	0.24	0.23	0.30	0.54	0.45
免疫增生性疾病	Immunoproliferative diseases	47	0.01	0.00	0.01	0.00	0.00	0.00	0.00	0.00	0.00	0.00
多发性骨髓瘤	Multiple myeloma	2 314	0.47	0.00	0.01	0.03	0.04	0.03	0.02	0.05	0.04	0.08
淋巴样白血病	Lymphoid leukemia	1 968	0.40	0.54	0.29	0.34	0.45	0.43	0.25	0.37	0.33	0.24
髓样白血病	Myeloid leukemia	3 855	0.78	0.17	0.35	0.22	0.28	0.25	0.27	0.41	0.48	0.54
白血病,未特指	Leukemia unspecified	4 818	0.98	1.22	0.61	0.58	0.61	0.68	0.46	0.63	0.67	0.67
其他或未指明部位	Other and unspecified	8 469	1.72	0.31	0.26	0.26	0.27	0.26	0.28	0.36	0.49	0.59
所有部位合计	All sites	492 226	100.00	5.06	3.43	3.26	3.44	4.18	4.59	8.42	15.25	23.78
所有部位除外 C44	All sites except C44	489 710	99.49	5.03	3.43	3.24	3.42	4.15	4.56	8.40	15.19	23.69

Age group										粗率 Crude rate/ 100 000⁻¹	中标率 ASR China/ 100 000⁻¹	世标率 ASR world/ 100 000⁻¹	累积率 Cum. Rate/%		ICD-10
40~44	45~49	50~54	55~59	60~64	65~69	70~74	75~79	80~84	85+				0~64	0~74	
0.01	0.01	0.04	0.06	0.13	0.20	0.30	0.50	0.74	1.27	0.07	0.04	0.04	0.00	0.00	C00
0.17	0.22	0.49	0.62	0.92	1.12	1.36	1.54	1.62	2.48	0.35	0.22	0.22	0.01	0.03	C01-C02
0.14	0.26	0.61	0.46	1.11	1.68	2.64	3.34	4.36	5.45	0.53	0.31	0.31	0.01	0.04	C03-C06
0.06	0.08	0.18	0.27	0.45	0.56	0.82	0.75	1.17	1.45	0.18	0.11	0.11	0.01	0.01	C07-C08
0.02	0.07	0.08	0.09	0.22	0.18	0.26	0.31	0.38	0.32	0.07	0.04	0.04	0.00	0.01	C09
0.02	0.04	0.20	0.16	0.32	0.59	0.66	0.90	0.81	0.78	0.14	0.09	0.09	0.00	0.01	C10
1.19	2.13	3.32	3.26	4.76	6.08	6.03	7.17	5.53	6.05	1.87	1.24	1.21	0.08	0.14	C11
0.03	0.13	0.29	0.40	0.69	0.84	0.97	0.81	0.88	0.85	0.21	0.13	0.13	0.01	0.02	C12-C13
0.04	0.08	0.19	0.21	0.47	0.58	1.10	1.38	1.43	1.56	0.20	0.12	0.12	0.01	0.01	C14
1.05	2.98	9.46	15.32	37.14	63.74	94.70	126.92	150.79	154.43	16.66	9.44	9.45	0.33	1.12	C15
3.15	7.26	15.09	20.87	45.73	76.40	112.62	149.73	186.97	179.33	21.13	12.29	12.16	0.48	1.42	C16
0.17	0.37	0.54	0.65	1.47	1.93	2.47	3.35	4.19	4.67	0.57	0.34	0.34	0.02	0.04	C17
1.17	2.10	3.82	4.83	9.57	14.90	21.53	33.34	48.47	62.80	4.97	2.88	2.85	0.12	0.30	C18
1.68	3.19	5.71	6.94	14.27	23.30	33.72	50.11	67.53	77.66	7.23	4.20	4.14	0.17	0.45	C19-C20
0.08	0.12	0.22	0.24	0.51	0.83	1.15	1.71	1.95	2.62	0.25	0.15	0.15	0.01	0.02	C21
13.17	23.01	37.42	39.29	62.92	80.04	95.41	110.36	127.99	130.51	25.19	15.99	15.69	0.94	1.82	C22
0.41	0.92	1.98	2.93	6.24	10.09	14.00	19.47	24.88	26.68	2.79	1.59	1.59	0.06	0.18	C23-C24
1.00	2.27	4.71	6.99	13.31	21.38	28.59	35.55	45.28	44.93	5.67	3.32	3.31	0.15	0.40	C25
0.09	0.15	0.34	0.35	0.43	0.57	1.00	1.02	1.22	1.66	0.22	0.14	0.14	0.01	0.02	C30-C31
0.08	0.31	0.90	1.41	2.37	3.71	5.20	6.24	8.24	6.44	0.99	0.58	0.58	0.03	0.07	C32
7.17	16.87	39.40	53.72	114.91	176.52	247.69	315.02	374.67	366.31	47.44	27.71	27.65	1.19	3.31	C33-C34
0.19	0.26	0.51	0.55	1.10	1.22	1.63	1.77	2.05	2.37	0.41	0.27	0.27	0.02	0.03	C37-C38
0.49	0.77	1.36	1.49	2.79	4.56	5.92	7.70	8.22	8.21	1.36	0.90	0.88	0.04	0.10	C40-C41
0.11	0.15	0.23	0.36	0.59	0.71	1.02	1.54	1.74	3.15	0.26	0.16	0.16	0.01	0.02	C43
0.14	0.26	0.45	0.58	0.96	1.76	2.84	5.14	10.63	26.29	0.88	0.45	0.47	0.01	0.04	C44
0.02	0.07	0.08	0.11	0.24	0.30	0.24	0.37	0.17	0.25	0.07	0.05	0.05	0.00	0.01	C45
0.01	0.02	0.01	0.02	0.05	0.03	0.05	0.08	0.14	0.21	0.02	0.01	0.01	0.00	0.00	C46
0.11	0.20	0.38	0.27	0.50	0.81	0.91	1.18	1.91	2.12	0.28	0.19	0.19	0.01	0.02	C47,C49
6.46	11.39	16.54	15.27	20.28	21.10	20.27	22.31	28.42	33.42	8.44	5.48	5.29	0.38	0.59	C50
0.07	0.10	0.17	0.26	0.28	0.38	0.94	1.16	1.25	1.45	0.18	0.10	0.10	0.00	0.01	C51
0.03	0.06	0.15	0.10	0.23	0.28	0.33	0.48	0.52	0.41	0.09	0.06	0.06	0.00	0.01	C52
4.32	7.34	12.21	10.28	12.33	16.62	18.39	19.99	22.45	18.71	6.01	3.86	3.72	0.25	0.43	C53
0.76	1.38	3.32	3.33	4.58	5.54	6.57	6.46	7.35	6.84	1.78	1.08	1.08	0.07	0.13	C54
0.49	0.76	1.41	1.25	1.70	2.55	3.12	4.08	3.85	4.98	0.86	0.53	0.51	0.03	0.06	C55
1.37	3.27	5.93	5.56	8.37	9.88	10.46	9.37	8.69	7.41	3.07	1.96	1.93	0.13	0.23	C56
0.06	0.11	0.29	0.26	0.36	0.61	0.68	0.59	0.56	0.70	0.16	0.10	0.10	0.01	0.01	C57
0.05	0.02	0.00	0.00	0.00	0.00	0.02	0.00	0.00	0.00	0.01	0.01	0.01	0.00	0.00	C58
0.11	0.19	0.29	0.11	0.50	0.76	1.15	1.66	3.29	4.00	0.27	0.17	0.16	0.01	0.02	C60
0.08	0.19	0.44	0.98	3.86	8.84	19.93	40.13	75.24	122.61	4.07	2.27	2.30	0.03	0.17	C61
0.05	0.10	0.06	0.08	0.18	0.30	0.33	0.55	0.90	1.55	0.11	0.09	0.08	0.00	0.01	C62
0.03	0.02	0.00	0.03	0.08	0.20	0.29	0.42	0.48	1.00	0.06	0.04	0.04	0.00	0.01	C63
0.26	0.55	0.97	1.33	2.39	3.63	5.22	5.95	7.91	9.06	1.08	0.65	0.66	0.03	0.08	C64
0.03	0.09	0.14	0.21	0.28	0.57	0.64	1.02	1.60	1.63	0.16	0.09	0.09	0.00	0.01	C65
0.02	0.02	0.09	0.16	0.32	0.66	1.07	1.34	1.69	1.77	0.18	0.10	0.10	0.00	0.01	C66
0.17	0.33	0.72	1.26	2.94	5.49	10.40	17.95	31.53	43.66	2.23	1.17	1.17	0.03	0.11	C67
0.00	0.00	0.02	0.03	0.09	0.11	0.16	0.33	0.64	0.53	0.04	0.02	0.02	0.00	0.00	C68
0.02	0.02	0.05	0.04	0.06	0.15	0.21	0.34	0.74	0.96	0.06	0.04	0.05	0.00	0.00	C69
2.34	3.35	5.30	5.74	9.51	13.06	16.13	18.52	22.30	22.43	4.37	3.00	3.00	0.17	0.32	C70-C72,D32-D33, D42-D43
0.22	0.44	0.64	0.87	1.20	1.79	1.95	2.79	3.29	4.07	0.55	0.35	0.34	0.02	0.04	C73
0.04	0.09	0.20	0.22	0.32	0.52	0.64	0.95	1.10	1.20	0.17	0.11	0.11	0.01	0.01	C74
0.06	0.04	0.12	0.13	0.20	0.36	0.38	0.65	0.71	1.10	0.11	0.07	0.07	0.00	0.01	C75
0.09	0.05	0.17	0.21	0.28	0.54	0.78	0.88	0.88	0.85	0.16	0.11	0.10	0.00	0.01	C81
0.81	1.32	2.40	2.73	5.63	7.81	10.80	13.30	15.06	13.59	2.35	1.51	1.48	0.08	0.17	C82-C86,C96
0.00	0.00	0.00	0.00	0.03	0.07	0.09	0.14	0.21	0.11	0.02	0.01	0.01	0.00	0.00	C88
0.17	0.34	0.79	1.16	2.08	3.47	4.10	4.83	4.62	2.79	0.81	0.50	0.49	0.02	0.06	C90
0.34	0.48	0.63	0.76	1.30	1.68	2.07	2.61	2.95	2.90	0.69	0.54	0.55	0.03	0.05	C91
0.62	0.91	1.54	1.60	2.74	4.04	5.14	6.66	6.91	6.16	1.34	0.94	0.92	0.05	0.10	C92-C94,D45-D47
0.80	1.04	1.67	1.83	3.17	4.71	6.41	7.53	8.70	6.65	1.68	1.24	1.25	0.07	0.12	C95
0.93	1.76	2.79	3.36	6.11	9.66	12.91	16.39	20.28	25.65	2.95	1.85	1.84	0.09	0.20	O&U
45.72	87.53	166.44	202.81	389.14	586.70	805.72	1 044.08	1 291.89	1 362.08	171.44	103.14	102.27	4.79	11.75	C00-C97,D32-D33, D42-D43,D45-D47
45.58	87.28	165.98	202.23	388.18	584.94	802.88	1 038.94	1 281.26	1 335.79	170.56	102.68	101.79	4.78	11.72	C00-C97,D32-D33, D42-D43,D45-D47 exc. C44

部位 Site		死亡数 No. deaths	构成 Freq. /%	年龄组								
				0~	1~4	5~9	10~14	15~19	20~24	25~29	30~34	35~39
唇	Lip	124	0.04	0.00	0.00	0.00	0.00	0.00	0.00	0.00	0.00	0.01
舌	Tongue	706	0.22	0.00	0.00	0.00	0.00	0.00	0.00	0.00	0.06	0.15
口	Mouth	1 026	0.32	0.00	0.00	0.00	0.00	0.00	0.00	0.03	0.05	0.09
唾液腺	Salivary glands	322	0.10	0.00	0.00	0.00	0.00	0.00	0.00	0.04	0.01	0.08
扁桃腺	Tonsil	145	0.05	0.00	0.00	0.00	0.00	0.00	0.00	0.00	0.01	0.00
其他口咽	Other oropharynx	331	0.10	0.00	0.00	0.01	0.01	0.00	0.01	0.01	0.02	0.08
鼻咽	Nasopharynx	3 990	1.26	0.00	0.01	0.01	0.02	0.09	0.10	0.18	0.44	1.05
下咽	Hypopharynx	552	0.17	0.00	0.00	0.00	0.00	0.01	0.01	0.00	0.00	0.02
咽,部位不明	Pharynx unspecified	435	0.14	0.00	0.00	0.00	0.00	0.00	0.00	0.02	0.02	0.02
食管	Esophagus	34 755	10.93	0.00	0.00	0.00	0.00	0.00	0.05	0.06	0.21	0.28
胃	Stomach	42 649	13.42	0.00	0.00	0.01	0.02	0.07	0.24	0.47	1.05	1.64
小肠	Small intestine	1 018	0.32	0.00	0.00	0.00	0.00	0.00	0.00	0.04	0.05	0.07
结肠	Colon	7 906	2.49	0.00	0.00	0.01	0.02	0.10	0.14	0.37	0.51	0.82
直肠	Rectum	12 788	4.02	0.00	0.01	0.01	0.01	0.07	0.11	0.31	0.68	0.95
肛门	Anus	420	0.13	0.00	0.00	0.00	0.00	0.00	0.02	0.03	0.01	0.08
肝脏	Liver	53 449	16.81	0.19	0.10	0.06	0.19	0.36	0.67	2.07	5.99	11.38
胆囊及其他	Gallbladder etc.	3 682	1.16	0.00	0.00	0.01	0.00	0.00	0.01	0.01	0.09	0.19
胰腺	Pancreas	9 592	3.02	0.00	0.01	0.00	0.00	0.01	0.01	0.11	0.26	0.47
鼻、鼻窦及其他	Nose, sinuses etc.	416	0.13	0.00	0.01	0.00	0.00	0.02	0.03	0.03	0.03	0.08
喉	Larynx	2 499	0.79	0.00	0.01	0.00	0.00	0.00	0.01	0.00	0.01	0.07
气管、支气管、肺	Trachea, bronchus & lung	95 858	30.15	0.00	0.07	0.03	0.08	0.13	0.36	0.97	2.06	3.79
其他胸腔器官	Other thoracic organs	752	0.24	0.00	0.04	0.04	0.04	0.15	0.12	0.13	0.12	0.11
骨	Bone	2 377	0.75	0.00	0.03	0.11	0.25	0.53	0.44	0.33	0.36	0.37
皮肤黑色素瘤	Melanoma of skin	425	0.13	0.00	0.00	0.01	0.00	0.00	0.00	0.04	0.06	0.09
皮肤其他	Other skin	1 332	0.42	0.00	0.00	0.01	0.04	0.02	0.03	0.02	0.06	0.09
间皮瘤	Mesothelioma	124	0.04	0.00	0.00	0.00	0.00	0.00	0.00	0.00	0.01	0.04
卡波氏肉瘤	Kaposi sarcoma	37	0.01	0.00	0.00	0.00	0.00	0.00	0.00	0.02	0.04	0.00
结缔组织、软组织	Connective & soft tissue	489	0.15	0.00	0.11	0.13	0.05	0.07	0.11	0.05	0.10	0.16
乳腺	Breast	294	0.09	0.00	0.00	0.00	0.01	0.00	0.00	0.03	0.02	0.04
外阴	Vulva	—	—	—	—	—	—	—	—	—	—	—
阴道	Vagina	—	—	—	—	—	—	—	—	—	—	—
子宫颈	Cervix uteri	—	—	—	—	—	—	—	—	—	—	—
子宫体	Corpus uteri	—	—	—	—	—	—	—	—	—	—	—
子宫,部位不明	Uterus unspecified	—	—	—	—	—	—	—	—	—	—	—
卵巢	Ovary	—	—	—	—	—	—	—	—	—	—	—
其他女性生殖器	Other female genital organs	—	—	—	—	—	—	—	—	—	—	—
胎盘	Placenta	—	—	—	—	—	—	—	—	—	—	—
阴茎	Penis	394	0.12	0.00	0.00	0.00	0.00	0.00	0.00	0.01	0.03	0.08
前列腺	Prostate	5 990	1.88	0.00	0.01	0.00	0.01	0.01	0.01	0.01	0.05	0.03
睾丸	Testis	169	0.05	0.00	0.03	0.01	0.00	0.05	0.03	0.06	0.07	0.09
其他男性生殖器	Other male genital organs	81	0.03	0.00	0.00	0.00	0.00	0.01	0.01	0.01	0.01	0.01
肾	Kidney	2 023	0.64	0.13	0.15	0.06	0.02	0.05	0.03	0.11	0.18	0.24
肾盂	Renal pelvis	310	0.10	0.00	0.00	0.00	0.00	0.00	0.00	0.02	0.01	0.00
输尿管	Ureter	290	0.09	0.00	0.00	0.00	0.00	0.00	0.00	0.00	0.00	0.00
膀胱	Bladder	5 066	1.59	0.00	0.01	0.00	0.00	0.00	0.01	0.04	0.01	0.09
其他泌尿器官	Other urinary organs	74	0.02	0.00	0.00	0.00	0.00	0.00	0.00	0.00	0.01	0.00
眼	Eye	96	0.03	0.00	0.13	0.03	0.00	0.00	0.02	0.00	0.01	0.00
脑、神经系统	Brain, nervous system	6 904	2.17	1.41	1.04	1.16	0.89	0.74	0.74	1.29	1.40	1.75
甲状腺	Thyroid	560	0.18	0.00	0.00	0.00	0.01	0.01	0.04	0.08	0.03	0.08
肾上腺	Adrenal gland	302	0.09	0.06	0.04	0.08	0.01	0.00	0.01	0.01	0.04	0.06
其他内分泌腺	Other endocrine	186	0.06	0.00	0.03	0.03	0.07	0.03	0.02	0.02	0.04	0.01
霍奇金淋巴瘤	Hodgkin lymphoma	295	0.09	0.00	0.00	0.01	0.01	0.06	0.07	0.05	0.05	0.09
非霍奇金淋巴瘤	Non-Hodgkin lymphoma	4 127	1.30	0.00	0.17	0.17	0.21	0.34	0.29	0.41	0.63	0.51
免疫增生性疾病	Immunoproliferative diseases	34	0.01	0.00	0.03	0.00	0.00	0.00	0.00	0.00	0.00	0.00
多发性骨髓瘤	Multiple myeloma	1 326	0.42	0.00	0.01	0.06	0.05	0.05	0.02	0.08	0.06	0.08
淋巴样白血病	Lymphoid leukemia	1 155	0.36	0.64	0.33	0.37	0.49	0.57	0.30	0.44	0.41	0.23
髓样白血病	Myeloid leukemia	2 240	0.70	0.32	0.35	0.19	0.33	0.22	0.28	0.49	0.49	0.65
白血病,未特指	Leukemia unspecified	2 829	0.89	1.09	0.60	0.66	0.73	0.80	0.65	0.82	0.78	0.81
其他或未指明部位	Other and unspecified	4 955	1.56	0.26	0.28	0.34	0.32	0.25	0.40	0.44	0.59	0.53
所有部位合计	All sites	317 899	100.00	4.09	3.64	3.65	3.97	4.82	5.39	9.74	17.20	27.55
所有部位除外 C44	All sites except C44	316 567	99.58	4.09	3.64	3.64	3.94	4.79	5.36	9.72	17.14	27.46

Appendix Table 1-17 Cancer mortality in rural registration areas of China, male in 2018

Age group										粗率 Crude rate/ 100 000⁻¹	中标率 ASR China/ 100 000⁻¹	世标率 ASR world/ 100 000⁻¹	累积率 Cum. Rate/%		ICD-10
40~44	45~49	50~54	55~59	60~64	65~69	70~74	75~79	80~84	85+				0~64	0~74	
0.01	0.02	0.04	0.10	0.20	0.29	0.35	0.65	0.96	1.45	0.08	0.05	0.05	0.00	0.01	C00
0.23	0.33	0.76	0.92	1.36	1.72	1.79	2.11	2.07	3.45	0.48	0.31	0.31	0.02	0.04	C01-C02
0.19	0.36	0.87	0.64	1.62	2.39	3.59	4.29	6.16	7.45	0.70	0.44	0.43	0.02	0.05	C03-C06
0.06	0.13	0.21	0.40	0.61	0.73	1.13	1.17	1.27	1.36	0.22	0.14	0.14	0.01	0.02	C07-C08
0.03	0.11	0.15	0.18	0.39	0.23	0.47	0.45	0.42	0.27	0.10	0.06	0.06	0.00	0.01	C09
0.03	0.06	0.31	0.29	0.59	0.99	1.04	1.40	1.38	1.27	0.23	0.15	0.14	0.01	0.02	C10
1.64	3.29	5.16	5.08	7.19	9.11	8.95	10.03	7.43	8.82	2.71	1.85	1.80	0.12	0.21	C11
0.05	0.26	0.53	0.74	1.29	1.54	1.73	1.43	1.70	1.82	0.38	0.24	0.24	0.01	0.03	C12-C13
0.08	0.15	0.32	0.34	0.75	0.94	1.73	2.14	2.07	2.36	0.30	0.19	0.18	0.01	0.02	C14
1.61	4.88	15.67	25.63	60.52	98.82	139.93	181.25	209.71	220.77	23.64	14.31	14.39	0.54	1.74	C15
3.60	9.42	21.10	30.35	68.85	115.24	168.19	220.56	269.14	254.21	29.01	17.79	17.68	0.68	2.10	C16
0.22	0.46	0.68	0.93	1.93	2.42	3.06	4.45	4.83	6.36	0.69	0.44	0.44	0.02	0.05	C17
1.25	2.26	4.24	5.26	11.31	17.46	24.92	39.44	57.79	72.71	5.38	3.32	3.29	0.13	0.34	C18
1.93	3.82	6.64	8.73	18.60	30.87	42.46	66.84	86.60	103.34	8.70	5.36	5.30	0.21	0.58	C19-C20
0.10	0.11	0.26	0.36	0.72	0.99	1.26	2.08	2.12	3.00	0.29	0.18	0.18	0.01	0.02	C21
22.39	38.39	60.77	63.08	95.57	116.09	131.87	149.46	171.08	175.96	36.36	24.23	23.71	1.51	2.74	C22
0.45	0.80	1.64	2.72	6.48	10.04	12.65	18.89	22.23	26.81	2.50	1.53	1.53	0.06	0.18	C23-C24
1.25	3.01	6.29	8.88	16.78	25.36	34.64	41.78	51.84	52.44	6.53	4.04	4.04	0.19	0.49	C25
0.10	0.22	0.40	0.50	0.66	0.75	1.35	1.36	1.96	2.09	0.28	0.19	0.18	0.01	0.02	C30-C31
0.12	0.58	1.56	2.62	4.35	6.83	9.37	10.81	15.60	11.82	1.70	1.04	1.04	0.05	0.13	C32
8.65	22.20	54.72	79.23	170.07	261.66	360.67	462.51	545.71	527.24	65.21	40.11	40.10	1.71	4.82	C33-C34
0.22	0.33	0.54	0.67	1.58	1.72	2.04	2.05	3.02	3.18	0.51	0.35	0.35	0.02	0.04	C37-C38
0.57	1.06	1.72	1.86	3.32	5.65	7.40	10.00	9.87	9.45	1.62	1.12	1.09	0.05	0.12	C40-C41
0.10	0.14	0.32	0.41	0.75	0.78	1.04	1.72	2.28	3.82	0.29	0.19	0.18	0.01	0.02	C43
0.20	0.26	0.59	0.73	1.23	2.38	3.43	6.27	12.10	25.63	0.91	0.53	0.55	0.02	0.05	C44
0.03	0.10	0.09	0.13	0.31	0.35	0.20	0.45	0.27	0.36	0.08	0.06	0.05	0.00	0.01	C45
0.02	0.01	0.01	0.03	0.08	0.03	0.07	0.13	0.21	0.36	0.03	0.02	0.02	0.00	0.00	C46
0.12	0.24	0.45	0.28	0.55	1.10	1.09	1.75	2.60	2.36	0.33	0.24	0.24	0.01	0.02	C47,C49
0.08	0.14	0.20	0.39	0.50	0.61	0.78	1.14	1.43	1.91	0.20	0.13	0.13	0.01	0.01	C50
—	—	—	—	—	—	—	—	—	—	—	—	—	—	—	C51
—	—	—	—	—	—	—	—	—	—	—	—	—	—	—	C52
—	—	—	—	—	—	—	—	—	—	—	—	—	—	—	C53
—	—	—	—	—	—	—	—	—	—	—	—	—	—	—	C54
—	—	—	—	—	—	—	—	—	—	—	—	—	—	—	C55
—	—	—	—	—	—	—	—	—	—	—	—	—	—	—	C56
—	—	—	—	—	—	—	—	—	—	—	—	—	—	—	C57
—	—	—	—	—	—	—	—	—	—	—	—	—	—	—	C58
0.11	0.19	0.29	0.11	0.50	0.76	1.15	1.66	3.29	4.00	0.27	0.17	0.16	0.01	0.02	C60
0.08	0.19	0.44	0.98	3.86	8.84	19.93	40.13	75.24	122.61	4.07	2.27	2.30	0.03	0.17	C61
0.05	0.10	0.06	0.08	0.18	0.30	0.33	0.55	0.90	1.55	0.11	0.09	0.08	0.00	0.01	C62
0.03	0.02	0.00	0.03	0.08	0.20	0.29	0.42	0.48	1.00	0.06	0.04	0.04	0.00	0.00	C63
0.29	0.69	1.38	1.79	3.19	5.23	7.15	7.76	10.56	12.09	1.38	0.88	0.88	0.04	0.10	C64
0.06	0.13	0.21	0.25	0.42	0.79	0.91	1.27	2.44	2.18	0.21	0.13	0.13	0.01	0.01	C65
0.03	0.05	0.12	0.20	0.41	0.76	1.22	1.53	2.28	1.91	0.20	0.12	0.12	0.00	0.01	C66
0.16	0.52	1.14	2.07	4.98	8.85	16.68	30.13	53.91	86.89	3.45	1.97	2.00	0.05	0.17	C67
0.01	0.00	0.03	0.07	0.08	0.14	0.22	0.45	0.64	1.00	0.05	0.03	0.03	0.00	0.00	C68
0.02	0.03	0.05	0.03	0.04	0.18	0.27	0.45	0.90	0.82	0.07	0.04	0.05	0.00	0.00	C69
2.62	3.76	5.73	6.45	10.71	14.98	17.47	20.35	24.46	23.45	4.70	3.37	3.35	0.19	0.35	C70-C72,D32-D33,D42-D43
0.19	0.22	0.35	0.63	0.94	1.36	1.59	1.88	2.65	3.64	0.38	0.25	0.25	0.01	0.03	C73
0.05	0.12	0.22	0.31	0.47	0.62	0.82	1.40	1.27	1.91	0.21	0.14	0.14	0.01	0.01	C74
0.05	0.02	0.15	0.14	0.16	0.46	0.55	0.81	1.01	1.18	0.13	0.09	0.09	0.00	0.01	C75
0.11	0.07	0.20	0.28	0.38	0.67	0.95	1.10	1.33	1.18	0.20	0.14	0.14	0.01	0.02	C81
1.02	1.68	3.00	3.49	7.02	9.81	13.16	16.52	18.36	18.09	2.81	1.87	1.84	0.09	0.21	C82-C86,C96
0.00	0.01	0.01	0.00	0.02	0.09	0.13	0.23	0.37	0.18	0.02	0.01	0.01	0.00	0.00	C88
0.18	0.36	0.89	1.33	2.45	3.67	4.65	5.65	6.37	4.64	0.90	0.58	0.57	0.03	0.07	C90
0.37	0.50	0.69	0.95	1.39	2.01	2.72	3.18	3.50	4.09	0.79	0.64	0.64	0.04	0.06	C91
0.69	1.05	1.75	1.83	3.13	4.42	6.40	8.08	9.18	9.73	1.52	1.09	1.07	0.06	0.11	C92-C94,D45-D47
0.98	1.18	1.96	2.06	3.70	5.03	7.44	9.90	11.04	9.09	1.92	1.47	1.46	0.08	0.14	C95
1.08	1.89	3.19	4.20	7.63	11.85	15.77	19.80	24.25	31.81	3.37	2.22	2.21	0.11	0.24	O&U
53.51	105.94	208.07	268.75	529.89	798.11	1 086.97	1 419.88	1 748.30	1 875.12	216.26	136.18	135.41	6.21	15.64	C00-C97,D32-D33,D42-D43,D45-D47
53.31	105.68	207.47	268.02	528.66	795.73	1 083.54	1 413.61	1 736.20	1 849.49	215.36	135.65	134.87	6.19	15.59	C00-C97,D32-D33,D42-D43,D45-D47 exc. C44

部位 Site		死亡数 No. deaths	构成 Freq./%	年龄组								
				0~	1~4	5~9	10~14	15~19	20~24	25~29	30~34	35~39
唇	Lip	75	0.04	0.00	0.00	0.00	0.00	0.00	0.00	0.00	0.01	0.00
舌	Tongue	308	0.18	0.07	0.00	0.00	0.00	0.00	0.02	0.06	0.06	0.07
口	Mouth	504	0.29	0.00	0.02	0.00	0.01	0.03	0.01	0.00	0.02	0.01
唾液腺	Salivary glands	181	0.10	0.00	0.00	0.00	0.00	0.01	0.01	0.00	0.02	0.03
扁桃腺	Tonsil	43	0.02	0.00	0.00	0.00	0.00	0.00	0.01	0.00	0.01	0.00
其他口咽	Other oropharynx	77	0.04	0.00	0.00	0.00	0.00	0.00	0.00	0.00	0.00	0.02
鼻咽	Nasopharynx	1 383	0.79	0.00	0.02	0.00	0.01	0.03	0.07	0.07	0.20	0.28
下咽	Hypopharynx	53	0.03	0.00	0.00	0.00	0.00	0.00	0.00	0.01	0.00	0.01
咽,部位不明	Pharynx unspecified	132	0.08	0.00	0.00	0.00	0.00	0.03	0.01	0.00	0.02	0.00
食管	Esophagus	13 078	7.50	0.65	0.00	0.00	0.00	0.00	0.00	0.07	0.06	0.15
胃	Stomach	18 018	10.34	0.44	0.00	0.01	0.00	0.06	0.20	0.73	1.22	1.65
小肠	Small intestine	620	0.36	0.00	0.02	0.01	0.00	0.00	0.01	0.01	0.04	0.04
结肠	Colon	6 377	3.66	0.07	0.00	0.00	0.01	0.09	0.09	0.23	0.42	0.60
直肠	Rectum	7 972	4.57	0.00	0.00	0.01	0.01	0.03	0.09	0.21	0.35	0.71
肛门	Anus	306	0.18	0.00	0.00	0.00	0.00	0.00	0.00	0.00	0.02	0.07
肝脏	Liver	18 880	10.83	0.87	0.16	0.11	0.08	0.25	0.36	0.67	1.28	1.95
胆囊及其他	Gallbladder etc.	4 316	2.48	0.00	0.00	0.00	0.00	0.00	0.00	0.00	0.04	0.06
胰腺	Pancreas	6 698	3.84	0.00	0.00	0.01	0.00	0.00	0.02	0.09	0.27	0.32
鼻,鼻窦及其他	Nose,sinuses etc.	219	0.13	0.00	0.03	0.04	0.00	0.03	0.00	0.02	0.04	0.04
喉	Larynx	342	0.20	0.00	0.00	0.00	0.00	0.00	0.00	0.00	0.04	0.03
气管、支气管、肺	Trachea,bronchus & lung	40 361	23.15	0.00	0.00	0.03	0.07	0.03	0.26	0.46	1.15	2.31
其他胸腔器官	Other thoracic organs	427	0.24	0.15	0.00	0.00	0.01	0.03	0.04	0.06	0.06	0.12
骨	Bone	1 520	0.87	0.07	0.02	0.09	0.23	0.32	0.22	0.16	0.13	0.25
皮肤黑色素瘤	Melanoma of skin	335	0.19	0.00	0.00	0.00	0.00	0.00	0.01	0.04	0.05	0.04
皮肤其他	Other skin	1 184	0.68	0.07	0.00	0.01	0.00	0.03	0.03	0.03	0.05	0.09
间皮瘤	Mesothelioma	84	0.05	0.00	0.00	0.00	0.00	0.00	0.01	0.01	0.00	0.03
卡波氏肉瘤	Kaposi sarcoma	20	0.01	0.00	0.00	0.00	0.03	0.00	0.01	0.00	0.00	0.01
结缔组织、软组织	Connective & soft tissue	313	0.18	0.07	0.02	0.05	0.04	0.06	0.02	0.05	0.08	0.06
乳腺	Breast	11 828	6.78	0.00	0.00	0.00	0.01	0.03	0.11	0.54	2.04	3.64
外阴	Vulva	250	0.14	0.00	0.00	0.00	0.00	0.00	0.00	0.01	0.01	0.03
阴道	Vagina	129	0.07	0.00	0.00	0.01	0.01	0.00	0.00	0.01	0.02	0.02
子宫颈	Cervix uteri	8 419	4.83	0.00	0.02	0.00	0.00	0.00	0.12	0.52	1.21	1.84
子宫体	Corpus uteri	2 497	1.43	0.00	0.00	0.00	0.00	0.01	0.01	0.06	0.19	0.26
子宫,部位不明	Uterus unspecified	1 212	0.70	0.00	0.00	0.00	0.00	0.00	0.00	0.12	0.10	0.21
卵巢	Ovary	4 304	2.47	0.00	0.00	0.00	0.01	0.18	0.17	0.30	0.46	0.65
其他女性生殖器	Other female genital organs	230	0.13	0.00	0.00	0.00	0.01	0.00	0.00	0.00	0.06	0.02
胎盘	Placenta	18	0.01	0.00	0.00	0.00	0.00	0.01	0.01	0.02	0.04	0.02
阴茎	Penis	—	—	—	—	—	—	—	—	—	—	—
前列腺	Prostate	—	—	—	—	—	—	—	—	—	—	—
睾丸	Testis	—	—	—	—	—	—	—	—	—	—	—
其他男性生殖器	Other male genital organs	—	—	—	—	—	—	—	—	—	—	—
肾	Kidney	1 066	0.61	0.15	0.13	0.08	0.01	0.00	0.02	0.07	0.07	0.10
肾盂	Renal pelvis	156	0.09	0.00	0.02	0.00	0.01	0.00	0.01	0.01	0.01	0.01
输尿管	Ureter	214	0.12	0.00	0.00	0.00	0.00	0.00	0.00	0.00	0.00	0.00
膀胱	Bladder	1 329	0.76	0.00	0.02	0.00	0.00	0.01	0.01	0.03	0.02	0.03
其他泌尿器官	Other urinary organs	46	0.03	0.00	0.00	0.00	0.00	0.00	0.00	0.00	0.00	0.00
眼	Eye	88	0.05	0.00	0.11	0.03	0.01	0.01	0.00	0.00	0.01	0.02
脑、神经系统	Brain,nervous system	5 637	3.23	1.23	0.93	0.92	0.62	0.61	0.63	0.74	0.87	1.22
甲状腺	Thyroid	1 029	0.59	0.00	0.00	0.00	0.01	0.00	0.07	0.06	0.20	0.32
肾上腺	Adrenal gland	179	0.10	0.15	0.08	0.04	0.01	0.00	0.00	0.01	0.06	0.04
其他内分泌腺	Other endocrine	136	0.08	0.00	0.00	0.01	0.03	0.00	0.00	0.00	0.00	0.06
霍奇金淋巴瘤	Hodgkin lymphoma	169	0.10	0.00	0.00	0.01	0.00	0.00	0.03	0.01	0.06	0.07
非霍奇金淋巴瘤	Non-Hodgkin lymphoma	2 633	1.51	0.00	0.13	0.09	0.19	0.14	0.16	0.18	0.46	0.39
免疫增生性疾病	Immunoproliferative diseases	13	0.01	0.00	0.00	0.00	0.00	0.00	0.00	0.00	0.00	0.00
多发性骨髓瘤	Multiple myeloma	988	0.57	0.00	0.02	0.00	0.00	0.03	0.01	0.02	0.02	0.08
淋巴样白血病	Lymphoid leukemia	813	0.47	0.44	0.24	0.31	0.40	0.29	0.20	0.30	0.23	0.25
髓样白血病	Myeloid leukemia	1 615	0.93	0.00	0.35	0.25	0.22	0.29	0.25	0.33	0.46	0.43
白血病,未特指	Leukemia unspecified	1 989	1.14	1.38	0.63	0.48	0.47	0.54	0.27	0.43	0.55	0.52
其他或未指明部位	Other and unspecified	3 514	2.02	0.36	0.24	0.18	0.21	0.27	0.16	0.27	0.38	0.65
所有部位合计	All sites	174 327	100.00	6.17	3.19	2.81	2.82	3.46	3.75	7.02	13.19	19.81
所有部位除外 C44	All sites except C44	173 143	99.32	6.10	3.19	2.80	2.82	3.44	3.72	6.99	13.14	19.72

Appendix Table 1-18　Cancer mortality in rural registration areas of China, female in 2018

Age group										粗率 Crude rate/ 100 000⁻¹	中标率 ASR China/ 100 000⁻¹	世标率 ASR world/ 100 000⁻¹	累积率 Cum. Rate/%		ICD-10
40~44	45~49	50~54	55~59	60~64	65~69	70~74	75~79	80~84	85+				0~64	0~74	
0.01	0.00	0.04	0.02	0.05	0.11	0.24	0.36	0.56	1.16	0.05	0.03	0.03	0.00	0.00	C00
0.11	0.12	0.21	0.32	0.47	0.51	0.94	1.01	1.25	1.85	0.22	0.13	0.13	0.01	0.01	C01-C02
0.08	0.14	0.33	0.27	0.58	0.97	1.70	2.47	2.90	4.17	0.36	0.20	0.19	0.01	0.02	C03-C06
0.06	0.03	0.15	0.14	0.28	0.38	0.52	0.36	1.08	1.51	0.13	0.07	0.07	0.00	0.01	C07-C08
0.00	0.03	0.01	0.01	0.04	0.14	0.07	0.18	0.35	0.35	0.03	0.02	0.02	0.00	0.00	C09
0.01	0.02	0.09	0.02	0.05	0.18	0.28	0.45	0.35	0.46	0.05	0.03	0.03	0.00	0.00	C10
0.73	0.95	1.41	1.39	2.26	3.04	3.15	4.55	3.98	4.29	0.99	0.62	0.60	0.04	0.07	C11
0.00	0.00	0.04	0.06	0.07	0.14	0.22	0.24	0.22	0.23	0.04	0.02	0.02	0.00	0.00	C12-C13
0.01	0.02	0.06	0.07	0.17	0.21	0.48	0.68	0.91	1.04	0.09	0.05	0.05	0.00	0.01	C14
0.46	1.03	3.03	4.78	13.07	28.45	50.09	77.14	102.77	112.15	9.33	4.74	4.69	0.11	0.51	C15
2.68	5.05	8.86	11.19	21.93	37.31	57.82	84.82	119.98	131.61	12.86	7.01	6.88	0.27	0.74	C16
0.12	0.28	0.39	0.36	1.00	1.44	1.90	2.35	3.68	3.59	0.44	0.25	0.25	0.01	0.03	C17
1.08	1.94	3.38	4.38	7.78	12.33	18.20	27.76	40.87	56.48	4.55	2.46	2.43	0.10	0.25	C18
1.42	2.54	4.74	5.10	9.82	15.69	25.10	34.78	51.99	61.29	5.69	3.09	3.05	0.13	0.33	C19-C20
0.06	0.14	0.17	0.11	0.31	0.66	1.05	1.37	1.82	2.38	0.22	0.12	0.12	0.00	0.01	C21
3.53	7.23	13.24	14.98	29.32	43.75	59.46	74.52	92.86	101.55	13.47	7.72	7.65	0.37	0.88	C22
0.37	1.05	2.34	3.15	5.98	10.14	15.33	19.99	27.03	26.59	3.08	1.66	1.65	0.06	0.19	C23-C24
0.73	1.51	3.06	5.05	9.74	17.39	22.63	29.84	39.92	40.14	4.78	2.61	2.60	0.10	0.30	C25
0.09	0.09	0.27	0.20	0.20	0.40	0.66	0.71	0.61	1.39	0.16	0.10	0.10	0.01	0.01	C30-C31
0.03	0.03	0.23	0.17	0.33	0.58	1.09	2.05	2.25	3.01	0.24	0.13	0.13	0.00	0.01	C32
5.63	11.40	23.54	27.64	58.16	90.84	136.26	179.86	235.25	263.74	28.81	15.75	15.65	0.65	1.79	C33-C34
0.16	0.18	0.48	0.42	0.61	0.71	1.22	1.52	1.25	1.85	0.30	0.19	0.19	0.01	0.02	C37-C38
0.41	0.46	0.98	1.11	2.25	3.47	4.46	5.59	6.88	7.41	1.08	0.68	0.67	0.03	0.07	C40-C41
0.11	0.16	0.14	0.32	0.42	0.64	1.00	1.37	1.30	2.72	0.24	0.14	0.14	0.01	0.01	C43
0.08	0.25	0.31	0.43	0.68	1.13	2.25	4.11	9.43	26.70	0.85	0.38	0.40	0.01	0.03	C44
0.01	0.05	0.08	0.08	0.16	0.25	0.28	0.30	0.09	0.17	0.06	0.04	0.04	0.00	0.00	C45
0.00	0.02	0.02	0.00	0.02	0.03	0.04	0.03	0.09	0.12	0.01	0.01	0.01	0.00	0.00	C46
0.10	0.16	0.31	0.26	0.44	0.52	0.74	0.65	1.34	1.97	0.22	0.15	0.14	0.01	0.01	C47, C49
6.46	11.39	16.54	15.27	20.28	21.10	20.27	22.31	28.42	33.42	8.44	5.48	5.29	0.38	0.59	C50
0.07	0.10	0.17	0.26	0.28	0.38	0.94	1.16	1.25	1.45	0.18	0.10	0.10	0.00	0.01	C51
0.03	0.06	0.15	0.10	0.23	0.28	0.33	0.48	0.52	0.41	0.09	0.06	0.06	0.00	0.01	C52
4.32	7.34	12.21	10.28	12.33	16.62	18.39	19.99	22.45	18.71	6.01	3.86	3.72	0.25	0.43	C53
0.76	1.38	3.32	3.33	4.58	5.54	6.57	6.46	7.36	6.84	1.78	1.08	1.08	0.07	0.13	C54
0.49	0.76	1.41	1.25	1.70	2.55	3.12	4.08	3.85	4.98	0.86	0.53	0.51	0.03	0.06	C55
1.37	3.27	5.93	5.56	8.37	9.88	10.46	9.37	8.69	7.41	3.07	1.96	1.93	0.13	0.23	C56
0.06	0.11	0.29	0.26	0.36	0.61	0.68	0.59	0.56	0.70	0.16	0.10	0.10	0.01	0.01	C57
0.05	0.02	0.00	0.00	0.00	0.02	0.00	0.02	0.00	0.00	0.01	0.01	0.01	0.00	0.00	C58
—	—	—	—	—	—	—	—	—	—	—	—	—	—	—	C60
—	—	—	—	—	—	—	—	—	—	—	—	—	—	—	C61
—	—	—	—	—	—	—	—	—	—	—	—	—	—	—	C62
—	—	—	—	—	—	—	—	—	—	—	—	—	—	—	C63
0.23	0.40	0.56	0.87	1.57	2.02	3.32	4.28	5.75	7.13	0.76	0.43	0.44	0.02	0.05	C64
0.00	0.05	0.08	0.17	0.15	0.34	0.37	0.80	0.91	1.27	0.11	0.06	0.06	0.00	0.01	C65
0.02	0.00	0.07	0.12	0.23	0.57	0.92	1.16	1.21	1.68	0.15	0.08	0.08	0.00	0.01	C66
0.18	0.14	0.29	0.43	0.84	2.10	4.22	6.78	13.28	16.10	0.95	0.46	0.46	0.01	0.04	C67
0.00	0.01	0.01	0.00	0.10	0.08	0.11	0.21	0.65	0.23	0.03	0.02	0.02	0.00	0.00	C68
0.03	0.00	0.06	0.05	0.09	0.11	0.15	0.24	0.61	1.04	0.06	0.04	0.04	0.00	0.01	C69
2.05	2.94	4.86	5.01	8.28	11.13	14.81	16.84	20.55	21.78	4.02	2.63	2.64	0.15	0.28	C70-C72, D32-D33, D42-D43
0.24	0.65	0.95	1.11	1.46	2.22	2.29	3.63	3.81	4.34	0.73	0.46	0.44	0.03	0.05	C73
0.04	0.06	0.19	0.12	0.17	0.41	0.46	0.54	0.95	0.75	0.13	0.08	0.09	0.00	0.01	C74
0.06	0.06	0.09	0.11	0.25	0.26	0.22	0.51	0.48	1.04	0.10	0.06	0.06	0.00	0.01	C75
0.06	0.03	0.13	0.14	0.17	0.40	0.61	0.68	0.52	0.64	0.12	0.08	0.07	0.00	0.01	C81
0.58	0.96	1.79	1.94	4.20	5.80	8.48	10.35	12.37	10.72	1.88	1.15	1.12	0.06	0.13	C82-C86, C96
0.00	0.00	0.00	0.00	0.04	0.05	0.04	0.06	0.09	0.06	0.01	0.00	0.01	0.00	0.00	C88
0.15	0.32	0.68	0.98	1.71	3.27	3.56	4.08	3.20	1.62	0.71	0.42	0.42	0.02	0.05	C90
0.30	0.46	0.58	0.56	1.22	1.35	1.42	2.08	2.51	2.14	0.58	0.45	0.45	0.03	0.04	C91
0.53	0.76	1.33	1.37	2.35	3.66	3.89	5.35	5.06	3.88	1.15	0.80	0.78	0.04	0.08	C92-C94, D45-D47
0.61	0.91	1.37	1.60	2.62	4.39	5.40	5.35	6.79	5.10	1.42	1.02	1.03	0.06	0.10	C95
0.78	1.63	2.39	2.50	4.55	7.45	10.09	13.27	17.04	21.72	2.51	1.50	1.49	0.07	0.16	O&U
37.57	68.65	123.34	135.41	244.30	373.94	528.32	699.70	919.86	1 035.10	124.42	71.30	70.43	3.33	7.84	C00-C97, D32-D33, D42-D43, D45-D47
37.49	68.40	123.03	134.98	243.62	372.81	526.07	695.60	910.43	1 008.39	123.57	70.92	70.03	3.32	7.81	C00-C97, D32-D33, D42-D43, D45-D47 exc. C44

附录2 2018年全国东中西部肿瘤登记地区癌症发病与死亡结果

附表 2-1 2018 年全国东部肿瘤登记地区癌症发病主要指标

Appendix Table 2-1 Cancer incidence in Eastern registration areas of China,2018

部位 Site		男性 Male						女性 Female						ICD-10
		病例数 No. cases	构成 Freq. /%	粗率 Crude rate/ $100\,000^{-1}$	世标率 ASR world/ $100\,000^{-1}$	累积率 Cum. Rate/%		病例数 No. cases	构成 Freq. /%	粗率 Crude rate/ $100\,000^{-1}$	世标率 ASR world/ $100\,000^{-1}$	累积率 Cum. Rate/%		
						0~64	0~74					0~64	0~74	
唇	Lip	284	0.07	0.26	0.15	0.01	0.02	221	0.06	0.20	0.10	0.00	0.01	C00
舌	Tongue	1 305	0.32	1.20	0.72	0.05	0.09	809	0.23	0.75	0.42	0.03	0.05	C01-C02
口	Mouth	1 526	0.37	1.40	0.81	0.05	0.10	958	0.27	0.89	0.46	0.02	0.05	C03-C06
唾液腺	Salivary glands	911	0.22	0.84	0.53	0.04	0.06	693	0.19	0.64	0.43	0.03	0.04	C07-C08
扁桃腺	Tonsil	315	0.08	0.29	0.18	0.01	0.02	112	0.03	0.10	0.06	0.00	0.01	C09
其他口咽	Other oropharynx	462	0.11	0.42	0.24	0.02	0.03	63	0.02	0.06	0.03	0.00	0.00	C10
鼻咽	Nasopharynx	5 537	1.35	5.08	3.33	0.26	0.36	2 122	0.59	1.96	1.26	0.10	0.13	C11
下咽	Hypopharynx	1 344	0.33	1.23	0.71	0.05	0.09	83	0.02	0.08	0.04	0.00	0.00	C12-C13
咽,部位不明	Pharynx unspecified	356	0.09	0.33	0.19	0.01	0.02	75	0.02	0.07	0.03	0.00	0.00	C14
食管	Esophagus	28 777	7.03	26.39	14.29	0.69	1.80	10 442	2.92	9.66	4.33	0.12	0.51	C15
胃	Stomach	47 463	11.60	43.52	23.81	1.13	2.97	20 862	5.83	19.30	9.71	0.49	1.12	C16
小肠	Small intestine	1 869	0.46	1.71	0.98	0.05	0.12	1 318	0.37	1.22	0.64	0.04	0.08	C17
结肠	Colon	25 465	6.23	23.35	12.95	0.67	1.54	19 602	5.48	18.13	9.11	0.48	1.05	C18
直肠	Rectum	22 913	5.60	21.01	11.77	0.65	1.45	14 215	3.97	13.15	6.78	0.37	0.81	C19-C20
肛门	Anus	366	0.09	0.34	0.19	0.01	0.02	302	0.08	0.28	0.14	0.01	0.02	C21
肝脏	Liver	40 969	10.02	37.57	22.08	1.48	2.56	14 811	4.14	13.70	6.85	0.34	0.79	C22
胆囊及其他	Gallbladder etc.	5 678	1.39	5.21	2.79	0.12	0.33	5 508	1.54	5.10	2.39	0.10	0.28	C23-C24
胰腺	Pancreas	11 514	2.81	10.56	5.73	0.28	0.68	8 912	2.49	8.24	3.89	0.16	0.45	C25
鼻、鼻窦及其他	Nose,sinuses etc.	611	0.15	0.56	0.34	0.02	0.04	357	0.10	0.33	0.20	0.01	0.02	C30-C31
喉	Larynx	4 374	1.07	4.01	2.26	0.14	0.29	344	0.10	0.32	0.16	0.01	0.02	C32
气管、支气管、肺	Trachea,bronchus & lung	101 041	24.70	92.65	50.68	2.45	6.31	62 488	17.45	57.81	30.15	1.75	3.57	C33-C34
其他胸腔器官	Other thoracic organs	1 543	0.38	1.41	0.92	0.06	0.10	1 011	0.28	0.94	0.60	0.04	0.06	C37-C38
骨	Bone	1 868	0.46	1.71	1.21	0.07	0.12	1 425	0.40	1.32	0.86	0.05	0.08	C40-C41
皮肤黑色素瘤	Melanoma of skin	778	0.19	0.71	0.42	0.02	0.05	782	0.22	0.72	0.40	0.02	0.04	C43
皮肤其他	Other skin	3 853	0.94	3.53	1.94	0.09	0.21	4 013	1.12	3.71	1.76	0.08	0.18	C44
间皮瘤	Mesothelioma	253	0.06	0.23	0.13	0.01	0.02	220	0.06	0.20	0.12	0.01	0.01	C45
卡波氏肉瘤	Kaposi sarcoma	52	0.01	0.05	0.03	0.00	0.00	21	0.01	0.02	0.01	0.00	0.00	C46
结缔组织、软组织	Connective & soft tissue	1 327	0.32	1.22	0.86	0.05	0.08	1 155	0.32	1.07	0.74	0.05	0.07	C47,C49
乳腺	Breast	600	0.15	0.55	0.32	0.02	0.04	60 022	16.76	55.53	34.62	2.80	3.77	C50
外阴	Vulva	—	—	—	—	—	—	595	0.17	0.55	0.29	0.02	0.03	C51
阴道	Vagina	—	—	—	—	—	—	335	0.09	0.31	0.18	0.01	0.02	C52
子宫颈	Cervix uteri	—	—	—	—	—	—	17 253	4.82	15.96	10.15	0.85	1.07	C53
子宫体	Corpus uteri	—	—	—	—	—	—	11 742	3.28	10.86	6.59	0.56	0.75	C54
子宫,部位不明	Uterus unspecified	—	—	—	—	—	—	1 758	0.49	1.63	0.96	0.08	0.10	C55
卵巢	Ovary	—	—	—	—	—	—	9 360	2.61	8.66	5.43	0.41	0.59	C56
其他女性生殖器	Other female genital organs	—	—	—	—	—	—	768	0.21	0.71	0.42	0.03	0.05	C57
胎盘	Placenta	—	—	—	—	—	—	78	0.02	0.07	0.06	0.00	0.00	C58
阴茎	Penis	916	0.22	0.84	0.47	0.03	0.06	—	—	—	—	—	—	C60
前列腺	Prostate	20 336	4.97	18.65	9.42	0.22	1.09	—	—	—	—	—	—	C61
睾丸	Testis	609	0.15	0.56	0.47	0.03	0.04	—	—	—	—	—	—	C62
其他男性生殖器	Other male genital organs	306	0.07	0.28	0.16	0.01	0.02	—	—	—	—	—	—	C63
肾	Kidney	8 422	2.06	7.72	4.69	0.32	0.56	4 418	1.23	4.09	2.37	0.15	0.28	C64
肾盂	Renal pelvis	892	0.22	0.82	0.45	0.02	0.05	669	0.19	0.62	0.29	0.01	0.03	C65
输尿管	Ureter	987	0.24	0.91	0.48	0.02	0.06	767	0.21	0.71	0.33	0.01	0.04	C66
膀胱	Bladder	12 756	3.12	11.70	6.26	0.28	0.71	3 377	0.94	3.12	1.48	0.06	0.17	C67
其他泌尿器官	Other urinary organs	220	0.05	0.20	0.11	0.00	0.01	132	0.04	0.12	0.06	0.00	0.01	C68
眼	Eye	187	0.05	0.17	0.17	0.01	0.01	146	0.04	0.14	0.14	0.01	0.01	C69
脑、神经系统	Brain,nervous system	8 801	2.15	8.07	5.51	0.35	0.56	10 865	3.03	10.05	6.26	0.41	0.67	C70-C72,D32-D33,D42-D43
甲状腺	Thyroid	14 316	3.50	13.13	9.89	0.80	0.91	41 135	11.49	38.06	27.59	2.32	2.60	C73
肾上腺	Adrenal gland	385	0.09	0.35	0.26	0.01	0.02	305	0.09	0.28	0.21	0.01	0.02	C74
其他内分泌腺	Other endocrine	591	0.14	0.54	0.40	0.03	0.04	640	0.18	0.59	0.42	0.03	0.04	C75
霍奇金淋巴瘤	Hodgkin lymphoma	411	0.10	0.38	0.29	0.02	0.03	270	0.08	0.25	0.20	0.01	0.02	C81
非霍奇金淋巴瘤	Non-Hodgkin lymphoma	7 531	1.84	6.91	4.31	0.25	0.48	5 802	1.62	5.37	3.09	0.18	0.35	C82-C86,C96
免疫增生性疾病	Immunoproliferative diseases	145	0.04	0.13	0.07	0.00	0.01	68	0.02	0.06	0.03	0.00	0.00	C88
多发性骨髓瘤	Multiple myeloma	2 460	0.60	2.26	1.26	0.06	0.16	2 035	0.57	1.88	1.01	0.06	0.13	C90
淋巴样白血病	Lymphoid leukemia	1 984	0.49	1.82	1.77	0.09	0.14	1 475	0.41	1.36	1.42	0.08	0.10	C91
髓样白血病	Myeloid leukemia	5 680	1.39	5.21	3.47	0.20	0.36	4 246	1.19	3.93	2.59	0.16	0.26	C92-C94,D45-D47
白血病,未特指	Leukemia unspecified	1 855	0.45	1.70	1.21	0.06	0.11	1 371	0.38	1.27	0.87	0.05	0.08	C95
其他或未指明部位	Other and unspecified	5 928	1.45	5.44	3.19	0.17	0.34	5 465	1.53	5.06	2.77	0.16	0.28	O&U
所有部位合计	All sites	409 072	100.00	375.12	214.86	11.49	25.27	358 021	100.00	331.22	191.52	12.79	20.94	C00-C97,D32-D33,D42-D43,D45-D47
所有部位除外 C44	All sites except C44	405 219	99.06	371.58	212.92	11.40	25.07	354 008	98.88	327.51	189.76	12.71	20.76	C00-C97,D32-D33,D42-D43,D45-D47 exc. C44

Appendix 2 Cancer incidence and mortality in Eastern, Central and Western registration areas of China, 2018

附表 2-2 2018 年全国东部城市肿瘤登记地区癌症发病主要指标

Appendix Table 2-2 Cancer incidence in Eastern urban registration areas of China, 2018

部位 Site		男性 Male						女性 Female						ICD-10
		病例数 No. cases	构成 Freq. /%	粗率 Crude rate/ $100\,000^{-1}$	世标率 ASR world/ $100\,000^{-1}$	累积率 Cum. Rate/%		病例数 No. cases	构成 Freq. /%	粗率 Crude rate/ $100\,000^{-1}$	世标率 ASR world/ $100\,000^{-1}$	累积率 Cum. Rate/%		
						0~64	0~74					0~64	0~74	
唇	Lip	110	0.05	0.20	0.11	0.01	0.01	102	0.05	0.18	0.09	0.00	0.01	C00
舌	Tongue	807	0.37	1.44	0.85	0.06	0.10	492	0.25	0.87	0.47	0.03	0.05	C01-C02
口	Mouth	880	0.40	1.57	0.88	0.06	0.10	577	0.29	1.02	0.51	0.02	0.06	C03-C06
唾液腺	Salivary glands	489	0.22	0.87	0.55	0.04	0.06	395	0.20	0.70	0.48	0.03	0.05	C07-C08
扁桃腺	Tonsil	206	0.09	0.37	0.22	0.02	0.03	73	0.04	0.13	0.07	0.01	0.01	C09
其他口咽	Other oropharynx	296	0.14	0.53	0.30	0.02	0.04	39	0.02	0.07	0.03	0.00	0.00	C11
鼻咽	Nasopharynx	3 277	1.50	5.84	3.82	0.30	0.42	1 272	0.63	2.25	1.45	0.11	0.15	C11
下咽	Hypopharynx	807	0.37	1.44	0.82	0.06	0.10	43	0.02	0.08	0.04	0.00	0.01	C12-C13
咽,部位不明	Pharynx unspecified	213	0.10	0.38	0.21	0.01	0.03	40	0.02	0.07	0.04	0.00	0.00	C14
食管	Esophagus	11 839	5.42	21.11	11.24	0.60	1.42	3 607	1.80	6.37	2.78	0.08	0.31	C15
胃	Stomach	22 769	10.43	40.59	21.59	1.04	2.67	10 521	5.25	18.58	9.26	0.48	1.06	C16
小肠	Small intestine	1 116	0.51	1.99	1.10	0.06	0.13	780	0.39	1.38	0.70	0.04	0.08	C17
结肠	Colon	15 769	7.22	28.11	15.09	0.77	1.80	12 229	6.10	21.60	10.58	0.55	1.21	C18
直肠	Rectum	12 987	5.95	23.15	12.66	0.71	1.56	8 047	4.02	14.21	7.19	0.40	0.85	C19-C20
肛门	Anus	198	0.09	0.35	0.19	0.01	0.02	109	0.05	0.19	0.10	0.01	0.02	C21
肝脏	Liver	20 742	9.50	36.98	21.24	1.44	2.46	7 420	3.70	13.10	6.35	0.31	0.72	C22
胆囊及其他	Gallbladder etc.	2 979	1.36	5.31	2.73	0.12	0.32	2 824	1.41	4.99	2.27	0.10	0.25	C23-C24
胰腺	Pancreas	6 127	2.81	10.92	5.74	0.28	0.68	4 878	2.43	8.61	3.97	0.17	0.45	C25
鼻、鼻窦及其他	Nose, sinuses etc.	345	0.16	0.62	0.37	0.02	0.04	199	0.10	0.35	0.21	0.01	0.02	C30-C31
喉	Larynx	2 512	1.15	4.48	2.47	0.16	0.32	192	0.10	0.34	0.16	0.01	0.02	C32
气管、支气管、肺	Trachea, bronchus & lung	52 608	24.09	93.79	49.95	2.49	6.19	34 588	17.26	61.08	31.41	1.87	3.67	C33-C34
其他胸腔器官	Other thoracic organs	897	0.41	1.60	1.02	0.07	0.11	584	0.29	1.03	0.65	0.04	0.07	C37-C38
骨	Bone	881	0.40	1.57	1.12	0.06	0.10	651	0.32	1.15	0.77	0.04	0.07	C40-C41
皮肤黑色素瘤	Melanoma of skin	431	0.20	0.77	0.44	0.02	0.05	435	0.22	0.77	0.42	0.02	0.05	C43
皮肤其他	Other skin	2 186	1.00	3.90	2.08	0.10	0.22	2 115	1.06	3.74	1.75	0.08	0.18	C44
间皮瘤	Mesothelioma	165	0.08	0.29	0.16	0.01	0.01	123	0.06	0.22	0.12	0.01	0.01	C45
卡波氏肉瘤	Kaposi sarcoma	35	0.02	0.06	0.04	0.00	0.00	13	0.01	0.02	0.02	0.00	0.00	C46
结缔组织、软组织	Connective & soft tissue	785	0.36	1.40	0.95	0.06	0.09	679	0.34	1.20	0.81	0.05	0.08	C47, C49
乳腺	Breast	325	0.15	0.58	0.32	0.02	0.04	36 280	18.11	64.07	39.28	3.15	4.30	C50
外阴	Vulva	—	—	—	—	—	—	336	0.17	0.59	0.30	0.01	0.03	C51
阴道	Vagina	—	—	—	—	—	—	183	0.09	0.32	0.19	0.01	0.02	C52
子宫颈	Cervix uteri	—	—	—	—	—	—	8 870	4.43	15.66	9.93	0.84	1.04	C53
子宫体	Corpus uteri	—	—	—	—	—	—	6 868	3.43	12.13	7.34	0.62	0.84	C54
子宫,部位不明	Uterus unspecified	—	—	—	—	—	—	898	0.45	1.59	0.93	0.07	0.10	C55
卵巢	Ovary	—	—	—	—	—	—	5 329	2.66	9.41	5.89	0.44	0.63	C56
其他女性生殖器	Other female genital organs	—	—	—	—	—	—	457	0.23	0.81	0.48	0.04	0.06	C57
胎盘	Placenta	—	—	—	—	—	—	44	0.02	0.08	0.06	0.00	0.01	C58
阴茎	Penis	440	0.20	0.78	0.43	0.02	0.05	—	—	—	—	—	—	C60
前列腺	Prostate	12 243	5.61	21.83	10.62	0.25	1.23	—	—	—	—	—	—	C61
睾丸	Testis	383	0.18	0.68	0.57	0.04	0.05	—	—	—	—	—	—	C62
其他男性生殖器	Other male genital organs	183	0.08	0.33	0.17	0.01	0.02	—	—	—	—	—	—	C63
肾	Kidney	5 202	2.38	9.27	5.53	0.37	0.65	2 570	1.28	4.54	2.55	0.16	0.30	C64
肾盂	Renal pelvis	553	0.25	0.99	0.53	0.03	0.06	447	0.22	0.79	0.36	0.01	0.04	C65
输尿管	Ureter	587	0.27	1.05	0.54	0.02	0.07	483	0.24	0.85	0.38	0.01	0.04	C66
膀胱	Bladder	7 214	3.30	12.86	6.66	0.29	0.75	2 011	1.00	3.55	1.63	0.07	0.18	C67
其他泌尿器官	Other urinary organs	125	0.06	0.22	0.11	0.00	0.01	80	0.04	0.14	0.06	0.00	0.01	C68
眼	Eye	80	0.04	0.14	0.14	0.01	0.01	76	0.04	0.13	0.14	0.01	0.01	C69
脑、神经系统	Brain, nervous system	4 567	2.09	8.14	5.48	0.35	0.56	5 826	2.91	10.29	6.27	0.42	0.67	C70-C72, D32-D33, D42-D43
甲状腺	Thyroid	9 001	4.12	16.05	12.05	0.98	1.09	24 538	12.25	43.33	31.35	2.62	2.92	C73
肾上腺	Adrenal gland	167	0.08	0.30	0.23	0.01	0.02	163	0.08	0.29	0.22	0.01	0.02	C74
其他内分泌腺	Other endocrine	254	0.12	0.45	0.35	0.02	0.03	233	0.12	0.41	0.29	0.02	0.03	C75
霍奇金淋巴瘤	Hodgkin lymphoma	212	0.10	0.38	0.30	0.02	0.03	146	0.07	0.26	0.22	0.01	0.02	C81
非霍奇金淋巴瘤	Non-Hodgkin lymphoma	4 285	1.96	7.64	4.67	0.27	0.50	3 357	1.68	5.93	3.34	0.20	0.37	C82-C86, C96
免疫增生性疾病	Immunoproliferative diseases	76	0.03	0.14	0.07	0.00	0.01	36	0.02	0.06	0.03	0.00	0.00	C88
多发性骨髓瘤	Multiple myeloma	1 417	0.65	2.53	1.37	0.07	0.17	1 141	0.57	2.02	1.07	0.06	0.14	C90
淋巴样白血病	Lymphoid leukemia	1 079	0.49	1.92	1.85	0.10	0.14	803	0.40	1.42	1.53	0.08	0.11	C91
髓样白血病	Myeloid leukemia	3 300	1.51	5.88	3.80	0.21	0.39	2 273	1.13	4.01	2.56	0.16	0.26	C92-C94, D45-D47
白血病,未特指	Leukemia unspecified	826	0.38	1.47	1.02	0.05	0.09	619	0.31	1.09	0.73	0.04	0.06	C95
其他或未指明部位	Other and unspecified	3 405	1.56	6.07	3.44	0.18	0.36	3 220	1.61	5.69	3.03	0.17	0.30	O&U
所有部位合计	All sites	218 380	100.00	389.33	218.19	11.96	25.42	200 374	100.00	353.86	202.94	13.75	21.98	C00-C97, D32-D33, D42-D43, D45-D47
所有部位除外 C44	All sites except C44	216 194	99.00	385.44	216.11	11.86	25.20	198 259	98.94	350.13	201.19	13.67	21.79	C00-C97, D32-D33, D42-D43, D45-D47 exc. C44

部位 Site		男性 Male						女性 Female						ICD-10
		病例数 No. cases	构成 Freq./%	粗率 Crude rate/ $100\,000^{-1}$	世标率 ASR world/ $100\,000^{-1}$	累积率 Cum. Rate/%		病例数 No. cases	构成 Freq./%	粗率 Crude rate/ $100\,000^{-1}$	世标率 ASR world/ $100\,000^{-1}$	累积率 Cum. Rate/%		
						0~64	0~74					0~64	0~74	
唇	Lip	174	0.09	0.33	0.19	0.01	0.02	119	0.08	0.23	0.11	0.01	0.01	C00
舌	Tongue	498	0.26	0.94	0.58	0.04	0.07	317	0.20	0.62	0.36	0.02	0.04	C01-C02
口	Mouth	646	0.34	1.22	0.73	0.04	0.09	381	0.24	0.74	0.40	0.02	0.05	C03-C06
唾液腺	Salivary glands	422	0.22	0.80	0.51	0.03	0.06	298	0.19	0.58	0.37	0.03	0.05	C07-C08
扁桃腺	Tonsil	109	0.06	0.21	0.13	0.01	0.01	39	0.02	0.08	0.05	0.00	0.01	C09
其他口咽	Other oropharynx	166	0.09	0.31	0.18	0.01	0.02	24	0.02	0.05	0.02	0.00	0.00	C10
鼻咽	Nasopharynx	2 260	1.19	4.27	2.80	0.22	0.31	850	0.54	1.65	1.06	0.08	0.11	C11
下咽	Hypopharynx	537	0.28	1.01	0.59	0.04	0.08	40	0.03	0.08	0.04	0.00	0.00	C12-C13
咽,部位不明	Pharynx unspecified	143	0.07	0.27	0.16	0.01	0.02	35	0.02	0.07	0.03	0.00	0.00	C14
食管	Esophagus	16 938	8.88	31.98	17.75	0.79	2.23	6 835	4.34	13.28	6.10	0.17	0.73	C15
胃	Stomach	24 694	12.95	46.63	26.28	1.23	3.30	10 341	6.56	20.09	10.25	0.50	1.20	C16
小肠	Small intestine	753	0.39	1.42	0.84	0.05	0.10	538	0.34	1.05	0.56	0.03	0.07	C17
结肠	Colon	9 696	5.08	18.31	10.56	0.55	1.26	7 373	4.68	14.33	7.45	0.39	0.87	C18
直肠	Rectum	9 926	5.21	18.74	10.80	0.59	1.33	6 168	3.91	11.98	6.31	0.34	0.76	C19-C20
肛门	Anus	168	0.09	0.32	0.18	0.01	0.02	133	0.08	0.26	0.13	0.01	0.02	C21
肝脏	Liver	20 227	10.61	38.19	23.01	1.52	2.67	7 391	4.69	14.36	7.40	0.38	0.87	C22
胆囊及其他	Gallbladder etc.	2 699	1.42	5.10	2.85	0.13	0.35	2 684	1.70	5.21	2.53	0.10	0.31	C23-C24
胰腺	Pancreas	5 387	2.82	10.17	5.72	0.27	0.68	4 034	2.56	7.84	3.81	0.16	0.45	C25
鼻、鼻窦及其他	Nose, sinuses etc.	266	0.14	0.50	0.31	0.02	0.03	158	0.10	0.31	0.18	0.01	0.02	C30-C31
喉	Larynx	1 862	0.98	3.52	2.03	0.12	0.26	152	0.10	0.30	0.15	0.01	0.02	C32
气管、支气管、肺	Trachea, bronchus & lung	48 433	25.40	91.45	51.50	2.41	6.44	27 900	17.70	54.21	28.77	1.62	3.46	C33-C34
其他胸腔器官	Other thoracic organs	646	0.34	1.22	0.82	0.05	0.09	427	0.27	0.83	0.54	0.04	0.06	C37-C38
骨	Bone	987	0.52	1.86	1.32	0.07	0.13	774	0.49	1.50	0.98	0.06	0.10	C40-C41
皮肤黑色素瘤	Melanoma of skin	347	0.18	0.66	0.40	0.02	0.05	347	0.22	0.67	0.37	0.02	0.04	C43
皮肤其他	Other skin	1 667	0.87	3.15	1.80	0.08	0.19	1 898	1.20	3.69	1.78	0.07	0.18	C44
间皮瘤	Mesothelioma	88	0.05	0.17	0.10	0.01	0.01	97	0.06	0.19	0.11	0.01	0.01	C45
卡波氏肉瘤	Kaposi sarcoma	17	0.01	0.03	0.02	0.00	0.00	8	0.01	0.02	0.01	0.00	0.00	C46
结缔组织、软组织	Connective & soft tissue	542	0.28	1.02	0.75	0.04	0.07	476	0.30	0.92	0.67	0.05	0.06	C47, C49
乳腺	Breast	275	0.14	0.52	0.32	0.02	0.04	23 742	15.06	46.13	29.39	2.41	3.18	C50
外阴	Vulva	—	—	—	—	—	—	259	0.16	0.50	0.28	0.02	0.03	C51
阴道	Vagina	—	—	—	—	—	—	152	0.10	0.30	0.16	0.01	0.02	C52
子宫颈	Cervix uteri	—	—	—	—	—	—	8 383	5.32	16.29	10.41	0.86	1.10	C53
子宫体	Corpus uteri	—	—	—	—	—	—	4 874	3.09	9.47	5.78	0.49	0.66	C54
子宫,部位不明	Uterus unspecified	—	—	—	—	—	—	860	0.55	1.67	1.00	0.08	0.11	C55
卵巢	Ovary	—	—	—	—	—	—	4 031	2.56	7.83	4.94	0.37	0.55	C56
其他女性生殖器	Other female genital organs	—	—	—	—	—	—	311	0.20	0.60	0.37	0.03	0.04	C57
胎盘	Placenta	—	—	—	—	—	—	34	0.02	0.07	0.06	0.00	0.00	C58
阴茎	Penis	476	0.25	0.90	0.52	0.03	0.06	—	—	—	—	—	—	C60
前列腺	Prostate	8 093	4.24	15.28	8.06	0.17	0.94	—	—	—	—	—	—	C61
睾丸	Testis	226	0.12	0.43	0.37	0.03	0.03	—	—	—	—	—	—	C62
其他男性生殖器	Other male genital organs	123	0.06	0.23	0.14	0.01	0.02	—	—	—	—	—	—	C63
肾	Kidney	3 220	1.69	6.08	3.76	0.25	0.45	1 848	1.17	3.59	2.15	0.14	0.25	C64
肾盂	Renal pelvis	339	0.18	0.64	0.37	0.02	0.05	222	0.14	0.43	0.21	0.01	0.03	C65
输尿管	Ureter	400	0.21	0.76	0.42	0.02	0.05	284	0.18	0.55	0.27	0.01	0.04	C66
膀胱	Bladder	5 542	2.91	10.46	5.81	0.26	0.66	1 366	0.87	2.65	1.31	0.06	0.16	C67
其他泌尿器官	Other urinary organs	95	0.05	0.18	0.10	0.00	0.01	52	0.03	0.10	0.05	0.00	0.01	C68
眼	Eye	107	0.06	0.20	0.21	0.01	0.01	70	0.04	0.14	0.13	0.01	0.01	C69
脑、神经系统	Brain, nervous system	4 234	2.22	7.99	5.55	0.35	0.57	5 039	3.20	9.79	6.26	0.41	0.67	C70-C72, D32-D33, D42-D43
甲状腺	Thyroid	5 315	2.79	10.04	7.57	0.62	0.71	16 597	10.53	32.25	23.40	1.97	2.23	C73
肾上腺	Adrenal gland	218	0.11	0.41	0.30	0.02	0.03	142	0.09	0.28	0.19	0.01	0.02	C74
其他内分泌腺	Other endocrine	337	0.18	0.64	0.45	0.03	0.05	407	0.26	0.79	0.55	0.04	0.06	C75
霍奇金淋巴瘤	Hodgkin lymphoma	199	0.10	0.38	0.28	0.02	0.03	124	0.08	0.24	0.19	0.01	0.02	C81
非霍奇金淋巴瘤	Non-Hodgkin lymphoma	3 246	1.70	6.13	3.91	0.23	0.45	2 445	1.55	4.75	2.81	0.16	0.32	C82-C86, C96
免疫增生性疾病	Immunoproliferative diseases	69	0.04	0.13	0.07	0.00	0.01	32	0.02	0.06	0.04	0.00	0.00	C88
多发性骨髓瘤	Multiple myeloma	1 043	0.55	1.97	1.13	0.06	0.15	894	0.57	1.74	0.94	0.05	0.12	C90
淋巴样白血病	Lymphoid leukemia	905	0.47	1.71	1.68	0.09	0.13	672	0.43	1.31	1.30	0.07	0.10	C91
髓样白血病	Myeloid leukemia	2 380	1.25	4.49	3.12	0.18	0.32	1 973	1.25	3.83	2.61	0.16	0.26	C92-C94, D45-D47
白血病,未特指	Leukemia unspecified	1 029	0.54	1.94	1.41	0.08	0.14	752	0.48	1.46	1.03	0.06	0.09	C95
其他或未指明部位	Other and unspecified	2 523	1.32	4.76	2.89	0.15	0.31	2 245	1.42	4.36	2.48	0.14	0.26	O&U
所有部位合计	All sites	190 692	100.00	360.06	211.36	10.98	25.12	157 647	100.00	306.31	178.86	11.71	19.80	C00-C97, D32-D33, D42-D43, D45-D47
所有部位除外 C44	All sites except C44	189 025	99.13	356.91	209.57	10.91	24.93	155 749	98.80	302.62	177.08	11.64	19.62	C00-C97, D32-D33, D42-D43, D45-D47 exc. C44

附表 2-4 2018 年全国中部肿瘤登记地区癌症发病主要指标
Appendix Table 2-4　Cancer incidence in Central registration areas of China, 2018

部位 Site		男性 Male						女性 Female						ICD-10
		病例数 No. cases	构成 Freq./%	粗率 Crude rate/ $100\,000^{-1}$	世标率 ASR world/ $100\,000^{-1}$	累积率 Cum. Rate/%		病例数 No. cases	构成 Freq./%	粗率 Crude rate/ $100\,000^{-1}$	世标率 ASR world/ $100\,000^{-1}$	累积率 Cum. Rate/%		
						0~64	0~74					0~64	0~74	
唇	Lip	119	0.06	0.18	0.12	0.00	0.01	82	0.05	0.13	0.07	0.00	0.01	C00
舌	Tongue	847	0.44	1.28	0.91	0.07	0.10	327	0.21	0.52	0.34	0.02	0.04	C01-C02
口	Mouth	940	0.49	1.42	0.98	0.07	0.11	446	0.28	0.70	0.45	0.02	0.04	C03-C06
唾液腺	Salivary glands	411	0.21	0.62	0.46	0.03	0.05	346	0.22	0.55	0.39	0.03	0.04	C07-C08
扁桃腺	Tonsil	163	0.09	0.25	0.19	0.01	0.02	67	0.04	0.11	0.07	0.00	0.01	C09
其他口咽	Other oropharynx	252	0.13	0.38	0.27	0.02	0.03	57	0.04	0.09	0.06	0.00	0.01	C10
鼻咽	Nasopharynx	2 938	1.54	4.43	3.20	0.25	0.36	1 226	0.77	1.93	1.34	0.10	0.15	C11
下咽	Hypopharynx	456	0.24	0.69	0.49	0.03	0.06	34	0.02	0.05	0.03	0.00	0.00	C12-C13
咽,部位不明	Pharynx unspecified	238	0.12	0.36	0.25	0.01	0.03	85	0.05	0.13	0.09	0.00	0.01	C14
食管	Esophagus	15 696	8.21	23.68	15.85	0.73	2.03	6 768	4.28	10.67	6.32	0.23	0.79	C15
胃	Stomach	24 911	13.02	37.59	25.33	1.24	3.24	10 857	6.86	17.12	10.59	0.54	1.24	C16
小肠	Small intestine	854	0.45	1.29	0.88	0.05	0.11	673	0.43	1.06	0.69	0.04	0.08	C17
结肠	Colon	8 516	4.45	12.85	8.75	0.48	1.05	6 709	4.24	10.58	6.66	0.37	0.79	C18
直肠	Rectum	9 621	5.03	14.52	9.84	0.55	1.20	6 479	4.10	10.22	6.47	0.37	0.77	C19-C20
肛门	Anus	239	0.12	0.36	0.25	0.01	0.03	203	0.13	0.32	0.20	0.01	0.03	C21
肝脏	Liver	24 743	12.93	37.33	25.81	1.65	3.04	9 400	5.94	14.82	9.23	0.47	1.09	C22
胆囊及其他	Gallbladder etc.	2 051	1.07	3.09	2.07	0.10	0.25	2 509	1.59	3.96	2.38	0.11	0.29	C23-C24
胰腺	Pancreas	4 174	2.18	6.30	4.21	0.22	0.50	3 090	1.95	4.87	2.96	0.14	0.35	C25
鼻、鼻窦及其他	Nose, sinuses etc.	321	0.17	0.48	0.34	0.02	0.04	201	0.13	0.32	0.22	0.01	0.02	C30-C31
喉	Larynx	2 115	1.11	3.19	2.17	0.13	0.28	277	0.18	0.44	0.27	0.01	0.03	C32
气管、支气管、肺	Trachea, bronchus & lung	51 430	26.89	77.60	51.94	2.51	6.52	23 196	14.66	36.58	22.53	1.18	2.68	C33-C34
其他胸腔器官	Other thoracic organs	736	0.38	1.11	0.83	0.05	0.09	496	0.31	0.78	0.57	0.04	0.06	C37-C38
骨	Bone	1 494	0.78	2.25	1.80	0.10	0.19	995	0.63	1.57	1.18	0.07	0.12	C40-C41
皮肤黑色素瘤	Melanoma of skin	305	0.16	0.46	0.33	0.02	0.03	244	0.15	0.38	0.28	0.02	0.03	C43
皮肤其他	Other skin	1 460	0.76	2.20	1.49	0.07	0.16	1 278	0.81	2.02	1.20	0.05	0.13	C44
间皮瘤	Mesothelioma	75	0.04	0.11	0.08	0.00	0.01	58	0.04	0.09	0.06	0.00	0.01	C45
卡波氏肉瘤	Kaposi sarcoma	19	0.01	0.03	0.02	0.00	0.00	5	0.00	0.01	0.01	0.00	0.00	C46
结缔组织、软组织	Connective & soft tissue	522	0.27	0.79	0.63	0.04	0.06	470	0.30	0.74	0.59	0.04	0.06	C47, C49
乳腺	Breast	345	0.18	0.52	0.36	0.02	0.04	25 677	16.23	40.49	28.17	2.33	3.02	C50
外阴	Vulva	—	—	—	—	—	—	253	0.16	0.40	0.25	0.01	0.03	C51
阴道	Vagina	—	—	—	—	—	—	204	0.13	0.32	0.22	0.02	0.02	C52
子宫颈	Cervix uteri	—	—	—	—	—	—	13 790	8.72	21.74	15.03	1.23	1.63	C53
子宫体	Corpus uteri	—	—	—	—	—	—	5 010	3.17	7.90	5.42	0.46	0.61	C54
子宫,部位不明	Uterus unspecified	—	—	—	—	—	—	1 039	0.66	1.64	1.12	0.09	0.12	C55
卵巢	Ovary	—	—	—	—	—	—	4 780	3.02	7.54	5.37	0.41	0.58	C56
其他女性生殖器	Other female genital organs	—	—	—	—	—	—	292	0.18	0.46	0.33	0.02	0.04	C57
胎盘	Placenta	—	—	—	—	—	—	36	0.02	0.06	0.05	0.00	0.00	C58
阴茎	Penis	471	0.25	0.71	0.49	0.03	0.06	—	—	—	—	—	—	C60
前列腺	Prostate	5 388	2.82	8.13	5.07	0.11	0.56	—	—	—	—	—	—	C61
睾丸	Testis	259	0.14	0.39	0.32	0.02	0.02	—	—	—	—	—	—	C62
其他男性生殖器	Other male genital organs	106	0.06	0.16	0.11	0.01	0.01	—	—	—	—	—	—	C63
肾	Kidney	2 670	1.40	4.03	2.86	0.18	0.34	1 591	1.01	2.51	1.71	0.11	0.20	C64
肾盂	Renal pelvis	292	0.15	0.44	0.30	0.02	0.03	185	0.12	0.29	0.18	0.01	0.02	C65
输尿管	Ureter	342	0.18	0.52	0.35	0.02	0.04	280	0.18	0.44	0.26	0.01	0.03	C66
膀胱	Bladder	4 788	2.50	7.22	4.78	0.21	0.55	1 309	0.83	2.06	1.22	0.05	0.14	C67
其他泌尿器官	Other urinary organs	72	0.04	0.11	0.07	0.00	0.00	46	0.03	0.07	0.04	0.00	0.00	C68
眼	Eye	117	0.06	0.18	0.17	0.01	0.01	113	0.07	0.18	0.18	0.01	0.01	C69
脑、神经系统	Brain, nervous system	4 381	2.29	6.61	5.15	0.33	0.53	4 682	2.96	7.38	5.44	0.36	0.57	C70-C72, D32-D33, D42-D43
甲状腺	Thyroid	3 778	1.97	5.70	4.35	0.36	0.41	12 463	7.88	19.65	14.61	1.24	1.39	C73
肾上腺	Adrenal gland	213	0.11	0.32	0.25	0.02	0.03	173	0.11	0.27	0.20	0.01	0.02	C74
其他内分泌腺	Other endocrine	199	0.10	0.30	0.24	0.02	0.02	233	0.15	0.37	0.27	0.02	0.03	C75
霍奇金淋巴瘤	Hodgkin lymphoma	239	0.12	0.36	0.30	0.02	0.03	149	0.09	0.23	0.18	0.01	0.02	C81
非霍奇金淋巴瘤	Non-Hodgkin lymphoma	2 968	1.55	4.48	3.34	0.20	0.37	2 114	1.34	3.33	2.34	0.15	0.26	C82-C86, C96
免疫增生性疾病	Immunoproliferative diseases	43	0.02	0.06	0.04	0.00	0.01	14	0.01	0.02	0.01	0.00	0.00	C88
多发性骨髓瘤	Multiple myeloma	985	0.51	1.49	1.04	0.06	0.13	707	0.45	1.11	0.73	0.05	0.09	C90
淋巴样白血病	Lymphoid leukemia	732	0.38	1.10	1.09	0.06	0.09	537	0.34	0.85	0.85	0.05	0.07	C91
髓样白血病	Myeloid leukemia	1 688	0.88	2.55	2.01	0.12	0.20	1 230	0.78	1.94	1.51	0.10	0.15	C92-C94, D45-D47
白血病,未特指	Leukemia unspecified	1 599	0.84	2.41	2.08	0.12	0.19	1 255	0.79	1.98	1.71	0.10	0.15	C95
其他或未指明部位	Other and unspecified	3 971	2.08	5.99	4.32	0.23	0.48	3 454	2.18	5.45	3.69	0.21	0.40	O&U
所有部位合计	All sites	191 292	100.00	288.64	198.53	10.62	23.82	158 197	100.00	249.44	166.30	10.96	18.48	C00-C97, D32-D33, D42-D43, D45-D47
所有部位除外 C44	All sites except C44	189 832	99.24	286.44	197.04	10.55	23.66	156 919	99.19	247.42	165.10	10.91	18.35	C00-C97, D32-D33, D42-D43, D45-D47 exc. C44

部位 Site		男性 Male 病例数 No. cases	构成 Freq./%	粗率 Crude rate/100 000⁻¹	世标率 ASR world/100 000⁻¹	累积率 Cum. Rate/% 0~64	0~74	女性 Female 病例数 No. cases	构成 Freq./%	粗率 Crude rate/100 000⁻¹	世标率 ASR world/100 000⁻¹	累积率 Cum. Rate/% 0~64	0~74	ICD-10
唇	Lip	39	0.05	0.16	0.10	0.00	0.01	21	0.03	0.09	0.05	0.00	0.01	C00
舌	Tongue	422	0.56	1.73	1.14	0.08	0.13	173	0.27	0.72	0.44	0.03	0.05	C01-C02
口	Mouth	448	0.59	1.84	1.17	0.08	0.13	176	0.27	0.74	0.44	0.03	0.05	C03-C06
唾液腺	Salivary glands	152	0.20	0.62	0.43	0.03	0.05	125	0.19	0.52	0.34	0.02	0.03	C07-C08
扁桃腺	Tonsil	70	0.09	0.29	0.19	0.01	0.02	24	0.04	0.10	0.06	0.00	0.01	C09
其他口咽	Other oropharynx	99	0.13	0.41	0.27	0.02	0.04	20	0.03	0.08	0.05	0.00	0.01	C10
鼻咽	Nasopharynx	967	1.28	3.97	2.72	0.21	0.31	385	0.59	1.61	1.06	0.08	0.12	C11
下咽	Hypopharynx	230	0.30	0.94	0.62	0.04	0.08	6	0.01	0.03	0.02	0.00	0.00	C12-C13
咽,部位不明	Pharynx unspecified	101	0.13	0.41	0.27	0.02	0.03	35	0.05	0.15	0.08	0.00	0.01	C14
食管	Esophagus	4 860	6.44	19.93	12.33	0.60	1.57	1 740	2.67	7.29	3.91	0.12	0.46	C15
胃	Stomach	7 791	10.32	31.95	19.78	0.94	2.50	3 645	5.60	15.27	8.70	0.43	0.98	C16
小肠	Small intestine	371	0.49	1.52	0.95	0.05	0.11	308	0.47	1.29	0.77	0.04	0.10	C17
结肠	Colon	4 151	5.50	17.02	10.61	0.55	1.26	3 235	4.97	13.55	7.86	0.42	0.91	C18
直肠	Rectum	4 089	5.42	16.77	10.54	0.60	1.28	2 607	4.01	10.92	6.45	0.36	0.76	C19-C20
肛门	Anus	84	0.11	0.34	0.21	0.01	0.02	77	0.12	0.32	0.19	0.01	0.02	C21
肝脏	Liver	9 011	11.93	36.96	23.77	1.53	2.79	3 356	5.16	14.06	8.12	0.40	0.94	C22
胆囊及其他	Gallbladder etc.	881	1.17	3.61	2.20	0.10	0.27	1 060	1.63	4.44	2.42	0.11	0.28	C23-C24
胰腺	Pancreas	1 855	2.46	7.61	4.67	0.25	0.54	1 386	2.13	5.81	3.23	0.15	0.37	C25
鼻、鼻窦及其他	Nose, sinuses etc.	131	0.17	0.54	0.35	0.02	0.04	70	0.11	0.29	0.19	0.01	0.02	C30-C31
喉	Larynx	905	1.20	3.71	2.36	0.15	0.31	127	0.20	0.53	0.31	0.02	0.05	C32
气管、支气管、肺	Trachea, bronchus & lung	20 649	27.35	84.69	52.26	2.53	6.55	9 762	15.00	40.89	23.54	1.25	2.76	C33-C34
其他胸腔器官	Other thoracic organs	318	0.42	1.30	0.91	0.06	0.11	221	0.34	0.93	0.63	0.04	0.07	C37-C38
骨	Bone	436	0.58	1.79	1.33	0.08	0.13	321	0.49	1.34	0.93	0.05	0.10	C40-C41
皮肤黑色素瘤	Melanoma of skin	125	0.17	0.51	0.34	0.02	0.04	100	0.15	0.42	0.30	0.02	0.03	C43
皮肤其他	Other skin	555	0.73	2.28	1.39	0.06	0.15	459	0.71	1.92	1.07	0.05	0.11	C44
间皮瘤	Mesothelioma	45	0.06	0.18	0.12	0.00	0.01	31	0.05	0.13	0.08	0.01	0.01	C45
卡波氏肉瘤	Kaposi sarcoma	3	0.00	0.01	0.01	0.00	0.00	4	0.01	0.02	0.01	0.00	0.00	C46
结缔组织、软组织	Connective & soft tissue	232	0.31	0.95	0.72	0.05	0.07	198	0.30	0.83	0.64	0.04	0.06	C47-C49
乳腺	Breast	112	0.15	0.46	0.30	0.02	0.03	11 458	17.61	48.00	31.56	2.58	3.44	C50
外阴	Vulva	—	—	—	—	—	—	115	0.18	0.48	0.28	0.01	0.03	C51
阴道	Vagina	—	—	—	—	—	—	68	0.10	0.28	0.18	0.01	0.02	C52
子宫颈	Cervix uteri	—	—	—	—	—	—	4 814	7.40	20.17	13.33	1.10	1.44	C53
子宫体	Corpus uteri	—	—	—	—	—	—	2 007	3.08	8.41	5.49	0.46	0.63	C54
子宫,部位不明	Uterus unspecified	—	—	—	—	—	—	282	0.43	1.18	0.76	0.06	0.08	C55
卵巢	Ovary	—	—	—	—	—	—	2 004	3.08	8.39	5.66	0.42	0.61	C56
其他女性生殖器	Other female genital organs	—	—	—	—	—	—	135	0.21	0.57	0.38	0.03	0.04	C57
胎盘	Placenta	—	—	—	—	—	—	9	0.01	0.04	0.03	0.00	0.00	C58
阴茎	Penis	189	0.25	0.78	0.49	0.02	0.06	—	—	—	—	—	—	C60
前列腺	Prostate	2 788	3.69	11.43	6.44	0.13	0.71	—	—	—	—	—	—	C61
睾丸	Testis	88	0.12	0.36	0.29	0.02	0.03	—	—	—	—	—	—	C62
其他男性生殖器	Other male genital organs	50	0.07	0.21	0.13	0.01	0.01	—	—	—	—	—	—	C63
肾	Kidney	1 344	1.78	5.51	3.62	0.23	0.44	723	1.11	3.03	1.90	0.12	0.22	C64
肾盂	Renal pelvis	153	0.20	0.63	0.39	0.02	0.05	115	0.18	0.48	0.26	0.01	0.03	C65
输尿管	Ureter	186	0.25	0.76	0.46	0.02	0.06	154	0.24	0.65	0.34	0.01	0.04	C66
膀胱	Bladder	2 248	2.98	9.22	5.57	0.24	0.63	620	0.95	2.60	1.39	0.06	0.15	C67
其他泌尿器官	Other urinary organs	35	0.05	0.14	0.08	0.00	0.01	19	0.03	0.08	0.04	0.00	0.00	C68
眼	Eye	32	0.04	0.13	0.13	0.01	0.01	35	0.05	0.15	0.12	0.00	0.01	C69
脑、神经系统	Brain, nervous system	1 546	2.05	6.34	4.64	0.30	0.49	1 649	2.53	6.91	4.82	0.32	0.51	C70-C72, D32-D33, D42-D43
甲状腺	Thyroid	2 207	2.92	9.05	6.71	0.55	0.62	6 897	10.60	28.89	20.74	1.77	1.97	C73
肾上腺	Adrenal gland	92	0.12	0.38	0.28	0.02	0.03	54	0.08	0.23	0.16	0.01	0.02	C74
其他内分泌腺	Other endocrine	92	0.12	0.38	0.28	0.02	0.03	123	0.19	0.52	0.37	0.03	0.04	C75
霍奇金淋巴瘤	Hodgkin lymphoma	89	0.12	0.37	0.31	0.02	0.03	50	0.08	0.21	0.16	0.01	0.01	C81
非霍奇金淋巴瘤	Non-Hodgkin lymphoma	1 279	1.69	5.25	3.55	0.21	0.40	977	1.50	4.09	2.65	0.17	0.30	C82-C86, C96
免疫增生性疾病	Immunoproliferative diseases	25	0.03	0.10	0.07	0.00	0.01	7	0.01	0.03	0.02	0.00	0.00	C88
多发性骨髓瘤	Multiple myeloma	460	0.61	1.89	1.25	0.07	0.15	343	0.53	1.44	0.87	0.05	0.10	C90
淋巴样白血病	Lymphoid leukemia	340	0.45	1.39	1.39	0.07	0.10	242	0.37	1.01	1.02	0.06	0.08	C91
髓样白血病	Myeloid leukemia	776	1.03	3.18	2.33	0.14	0.24	525	0.81	2.20	1.60	0.10	0.16	C92-C94, D45-D47
白血病,未特指	Leukemia unspecified	454	0.60	1.86	1.45	0.08	0.13	369	0.57	1.55	1.18	0.06	0.11	C95
其他或未指明部位	Other and unspecified	1 906	2.52	7.82	5.23	0.27	0.58	1 603	2.46	6.71	4.19	0.24	0.44	O&U
所有部位合计	All sites	75 511	100.00	309.70	197.15	10.58	23.40	65 069	100.00	272.56	171.38	11.38	18.80	C00-C97, D32-D33, D42-D43, D45-D47
所有部位除外 C44	All sites except C44	74 956	99.27	307.42	195.75	10.52	23.25	64 610	99.29	270.64	170.31	11.33	18.68	C00-C97, D32-D33, D42-D43, D45-D47 exc. C44

附表 2-6　2018 年全国中部农村肿瘤登记地区癌症发病主要指标

Appendix Table 2-6　Cancer incidence in Central rural registration areas of China, 2018

部位 Site		男性 Male						女性 Female						ICD-10
		病例数 No. cases	构成 Freq./%	粗率 Crude rate/ $100\,000^{-1}$	世标率 ASR world/ $100\,000^{-1}$	累积率 Cum. Rate/%		病例数 No. cases	构成 Freq./%	粗率 Crude rate/ $100\,000^{-1}$	世标率 ASR world/ $100\,000^{-1}$	累积率 Cum. Rate/%		
						0~64	0~74					0~64	0~74	
唇	Lip	80	0.07	0.19	0.13	0.01	0.01	61	0.07	0.15	0.09	0.00	0.01	C00
舌	Tongue	425	0.37	1.01	0.75	0.06	0.08	154	0.17	0.39	0.27	0.02	0.03	C01-C02
口	Mouth	492	0.42	1.17	0.86	0.06	0.10	270	0.29	0.68	0.46	0.02	0.06	C03-C06
唾液腺	Salivary glands	259	0.22	0.62	0.48	0.03	0.05	221	0.24	0.56	0.42	0.03	0.04	C07-C08
扁桃腺	Tonsil	93	0.08	0.22	0.18	0.01	0.02	43	0.05	0.11	0.08	0.01	0.01	C09
其他口咽	Other oropharynx	153	0.13	0.37	0.27	0.02	0.03	37	0.04	0.09	0.06	0.00	0.01	C10
鼻咽	Nasopharynx	1 971	1.70	4.71	3.50	0.27	0.40	841	0.90	2.13	1.52	0.12	0.17	C11
下咽	Hypopharynx	226	0.20	0.54	0.40	0.03	0.05	28	0.03	0.07	0.05	0.00	0.01	C12-C13
咽,部位不明	Pharynx unspecified	137	0.12	0.33	0.23	0.01	0.03	50	0.05	0.13	0.09	0.01	0.01	C14
食管	Esophagus	10 836	9.36	25.87	18.18	0.81	2.33	5 028	5.40	12.71	7.94	0.30	1.01	C15
胃	Stomach	17 120	14.79	40.87	28.93	1.44	3.72	7 212	7.74	18.24	11.85	0.61	1.41	C16
小肠	Small intestine	483	0.42	1.15	0.83	0.05	0.10	365	0.39	0.92	0.63	0.04	0.08	C17
结肠	Colon	4 365	3.77	10.42	7.50	0.43	0.92	3 474	3.73	8.78	5.85	0.33	0.71	C18
直肠	Rectum	5 532	4.78	13.21	9.36	0.52	1.15	3 872	4.16	9.79	6.47	0.37	0.78	C19-C20
肛门	Anus	155	0.13	0.37	0.27	0.01	0.03	126	0.14	0.32	0.20	0.01	0.02	C21
肝脏	Liver	15 732	13.59	37.55	27.10	1.73	3.20	6 044	6.49	15.28	9.97	0.52	1.20	C22
胆囊及其他	Gallbladder etc.	1 170	1.01	2.79	1.98	0.09	0.24	1 449	1.56	3.66	2.36	0.12	0.29	C23-C24
胰腺	Pancreas	2 319	2.00	5.54	3.89	0.20	0.48	1 704	1.83	4.31	2.77	0.13	0.34	C25
鼻、鼻窦及其他	Nose, sinuses etc.	190	0.16	0.45	0.33	0.02	0.04	131	0.14	0.33	0.24	0.02	0.03	C30-C31
喉	Larynx	1 210	1.05	2.89	2.04	0.11	0.26	150	0.16	0.38	0.24	0.01	0.03	C32
气管、支气管、肺	Trachea, bronchus & lung	30 781	26.59	73.48	51.69	2.49	6.50	13 437	14.43	33.98	21.85	1.14	2.62	C33-C34
其他胸腔器官	Other thoracic organs	418	0.36	1.00	0.78	0.05	0.08	275	0.30	0.70	0.53	0.04	0.05	C37-C38
骨	Bone	1 058	0.91	2.53	2.08	0.11	0.23	674	0.72	1.70	1.33	0.08	0.13	C40-C41
皮肤黑色素瘤	Melanoma of skin	180	0.16	0.43	0.33	0.02	0.03	144	0.15	0.36	0.26	0.02	0.03	C43
皮肤其他	Other skin	905	0.78	2.16	1.55	0.07	0.16	819	0.88	2.07	1.29	0.05	0.13	C44
间皮瘤	Mesothelioma	30	0.03	0.07	0.05	0.00	0.01	27	0.03	0.07	0.05	0.00	0.01	C45
卡波氏肉瘤	Kaposi sarcoma	16	0.01	0.04	0.03	0.00	0.00	1	0.00	0.00	0.00	0.00	0.00	C46
结缔组织、软组织	Connective & soft tissue	290	0.25	0.69	0.57	0.04	0.06	272	0.29	0.69	0.56	0.04	0.05	C47, C49
乳腺	Breast	233	0.20	0.56	0.40	0.02	0.05	14 219	15.27	35.95	25.88	2.15	2.73	C50
外阴	Vulva	—	—	—	—	—	—	138	0.15	0.35	0.23	0.01	0.03	C51
阴道	Vagina	—	—	—	—	—	—	136	0.15	0.34	0.24	0.02	0.03	C52
子宫颈	Cervix uteri	—	—	—	—	—	—	8 976	9.64	22.70	16.15	1.31	1.75	C53
子宫体	Corpus uteri	—	—	—	—	—	—	3 003	3.22	7.59	5.37	0.46	0.60	C54
子宫,部位不明	Uterus unspecified	—	—	—	—	—	—	757	0.81	1.91	1.35	0.11	0.14	C55
卵巢	Ovary	—	—	—	—	—	—	2 776	2.98	7.02	5.17	0.40	0.56	C56
其他女性生殖器	Other female genital organs	—	—	—	—	—	—	157	0.17	0.40	0.29	0.02	0.03	C57
胎盘	Placenta	—	—	—	—	—	—	27	0.03	0.07	0.06	0.00	0.00	C58
阴茎	Penis	282	0.24	0.67	0.49	0.03	0.06	—	—	—	—	—	—	C60
前列腺	Prostate	2 600	2.25	6.21	4.13	0.09	0.46	—	—	—	—	—	—	C61
睾丸	Testis	171	0.15	0.41	0.34	0.02	0.03	—	—	—	—	—	—	C62
其他男性生殖器	Other male genital organs	56	0.05	0.13	0.10	0.01	0.01	—	—	—	—	—	—	C63
肾	Kidney	1 326	1.15	3.17	2.36	0.15	0.28	868	0.93	2.19	1.58	0.11	0.18	C64
肾盂	Renal pelvis	139	0.12	0.33	0.24	0.01	0.03	70	0.08	0.18	0.12	0.01	0.02	C65
输尿管	Ureter	156	0.13	0.37	0.27	0.01	0.04	126	0.14	0.32	0.21	0.01	0.03	C66
膀胱	Bladder	2 540	2.19	6.06	4.24	0.20	0.50	689	0.74	1.74	1.10	0.05	0.13	C67
其他泌尿器官	Other urinary organs	37	0.03	0.09	0.07	0.00	0.01	27	0.03	0.07	0.05	0.00	0.01	C68
眼	Eye	85	0.07	0.20	0.20	0.01	0.02	78	0.08	0.20	0.21	0.01	0.01	C69
脑、神经系统	Brain, nervous system	2 835	2.45	6.77	5.45	0.34	0.56	3 033	3.26	7.67	5.82	0.39	0.61	C70-C72, D32-D33, D42-D43
甲状腺	Thyroid	1 571	1.36	3.75	2.92	0.23	0.29	5 566	5.98	14.07	10.68	0.90	1.02	C73
肾上腺	Adrenal gland	121	0.10	0.29	0.22	0.01	0.02	119	0.13	0.30	0.22	0.02	0.03	C74
其他内分泌腺	Other endocrine	107	0.09	0.26	0.21	0.01	0.02	110	0.12	0.28	0.21	0.02	0.02	C75
霍奇金淋巴瘤	Hodgkin lymphoma	150	0.13	0.36	0.29	0.02	0.03	99	0.11	0.25	0.19	0.01	0.02	C81
非霍奇金淋巴瘤	Non-Hodgkin lymphoma	1 689	1.46	4.03	3.18	0.20	0.35	1 137	1.22	2.87	2.13	0.13	0.24	C82-C86, C96
免疫增生性疾病	Immunoproliferative diseases	18	0.02	0.04	0.03	0.00	0.00	7	0.01	0.02	0.01	0.00	0.00	C88
多发性骨髓瘤	Multiple myeloma	525	0.45	1.25	0.91	0.05	0.11	364	0.39	0.92	0.63	0.04	0.07	C90
淋巴样白血病	Lymphoid leukemia	392	0.34	0.94	0.93	0.05	0.08	295	0.32	0.75	0.75	0.04	0.06	C91
髓样白血病	Myeloid leukemia	912	0.79	2.18	1.79	0.11	0.18	705	0.76	1.78	1.44	0.10	0.14	C92-C94, D45-D47
白血病,未特指	Leukemia unspecified	1 145	0.99	2.73	2.43	0.14	0.22	886	0.95	2.24	2.01	0.12	0.18	C95
其他或未指明部位	Other and unspecified	2 065	1.78	4.93	3.72	0.20	0.42	1 851	1.99	4.68	3.36	0.20	0.37	O&U
所有部位合计	All sites	115 781	100.00	276.38	199.20	10.64	24.08	93 128	100.00	235.48	162.90	10.69	18.27	C00-C97, D32-D33, D42-D43, D45-D47
所有部位除外 C44	All sites except C44	114 876	99.22	274.22	197.65	10.57	23.92	92 309	99.12	233.41	161.61	10.63	18.13	C00-C97, D32-D33, D42-D43, D45-D47 exc. C44

部位 Site		男性 Male						女性 Female						ICD-10
		病例数 No. cases	构成 Freq./%	粗率 Crude rate/ 100 000⁻¹	世标率 ASR world/ 100 000⁻¹	累积率 Cum. Rate/% 0~64	0~74	病例数 No. cases	构成 Freq./%	粗率 Crude rate/ 100 000⁻¹	世标率 ASR world/ 100 000⁻¹	累积率 Cum. Rate/% 0~64	0~74	
唇	Lip	167	0.06	0.19	0.12	0.01	0.01	103	0.05	0.12	0.08	0.00	0.01	C00
舌	Tongue	876	0.34	0.97	0.66	0.04	0.08	451	0.24	0.52	0.34	0.02	0.04	C01-C02
口	Mouth	1 399	0.54	1.55	1.03	0.05	0.12	679	0.36	0.79	0.50	0.03	0.06	C03-C06
唾液腺	Salivary glands	470	0.18	0.52	0.36	0.02	0.04	389	0.21	0.45	0.32	0.02	0.03	C07-C08
扁桃腺	Tonsil	183	0.07	0.20	0.14	0.01	0.02	67	0.04	0.08	0.06	0.00	0.01	C09
其他口咽	Other oropharynx	457	0.18	0.51	0.34	0.02	0.04	84	0.04	0.10	0.06	0.00	0.01	C10
鼻咽	Nasopharynx	5 437	2.09	6.03	4.25	0.33	0.46	2 304	1.23	2.67	1.85	0.14	0.20	C11
下咽	Hypopharynx	669	0.26	0.74	0.50	0.03	0.06	66	0.04	0.08	0.05	0.00	0.01	C12-C13
咽,部位不明	Pharynx unspecified	457	0.18	0.51	0.33	0.02	0.04	143	0.08	0.17	0.10	0.00	0.01	C14
食管	Esophagus	25 348	9.75	28.11	18.27	0.89	2.35	6 914	3.69	8.02	4.62	0.17	0.55	C15
胃	Stomach	26 168	10.06	29.02	18.96	0.99	2.37	11 154	5.96	12.95	7.85	0.41	0.90	C16
小肠	Small intestine	1 006	0.39	1.12	0.74	0.04	0.09	723	0.39	0.84	0.52	0.03	0.06	C17
结肠	Colon	10 301	3.96	11.42	7.48	0.41	0.86	7 867	4.20	9.13	5.61	0.30	0.66	C18
直肠	Rectum	15 872	6.10	17.60	11.49	0.59	1.40	10 181	5.44	11.82	7.22	0.39	0.85	C19-C20
肛门	Anus	472	0.18	0.52	0.34	0.02	0.04	312	0.17	0.36	0.22	0.01	0.02	C21
肝脏	Liver	40 536	15.59	44.96	30.50	2.08	3.52	12 979	6.93	15.06	9.30	0.50	1.08	C22
胆囊及其他	Gallbladder etc.	2 564	0.99	2.84	1.82	0.09	0.21	2 950	1.58	3.42	2.02	0.10	0.24	C23-C24
胰腺	Pancreas	5 877	2.26	6.52	4.24	0.23	0.51	4 050	2.16	4.70	2.80	0.13	0.33	C25
鼻、鼻窦及其他	Nose,sinuses etc.	504	0.19	0.56	0.39	0.03	0.04	275	0.15	0.32	0.21	0.01	0.02	C30-C31
喉	Larynx	2 505	0.96	2.78	1.83	0.11	0.23	283	0.15	0.33	0.20	0.01	0.02	C32
气管、支气管、肺	Trachea,bronchus & lung	69 082	26.56	76.62	50.01	2.68	6.16	33 092	17.67	38.41	23.47	1.26	2.78	C33-C34
其他胸腔器官	Other thoracic organs	873	0.34	0.97	0.71	0.05	0.08	532	0.28	0.62	0.42	0.03	0.04	C37-C38
骨	Bone	2 019	0.78	2.24	1.65	0.09	0.17	1 407	0.75	1.63	1.19	0.07	0.12	C40-C41
皮肤黑色素瘤	Melanoma of skin	382	0.15	0.42	0.29	0.02	0.03	369	0.20	0.43	0.28	0.02	0.03	C43
皮肤其他	Other skin	2 025	0.78	2.25	1.49	0.07	0.16	2 050	1.09	2.38	1.44	0.07	0.15	C44
间皮瘤	Mesothelioma	101	0.04	0.11	0.08	0.01	0.01	83	0.04	0.10	0.07	0.00	0.01	C45
卡波氏肉瘤	Kaposi sarcoma	52	0.02	0.06	0.04	0.00	0.00	26	0.01	0.03	0.02	0.00	0.00	C46
结缔组织、软组织	Connective & soft tissue	852	0.33	0.94	0.74	0.05	0.07	656	0.35	0.76	0.56	0.04	0.06	C47,C49
乳腺	Breast	567	0.22	0.63	0.43	0.03	0.05	25 164	13.44	29.21	20.12	1.68	2.12	C50
外阴	Vulva	—	—	—	—	—	—	413	0.22	0.48	0.31	0.02	0.04	C51
阴道	Vagina	—	—	—	—	—	—	256	0.14	0.30	0.19	0.01	0.02	C52
子宫颈	Cervix uteri	—	—	—	—	—	—	15 583	8.32	18.09	12.45	1.01	1.34	C53
子宫体	Corpus uteri	—	—	—	—	—	—	6 104	3.26	7.08	4.84	0.41	0.53	C54
子宫,部位不明	Uterus unspecified	—	—	—	—	—	—	1 564	0.84	1.82	1.22	0.09	0.13	C55
卵巢	Ovary	—	—	—	—	—	—	6 053	3.23	7.03	4.97	0.38	0.53	C56
其他女性生殖器	Other female genital organs	—	—	—	—	—	—	388	0.21	0.45	0.31	0.02	0.04	C57
胎盘	Placenta	—	—	—	—	—	—	90	0.05	0.10	0.09	0.01	0.01	C58
阴茎	Penis	661	0.25	0.73	0.49	0.03	0.06	—	—	—	—	—	—	C60
前列腺	Prostate	8 132	3.13	9.02	5.35	0.10	0.56	—	—	—	—	—	—	C61
睾丸	Testis	388	0.15	0.43	0.36	0.02	0.03	—	—	—	—	—	—	C62
其他男性生殖器	Other male genital organs	90	0.03	0.10	0.07	0.00	0.01	—	—	—	—	—	—	C63
肾	Kidney	2 493	0.96	2.77	1.90	0.13	0.21	1 545	0.82	1.79	1.18	0.08	0.13	C64
肾盂	Renal pelvis	361	0.14	0.40	0.26	0.01	0.03	239	0.13	0.28	0.17	0.01	0.02	C65
输尿管	Ureter	326	0.13	0.36	0.23	0.01	0.03	281	0.15	0.33	0.19	0.01	0.02	C66
膀胱	Bladder	6 588	2.53	7.31	4.61	0.20	0.51	1 798	0.96	2.09	1.24	0.06	0.14	C67
其他泌尿器官	Other urinary organs	77	0.03	0.09	0.06	0.00	0.01	68	0.04	0.08	0.05	0.00	0.01	C68
眼	Eye	159	0.06	0.18	0.15	0.01	0.01	134	0.07	0.16	0.12	0.01	0.01	C69
脑、神经系统	Brain,nervous system	5 486	2.11	6.08	4.55	0.29	0.47	5 973	3.19	6.93	4.87	0.32	0.52	C70-C72,D32, D33,D42-D43
甲状腺	Thyroid	3 104	1.19	3.44	2.62	0.21	0.25	9 797	5.23	11.37	8.56	0.71	0.81	C73
肾上腺	Adrenal gland	229	0.09	0.25	0.19	0.01	0.02	189	0.10	0.22	0.15	0.01	0.02	C74
其他内分泌腺	Other endocrine	260	0.10	0.29	0.22	0.02	0.02	293	0.16	0.34	0.25	0.02	0.03	C75
霍奇金淋巴瘤	Hodgkin lymphoma	337	0.13	0.37	0.29	0.02	0.03	202	0.11	0.23	0.18	0.01	0.02	C81
非霍奇金淋巴瘤	Non-Hodgkin lymphoma	3 358	1.29	3.72	2.64	0.16	0.29	2 375	1.27	2.76	1.89	0.12	0.22	C82-C86,C96
免疫增生性疾病	Immunoproliferative diseases	71	0.03	0.08	0.06	0.00	0.01	50	0.03	0.06	0.04	0.00	0.00	C88
多发性骨髓瘤	Multiple myeloma	1 200	0.46	1.33	0.89	0.05	0.11	906	0.48	1.05	0.69	0.04	0.09	C90
淋巴样白血病	Lymphoid leukemia	813	0.31	0.90	0.83	0.04	0.07	605	0.32	0.70	0.66	0.04	0.05	C91
髓样白血病	Myeloid leukemia	1 940	0.75	2.15	1.65	0.10	0.16	1 495	0.80	1.74	1.31	0.08	0.13	C92-C94,D45- D47
白血病,未特指	Leukemia unspecified	1 823	0.70	2.02	1.71	0.10	0.16	1 460	0.78	1.69	1.42	0.08	0.13	C95
其他或未指明部位	Other and unspecified	4 936	1.90	5.47	3.90	0.22	0.42	4 074	2.18	4.73	3.19	0.18	0.34	O&U
所有部位合计	All sites	260 053	100.00	288.43	192.26	10.76	22.70	187 288	100.00	217.38	142.11	9.21	15.75	C00-C97,D32- D33,D42-D43, D45-D47
所有部位除外 C44	All sites except C44	258 028	99.22	286.18	190.76	10.68	22.54	185 238	98.91	215.00	140.66	9.14	15.61	C00-C97,D32- D33,D42-D43, D45-D47 exc. C44

部位 Site		男性 Male						女性 Female						ICD-10
		病例数 No. cases	构成率 Freq. /%	粗率 Crude rate/ $100\,000^{-1}$	世标率 ASR world/ $100\,000^{-1}$	累积率 Cum. Rate/% 0~64	0~74	病例数 No. cases	构成率 Freq. /%	粗率 Crude rate/ $100\,000^{-1}$	世标率 ASR world/ $100\,000^{-1}$	累积率 Cum. Rate/% 0~64	0~74	
唇	Lip	60	0.05	0.16	0.10	0.00	0.01	46	0.05	0.12	0.08	0.00	0.01	C00
舌	Tongue	381	0.34	1.00	0.68	0.04	0.08	200	0.23	0.54	0.34	0.02	0.04	C01-C02
口	Mouth	522	0.46	1.37	0.91	0.05	0.11	296	0.35	0.80	0.49	0.02	0.06	C03-C06
唾液腺	Salivary glands	190	0.17	0.50	0.35	0.02	0.04	174	0.20	0.47	0.33	0.02	0.04	C07-C08
扁桃腺	Tonsil	82	0.07	0.22	0.15	0.01	0.02	25	0.03	0.07	0.05	0.00	0.01	C09
其他口咽	Other oropharynx	205	0.18	0.54	0.35	0.02	0.04	32	0.04	0.09	0.06	0.00	0.01	C10
鼻咽	Nasopharynx	2 234	1.98	5.88	4.10	0.32	0.45	969	1.13	2.61	1.78	0.14	0.19	C11
下咽	Hypopharynx	343	0.30	0.90	0.61	0.04	0.08	23	0.03	0.06	0.04	0.00	0.01	C12-C13
咽,部位不明	Pharynx unspecified	172	0.15	0.45	0.30	0.02	0.04	61	0.07	0.16	0.09	0.00	0.01	C14
食管	Esophagus	9 110	8.09	23.96	15.75	0.79	2.02	2 445	2.86	6.60	3.86	0.14	0.47	C15
胃	Stomach	10 582	9.40	27.83	18.34	0.96	2.27	4 671	5.47	12.60	7.72	0.41	0.88	C16
小肠	Small intestine	507	0.45	1.33	0.88	0.05	0.11	373	0.44	1.01	0.63	0.04	0.07	C17
结肠	Colon	5 464	4.85	14.37	9.37	0.49	1.07	4 203	4.92	11.34	6.93	0.35	0.81	C18
直肠	Rectum	6 952	6.18	18.29	12.02	0.61	1.49	4 371	5.12	11.80	7.22	0.38	0.84	C19-C20
肛门	Anus	196	0.17	0.52	0.34	0.02	0.04	139	0.16	0.38	0.23	0.01	0.04	C21
肝脏	Liver	16 077	14.28	42.29	28.65	1.93	3.32	5 397	6.32	14.56	8.97	0.46	1.03	C22
胆囊及其他	Gallbladder etc.	1 224	1.09	3.22	2.07	0.10	0.24	1 395	1.63	3.76	2.22	0.10	0.26	C23-C24
胰腺	Pancreas	2 729	2.42	7.18	4.68	0.25	0.57	1 957	2.29	5.28	3.13	0.14	0.37	C25
鼻、鼻窦及其他	Nose,sinuses etc.	214	0.19	0.56	0.39	0.02	0.05	106	0.12	0.29	0.19	0.01	0.02	C30-C31
喉	Larynx	1 245	1.11	3.27	2.18	0.12	0.28	136	0.16	0.37	0.22	0.01	0.03	C32
气管、支气管、肺	Trachea,bronchus & lung	30 102	26.74	79.18	51.90	2.70	6.41	14 263	16.70	38.49	23.63	1.24	2.80	C33-C34
其他胸腔器官	Other thoracic organs	401	0.36	1.05	0.76	0.05	0.08	235	0.28	0.63	0.44	0.03	0.05	C37-C38
骨	Bone	782	0.69	2.06	1.52	0.08	0.15	527	0.62	1.42	1.04	0.06	0.11	C40-C41
皮肤黑色素瘤	Melanoma of skin	186	0.17	0.49	0.32	0.02	0.03	183	0.21	0.49	0.33	0.02	0.04	C43
皮肤其他	Other skin	935	0.83	2.46	1.60	0.08	0.17	959	1.12	2.59	1.58	0.07	0.17	C44
间皮瘤	Mesothelioma	40	0.04	0.11	0.07	0.00	0.01	25	0.03	0.07	0.05	0.00	0.01	C45
卡波氏肉瘤	Kaposi sarcoma	36	0.03	0.09	0.07	0.00	0.01	23	0.03	0.06	0.04	0.00	0.01	C46
结缔组织、软组织	Connective & soft tissue	384	0.34	1.01	0.78	0.05	0.08	323	0.38	0.87	0.64	0.04	0.06	C47,C49
乳腺	Breast	336	0.30	0.88	0.61	0.04	0.06	12 657	14.82	34.16	23.22	1.93	2.50	C50
外阴	Vulva	—	—	—	—	—	—	187	0.22	0.50	0.33	0.02	0.04	C51
阴道	Vagina	—	—	—	—	—	—	109	0.13	0.29	0.19	0.01	0.02	C52
子宫颈	Cervix uteri	—	—	—	—	—	—	6 425	7.52	17.34	11.85	0.97	1.29	C53
子宫体	Corpus uteri	—	—	—	—	—	—	2 822	3.30	7.62	5.17	0.44	0.57	C54
子宫,部位不明	Uterus unspecified	—	—	—	—	—	—	491	0.57	1.32	0.88	0.07	0.10	C55
卵巢	Ovary	—	—	—	—	—	—	3 048	3.57	8.23	5.76	0.44	0.62	C56
其他女性生殖器	Other female genital organs	—	—	—	—	—	—	177	0.21	0.48	0.33	0.03	0.04	C57
胎盘	Placenta	—	—	—	—	—	—	38	0.04	0.10	0.09	0.01	0.01	C58
阴茎	Penis	258	0.23	0.68	0.46	0.03	0.05	—	—	—	—	—	—	C60
前列腺	Prostate	4 417	3.92	11.62	6.92	0.14	0.70	—	—	—	—	—	—	C61
睾丸	Testis	163	0.14	0.43	0.36	0.02	0.03	—	—	—	—	—	—	C62
其他男性生殖器	Other male genital organs	53	0.05	0.14	0.09	0.01	0.01	—	—	—	—	—	—	C63
肾	Kidney	1 378	1.22	3.62	2.48	0.17	0.28	888	1.04	2.40	1.60	0.10	0.18	C64
肾盂	Renal pelvis	200	0.18	0.53	0.34	0.02	0.04	132	0.15	0.36	0.21	0.01	0.02	C65
输尿管	Ureter	169	0.15	0.44	0.27	0.01	0.03	150	0.18	0.40	0.23	0.01	0.03	C66
膀胱	Bladder	3 022	2.68	7.95	5.02	0.21	0.54	926	1.08	2.50	1.51	0.07	0.18	C67
其他泌尿器官	Other urinary organs	39	0.03	0.10	0.07	0.00	0.01	34	0.04	0.09	0.06	0.00	0.01	C68
眼	Eye	65	0.06	0.17	0.15	0.01	0.01	62	0.07	0.17	0.15	0.01	0.01	C69
脑、神经系统	Brain,nervous system	2 251	2.00	5.92	4.45	0.28	0.46	2 553	2.99	6.89	4.80	0.32	0.51	C70-C72,D32-D33,D42-D43
甲状腺	Thyroid	1 975	1.75	5.19	3.87	0.31	0.37	5 712	6.69	15.41	11.35	0.94	1.08	C73
肾上腺	Adrenal gland	110	0.10	0.29	0.22	0.01	0.02	85	0.10	0.23	0.15	0.01	0.01	C74
其他内分泌腺	Other endocrine	120	0.11	0.32	0.25	0.02	0.02	147	0.17	0.40	0.29	0.02	0.03	C75
霍奇金淋巴瘤	Hodgkin lymphoma	162	0.14	0.43	0.33	0.02	0.03	86	0.10	0.23	0.18	0.01	0.02	C81
非霍奇金淋巴瘤	Non-Hodgkin lymphoma	1 636	1.45	4.30	3.03	0.18	0.34	1 182	1.38	3.19	2.14	0.13	0.25	C82-C86,C96
免疫增生性疾病	Immunoproliferative diseases	61	0.05	0.16	0.13	0.01	0.01	40	0.05	0.11	0.09	0.00	0.01	C88
多发性骨髓瘤	Multiple myeloma	581	0.52	1.53	1.00	0.05	0.13	459	0.54	1.24	0.80	0.04	0.10	C90
淋巴样白血病	Lymphoid leukemia	400	0.36	1.05	0.98	0.05	0.08	323	0.38	0.87	0.84	0.05	0.07	C91
髓样白血病	Myeloid leukemia	877	0.78	2.31	1.75	0.11	0.17	723	0.85	1.95	1.44	0.09	0.15	C92-C94,D45-D47
白血病,未特指	Leukemia unspecified	658	0.58	1.73	1.50	0.08	0.14	501	0.59	1.35	1.10	0.06	0.10	C95
其他或未指明部位	Other and unspecified	2 270	2.02	5.97	4.23	0.23	0.45	1 903	2.23	5.14	3.46	0.19	0.36	O&U
所有部位合计	All sites	112 556	100.00	296.05	197.75	10.85	23.25	85 417	100.00	230.50	150.54	9.72	16.68	C00-C97、D32-D33、D42-D43、D45-D47
所有部位除外 C44	All sites except C44	111 621	99.17	293.59	196.15	10.77	23.08	84 458	98.88	227.91	148.96	9.65	16.51	C00-C97、D32-D33、D42-D43、D45-D47 exc. C44

附表 2-9　2018 年全国西部农村肿瘤登记地区癌症发病主要指标
Appendix Table 2-9　Cancer incidence in Western rural registration areas of China,2018

部位 Site		男性 Male						女性 Female						ICD-10
		病例数 No. cases	构成 Freq. /%	粗率 Crude rate/ $100\,000^{-1}$	世标率 ASR world/ $100\,000^{-1}$	累积率 Cum. Rate/%		病例数 No. cases	构成 Freq. /%	粗率 Crude rate/ $100\,000^{-1}$	世标率 ASR world/ $100\,000^{-1}$	累积率 Cum. Rate/%		
						0~64	0~74					0~64	0~74	
唇	Lip	107	0.07	0.21	0.14	0.01	0.02	57	0.06	0.12	0.08	0.00	0.01	C00
舌	Tongue	495	0.34	0.95	0.64	0.04	0.08	251	0.25	0.51	0.33	0.02	0.04	C01-C02
口	Mouth	877	0.59	1.68	1.11	0.06	0.13	383	0.38	0.78	0.51	0.03	0.06	C03-C06
唾液腺	Salivary glands	280	0.19	0.54	0.38	0.02	0.04	215	0.21	0.44	0.32	0.02	0.03	C07-C08
扁桃腺	Tonsil	101	0.07	0.19	0.14	0.01	0.02	42	0.04	0.09	0.06	0.00	0.01	C09
其他口咽	Other oropharynx	252	0.17	0.48	0.32	0.02	0.04	52	0.05	0.11	0.07	0.00	0.01	C10
鼻咽	Nasopharynx	3 203	2.17	6.14	4.36	0.34	0.47	1 335	1.31	2.72	1.91	0.15	0.21	C11
下咽	Hypopharynx	326	0.22	0.63	0.42	0.03	0.05	43	0.04	0.09	0.06	0.00	0.01	C12-C13
咽,部位不明	Pharynx unspecified	285	0.19	0.55	0.36	0.02	0.04	82	0.08	0.17	0.10	0.01	0.01	C14
食管	Esophagus	16 238	11.01	31.14	20.07	0.97	2.58	4 469	4.39	9.10	5.19	0.19	0.62	C15
胃	Stomach	15 586	10.57	29.89	19.42	1.02	2.44	6 483	6.36	13.20	7.95	0.42	0.91	C16
小肠	Small intestine	499	0.34	0.96	0.64	0.04	0.08	350	0.34	0.71	0.45	0.03	0.05	C17
结肠	Colon	4 837	3.28	9.28	6.12	0.35	0.71	3 664	3.60	7.46	4.65	0.27	0.55	C18
直肠	Rectum	8 920	6.05	17.11	11.11	0.58	1.34	5 810	5.70	11.83	7.23	0.39	0.86	C19-C20
肛门	Anus	276	0.19	0.53	0.35	0.02	0.04	173	0.17	0.35	0.22	0.01	0.02	C21
肝脏	Liver	24 459	16.58	46.91	31.88	2.20	3.67	7 582	7.44	15.44	9.56	0.53	1.12	C22
胆囊及其他	Gallbladder etc.	1 340	0.91	2.57	1.65	0.08	0.20	1 555	1.53	3.17	1.87	0.09	0.23	C23-C24
胰腺	Pancreas	3 148	2.13	6.04	3.92	0.21	0.47	2 093	2.05	4.26	2.56	0.13	0.	C25
鼻、鼻窦及其他	Nose,sinuses etc.	290	0.20	0.56	0.39	0.03	0.04	169	0.17	0.34	0.23	0.01	0.03	C30-C31
喉	Larynx	1 260	0.85	2.42	1.58	0.10	0.20	147	0.14	0.30	0.19	0.01	0.02	C32
气管、支气管、肺	Trachea,bronchus & lung	38 980	26.43	74.76	48.72	2.68	5.99	18 829	18.48	38.35	23.36	1.27	2.77	C33-C34
其他胸腔器官	Other thoracic organs	472	0.32	0.91	0.67	0.04	0.07	297	0.29	0.60	0.40	0.03	0.04	C37-C38
骨	Bone	1 237	0.84	2.37	1.74	0.10	0.18	880	0.86	1.79	1.31	0.08	0.13	C40-C41
皮肤黑色素瘤	Melanoma of skin	196	0.13	0.38	0.26	0.02	0.03	186	0.18	0.38	0.25	0.02	0.03	C43
皮肤其他	Other skin	1 090	0.74	2.09	1.41	0.07	0.15	1 091	1.07	2.22	1.35	0.07	0.13	C44
间皮瘤	Mesothelioma	61	0.04	0.12	0.08	0.01	0.01	58	0.06	0.12	0.08	0.01	0.01	C45
卡波氏肉瘤	Kaposi sarcoma	16	0.01	0.03	0.02	0.00	0.00	3	0.00	0.01	0.00	0.00	0.00	C46
结缔组织、软组织	Connective & soft tissue	468	0.32	0.90	0.71	0.05	0.07	333	0.33	0.68	0.51	0.03	0.05	C47,C49
乳腺	Breast	231	0.16	0.44	0.30	0.02	0.03	12 507	12.28	25.47	17.80	1.50	1.85	C50
外阴	Vulva	—	—	—	—	—	—	226	0.22	0.46	0.30	0.02	0.03	C51
阴道	Vagina	—	—	—	—	—	—	147	0.14	0.30	0.20	0.01	0.02	C52
子宫颈	Cervix uteri	—	—	—	—	—	—	9 158	8.99	18.65	12.91	1.04	1.39	C53
子宫体	Corpus uteri	—	—	—	—	—	—	3 282	3.22	6.68	4.58	0.39	0.51	C54
子宫,部位不明	Uterus unspecified	—	—	—	—	—	—	1 073	1.05	2.19	1.48	0.12	0.16	C55
卵巢	Ovary	—	—	—	—	—	—	3 005	2.95	6.12	4.38	0.34	0.47	C56
其他女性生殖器	Other female genital organs	—	—	—	—	—	—	211	0.21	0.43	0.30	0.02	0.03	C57
胎盘	Placenta	—	—	—	—	—	—	52	0.05	0.11	0.09	0.01	0.01	C58
阴茎	Penis	403	0.27	0.77	0.52	0.03	0.06	—	—	—	—	—	—	C60
前列腺	Prostate	3 715	2.52	7.12	4.21	0.08	0.45	—	—	—	—	—	—	C61
睾丸	Testis	225	0.15	0.43	0.36	0.02	0.03	—	—	—	—	—	—	C62
其他男性生殖器	Other male genital organs	37	0.03	0.07	0.05	0.00	0.01	—	—	—	—	—	—	C63
肾	Kidney	1 115	0.76	2.14	1.47	0.10	0.17	657	0.64	1.34	0.88	0.06	0.10	C64
肾盂	Renal pelvis	161	0.11	0.31	0.20	0.01	0.02	107	0.11	0.22	0.14	0.01	0.02	C65
输尿管	Ureter	157	0.11	0.30	0.20	0.01	0.03	131	0.13	0.27	0.16	0.01	0.02	C66
膀胱	Bladder	3 566	2.42	6.84	4.31	0.19	0.48	872	0.86	1.78	1.04	0.05	0.12	C67
其他泌尿器官	Other urinary organs	38	0.03	0.07	0.05	0.00	0.01	34	0.03	0.07	0.04	0.00	0.01	C68
眼	Eye	94	0.06	0.18	0.16	0.01	0.02	72	0.07	0.15	0.11	0.01	0.01	C69
脑、神经系统	Brain,nervous system	3 235	2.19	6.20	4.64	0.30	0.47	3 420	3.36	6.97	4.93	0.33	0.53	C70-C72,D32-D33,D42-D43
甲状腺	Thyroid	1 129	0.77	2.17	1.67	0.13	0.16	4 085	4.01	8.32	6.36	0.52	0.59	C73
肾上腺	Adrenal gland	119	0.08	0.23	0.17	0.01	0.02	104	0.10	0.21	0.14	0.01	0.02	C74
其他内分泌腺	Other endocrine	140	0.09	0.27	0.19	0.01	0.02	146	0.14	0.30	0.22	0.02	0.02	C75
霍奇金淋巴瘤	Hodgkin lymphoma	175	0.12	0.34	0.26	0.02	0.03	116	0.11	0.24	0.18	0.01	0.02	C81
非霍奇金淋巴瘤	Non-Hodgkin lymphoma	1 722	1.17	3.30	2.36	0.14	0.27	1 193	1.17	2.43	1.71	0.11	0.19	C82-C86,C96
免疫增生性疾病	Immunoproliferative diseases	10	0.01	0.02	0.02	0.00	0.00	10	0.01	0.02	0.01	0.00	0.00	C88
多发性骨髓瘤	Multiple myeloma	619	0.42	1.19	0.81	0.05	0.10	447	0.44	0.91	0.61	0.04	0.08	C90
淋巴样白血病	Lymphoid leukemia	413	0.28	0.79	0.73	0.04	0.06	282	0.28	0.57	0.54	0.03	0.04	C91
髓样白血病	Myeloid leukemia	1 063	0.72	2.04	1.59	0.10	0.16	772	0.76	1.57	1.22	0.08	0.12	C92-C94,D45-D47
白血病,未特指	Leukemia unspecified	1 165	0.79	2.23	1.87	0.10	0.17	959	0.94	1.95	1.65	0.10	0.15	C95
其他或未指明部位	Other and unspecified	2 666	1.81	5.11	3.66	0.21	0.40	2 171	2.13	4.42	2.99	0.18	0.33	O&U
所有部位合计	All sites	147 497	100.00	282.87	188.39	10.70	22.32	101 871	100.00	207.47	135.80	8.82	15.06	C00-C97、D32-D33,D42-D43,D45-D47
所有部位除外 C44	All sites except C44	146 407	99.26	280.78	186.98	10.63	22.17	100 780	98.93	205.25	134.45	8.76	14.93	C00-C97、D32-D33,D42-D43,D45-D47 exc. C44

附表 2-10　2018 年全国东部肿瘤登记地区癌症死亡主要指标
Appendix Table 2-10　Cancer mortality in Eastern registration areas of China,2018

部位 Site		男性 Male						女性 Female						ICD-10
		死亡数 No. deaths	构成 Freq./%	粗率 Crude rate/ 100 000^{-1}	世标率 ASR world/ 100 000^{-1}	累积率 Cum. Rate/%		死亡数 No. deaths	构成 Freq./%	粗率 Crude rate/ 100 000^{-1}	世标率 ASR world/ 100 000^{-1}	累积率 Cum. Rate/%		
						0~64	0~74					0~64	0~74	
唇	Lip	92	0.03	0.08	0.04	0.00	0.00	55	0.04	0.05	0.02	0.00	0.00	C00
舌	Tongue	679	0.26	0.62	0.35	0.02	0.04	370	0.24	0.34	0.16	0.01	0.02	C01-C02
口	Mouth	862	0.33	0.79	0.42	0.02	0.05	519	0.33	0.48	0.20	0.01	0.02	C03-C06
唾液腺	Salivary glands	325	0.12	0.30	0.16	0.01	0.02	179	0.12	0.17	0.08	0.00	0.01	C07-C08
扁桃腺	Tonsil	130	0.05	0.12	0.07	0.00	0.01	37	0.02	0.03	0.02	0.00	0.00	C09
其他口咽	Other oropharynx	262	0.10	0.24	0.14	0.01	0.02	61	0.04	0.06	0.03	0.00	0.00	C10
鼻咽	Nasopharynx	3 159	1.20	2.90	1.72	0.11	0.21	1 079	0.70	1.00	0.54	0.03	0.06	C11
下咽	Hypopharynx	661	0.25	0.61	0.34	0.02	0.04	45	0.03	0.04	0.02	0.00	0.00	C12-C13
咽,部位不明	Pharynx unspecified	230	0.09	0.21	0.12	0.01	0.01	69	0.04	0.06	0.03	0.00	0.00	C14
食管	Esophagus	23 810	9.03	21.83	11.47	0.46	1.36	8 806	5.68	8.15	3.36	0.07	0.34	C15
胃	Stomach	34 141	12.95	31.31	16.32	0.58	1.86	14 798	9.55	13.69	6.24	0.24	0.65	C16
小肠	Small intestine	1 131	0.43	1.04	0.56	0.02	0.06	692	0.45	0.64	0.29	0.01	0.03	C17
结肠	Colon	11 003	4.17	10.09	5.21	0.18	0.52	8 839	5.70	8.18	3.54	0.13	0.34	C18
直肠	Rectum	10 835	4.11	9.94	5.17	0.20	0.54	6 661	4.30	6.16	2.74	0.10	0.28	C19-C20
肛门	Anus	186	0.07	0.17	0.09	0.00	0.01	158	0.10	0.15	0.07	0.00	0.01	C21
肝脏	Liver	35 506	13.46	32.56	18.73	1.17	2.17	13 526	8.73	12.51	5.96	0.27	0.66	C22
胆囊及其他	Gallbladder etc.	4 201	1.59	3.85	2.00	0.07	0.22	4 351	2.81	4.03	1.78	0.06	0.19	C23-C24
胰腺	Pancreas	10 596	4.02	9.72	5.18	0.23	0.60	8 042	5.19	7.44	3.39	0.12	0.38	C25
鼻、鼻窦及其他	Nose,sinuses etc.	340	0.13	0.31	0.18	0.01	0.02	173	0.11	0.16	0.09	0.00	0.01	C30-C31
喉	Larynx	2 132	0.81	1.96	1.03	0.05	0.12	277	0.18	0.26	0.11	0.00	0.01	C32
气管、支气管、肺	Trachea,bronchus & lung	78 878	29.91	72.33	38.06	1.47	4.50	35 696	23.04	33.02	14.94	0.57	1.61	C33-C34
其他胸腔器官	Other thoracic organs	836	0.32	0.77	0.45	0.03	0.05	447	0.29	0.41	0.22	0.01	0.02	C37-C38
骨	Bone	1 520	0.58	1.39	0.85	0.04	0.08	1 053	0.68	0.97	0.54	0.03	0.05	C40-C41
皮肤黑色素瘤	Melanoma of skin	421	0.16	0.39	0.21	0.01	0.02	382	0.25	0.35	0.17	0.01	0.02	C43
皮肤其他	Other skin	965	0.37	0.88	0.43	0.01	0.03	936	0.60	0.87	0.32	0.01	0.02	C44
间皮瘤	Mesothelioma	208	0.08	0.19	0.11	0.01	0.01	143	0.09	0.13	0.07	0.00	0.01	C45
卡波氏肉瘤	Kaposi sarcoma	28	0.01	0.03	0.02	0.00	0.00	28	0.02	0.03	0.02	0.00	0.00	C46
结缔组织、软组织	Connective & soft tissue	523	0.20	0.48	0.29	0.01	0.03	370	0.24	0.34	0.20	0.01	0.02	C47,C49
乳腺	Breast	223	0.08	0.20	0.11	0.01	0.01	12 618	8.14	11.67	6.29	0.42	0.69	C50
外阴	Vulva	—	—	—	—	—	—	249	0.16	0.23	0.10	0.00	0.01	C51
阴道	Vagina	—	—	—	—	—	—	114	0.07	0.11	0.05	0.00	0.01	C52
子宫颈	Cervix uteri	—	—	—	—	—	—	5 202	3.36	4.81	2.73	0.19	0.30	C53
子宫体	Corpus uteri	—	—	—	—	—	—	2 030	1.31	1.88	0.97	0.06	0.11	C54
子宫,部位不明	Uterus unspecified	—	—	—	—	—	—	829	0.54	0.77	0.39	0.02	0.04	C55
卵巢	Ovary	—	—	—	—	—	—	4 698	3.03	4.35	2.37	0.15	0.28	C56
其他女性生殖器	Other female genital organs	—	—	—	—	—	—	255	0.16	0.24	0.12	0.01	0.01	C57
胎盘	Placenta	—	—	—	—	—	—	8	0.01	0.01	0.01	0.00	0.00	C58
阴茎	Penis	306	0.12	0.28	0.15	0.01	0.01	—	—	—	—	—	—	C60
前列腺	Prostate	7 250	2.75	6.65	3.07	0.03	0.20	—	—	—	—	—	—	C61
睾丸	Testis	96	0.04	0.09	0.06	0.00	0.01	—	—	—	—	—	—	C62
其他男性生殖器	Other male genital organs	96	0.04	0.09	0.05	0.00	0.00	—	—	—	—	—	—	C63
肾	Kidney	2 728	1.03	2.50	1.36	0.06	0.15	1 293	0.83	1.20	0.56	0.02	0.06	C64
肾盂	Renal pelvis	372	0.14	0.34	0.18	0.01	0.02	239	0.15	0.22	0.09	0.00	0.01	C65
输尿管	Ureter	426	0.16	0.39	0.19	0.01	0.02	370	0.24	0.34	0.14	0.00	0.01	C66
膀胱	Bladder	5 442	2.06	4.99	2.39	0.05	0.19	1 549	1.00	1.43	0.54	0.01	0.04	C67
其他泌尿器官	Other urinary organs	115	0.04	0.11	0.05	0.00	0.00	64	0.04	0.06	0.03	0.00	0.00	C68
眼	Eye	71	0.03	0.07	0.05	0.00	0.00	70	0.05	0.06	0.04	0.00	0.00	C69
脑、神经系统	Brain,nervous system	5 390	2.04	4.94	3.16	0.17	0.33	4 419	2.85	4.09	2.35	0.12	0.24	C70-C72,D32-D33,D42-D43
甲状腺	Thyroid	576	0.22	0.53	0.29	0.01	0.03	963	0.62	0.89	0.45	0.02	0.05	C73
肾上腺	Adrenal gland	276	0.10	0.25	0.15	0.01	0.02	169	0.11	0.16	0.09	0.00	0.01	C74
其他内分泌腺	Other endocrine	186	0.07	0.17	0.10	0.00	0.01	142	0.09	0.13	0.08	0.00	0.01	C75
霍奇金淋巴瘤	Hodgkin lymphoma	244	0.09	0.22	0.13	0.01	0.01	118	0.08	0.11	0.06	0.00	0.01	C81
非霍奇金淋巴瘤	Non-Hodgkin lymphoma	4 421	1.68	4.05	2.28	0.10	0.25	2 937	1.90	2.72	1.35	0.06	0.15	C82-C86,C96
免疫增生性疾病	Immunoproliferative diseases	51	0.02	0.05	0.02	0.00	0.00	17	0.01	0.02	0.01	0.00	0.00	C88
多发性骨髓瘤	Multiple myeloma	1 573	0.60	1.44	0.78	0.03	0.09	1 145	0.74	1.06	0.54	0.02	0.07	C90
淋巴样白血病	Lymphoid leukemia	1 093	0.41	1.00	0.75	0.04	0.07	797	0.51	0.74	0.55	0.03	0.05	C91
髓样白血病	Myeloid leukemia	2 853	1.08	2.62	1.54	0.07	0.16	1 997	1.29	1.85	1.05	0.05	0.11	C92-C94,D45-D47
白血病,未特指	Leukemia unspecified	1 858	0.70	1.70	1.08	0.05	0.11	1 381	0.89	1.28	0.77	0.04	0.08	D95
其他或未指明部位	Other and unspecified	4 417	1.67	4.05	2.23	0.10	0.24	3 471	2.24	3.21	1.55	0.07	0.15	O&U
所有部位合计	All sites	263 723	100.00	241.83	129.89	5.53	14.56	154 936	100.00	143.34	68.37	3.05	7.25	C00-C97,D32-D33,D42-D43,D45-D47
所有部位除外 C44	All sites except C44	262 758	99.63	240.95	129.45	5.53	14.52	154 000	99.40	142.47	68.05	3.04	7.23	C00-C97,D32-D33,D42-D43,D45-D47 exc.C44

附表 2-11　2018 年全国东部城市肿瘤登记地区癌症死亡主要指标
Appendix Table 2-11　Cancer mortality in Eastern urban registration areas of China, 2018

部位 Site		男性 Male						女性 Female						ICD-10
		死亡数 No. deaths	构成 Freq./%	粗率 Crude rate/ $100\,000^{-1}$	世标率 ASR world/ $100\,000^{-1}$	累积率 Cum. Rate/% 0~64	0~74	死亡数 No. deaths	构成 Freq./%	粗率 Crude rate/ $100\,000^{-1}$	世标率 ASR world/ $100\,000^{-1}$	累积率 Cum. Rate/% 0~64	0~74	
唇	Lip	27	0.02	0.05	0.02	0.00	0.00	23	0.03	0.04	0.02	0.00	0.00	C00
舌	Tongue	397	0.29	0.71	0.39	0.02	0.05	237	0.29	0.42	0.19	0.01	0.02	C01-C02
口	Mouth	498	0.37	0.89	0.46	0.03	0.05	297	0.36	0.52	0.21	0.01	0.02	C03-C06
唾液腺	Salivary glands	181	0.13	0.32	0.17	0.01	0.02	107	0.13	0.19	0.09	0.00	0.01	C07-C08
扁桃腺	Tonsil	76	0.06	0.14	0.08	0.01	0.01	19	0.02	0.03	0.02	0.00	0.00	C09
其他口咽	Other oropharynx	179	0.13	0.32	0.18	0.01	0.02	36	0.04	0.06	0.03	0.00	0.00	C10
鼻咽	Nasopharynx	1 797	1.33	3.20	1.87	0.12	0.23	585	0.72	1.03	0.55	0.03	0.07	C11
下咽	Hypopharynx	424	0.31	0.76	0.42	0.03	0.05	24	0.03	0.04	0.02	0.00	0.00	C12-C13
咽,部位不明	Pharynx unspecified	115	0.08	0.21	0.11	0.01	0.01	33	0.04	0.06	0.03	0.00	0.00	C14
食管	Esophagus	9 990	7.38	17.81	9.19	0.43	1.10	3 047	3.73	5.38	2.09	0.04	0.19	C15
胃	Stomach	16 057	11.86	28.63	14.42	0.52	1.63	7 152	8.75	12.63	5.61	0.22	0.57	C16
小肠	Small intestine	653	0.48	1.16	0.61	0.03	0.07	427	0.52	0.75	0.33	0.01	0.04	C17
结肠	Colon	6 890	5.09	12.28	6.07	0.21	0.61	5 438	6.66	9.60	3.99	0.14	0.38	C18
直肠	Rectum	6 004	4.44	10.70	5.36	0.22	0.56	3 682	4.51	6.50	2.81	0.11	0.28	C19-C20
肛门	Anus	97	0.07	0.17	0.09	0.00	0.01	79	0.10	0.14	0.06	0.00	0.01	C21
肝脏	Liver	17 769	13.13	31.68	17.73	1.11	2.06	6 758	8.27	11.93	5.43	0.23	0.59	C22
胆囊及其他	Gallbladder etc.	2 327	1.72	4.15	2.06	0.08	0.22	2 291	2.80	4.05	1.72	0.06	0.18	C23-C24
胰腺	Pancreas	5 696	4.21	10.15	5.24	0.24	0.60	4 456	5.45	7.87	3.48	0.13	0.38	C25
鼻、鼻窦及其他	Nose, sinuses etc.	172	0.13	0.31	0.17	0.01	0.02	83	0.10	0.15	0.07	0.00	0.01	C30-C31
喉	Larynx	1 168	0.86	2.08	1.07	0.05	0.12	150	0.18	0.26	0.10	0.00	0.01	C32
气管、支气管、肺	Trachea, bronchus & lung	40 225	29.72	71.71	36.43	1.44	4.25	188 49	23.07	33.29	14.41	0.54	1.48	C33-C34
其他胸腔器官	Other thoracic organs	514	0.38	0.92	0.53	0.03	0.06	267	0.33	0.47	0.24	0.01	0.03	C37-C38
骨	Bone	676	0.50	1.21	0.72	0.04	0.07	476	0.58	0.84	0.45	0.02	0.04	C40-C41
皮肤黑色素瘤	Melanoma of skin	203	0.15	0.36	0.19	0.01	0.02	201	0.25	0.35	0.17	0.01	0.02	C43
皮肤其他	Other skin	461	0.34	0.82	0.39	0.01	0.03	400	0.49	0.71	0.25	0.01	0.02	C44
间皮瘤	Mesothelioma	142	0.10	0.25	0.14	0.01	0.02	100	0.12	0.18	0.09	0.00	0.01	C45
卡波氏肉瘤	Kaposi sarcoma	20	0.01	0.04	0.02	0.00	0.00	18	0.02	0.03	0.02	0.00	0.00	C46
结缔组织、软组织	Connective & soft tissue	280	0.21	0.50	0.29	0.02	0.03	227	0.28	0.40	0.25	0.01	0.02	C47, C49
乳腺	Breast	121	0.09	0.22	0.11	0.00	0.01	7 359	9.01	13.00	6.84	0.46	0.74	C50
外阴	Vulva	—	—	—	—	—	—	141	0.17	0.25	0.11	0.00	0.01	C51
阴道	Vagina	—	—	—	—	—	—	72	0.09	0.13	0.06	0.00	0.01	C52
子宫颈	Cervix uteri	—	—	—	—	—	—	2 577	3.15	4.55	2.57	0.19	0.28	C53
子宫体	Corpus uteri	—	—	—	—	—	—	1171	1.43	2.07	1.05	0.07	0.12	C54
子宫,部位不明	Uterus unspecified	—	—	—	—	—	—	407	0.50	0.72	0.36	0.02	0.04	C55
卵巢	Ovary	—	—	—	—	—	—	2 767	3.39	4.89	2.61	0.17	0.31	C56
其他女性生殖器	Other female genital organs	—	—	—	—	—	—	159	0.19	0.28	0.14	0.01	0.02	C57
胎盘	Placenta	—	—	—	—	—	—	3	0.00	0.01	0.00	0.00	0.00	C58
阴茎	Penis	135	0.10	0.24	0.12	0.01	0.01	—	—	—	—	—	—	C60
前列腺	Prostate	4 205	3.11	7.50	3.26	0.03	0.21	—	—	—	—	—	—	C61
睾丸	Testis	46	0.03	0.08	0.06	0.00	0.00	—	—	—	—	—	—	C62
其他男性生殖器	Other male genital organs	55	0.04	0.10	0.05	0.00	0.00	—	—	—	—	—	—	C63
肾	Kidney	1 679	1.24	2.99	1.56	0.07	0.17	772	0.94	1.36	0.59	0.02	0.06	C64
肾盂	Renal pelvis	226	0.17	0.40	0.20	0.01	0.01	162	0.20	0.29	0.11	0.00	0.01	C65
输尿管	Ureter	259	0.19	0.46	0.21	0.01	0.02	245	0.30	0.43	0.16	0.00	0.01	C66
膀胱	Bladder	3 047	2.25	5.43	2.47	0.05	0.19	930	1.14	1.64	0.58	0.01	0.04	C67
其他泌尿器官	Other urinary organs	79	0.06	0.14	0.06	0.00	0.00	45	0.06	0.08	0.03	0.00	0.00	C68
眼	Eye	34	0.03	0.06	0.04	0.00	0.00	39	0.05	0.07	0.04	0.00	0.00	C69
脑、神经系统	Brain, nervous system	2 663	1.97	4.75	2.97	0.17	0.31	2 169	2.65	3.83	2.15	0.12	0.22	C70-C72, D32-D33, D42-D43
甲状腺	Thyroid	320	0.24	0.57	0.30	0.02	0.03	507	0.62	0.90	0.44	0.02	0.04	C73
肾上腺	Adrenal gland	136	0.10	0.24	0.15	0.01	0.02	86	0.11	0.15	0.08	0.00	0.01	C74
其他内分泌腺	Other endocrine	77	0.06	0.14	0.08	0.00	0.01	68	0.08	0.12	0.07	0.00	0.01	C75
霍奇金淋巴瘤	Hodgkin lymphoma	121	0.09	0.22	0.12	0.00	0.01	49	0.06	0.09	0.05	0.00	0.01	C81
非霍奇金淋巴瘤	Non-Hodgkin lymphoma	2 430	1.80	4.33	2.37	0.11	0.25	1 571	1.92	2.77	1.32	0.06	0.14	C82-C86, C96
免疫增生性疾病	Immunoproliferative diseases	29	0.02	0.05	0.03	0.00	0.00	7	0.01	0.01	0.01	0.00	0.00	C88
多发性骨髓瘤	Multiple myeloma	900	0.66	1.60	0.83	0.04	0.10	619	0.76	1.09	0.55	0.03	0.07	C90
淋巴样白血病	Lymphoid leukemia	570	0.42	1.02	0.74	0.04	0.07	420	0.51	0.74	0.55	0.03	0.05	C91
髓样白血病	Myeloid leukemia	1 693	1.25	3.02	1.70	0.08	0.18	1 125	1.38	1.99	1.06	0.05	0.11	C92-C94, D45-D47
白血病,未特指	Leukemia unspecified	868	0.64	1.55	0.93	0.04	0.09	641	0.78	1.13	0.64	0.03	0.06	C95
其他或未指明部位	Other and unspecified	2 609	1.93	4.65	2.45	0.11	0.26	2 136	2.61	3.77	1.75	0.08	0.17	O&U
所有部位合计	All sites	135 340	100.00	241.29	125.23	5.45	13.91	81 709	100.00	144.30	66.68	3.00	6.89	C00-C97, D32-D33, D42-D43, D45-D47
所有部位除外 C44	All sites except C44	134 879	99.66	240.47	124.84	5.44	13.88	81 309	99.51	143.59	66.43	3.00	6.87	C00-C97, D32-D33, D42-D43, D45-D47 exc. C44

附表 2-12 2018 年全国东部农村肿瘤登记地区癌症死亡主要指标
Appendix Table 2-12 Cancer mortality in Eastern rural registration areas of China, 2018

部位 Site		男性 Male						女性 Female						ICD-10
		死亡数 No. deaths	构成 Freq. /%	粗率 Crude rate/ $100\,000^{-1}$	世标率 ASR world/ $100\,000^{-1}$	累积率 Cum. Rate/%		死亡数 No. deaths	构成 Freq. /%	粗率 Crude rate/ $100\,000^{-1}$	世标率 ASR world/ $100\,000^{-1}$	累积率 Cum. Rate/%		
						0~64	0~74					0~64	0~74	
唇	Lip	65	0.05	0.12	0.07	0.00	0.01	32	0.04	0.06	0.03	0.00	0.00	C00
舌	Tongue	282	0.22	0.53	0.31	0.02	0.04	133	0.18	0.26	0.13	0.01	0.01	C01-C02
口	Mouth	364	0.28	0.69	0.38	0.02	0.04	222	0.30	0.43	0.20	0.01	0.02	C03-C06
唾液腺	Salivary glands	144	0.11	0.27	0.16	0.01	0.02	72	0.10	0.14	0.07	0.00	0.01	C07-C08
扁桃腺	Tonsil	54	0.04	0.10	0.06	0.00	0.01	18	0.02	0.03	0.02	0.00	0.00	C09
其他口咽	Other oropharynx	83	0.06	0.16	0.09	0.00	0.01	25	0.03	0.05	0.02	0.00	0.00	C10
鼻咽	Nasopharynx	1 362	1.06	2.57	1.55	0.10	0.18	494	0.67	0.96	0.52	0.03	0.06	C11
下咽	Hypopharynx	237	0.18	0.45	0.26	0.01	0.03	21	0.03	0.04	0.02	0.00	0.00	C12-C13
咽,部位不明	Pharynx unspecified	115	0.09	0.22	0.12	0.00	0.01	36	0.05	0.07	0.03	0.00	0.00	C14
食管	Esophagus	13 820	10.76	26.09	14.09	0.50	1.66	5 759	7.86	11.19	4.82	0.10	0.50	C15
胃	Stomach	18 084	14.09	34.15	18.47	0.65	2.12	7 646	10.44	14.86	6.98	0.26	0.74	C16
小肠	Small intestine	478	0.37	0.90	0.51	0.02	0.06	265	0.36	0.51	0.25	0.01	0.03	C17
结肠	Colon	4 113	3.20	7.77	4.22	0.15	0.42	3 401	4.64	6.61	3.01	0.11	0.29	C18
直肠	Rectum	4 831	3.76	9.12	4.95	0.18	0.51	2 979	4.07	5.79	2.65	0.10	0.28	C19-C20
肛门	Anus	89	0.07	0.17	0.09	0.00	0.01	79	0.11	0.15	0.07	0.00	0.01	C21
肝脏	Liver	17 737	13.82	33.49	19.81	1.23	2.28	6 768	9.24	13.15	6.55	0.31	0.74	C22
胆囊及其他	Gallbladder etc.	1 874	1.46	3.54	1.92	0.07	0.22	2 060	2.81	4.00	1.83	0.06	0.21	C23-C24
胰腺	Pancreas	4 900	3.82	9.25	5.11	0.22	0.61	3 586	4.90	6.97	3.28	0.12	0.37	C25
鼻、鼻窦及其他	Nose, sinuses etc.	168	0.13	0.32	0.18	0.01	0.02	90	0.12	0.17	0.10	0.01	0.01	C30-C31
喉	Larynx	964	0.75	1.82	0.99	0.04	0.12	127	0.17	0.25	0.11	0.00	0.01	C32
气管、支气管、肺	Trachea, bronchus & lung	38 653	30.11	72.98	39.85	1.52	4.77	16 847	23.01	32.73	15.52	0.61	1.76	C33-C34
其他胸腔器官	Other thoracic organs	322	0.25	0.61	0.37	0.02	0.04	180	0.25	0.35	0.20	0.01	0.02	C37-C38
骨	Bone	844	0.66	1.59	1.00	0.05	0.10	577	0.79	1.12	0.64	0.03	0.07	C40-C41
皮肤黑色素瘤	Melanoma of skin	218	0.17	0.41	0.23	0.01	0.02	181	0.25	0.35	0.17	0.01	0.02	C43
皮肤其他	Other skin	504	0.39	0.95	0.50	0.01	0.04	536	0.73	1.04	0.40	0.01	0.02	C44
间皮瘤	Mesothelioma	66	0.05	0.12	0.07	0.00	0.01	43	0.06	0.08	0.05	0.00	0.01	C45
卡波氏肉瘤	Kaposi sarcoma	8	0.01	0.02	0.01	0.00	0.00	10	0.01	0.02	0.01	0.00	0.00	C46
结缔组织、软组织	Connective & soft tissue	243	0.19	0.46	0.29	0.01	0.03	143	0.20	0.28	0.16	0.01	0.02	C47, C49
乳腺	Breast	102	0.08	0.19	0.11	0.01	0.01	5 259	7.18	10.22	5.67	0.38	0.63	C50
外阴	Vulva	—	—	—	—	—	—	108	0.15	0.21	0.10	0.00	0.01	C51
阴道	Vagina	—	—	—	—	—	—	42	0.06	0.08	0.04	0.00	0.01	C52
子宫颈	Cervix uteri	—	—	—	—	—	—	2 625	3.58	5.10	2.90	0.20	0.33	C53
子宫体	Corpus uteri	—	—	—	—	—	—	859	1.17	1.67	0.88	0.05	0.11	C54
子宫,部位不明	Uterus unspecified	—	—	—	—	—	—	422	0.58	0.82	0.43	0.02	0.05	C55
卵巢	Ovary	—	—	—	—	—	—	1 931	2.64	3.75	2.11	0.14	0.26	C56
其他女性生殖器	Other female genital organs	—	—	—	—	—	—	96	0.13	0.19	0.10	0.01	0.01	C57
胎盘	Placenta	—	—	—	—	—	—	5	0.01	0.01	0.01	0.00	0.00	C58
阴茎	Penis	171	0.13	0.32	0.18	0.01	0.02	—	—	—	—	—	—	C60
前列腺	Prostate	3 045	2.37	5.75	2.84	0.03	0.19	—	—	—	—	—	—	C61
睾丸	Testis	50	0.04	0.09	0.06	0.00	0.01	—	—	—	—	—	—	C62
其他男性生殖器	Other male genital organs	41	0.03	0.08	0.04	0.00	0.00	—	—	—	—	—	—	C63
肾	Kidney	1 049	0.82	1.98	1.13	0.05	0.13	521	0.71	1.01	0.52	0.02	0.05	C64
肾盂	Renal pelvis	146	0.11	0.28	0.14	0.01	0.01	77	0.11	0.15	0.07	0.00	0.01	C65
输尿管	Ureter	167	0.13	0.32	0.17	0.01	0.02	125	0.17	0.24	0.11	0.00	0.01	C66
膀胱	Bladder	2 395	1.87	4.52	2.30	0.04	0.18	619	0.85	1.20	0.48	0.01	0.04	C67
其他泌尿器官	Other urinary organs	36	0.03	0.07	0.04	0.00	0.00	19	0.03	0.04	0.02	0.00	0.00	C68
眼	Eye	37	0.03	0.07	0.05	0.00	0.00	31	0.04	0.06	0.04	0.00	0.00	C69
脑、神经系统	Brain, nervous system	2 727	2.12	5.15	3.37	0.18	0.36	2 250	3.07	4.37	2.57	0.13	0.26	C70-C72, D32-D33, D42-D43
甲状腺	Thyroid	256	0.20	0.48	0.28	0.01	0.03	456	0.62	0.89	0.46	0.02	0.05	C73
肾上腺	Adrenal gland	140	0.11	0.26	0.16	0.01	0.02	83	0.11	0.16	0.10	0.00	0.01	C74
其他内分泌腺	Other endocrine	109	0.08	0.21	0.13	0.01	0.01	74	0.10	0.14	0.08	0.00	0.01	C75
霍奇金淋巴瘤	Hodgkin lymphoma	123	0.10	0.23	0.14	0.01	0.02	69	0.09	0.13	0.07	0.00	0.01	C81
非霍奇金淋巴瘤	Non-Hodgkin lymphoma	1 991	1.55	3.76	2.18	0.10	0.24	1 366	1.87	2.65	1.38	0.06	0.16	C82-C86, C96
免疫增生性疾病	Immunoproliferative diseases	22	0.02	0.04	0.02	0.00	0.00	10	0.01	0.02	0.01	0.00	0.00	C88
多发性骨髓瘤	Multiple myeloma	673	0.52	1.27	0.72	0.03	0.09	526	0.72	1.02	0.53	0.02	0.07	C90
淋巴样白血病	Lymphoid leukemia	523	0.41	0.99	0.76	0.04	0.07	377	0.51	0.73	0.55	0.03	0.05	C91
髓样白血病	Myeloid leukemia	1 160	0.90	2.19	1.36	0.07	0.14	872	1.19	1.69	1.02	0.05	0.11	C92-C94, D45-D47
白血病,未特指	Leukemia unspecified	990	0.77	1.87	1.24	0.06	0.12	740	1.01	1.44	0.91	0.05	0.09	C95
其他或未特指部位	Other and unspecified	1 808	1.41	3.41	1.98	0.09	0.21	1 335	1.82	2.59	1.31	0.06	0.13	O&U
所有部位合计	All sites	128 383	100.00	242.41	135.06	5.64	15.27	73 227	100.00	142.28	70.28	3.10	7.66	C00-C97, D32-D33, D42-D43, D45-D47
所有部位除外 C44	All sites except C44	127 879	99.61	241.46	134.56	5.63	15.24	72 691	99.27	141.24	69.89	3.09	7.64	C00-C97, D32-D33, D42-D43, D45-D47 exc. C44

附表 2-13　2018 年全国中部肿瘤登记地区癌症死亡主要指标
Appendix Table 2-13　Cancer mortality in Central registration areas of China, 2018

部位 Site		男性 Male						女性 Female						ICD-10
		死亡数 No. deaths	构成 Freq./%	粗率 Crude rate/ $100\,000^{-1}$	世标率 ASR world/ $100\,000^{-1}$	累积率 Cum. Rate/% 0~64	0~74	死亡数 No. deaths	构成 Freq./%	粗率 Crude rate/ $100\,000^{-1}$	世标率 ASR world/ $100\,000^{-1}$	累积率 Cum. Rate/% 0~64	0~74	
唇	Lip	50	0.04	0.08	0.05	0.00	0.01	30	0.04	0.05	0.02	0.00	0.00	C00
舌	Tongue	389	0.29	0.59	0.40	0.03	0.04	144	0.19	0.23	0.14	0.01	0.02	C01-C02
口	Mouth	496	0.37	0.75	0.50	0.03	0.06	215	0.28	0.34	0.20	0.01	0.02	C03-C06
唾液腺	Salivary glands	138	0.10	0.21	0.14	0.01	0.02	90	0.12	0.14	0.09	0.00	0.01	C07-C08
扁桃腺	Tonsil	71	0.05	0.11	0.07	0.01	0.01	23	0.03	0.04	0.02	0.00	0.00	C09
其他口咽	Other oropharynx	174	0.13	0.26	0.18	0.01	0.02	40	0.05	0.06	0.04	0.00	0.00	C10
鼻咽	Nasopharynx	1 556	1.16	2.35	1.64	0.11	0.20	555	0.73	0.88	0.56	0.03	0.07	C11
下咽	Hypopharynx	266	0.20	0.40	0.28	0.02	0.03	16	0.02	0.03	0.01	0.00	0.00	C12-C13
咽,部位不明	Pharynx unspecified	168	0.13	0.25	0.17	0.01	0.02	52	0.07	0.08	0.04	0.00	0.00	C14
食管	Esophagus	12 387	9.23	18.69	12.18	0.46	1.49	5 107	6.70	8.05	4.44	0.11	0.50	C15
胃	Stomach	18 407	13.71	27.77	18.11	0.69	2.19	8 033	10.53	12.67	7.38	0.30	0.81	C16
小肠	Small intestine	540	0.40	0.81	0.55	0.03	0.06	377	0.49	0.59	0.36	0.02	0.04	C17
结肠	Colon	3 897	2.90	5.88	3.83	0.16	0.41	3 045	3.99	4.80	2.79	0.12	0.30	C18
直肠	Rectum	5 005	3.73	7.55	4.91	0.21	0.55	3 176	4.16	5.01	2.90	0.13	0.32	C19-C20
肛门	Anus	189	0.14	0.29	0.19	0.01	0.02	124	0.16	0.20	0.12	0.00	0.01	C21
肝脏	Liver	21 502	16.02	32.44	22.19	1.34	2.60	8 134	10.67	12.83	7.74	0.35	0.90	C22
胆囊及其他	Gallbladder etc.	1 573	1.17	2.37	1.56	0.06	0.18	1 970	2.58	3.11	1.81	0.08	0.21	C23-C24
胰腺	Pancreas	3 757	2.80	5.67	3.74	0.18	0.44	2 649	3.47	4.18	2.46	0.10	0.28	C25
鼻、鼻窦及其他	Nose, sinuses etc.	162	0.12	0.24	0.16	0.01	0.02	92	0.12	0.15	0.10	0.00	0.01	C30-C31
喉	Larynx	1 278	0.95	1.93	1.26	0.06	0.15	170	0.22	0.27	0.15	0.00	0.02	C32
气管、支气管、肺	Trachea, bronchus & lung	42 251	31.48	63.75	41.79	1.74	5.08	16 643	21.82	26.24	15.25	0.62	1.72	C33-C34
其他胸腔器官	Other thoracic organs	378	0.28	0.57	0.42	0.02	0.05	219	0.29	0.35	0.23	0.01	0.03	C37-C38
骨	Bone	905	0.67	1.37	0.98	0.05	0.10	631	0.83	0.99	0.64	0.03	0.07	C40-C41
皮肤黑色素瘤	Melanoma of skin	168	0.13	0.25	0.17	0.01	0.02	141	0.18	0.22	0.14	0.01	0.02	C43
皮肤其他	Other skin	597	0.44	0.90	0.57	0.02	0.05	463	0.61	0.73	0.37	0.01	0.03	C44
间皮瘤	Mesothelioma	55	0.04	0.08	0.06	0.00	0.01	43	0.06	0.07	0.04	0.00	0.01	C45
卡波氏肉瘤	Kaposi sarcoma	16	0.01	0.02	0.02	0.00	0.00	10	0.01	0.02	0.01	0.00	0.00	C46
结缔组织、软组织	Connective & soft tissue	209	0.16	0.32	0.24	0.01	0.03	150	0.20	0.24	0.17	0.01	0.02	C47, C49
乳腺	Breast	158	0.12	0.24	0.16	0.01	0.02	5 917	7.76	9.33	6.14	0.44	0.69	C50
外阴	Vulva	—	—	—	—	—	—	97	0.13	0.15	0.09	0.00	0.01	C51
阴道	Vagina	—	—	—	—	—	—	51	0.07	0.08	0.05	0.00	0.01	C52
子宫颈	Cervix uteri	—	—	—	—	—	—	4 235	5.55	6.68	4.31	0.28	0.50	C53
子宫体	Corpus uteri	—	—	—	—	—	—	1 190	1.56	1.88	1.22	0.08	0.15	C54
子宫,部位不明	Uterus unspecified	—	—	—	—	—	—	391	0.51	0.62	0.39	0.02	0.05	C55
卵巢	Ovary	—	—	—	—	—	—	2 165	2.84	3.41	2.27	0.15	0.27	C56
其他女性生殖器	Other female genital organs	—	—	—	—	—	—	112	0.15	0.18	0.12	0.01	0.01	C57
胎盘	Placenta	—	—	—	—	—	—	8	0.01	0.01	0.01	0.00	0.00	C58
阴茎	Penis	164	0.12	0.25	0.16	0.01	0.02	—	—	—	—	—	—	C60
前列腺	Prostate	2 506	1.87	3.78	2.25	0.03	0.18	—	—	—	—	—	—	C61
睾丸	Testis	64	0.05	0.10	0.07	0.01	0.01	—	—	—	—	—	—	C62
其他男性生殖器	Other male genital organs	36	0.03	0.05	0.04	0.00	0.00	—	—	—	—	—	—	C63
肾	Kidney	1 006	0.75	1.52	1.04	0.05	0.12	538	0.71	0.85	0.51	0.02	0.05	C64
肾盂	Renal pelvis	162	0.12	0.24	0.16	0.01	0.02	95	0.12	0.15	0.08	0.00	0.01	C65
输尿管	Ureter	138	0.10	0.21	0.13	0.00	0.01	99	0.13	0.16	0.09	0.00	0.01	C66
膀胱	Bladder	2 071	1.54	3.12	1.92	0.04	0.17	631	0.83	0.99	0.52	0.01	0.05	C67
其他泌尿器官	Other urinary organs	43	0.03	0.06	0.04	0.00	0.01	23	0.03	0.04	0.02	0.00	0.00	C68
眼	Eye	35	0.03	0.05	0.05	0.00	0.00	33	0.04	0.05	0.04	0.00	0.00	C69
脑、神经系统	Brain, nervous system	3 062	2.28	4.62	3.42	0.20	0.37	2 433	3.19	3.84	2.65	0.15	0.28	C70-C72, D32-D33, D42-D43
甲状腺	Thyroid	282	0.21	0.43	0.29	0.02	0.03	501	0.66	0.79	0.50	0.03	0.05	C73
肾上腺	Adrenal gland	162	0.12	0.24	0.17	0.01	0.02	85	0.11	0.13	0.09	0.00	0.01	C74
其他内分泌腺	Other endocrine	61	0.05	0.09	0.07	0.00	0.01	55	0.07	0.09	0.06	0.00	0.01	C75
霍奇金淋巴瘤	Hodgkin lymphoma	99	0.07	0.15	0.10	0.01	0.01	82	0.11	0.13	0.08	0.00	0.01	C81
非霍奇金淋巴瘤	Non-Hodgkin lymphoma	1 768	1.32	2.67	1.86	0.10	0.21	1 085	1.42	1.71	1.09	0.05	0.12	C82-C86, C96
免疫增生性疾病	Immunoproliferative diseases	9	0.01	0.01	0.01	0.00	0.00	2	0.00	0.00	0.00	0.00	0.00	C88
多发性骨髓瘤	Multiple myeloma	632	0.47	0.95	0.65	0.03	0.08	434	0.57	0.68	0.44	0.02	0.06	C90
淋巴样白血病	Lymphoid leukemia	505	0.38	0.76	0.63	0.03	0.06	335	0.44	0.53	0.41	0.02	0.04	C91
髓样白血病	Myeloid leukemia	963	0.72	1.45	1.07	0.06	0.11	599	0.79	0.94	0.68	0.04	0.07	C92-C94, D45-D47
白血病,未特指	Leukemia unspecified	1 234	0.92	1.86	1.48	0.08	0.14	843	1.11	1.33	0.99	0.05	0.10	C95
其他或未指明部位	Other and unspecified	2 483	1.85	3.75	2.56	0.12	0.28	1 876	2.46	2.96	1.85	0.09	0.20	O&U
所有部位合计	All sites	134 227	100.00	202.53	134.67	6.07	15.73	76 257	100.00	120.24	72.90	3.47	8.17	C00-C97、D32-D33、D42-D43、D45-D47
所有部位除外 C44	All sites except C44	133 630	99.56	201.63	134.09	6.06	15.67	75 794	99.39	119.51	72.53	3.46	8.14	C00-C97、D32-D33、D42-D43、D45-D47 exc. C44

附表 2-14　2018 年全国中部城市肿瘤登记地区癌症死亡主要指标
Appendix Table 2-14　Cancer mortality in Central urban registration areas of China, 2018

部位 Site		男性 Male						女性 Female						ICD-10
		死亡数 No. deaths	构成 Freq./%	粗率 Crude rate/ $100\,000^{-1}$	世标率 ASR world/ $100\,000^{-1}$	累积率 Cum. Rate/% 0~64	0~74	死亡数 No. deaths	构成 Freq./%	粗率 Crude rate/ $100\,000^{-1}$	世标率 ASR world/ $100\,000^{-1}$	累积率 Cum. Rate/% 0~64	0~74	
唇	Lip	20	0.04	0.08	0.05	0.00	0.00	8	0.03	0.03	0.02	0.00	0.00	C00
舌	Tongue	206	0.40	0.84	0.52	0.03	0.06	73	0.25	0.31	0.16	0.01	0.01	C01-C02
口	Mouth	223	0.44	0.91	0.57	0.03	0.07	95	0.33	0.40	0.20	0.01	0.02	C03-C06
唾液腺	Salivary glands	44	0.09	0.18	0.11	0.01	0.01	29	0.10	0.12	0.07	0.00	0.01	C07-C08
扁桃腺	Tonsil	30	0.06	0.12	0.08	0.01	0.01	10	0.03	0.04	0.02	0.00	0.00	C09
其他口咽	Other oropharynx	76	0.15	0.31	0.20	0.01	0.03	17	0.06	0.07	0.04	0.00	0.00	C10
鼻咽	Nasopharynx	546	1.07	2.24	1.46	0.10	0.18	193	0.66	0.81	0.48	0.03	0.06	C11
下咽	Hypopharynx	130	0.26	0.53	0.34	0.02	0.04	8	0.03	0.03	0.02	0.00	0.00	C12-C13
咽,部位不明	Pharynx unspecified	78	0.15	0.32	0.20	0.01	0.02	26	0.09	0.11	0.05	0.00	0.00	C14
食管	Esophagus	3 932	7.72	16.13	9.73	0.43	1.18	1 312	4.49	5.50	2.78	0.07	0.28	C15
胃	Stomach	5 680	11.16	23.30	13.81	0.53	1.59	2 586	8.86	10.83	5.86	0.24	0.61	C16
小肠	Small intestine	251	0.49	1.03	0.63	0.03	0.07	177	0.61	0.74	0.41	0.02	0.05	C17
结肠	Colon	2 025	3.98	8.31	4.88	0.19	0.52	1 485	5.09	6.22	3.29	0.13	0.34	C18
直肠	Rectum	2 088	4.10	8.56	5.07	0.22	0.55	1 229	4.21	5.15	2.71	0.11	0.28	C19-C20
肛门	Anus	64	0.14	0.26	0.16	0.01	0.02	55	0.19	0.23	0.13	0.00	0.01	C21
肝脏	Liver	7 525	14.78	30.86	19.61	1.20	2.28	2 808	9.62	11.76	6.53	0.28	0.73	C22
胆囊及其他	Gallbladder etc.	709	1.39	2.91	1.74	0.06	0.20	852	2.92	3.57	1.87	0.07	0.20	C23-C24
胰腺	Pancreas	1 653	3.25	6.78	4.08	0.20	0.46	1 204	4.12	5.04	2.72	0.12	0.30	C25
鼻、鼻窦及其他	Nose, sinuses etc.	65	0.13	0.27	0.16	0.01	0.02	31	0.11	0.13	0.08	0.00	0.01	C30-C31
喉	Larynx	544	1.07	2.23	1.36	0.07	0.16	75	0.26	0.31	0.16	0.00	0.02	C32
气管、支气管、肺	Trachea, bronchus & lung	16 614	32.64	68.14	40.85	1.69	4.89	6 683	22.89	27.99	14.96	0.59	1.63	C33-C34
其他胸腔器官	Other thoracic organs	178	0.35	0.73	0.50	0.03	0.06	102	0.35	0.43	0.26	0.01	0.03	C37-C38
骨	Bone	325	0.64	1.33	0.87	0.04	0.09	227	0.78	0.95	0.55	0.02	0.06	C40-C41
皮肤黑色素瘤	Melanoma of skin	71	0.14	0.29	0.17	0.01	0.02	64	0.22	0.27	0.17	0.01	0.02	C43
皮肤其他	Other skin	193	0.38	0.79	0.47	0.02	0.05	143	0.49	0.60	0.29	0.01	0.02	C44
间皮瘤	Mesothelioma	31	0.06	0.13	0.08	0.00	0.01	28	0.10	0.12	0.07	0.00	0.01	C45
卡波氏肉瘤	Kaposi sarcoma	4	0.01	0.02	0.01	0.00	0.00	6	0.02	0.03	0.02	0.00	0.00	C46
结缔组织、软组织	Connective & soft tissue	98	0.19	0.40	0.29	0.02	0.03	65	0.22	0.27	0.18	0.01	0.02	C47, C49
乳腺	Breast	68	0.13	0.28	0.17	0.01	0.02	2 482	8.50	10.40	6.33	0.43	0.71	C50
外阴	Vulva	—	—	—	—	—	—	45	0.15	0.19	0.10	0.00	0.01	C51
阴道	Vagina	—	—	—	—	—	—	19	0.07	0.08	0.04	0.00	0.01	C52
子宫颈	Cervix uteri	—	—	—	—	—	—	1 475	5.05	6.18	3.77	0.26	0.43	C53
子宫体	Corpus uteri	—	—	—	—	—	—	397	1.36	1.66	1.01	0.07	0.12	C54
子宫,部位不明	Uterus unspecified	—	—	—	—	—	—	131	0.45	0.55	0.33	0.02	0.04	C55
卵巢	Ovary	—	—	—	—	—	—	963	3.30	4.03	2.48	0.17	0.29	C56
其他女性生殖器	Other female genital organs	—	—	—	—	—	—	52	0.18	0.22	0.13	0.01	0.02	C57
胎盘	Placenta	—	—	—	—	—	—	2	0.01	0.01	0.01	0.00	0.00	C58
阴茎	Penis	50	0.10	0.21	0.11	0.00	0.01	—	—	—	—	—	—	C60
前列腺	Prostate	1 213	2.38	4.97	2.60	0.03	0.18	—	—	—	—	—	—	C61
睾丸	Testis	20	0.04	0.08	0.05	0.00	0.00	—	—	—	—	—	—	C62
其他男性生殖器	Other male genital organs	18	0.04	0.07	0.05	0.00	0.00	—	—	—	—	—	—	C63
肾	Kidney	501	0.98	2.05	1.27	0.05	0.14	242	0.83	1.01	0.54	0.02	0.05	C64
肾盂	Renal pelvis	69	0.14	0.28	0.17	0.01	0.02	69	0.24	0.29	0.14	0.00	0.01	C65
输尿管	Ureter	74	0.15	0.30	0.17	0.01	0.02	54	0.18	0.23	0.11	0.00	0.01	C66
膀胱	Bladder	952	1.87	3.90	2.13	0.05	0.16	291	1.00	1.22	0.58	0.01	0.05	C67
其他泌尿器官	Other urinary organs	23	0.05	0.09	0.06	0.00	0.01	7	0.02	0.03	0.02	0.00	0.00	C68
眼	Eye	11	0.02	0.05	0.05	0.00	0.00	15	0.05	0.06	0.04	0.00	0.00	C69
脑、神经系统	Brain, nervous system	1 072	2.11	4.40	3.06	0.18	0.33	797	2.73	3.34	2.14	0.12	0.23	C70-C72, D32-D33, D42-D43
甲状腺	Thyroid	122	0.24	0.50	0.31	0.02	0.03	196	0.67	0.82	0.48	0.03	0.05	C73
肾上腺	Adrenal gland	84	0.17	0.34	0.23	0.01	0.02	40	0.14	0.17	0.11	0.01	0.01	C74
其他内分泌腺	Other endocrine	30	0.06	0.12	0.10	0.00	0.01	32	0.11	0.13	0.09	0.00	0.01	C75
霍奇金淋巴瘤	Hodgkin lymphoma	28	0.06	0.11	0.07	0.01	0.01	27	0.09	0.11	0.07	0.00	0.01	C81
非霍奇金淋巴瘤	Non-Hodgkin lymphoma	713	1.40	2.92	1.84	0.09	0.20	476	1.63	1.99	1.16	0.05	0.13	C82-C86, C96
免疫增生性疾病	Immunoproliferative diseases	2	0.00	0.01	0.01	0.00	0.00	1	0.00	0.00	0.00	0.00	0.00	C88
多发性骨髓瘤	Multiple myeloma	284	0.56	1.16	0.73	0.03	0.09	199	0.68	0.83	0.50	0.02	0.06	C90
淋巴样白血病	Lymphoid leukemia	240	0.47	0.98	0.74	0.04	0.06	148	0.51	0.62	0.48	0.02	0.05	C91
髓样白血病	Myeloid leukemia	393	0.77	1.61	1.07	0.05	0.11	261	0.89	1.09	0.73	0.04	0.07	C92-C94, D45-D47
白血病,未特指	Leukemia unspecified	285	0.56	1.17	0.82	0.04	0.07	242	0.83	1.01	0.66	0.03	0.07	D95
其他或未指明部位	Other and unspecified	1 248	2.45	5.12	3.20	0.15	0.34	945	3.24	3.96	2.27	0.10	0.24	O&U
所有部位合计	All sites	50 908	100.00	208.79	127.01	5.76	14.47	29 199	100.00	122.31	68.40	3.18	7.40	C00-C97, D32-D33, D42-D43, D45-D47
所有部位除外 C44	All sites except C44	50 715	99.62	208.00	126.54	5.75	14.42	29 056	99.51	121.71	68.12	3.17	7.38	C00-C97, D32-D33, D42-D43, D45-D47 exc. C44

部位 Site		男性 Male 死亡数 No. deaths	构成 Freq./%	粗率 Crude rate/ 100 000⁻¹	世标率 ASR world/ 100 000⁻¹	累积率 Cum. Rate/% 0~64	0~74	女性 Female 死亡数 No. deaths	构成 Freq./%	粗率 Crude rate/ 100 000⁻¹	世标率 ASR world/ 100 000⁻¹	累积率 Cum. Rate/% 0~64	0~74	ICD-10
唇	Lip	30	0.04	0.07	0.05	0.00	0.01	22	0.05	0.06	0.03	0.00	0.00	C00
舌	Tongue	183	0.22	0.44	0.31	0.02	0.04	71	0.15	0.18	0.12	0.01	0.02	C01-C02
口	Mouth	273	0.33	0.65	0.46	0.02	0.05	120	0.26	0.30	0.19	0.01	0.02	C03-C06
唾液腺	Salivary glands	94	0.11	0.22	0.16	0.01	0.02	61	0.13	0.15	0.10	0.01	0.01	C07-C08
扁桃腺	Tonsil	41	0.05	0.10	0.07	0.00	0.01	13	0.03	0.03	0.02	0.00	0.00	C09
其他口咽	Other oropharynx	98	0.12	0.23	0.17	0.01	0.02	23	0.05	0.06	0.04	0.00	0.00	C10
鼻咽	Nasopharynx	1 010	1.21	2.41	1.75	0.12	0.21	362	0.77	0.92	0.61	0.04	0.07	C11
下咽	Hypopharynx	136	0.16	0.32	0.24	0.02	0.03	8	0.02	0.02	0.01	0.00	0.00	C12-C13
咽,部位不明	Pharynx unspecified	90	0.11	0.21	0.15	0.01	0.02	26	0.06	0.07	0.04	0.00	0.00	C14
食管	Esophagus	8 455	10.15	20.18	13.83	0.48	1.68	3 795	8.06	9.60	5.56	0.14	0.65	C15
胃	Stomach	12 727	15.28	30.38	20.93	0.79	2.58	5 447	11.58	13.77	8.40	0.34	0.95	C16
小肠	Small intestine	289	0.35	0.69	0.49	0.02	0.06	200	0.43	0.51	0.32	0.01	0.04	C17
结肠	Colon	1 872	2.25	4.47	3.10	0.14	0.35	1 560	3.32	3.94	2.45	0.11	0.27	C18
直肠	Rectum	2 917	3.50	6.96	4.78	0.20	0.54	1 947	4.14	4.92	3.03	0.14	0.35	C19-C20
肛门	Anus	120	0.14	0.29	0.20	0.01	0.02	69	0.15	0.17	0.11	0.00	0.01	C21
肝脏	Liver	13 977	16.78	33.36	23.85	1.43	2.81	5 326	11.32	13.47	8.55	0.39	1.01	C22
胆囊及其他	Gallbladder etc.	864	1.04	2.06	1.43	0.06	0.17	1 118	2.38	2.83	1.76	0.08	0.21	C23-C24
胰腺	Pancreas	2 104	2.53	5.02	3.51	0.17	0.43	1 445	3.07	3.65	2.29	0.10	0.28	C25
鼻、鼻窦及其他	Nose,sinuses etc.	97	0.12	0.23	0.16	0.01	0.02	61	0.13	0.15	0.11	0.01	0.01	C30-C31
喉	Larynx	734	0.88	1.75	1.20	0.05	0.15	95	0.20	0.24	0.14	0.00	0.01	C32
气管、支气管、肺	Trachea,bronchus & lung	25 637	30.77	61.20	42.35	1.77	5.20	9 960	21.17	25.18	15.44	0.64	1.78	C33-C34
其他胸腔器官	Other thoracic organs	200	0.24	0.48	0.37	0.02	0.04	117	0.25	0.30	0.21	0.01	0.02	C37-C38
骨	Bone	580	0.70	1.38	1.04	0.05	0.12	404	0.86	1.02	0.69	0.03	0.08	C40-C41
皮肤黑色素瘤	Melanoma of skin	97	0.12	0.23	0.17	0.01	0.02	77	0.16	0.19	0.13	0.01	0.01	C43
皮肤其他	Other skin	404	0.48	0.96	0.65	0.02	0.06	320	0.68	0.81	0.43	0.01	0.03	C44
间皮瘤	Mesothelioma	24	0.03	0.06	0.04	0.00	0.00	15	0.03	0.04	0.03	0.00	0.00	C45
卡波氏肉瘤	Kaposi sarcoma	12	0.01	0.03	0.02	0.00	0.00	4	0.01	0.01	0.01	0.00	0.00	C46
结缔组织、软组织	Connective & soft tissue	111	0.13	0.26	0.21	0.01	0.02	85	0.18	0.21	0.16	0.01	0.02	C47,C49
乳腺	Breast	90	0.11	0.21	0.15	0.01	0.02	3 435	7.30	8.69	6.00	0.45	0.68	C50
外阴	Vulva	—	—	—	—	—	—	52	0.11	0.13	0.09	0.00	0.01	C51
阴道	Vagina	—	—	—	—	—	—	32	0.07	0.08	0.06	0.00	0.01	C52
子宫颈	Cervix uteri	—	—	—	—	—	—	2 760	5.87	6.98	4.67	0.30	0.54	C53
子宫体	Corpus uteri	—	—	—	—	—	—	793	1.69	2.01	1.36	0.09	0.16	C54
子宫,部位不明	Uterus unspecified	—	—	—	—	—	—	260	0.55	0.66	0.43	0.02	0.05	C55
卵巢	Ovary	—	—	—	—	—	—	1 202	2.55	3.04	2.12	0.14	0.26	C56
其他女性生殖器	Other female genital organs	—	—	—	—	—	—	60	0.13	0.15	0.10	0.01	0.01	C57
胎盘	Placenta	—	—	—	—	—	—	6	0.01	0.02	0.01	0.00	0.00	C58
阴茎	Penis	114	0.14	0.27	0.18	0.01	0.02	—	—	—	—	—	—	C60
前列腺	Prostate	1 293	1.55	3.09	1.98	0.03	0.17	—	—	—	—	—	—	C61
睾丸	Testis	44	0.05	0.11	0.08	0.00	0.01	—	—	—	—	—	—	C62
其他男性生殖器	Other male genital organs	18	0.02	0.04	0.03	0.00	0.00	—	—	—	—	—	—	C63
肾	Kidney	505	0.61	1.21	0.88	0.04	0.11	296	0.63	0.75	0.48	0.02	0.05	C64
肾盂	Renal pelvis	93	0.11	0.22	0.16	0.01	0.02	26	0.06	0.07	0.05	0.00	0.01	C65
输尿管	Ureter	64	0.08	0.15	0.11	0.00	0.01	45	0.10	0.11	0.07	0.00	0.01	C66
膀胱	Bladder	1 119	1.34	2.67	1.76	0.04	0.17	340	0.72	0.86	0.48	0.01	0.05	C67
其他泌尿器官	Other urinary organs	20	0.02	0.05	0.03	0.00	0.00	16	0.03	0.04	0.02	0.00	0.00	C68
眼	Eye	24	0.03	0.06	0.05	0.00	0.00	18	0.04	0.05	0.03	0.00	0.00	C69
脑、神经系统	Brain,nervous system	1 990	2.39	4.75	3.65	0.21	0.40	1 636	3.48	4.14	2.98	0.17	0.32	C70-C72,D32,D33,D42-D43
甲状腺	Thyroid	160	0.19	0.38	0.27	0.01	0.03	305	0.65	0.77	0.52	0.03	0.06	C73
肾上腺	Adrenal gland	78	0.09	0.19	0.14	0.01	0.01	45	0.10	0.11	0.08	0.00	0.01	C74
其他内分泌腺	Other endocrine	31	0.04	0.07	0.06	0.00	0.01	23	0.05	0.06	0.04	0.00	0.00	C75
霍奇金淋巴瘤	Hodgkin lymphoma	71	0.09	0.17	0.12	0.01	0.01	55	0.12	0.14	0.09	0.01	0.01	C81
非霍奇金淋巴瘤	Non-Hodgkin lymphoma	1 055	1.27	2.52	1.85	0.10	0.22	609	1.29	1.54	1.04	0.05	0.12	C82-C86,C96
免疫增生性疾病	Immunoproliferative diseases	7	0.01	0.02	0.01	0.00	0.00	1	0.00	0.00	0.00	0.00	0.00	C88
多发性骨髓瘤	Multiple myeloma	348	0.42	0.83	0.59	0.03	0.07	235	0.50	0.59	0.39	0.02	0.05	C90
淋巴样白血病	Lymphoid leukemia	265	0.32	0.63	0.55	0.03	0.05	187	0.40	0.47	0.38	0.02	0.04	C91
髓样白血病	Myeloid leukemia	570	0.68	1.36	1.05	0.06	0.11	338	0.72	0.85	0.64	0.04	0.07	C92-C94,D45-D47
白血病,未特指	Leukemia unspecified	949	1.14	2.27	1.86	0.10	0.18	601	1.28	1.52	1.19	0.06	0.12	C95
其他或未指明部位	Other and unspecified	1 235	1.48	2.95	2.14	0.10	0.24	931	1.98	2.35	1.56	0.07	0.16	O&U
所有部位合计	All sites	83 319	100.00	198.89	139.42	6.27	16.53	47 058	100.00	118.99	75.85	3.66	8.69	C00-C97,D32-D33,D42-D43,D45-D47
所有部位除外 C44	All sites except C44	82 915	99.52	197.93	138.77	6.25	16.47	46 738	99.32	118.18	75.42	3.64	8.65	C00-C97,D32-D33,D42-D43,D45-D47 exc.C44

附表 2-16　2018 年全国西部肿瘤登记地区癌症死亡主要指标
Appendix Table 2-16　Cancer mortality in Western registration areas of China, 2018

部位 Site		男性 Male						女性 Female						ICD-10
		死亡数 No. deaths	构成 Freq./%	粗率 Crude rate/ 100 000⁻¹	世标率 ASR world/ 100 000⁻¹	累积率 Cum. Rate/% 0~64	0~74	死亡数 No. deaths	构成 Freq./%	粗率 Crude rate/ 100 000⁻¹	世标率 ASR world/ 100 000⁻¹	累积率 Cum. Rate/% 0~64	0~74	
唇	Lip	48	0.03	0.05	0.03	0.00	0.00	34	0.04	0.04	0.02	0.00	0.00	C00
舌	Tongue	507	0.27	0.56	0.37	0.02	0.04	223	0.23	0.26	0.16	0.01	0.02	C01-C02
口	Mouth	686	0.37	0.76	0.49	0.02	0.06	314	0.32	0.36	0.21	0.01	0.02	C03-C06
唾液腺	Salivary glands	167	0.09	0.19	0.12	0.01	0.01	93	0.10	0.11	0.07	0.00	0.01	C07-C08
扁桃腺	Tonsil	97	0.05	0.11	0.07	0.00	0.01	26	0.03	0.03	0.02	0.00	0.00	C09
其他口咽	Other oropharynx	267	0.14	0.30	0.19	0.01	0.02	46	0.05	0.05	0.03	0.00	0.00	C10
鼻咽	Nasopharynx	2 777	1.49	3.08	2.10	0.15	0.24	973	1.00	1.13	0.73	0.05	0.08	C11
下咽	Hypopharynx	397	0.21	0.44	0.29	0.02	0.04	41	0.04	0.05	0.03	0.00	0.00	C12-C13
咽, 部位不明	Pharynx unspecified	376	0.20	0.42	0.27	0.01	0.03	129	0.13	0.15	0.08	0.00	0.01	C14
食管	Esophagus	19 452	10.43	21.57	13.78	0.60	1.71	5 340	5.51	6.20	3.38	0.10	0.37	C15
胃	Stomach	19 608	10.52	21.75	13.87	0.62	1.67	8 391	8.67	9.74	5.55	0.23	0.60	C16
小肠	Small intestine	533	0.29	0.59	0.38	0.02	0.04	362	0.37	0.42	0.25	0.01	0.03	C17
结肠	Colon	4 493	2.41	4.98	3.13	0.13	0.33	3 294	3.40	3.82	2.18	0.09	0.23	C18
直肠	Rectum	9 021	4.84	10.01	6.30	0.26	0.70	5 426	5.60	6.30	3.57	0.15	0.38	C19-C20
肛门	Anus	362	0.19	0.40	0.26	0.01	0.02	249	0.26	0.29	0.16	0.01	0.02	C21
肝脏	Liver	35 898	19.25	39.81	26.75	1.75	3.08	11 556	11.93	13.41	8.04	0.39	0.91	C22
胆囊及其他	Gallbladder etc.	1 827	0.98	2.03	1.29	0.06	0.15	2 218	2.29	2.57	1.48	0.06	0.17	C23-C24
胰腺	Pancreas	5 056	2.71	5.61	3.61	0.18	0.43	3 355	3.46	3.89	2.25	0.09	0.26	C25
鼻、鼻窦及其他	Nose, sinuses etc.	262	0.14	0.29	0.19	0.01	0.02	120	0.12	0.14	0.09	0.00	0.01	C30-C31
喉	Larynx	1 583	0.85	1.76	1.12	0.05	0.14	212	0.22	0.25	0.14	0.01	0.01	C32
气管、支气管、肺	Trachea, bronchus & lung	56 912	30.52	63.12	40.51	1.92	4.84	23 321	24.08	27.07	15.66	0.68	1.76	C33-C34
其他胸腔器官	Other thoracic organs	465	0.25	0.52	0.36	0.02	0.04	245	0.25	0.28	0.18	0.01	0.02	C37-C38
骨	Bone	1 558	0.84	1.73	1.19	0.06	0.13	926	0.96	1.07	0.70	0.03	0.08	C40-C41
皮肤黑色素瘤	Melanoma of skin	203	0.11	0.23	0.15	0.01	0.02	144	0.15	0.17	0.10	0.01	0.01	C43
皮肤其他	Other skin	788	0.42	0.87	0.55	0.02	0.05	565	0.58	0.66	0.36	0.01	0.03	C44
间皮瘤	Mesothelioma	68	0.04	0.08	0.05	0.00	0.01	43	0.04	0.05	0.03	0.00	0.00	C45
卡波氏肉瘤	Kaposi sarcoma	42	0.02	0.05	0.03	0.00	0.00	23	0.02	0.03	0.02	0.00	0.00	C46
结缔组织、软组织	Connective & soft tissue	271	0.15	0.30	0.23	0.01	0.02	187	0.19	0.22	0.15	0.01	0.02	C47, C49
乳腺	Breast	208	0.11	0.23	0.15	0.01	0.02	6 348	6.56	7.37	4.83	0.37	0.53	C50
外阴	Vulva	—	—	—	—	—	—	188	0.19	0.22	0.13	0.01	0.01	C51
阴道	Vagina	—	—	—	—	—	—	102	0.11	0.12	0.07	0.00	0.01	C52
子宫颈	Cervix uteri	—	—	—	—	—	—	5 300	5.47	6.15	4.01	0.28	0.46	C53
子宫体	Corpus uteri	—	—	—	—	—	—	1 540	1.59	1.79	1.14	0.08	0.13	C54
子宫, 部位不明	Uterus unspecified	—	—	—	—	—	—	816	0.84	0.95	0.60	0.04	0.07	C55
卵巢	Ovary	—	—	—	—	—	—	2 541	2.62	2.95	1.93	0.13	0.23	C56
其他女性生殖器	Other female genital organs	—	—	—	—	—	—	136	0.14	0.16	0.10	0.01	0.01	C57
胎盘	Placenta	—	—	—	—	—	—	10	0.01	0.01	0.01	0.00	0.00	C58
阴茎	Penis	205	0.11	0.23	0.15	0.01	0.01	—	—	—	—	—	—	C60
前列腺	Prostate	3 695	1.98	4.10	2.37	0.03	0.18	—	—	—	—	—	—	C61
睾丸	Testis	125	0.07	0.14	0.11	0.01	0.01	—	—	—	—	—	—	C62
其他男性生殖器	Other male genital organs	39	0.02	0.04	0.03	0.00	0.00	—	—	—	—	—	—	C63
肾	Kidney	1 048	0.56	1.16	0.77	0.04	0.09	534	0.55	0.62	0.40	0.02	0.04	C64
肾盂	Renal pelvis	175	0.09	0.19	0.12	0.01	0.01	106	0.11	0.12	0.07	0.00	0.01	C65
输尿管	Ureter	141	0.08	0.16	0.10	0.00	0.01	131	0.14	0.15	0.08	0.00	0.01	C66
膀胱	Bladder	2 895	1.55	3.21	1.93	0.05	0.18	734	0.76	0.85	0.45	0.01	0.04	C67
其他泌尿器官	Other urinary organs	30	0.02	0.03	0.02	0.00	0.00	24	0.02	0.03	0.02	0.00	0.00	C68
眼	Eye	54	0.03	0.06	0.05	0.00	0.00	61	0.06	0.07	0.05	0.00	0.00	C69
脑、神经系统	Brain, nervous system	3 772	2.02	4.18	3.07	0.18	0.32	3 048	3.15	3.54	2.46	0.14	0.26	C70-C72, D32-D33, D42-D43
甲状腺	Thyroid	329	0.18	0.36	0.25	0.01	0.03	581	0.60	0.67	0.42	0.03	0.04	C73
肾上腺	Adrenal gland	159	0.09	0.18	0.13	0.01	0.01	99	0.10	0.11	0.08	0.00	0.01	C74
其他内分泌腺	Other endocrine	84	0.05	0.09	0.07	0.00	0.01	74	0.08	0.09	0.06	0.00	0.01	C75
霍奇金淋巴瘤	Hodgkin lymphoma	192	0.10	0.21	0.15	0.01	0.02	90	0.09	0.10	0.07	0.00	0.01	C81
非霍奇金淋巴瘤	Non-Hodgkin lymphoma	2 058	1.10	2.28	1.57	0.09	0.17	1 205	1.24	1.40	0.90	0.05	0.10	C82-C86, C96
免疫增生性疾病	Immunoproliferative diseases	14	0.01	0.02	0.01	0.00	0.00	4	0.00	0.00	0.00	0.00	0.00	C88
多发性骨髓瘤	Multiple myeloma	690	0.37	0.77	0.51	0.02	0.06	502	0.52	0.58	0.36	0.02	0.04	C90
淋巴样白血病	Lymphoid leukemia	675	0.36	0.75	0.62	0.03	0.05	466	0.48	0.54	0.44	0.02	0.04	C91
髓样白血病	Myeloid leukemia	1 017	0.55	1.13	0.83	0.05	0.09	815	0.84	0.95	0.69	0.04	0.07	C92-C94, D45-D47
白血病, 未特指	Leukemia unspecified	1 525	0.82	1.69	1.34	0.07	0.13	1 082	1.12	1.26	0.98	0.05	0.10	C95
其他或未指明部位	Other and unspecified	3 593	1.93	3.99	2.71	0.14	0.30	2 442	2.52	2.83	1.77	0.09	0.19	O&U
所有部位合计	All sites	186 447	100.00	206.79	134.74	6.75	15.57	96 835	100.00	112.39	67.78	3.37	7.49	C00-C97, D32-D33, D42-D43, D45-D47
所有部位除外 C44	All sites except C44	185 659	99.58	205.92	134.19	6.73	15.51	96 270	99.42	111.74	67.42	3.36	7.46	C00-C97, D32-D33, D42-D43, D45-D47 exc. C44

附表 2-17　2018 年全国西部城市肿瘤登记地区癌症死亡主要指标

Appendix Table 2-17　Cancer mortality in Western urban registration areas of China, 2018

部位 Site		男性 Male						女性 Female						ICD-10
		死亡数 No. deaths	构成 Freq./%	粗率 Crude rate/ 100 000⁻¹	世标率 ASR world/ 100 000⁻¹	累积率 Cum. Rate/%		死亡数 No. deaths	构成 Freq./%	粗率 Crude rate/ 100 000⁻¹	世标率 ASR world/ 100 000⁻¹	累积率 Cum. Rate/%		
						0~64	0~74					0~64	0~74	
唇	Lip	19	0.02	0.05	0.03	0.00	0.00	13	0.03	0.04	0.02	0.00	0.00	C00
舌	Tongue	266	0.33	0.70	0.46	0.02	0.05	119	0.28	0.32	0.19	0.01	0.02	C01-C02
口	Mouth	297	0.37	0.78	0.51	0.02	0.06	152	0.36	0.41	0.23	0.01	0.02	C03-C06
唾液腺	Salivary glands	83	0.10	0.22	0.14	0.01	0.02	45	0.11	0.12	0.08	0.00	0.01	C07-C08
扁桃腺	Tonsil	47	0.06	0.12	0.08	0.00	0.01	14	0.03	0.04	0.03	0.00	0.00	C09
其他口咽	Other oropharynx	117	0.15	0.31	0.20	0.01	0.02	17	0.04	0.05	0.03	0.00	0.00	C10
鼻咽	Nasopharynx	1 159	1.44	3.05	2.08	0.14	0.24	446	1.04	1.20	0.79	0.05	0.09	C11
下咽	Hypopharynx	218	0.27	0.57	0.38	0.02	0.05	17	0.04	0.05	0.03	0.00	0.00	C12-C13
咽,部位不明	Pharynx unspecified	146	0.18	0.38	0.26	0.01	0.03	59	0.14	0.16	0.08	0.00	0.01	C14
食管	Esophagus	6 972	8.69	18.34	11.86	0.54	1.47	1 816	4.24	4.90	2.69	0.07	0.29	C15
胃	Stomach	7 770	9.68	20.44	13.15	0.59	1.57	3 466	8.10	9.35	5.42	0.23	0.58	C16
小肠	Small intestine	282	0.35	0.74	0.47	0.02	0.05	207	0.48	0.56	0.33	0.01	0.04	C17
结肠	Colon	2 572	3.20	6.76	4.25	0.17	0.45	1 878	4.39	5.07	2.86	0.11	0.29	C18
直肠	Rectum	3 981	4.96	10.47	6.63	0.27	0.73	2 380	5.56	6.42	3.65	0.14	0.38	C19-C20
肛门	Anus	151	0.19	0.40	0.25	0.01	0.03	91	0.21	0.25	0.14	0.01	0.01	C21
肝脏	Liver	14 163	17.65	37.25	25.01	1.59	2.88	4 770	11.15	12.87	7.68	0.36	0.86	C22
胆囊及其他	Gallbladder etc.	883	1.10	2.32	1.48	0.06	0.16	1 080	2.52	2.91	1.66	0.07	0.18	C23-C24
胰腺	Pancreas	2 468	3.08	6.49	4.19	0.20	0.48	1 688	3.94	4.56	2.61	0.10	0.29	C25
鼻、鼻窦及其他	Nose, sinuses etc.	111	0.14	0.29	0.19	0.01	0.02	52	0.12	0.14	0.09	0.00	0.01	C30-C31
喉	Larynx	782	0.97	2.06	1.31	0.06	0.15	92	0.21	0.25	0.15	0.01	0.02	C32
气管、支气管、肺	Trachea, bronchus & lung	25 344	31.58	66.66	42.95	1.96	5.13	9 767	22.82	26.36	15.26	0.64	1.67	C33-C34
其他胸腔器官	Other thoracic organs	235	0.29	0.62	0.42	0.02	0.05	115	0.27	0.31	0.19	0.01	0.02	C37-C38
骨	Bone	605	0.75	1.59	1.12	0.05	0.12	387	0.90	1.04	0.68	0.03	0.08	C40-C41
皮肤黑色素瘤	Melanoma of skin	93	0.12	0.24	0.16	0.01	0.02	67	0.16	0.18	0.11	0.00	0.01	C43
皮肤其他	Other skin	364	0.45	0.96	0.60	0.02	0.06	237	0.55	0.64	0.35	0.01	0.03	C44
间皮瘤	Mesothelioma	34	0.04	0.09	0.06	0.00	0.01	17	0.04	0.05	0.03	0.00	0.00	C45
卡波氏肉瘤	Kaposi sarcoma	25	0.03	0.07	0.04	0.00	0.00	17	0.04	0.05	0.03	0.00	0.00	C46
结缔组织、软组织	Connective & soft tissue	136	0.17	0.36	0.27	0.02	0.02	102	0.24	0.28	0.20	0.01	0.02	C47, C49
乳腺	Breast	106	0.13	0.28	0.18	0.01	0.02	3 214	7.51	8.67	5.59	0.41	0.60	C50
外阴	Vulva	—	—	—	—	—	—	98	0.23	0.26	0.16	0.01	0.02	C51
阴道	Vagina	—	—	—	—	—	—	47	0.11	0.13	0.08	0.00	0.01	C52
子宫颈	Cervix uteri	—	—	—	—	—	—	2 266	5.30	6.11	3.98	0.28	0.45	C53
子宫体	Corpus uteri	—	—	—	—	—	—	695	1.62	1.88	1.19	0.08	0.14	C54
子宫,部位不明	Uterus unspecified	—	—	—	—	—	—	286	0.67	0.77	0.49	0.03	0.06	C55
卵巢	Ovary	—	—	—	—	—	—	1 370	3.20	3.70	2.41	0.16	0.28	C56
其他女性生殖器	Other female genital organs	—	—	—	—	—	—	62	0.14	0.17	0.11	0.01	0.01	C57
胎盘	Placenta	—	—	—	—	—	—	3	0.01	0.01	0.01	0.00	0.00	C58
阴茎	Penis	96	0.12	0.25	0.16	0.01	0.02	—	—	—	—	—	—	C60
前列腺	Prostate	2 043	2.55	5.37	3.08	0.04	0.22	—	—	—	—	—	—	C61
睾丸	Testis	50	0.06	0.13	0.10	0.00	0.01	—	—	—	—	—	—	C62
其他男性生殖器	Other male genital organs	17	0.02	0.04	0.03	0.00	0.00	—	—	—	—	—	—	C63
肾	Kidney	579	0.72	1.52	1.00	0.05	0.11	285	0.67	0.77	0.51	0.02	0.05	C64
肾盂	Renal pelvis	104	0.13	0.27	0.17	0.01	0.02	53	0.12	0.14	0.08	0.00	0.01	C65
输尿管	Ureter	82	0.10	0.22	0.13	0.01	0.01	87	0.20	0.23	0.12	0.00	0.01	C66
膀胱	Bladder	1 343	1.67	3.53	2.12	0.05	0.19	364	0.85	0.98	0.52	0.01	0.04	C67
其他泌尿器官	Other urinary organs	12	0.01	0.03	0.02	0.00	0.00	13	0.03	0.04	0.02	0.00	0.00	C68
眼	Eye	19	0.02	0.05	0.04	0.00	0.00	22	0.05	0.06	0.04	0.00	0.00	C69
脑、神经系统	Brain, nervous system	1 585	1.98	4.17	3.03	0.18	0.32	1 297	3.03	3.50	2.46	0.14	0.26	C70-C72, D32- D33, D42-D43
甲状腺	Thyroid	185	0.23	0.49	0.33	0.02	0.03	313	0.73	0.84	0.53	0.03	0.05	C73
肾上腺	Adrenal gland	75	0.09	0.20	0.14	0.01	0.01	48	0.11	0.13	0.08	0.00	0.01	C74
其他内分泌腺	Other endocrine	38	0.05	0.10	0.07	0.00	0.01	35	0.08	0.09	0.06	0.00	0.01	C75
霍奇金淋巴瘤	Hodgkin lymphoma	91	0.11	0.24	0.16	0.01	0.02	45	0.11	0.12	0.09	0.00	0.01	C81
非霍奇金淋巴瘤	Non-Hodgkin lymphoma	977	1.22	2.57	1.74	0.09	0.19	547	1.28	1.48	0.96	0.04	0.11	C82-C86, C96
免疫增生性疾病	Immunoproliferative diseases	9	0.01	0.02	0.01	0.00	0.00	2	0.00	0.01	0.00	0.00	0.00	C88
多发性骨髓瘤	Multiple myeloma	385	0.48	1.01	0.67	0.03	0.08	275	0.64	0.74	0.46	0.02	0.06	C90
淋巴样白血病	Lymphoid leukemia	308	0.38	0.81	0.66	0.03	0.06	217	0.51	0.59	0.47	0.02	0.04	C91
髓样白血病	Myeloid leukemia	507	0.63	1.33	0.97	0.05	0.10	410	0.96	1.11	0.79	0.04	0.08	C92-C94, D45- D47
白血病,未特指	Leukemia unspecified	635	0.79	1.67	1.32	0.07	0.13	434	1.01	1.17	0.91	0.05	0.09	C95
其他或未指明部位	Other and unspecified	1 681	2.09	4.42	2.98	0.15	0.32	1 194	2.79	3.22	2.00	0.10	0.20	O&U
所有部位合计	All sites	80 250	100.00	211.08	137.65	6.66	15.75	42 793	100.00	115.48	69.72	3.39	7.53	C00-C97、D32- D33、D42-D43, D45-D47
所有部位除外 C44	All sites except C44	79 886	99.55	210.12	137.05	6.64	15.70	42 556	99.45	114.84	69.37	3.38	7.50	C00-C97、D32- D33、D42-D43, D45-D47 exc. C44

附表 2-18　2018 年全国西部农村肿瘤登记地区癌症死亡主要指标

Appendix Table 2-18　Cancer mortality in Western rural registration areas of China, 2018

部位 Site		男性 Male						女性 Female						ICD-10
		死亡数 No. deaths	构成 Freq. /%	粗率 Crude rate/ $100\,000^{-1}$	世标率 ASR world/ $100\,000^{-1}$	累积率 Cum. Rate/% 0~64	0~74	死亡数 No. deaths	构成 Freq. /%	粗率 Crude rate/ $100\,000^{-1}$	世标率 ASR world/ $100\,000^{-1}$	累积率 Cum. Rate/% 0~64	0~74	
唇	Lip	29	0.03	0.06	0.03	0.00	0.00	21	0.04	0.04	0.02	0.00	0.00	C00
舌	Tongue	241	0.23	0.46	0.30	0.02	0.04	104	0.19	0.21	0.14	0.01	0.01	C01-C02
口	Mouth	389	0.37	0.75	0.47	0.02	0.06	162	0.30	0.33	0.19	0.01	0.02	C03-C06
唾液腺	Salivary glands	84	0.08	0.16	0.10	0.00	0.01	48	0.09	0.10	0.06	0.00	0.01	C07-C08
扁桃腺	Tonsil	50	0.05	0.10	0.06	0.00	0.01	12	0.02	0.02	0.01	0.00	0.00	C09
其他口咽	Other oropharynx	150	0.14	0.29	0.19	0.01	0.02	29	0.05	0.06	0.03	0.00	0.00	C10
鼻咽	Nasopharynx	1 618	1.52	3.10	2.13	0.15	0.25	527	0.98	1.07	0.70	0.05	0.08	C11
下咽	Hypopharynx	179	0.17	0.34	0.23	0.01	0.03	24	0.04	0.05	0.03	0.00	0.00	C12-C13
咽,部位不明	Pharynx unspecified	230	0.22	0.44	0.28	0.01	0.03	70	0.13	0.14	0.08	0.00	0.01	C14
食管	Esophagus	12 480	11.75	23.93	15.16	0.64	1.88	3 524	6.52	7.18	3.88	0.11	0.42	C15
胃	Stomach	11 838	11.15	22.70	14.39	0.65	1.74	4 925	9.11	10.03	5.64	0.23	0.61	C16
小肠	Small intestine	251	0.24	0.48	0.31	0.02	0.04	155	0.29	0.32	0.19	0.01	0.02	C17
结肠	Colon	1 921	1.81	3.68	2.33	0.10	0.25	1 416	2.62	2.88	1.68	0.08	0.19	C18
直肠	Rectum	5 040	4.75	9.67	6.07	0.25	0.67	3 046	5.64	6.20	3.52	0.15	0.38	C19-C20
肛门	Anus	211	0.20	0.40	0.26	0.01	0.03	158	0.29	0.32	0.18	0.01	0.02	C21
肝脏	Liver	21 735	20.47	41.68	28.05	1.87	3.23	6 786	12.56	13.82	8.31	0.42	0.95	C22
胆囊及其他	Gallbladder etc.	944	0.89	1.81	1.15	0.06	0.13	1 138	2.11	2.32	1.34	0.06	0.16	C23-C24
胰腺	Pancreas	2 588	2.44	4.96	3.20	0.16	0.39	1 667	3.08	3.39	1.99	0.09	0.24	C25
鼻、鼻窦及其他	Nose, sinuses etc.	151	0.14	0.29	0.20	0.01	0.02	68	0.13	0.14	0.09	0.01	0.01	C30-C31
喉	Larynx	801	0.75	1.54	0.99	0.05	0.12	120	0.22	0.24	0.14	0.01	0.01	C32
气管、支气管、肺	Trachea, bronchus & lung	31 568	29.73	60.54	38.80	1.90	4.63	13 554	25.08	27.60	15.97	0.71	1.83	C33-C34
其他胸腔器官	Other thoracic organs	230	0.22	0.44	0.31	0.02	0.03	130	0.24	0.26	0.17	0.01	0.02	C37-C38
骨	Bone	953	0.90	1.83	1.25	0.07	0.14	539	1.00	1.10	0.70	0.04	0.08	C40-C41
皮肤黑色素瘤	Melanoma of skin	110	0.10	0.21	0.14	0.01	0.01	77	0.14	0.16	0.10	0.00	0.01	C43
皮肤其他	Other skin	424	0.40	0.81	0.51	0.02	0.05	328	0.61	0.67	0.36	0.01	0.03	C44
间皮瘤	Mesothelioma	34	0.03	0.07	0.04	0.00	0.00	26	0.05	0.05	0.03	0.00	0.00	C45
卡波氏肉瘤	Kaposi sarcoma	17	0.02	0.03	0.02	0.00	0.00	6	0.01	0.01	0.01	0.00	0.00	C46
结缔组织、软组织	Connective & soft tissue	135	0.13	0.26	0.20	0.01	0.02	85	0.16	0.17	0.11	0.01	0.01	C47, C49
乳腺	Breast	102	0.10	0.20	0.13	0.01	0.01	3 134	5.80	6.38	4.26	0.33	0.47	C50
外阴	Vulva	—	—	—	—	—	—	90	0.17	0.18	0.11	0.01	0.01	C51
阴道	Vagina	—	—	—	—	—	—	55	0.10	0.11	0.07	0.00	0.01	C52
子宫颈	Cervix uteri	—	—	—	—	—	—	3 034	5.61	6.18	4.02	0.28	0.47	C53
子宫体	Corpus uteri	—	—	—	—	—	—	845	1.56	1.72	1.11	0.08	0.13	C54
子宫,部位不明	Uterus unspecified	—	—	—	—	—	—	530	0.98	1.08	0.68	0.04	0.08	C55
卵巢	Ovary	—	—	—	—	—	—	1 171	2.17	2.38	1.57	0.11	0.19	C56
其他女性生殖器	Other female genital organs	—	—	—	—	—	—	74	0.14	0.15	0.10	0.01	0.01	C57
胎盘	Placenta	—	—	—	—	—	—	7	0.01	0.01	0.01	0.00	0.00	C58
阴茎	Penis	109	0.10	0.21	0.13	0.01	0.01	—	—	—	—	—	—	C60
前列腺	Prostate	1 652	1.56	3.17	1.85	0.03	0.16	—	—	—	—	—	—	C61
睾丸	Testis	75	0.07	0.14	0.11	0.01	0.01	—	—	—	—	—	—	C62
其他男性生殖器	Other male genital organs	22	0.02	0.04	0.04	0.00	0.00	—	—	—	—	—	—	C63
肾	Kidney	469	0.44	0.90	0.60	0.03	0.07	249	0.46	0.51	0.31	0.01	0.03	C64
肾盂	Renal pelvis	71	0.07	0.14	0.09	0.00	0.01	53	0.10	0.11	0.07	0.00	0.01	C65
输尿管	Ureter	59	0.06	0.11	0.07	0.00	0.01	44	0.08	0.09	0.05	0.00	0.01	C66
膀胱	Bladder	1 552	1.46	2.98	1.79	0.05	0.17	370	0.68	0.75	0.40	0.01	0.04	C67
其他泌尿器官	Other urinary organs	18	0.02	0.03	0.02	0.00	0.00	11	0.02	0.02	0.01	0.00	0.00	C68
眼	Eye	35	0.03	0.07	0.05	0.00	0.00	39	0.07	0.08	0.06	0.00	0.00	C69
脑、神经系统	Brain, nervous system	2 187	2.06	4.19	3.10	0.19	0.32	1 751	3.24	3.57	2.47	0.15	0.27	C70-C72, D32-D33, D42-D43
甲状腺	Thyroid	144	0.14	0.28	0.19	0.01	0.02	268	0.50	0.55	0.34	0.02	0.04	C73
肾上腺	Adrenal gland	84	0.08	0.16	0.12	0.01	0.01	51	0.09	0.10	0.08	0.00	0.01	C74
其他内分泌腺	Other endocrine	46	0.04	0.09	0.07	0.00	0.01	39	0.07	0.08	0.05	0.00	0.00	C75
霍奇金淋巴瘤	Hodgkin lymphoma	101	0.10	0.19	0.14	0.01	0.01	45	0.08	0.09	0.06	0.00	0.00	C81
非霍奇金淋巴瘤	Non-Hodgkin lymphoma	1 081	1.02	2.07	1.44	0.08	0.16	658	1.22	1.34	0.86	0.05	0.10	C82-C86, C96
免疫增生性疾病	Immunoproliferative diseases	5	0.00	0.01	0.01	0.00	0.00	2	0.00	0.00	0.00	0.00	0.00	C88
多发性骨髓瘤	Multiple myeloma	305	0.29	0.58	0.39	0.02	0.05	227	0.42	0.46	0.30	0.02	0.04	C90
淋巴样白血病	Lymphoid leukemia	367	0.35	0.70	0.59	0.03	0.05	249	0.46	0.51	0.42	0.03	0.04	C91
髓样白血病	Myeloid leukemia	510	0.48	0.98	0.73	0.04	0.08	405	0.75	0.82	0.62	0.04	0.06	C92-C94, D45-D47
白血病,未特指	Leukemia unspecified	890	0.84	1.71	1.35	0.08	0.13	648	1.20	1.32	1.03	0.06	0.10	C95
其他或未指明部位	Other and unspecified	1 912	1.80	3.67	2.52	0.13	0.29	1 248	2.31	2.54	1.61	0.08	0.18	O&U
所有部位合计	All sites	106 197	100.00	203.66	132.70	6.83	15.45	54 042	100.00	110.06	66.37	3.36	7.45	C00-C97, D32-D33, D42-D43, D45-D47
所有部位除外 C44	All sites except C44	105 773	99.60	202.85	132.19	6.81	15.40	53 714	99.39	109.39	66.01	3.35	7.42	C00-C97, D32-D33, D42-D43, D45-D47 exc. C44

鸣　谢

　　《中国肿瘤登记年报》编委会对各肿瘤登记处的相关工作人员在本年报出版过程中给予的大力协助,尤其在整理、补充、审核登记资料,以及建档建库等方面所做出的贡献表示感谢。衷心感谢编写组成员在年报撰写工作中付出的辛苦努力。

Acknowledgement

　　The editorial committee of *Chinese Cancer Registry Annual Report* would like to express their gratitude to all staff of cancer registries who have made a great contribution for the report, especially on data reduction, supplements, auditing and cancer registration database management. Sincere thanks go to all members of the contributors for their great efforts.

肿瘤登记处名单 List of Cancer Registries and Registrars

省(自治区、直辖市) Province (autonomous region, municipality)	肿瘤登记处 Cancer Registry	登记处所在单位 Affiliation	主要工作人员 Staff				
北京市	北京市	北京大学肿瘤医院暨北京市肿瘤防治研究所	季加孚　王　宁　杨　雷　刘　硕　李慧超　张　希　李晴雨　程杨杨				
天津市	天津市	天津市疾病预防控制中心	江国虹　王德征　沈成凤　王　冲　孙　坤　张　爽　张　辉　宋桂德				
河北省	河北省	河北医科大学第四医院	单保恩　贺宇彤　李道娟　刘言玉　梁　迪　温登瑰　靳　晶　师　金　瞿　峰				
	石家庄市	石家庄市疾病预防控制中心	马新颜　梁震宇　高　从　范志磊　张幸岩　曹朴芳　赵　炜				
	石家庄市郊区	石家庄市疾病预防控制中心	高　从　梁震宇　马新颜　田密格　任军辉　张玉峰　张玉伟　邓莉莉				
	赞皇县	赞皇县疾病预防控制中心	王树革　李　丽　郝月红　吕晓红				
	迁西县	迁西县疾病预防控制中心	盛振海　赵金鸽　陈晓东　王伟光　赵　珊　赵　丹				
	迁安市	迁安市疾病预防控制中心	刘　芳　王翠玲　邵舰伟　谌华卿				
	秦皇岛市	秦皇岛市第四医院	熊润红　赵　月　杨　晋　窦雅琳				
	邯郸市邯山区	邯郸市邯山区疾病预防控制中心	张瑞欣　李金娥　王晓燕　白银燕				
	大名县	大名县疾病预防控制中心	任永彪　刘肖单　孙成旭　孙建冰　杨永华　张　赛　李欣欣				
	涉县	涉县肿瘤防治所	李永伟　温登瑰　杨保证　张书宾　贾瑞强　张　喻				
	磁县	磁县肿瘤防治研究所	宋国慧　陈　超　孟凡书　龚妍玮　冀鸿新　张　金　路晓雪　高志光				
	武安市	武安市疾病预防控制中心	杨　慧　魏延其　郭秀杰　崔亚宁				
	邢台市	邢台市人民医院	刘登湘　王军辉　贾丹丹　张亚琛　刘淑娴　韩　蕾　孟亚飞　王艳霞				
	邢台县	邢台县疾病预防控制中心	董　玲　贾丹丹　刘淑娴　王德旗　赵书云				

省（自治区、直辖市）Province（autonomous region，municipality）	肿瘤登记处 Cancer Registry	登记处所在单位 Affiliation	主要工作人员 Staff
	临城县	临城县人民医院	和丽娜　王　童
	内丘县	内丘县疾病预防控制中心	龙　云　石胜民　智　玉　房晓芳
	邢台市任泽区	河北省任县医院	赵雅芳　吉国强　孟　飞
	保定市	保定市疾病预防控制中心	张　雁　赵凤芹　侯　烨　和丽娜　张卫君 曹　帅　孙　明　张　利
	望都县	望都县疾病预防控制中心	梁鹏涛　田红梅　谷朝华
	安国市	安国市疾病预防控制中心	刘树生　李　辉　魏泽永
	张家口市宣化区	张家口市宣化区疾病预防控制中心	左存锐　李少英　支　雯
	张北县	张北县疾病预防控制中心	刘　会　刘东雍
	承德市双桥区	承德市双桥区疾病预防控制中心	管丽娟　李广鲲　王明慧　平　萍　彭媛媛
	丰宁满族自治县	丰宁满族自治县医院	梁树军　颜学文　付杨健娇
	沧州市	沧州市疾病预防控制中心	杨希晨　鲁文慧　安连芹　高哲敏　李文娟 仝建玲　付素红　杨秀敏
	海兴县	海兴县疾病预防控制中心	韩明明　张　策
	盐山县	盐山县疾病预防控制中心	巩吉良　陈清彦　边梅芳　侯美娟
	衡水市冀州区	衡水市冀州区疾病预防控制中心	魏　丹　郭志超　贾向勇　酒梅洁　王英林
	辛集市	辛集市疾病预防控制中心	郝士卿　万真真　耿　兵
山西省	山西省	山西省肿瘤医院	张永贞　郭雪蓉　马朝辉　曹　凌　王昕琛 崔王飞
	太原市杏花岭区	太原市杏花岭区疾病预防控制中心	荆国旗　倪　芳　薛秀丽　赵　虹　李芝玲
	阳泉市	阳泉市肿瘤防治研究所	高秋生　吕利成　冯俊青　蒋书琼
	平定县	平定县疾病预防控制中心	贾源瑶　李春霞
	盂县	盂县疾病预防控制中心	李俊才　郭长青　韩瑞贞
	平顺县	平顺县疾病预防控制中心	贾艳芳　王丽娟
	沁源县	沁源县疾病预防控制中心	关鹏飞
	阳城县	阳城县肿瘤医院	王新正　元芳梅　李　阳
	晋中市榆次区	晋中市榆次区疾病预防控制中心	郑永萍　郭秀峰　董小平　智　伟　李巧凤 闫梦娇　郭　磊
	昔阳县	昔阳县疾病预防控制中心	王晓霞
	寿阳县	寿阳县疾病预防控制中心	张慧玲　郝佐文　霍志强　杨晓静　胡旭强 王俊红

省(自治区、直辖市) Province (autonomous region, municipality)	肿瘤登记处 Cancer Registry	登记处所在单位 Affiliation	主要工作人员 Staff			
	稷山县	稷山县疾病预防控制中心	谭万霞	赵夏娟		
	绛县	绛县疾病预防控制中心	李姣霞	高丽莉		
	垣曲县	垣曲县疾病预防控制中心	张红霞	武茹燕		
	芮城县	芮城县疾病预防控制中心	范夏莉	王康宁		
	洪洞县	洪洞县疾病预防控制中心	侯晓艳	焦燕燕		
	临县	临县疾病预防控制中心	刘秀娥	高旭亮		
	孝义市	孝义市疾病预防控制中心	冀德恩	张学慧	黄 丽	张剑荣
内蒙古自治区	内蒙古自治区	内蒙古自治区综合疾病预防控制中心	席云峰	乔丽颖		
	呼和浩特市	呼和浩特市疾病预防控制中心	汪洋杰	李 娜	董连英	
	呼伦贝尔市	呼伦贝尔市疾病预防控制中心	王 勇	蔡静明		
	通辽市	通辽市疾病预防控制中心	李智慧			
	赤峰市	赤峰市疾病预防控制中心	张竞丹	谢景学	王化彬	迟艳玲
	锡林郭勒盟	锡林郭勒盟疾病预防控制中心	彭爱云	格日勒	王树丽	
	巴彦淖尔市	巴彦淖尔市疾病预防控制中心	张 琳	韩爱英	邓海凤	
	武川县	武川县疾病预防控制中心	郭建平	赵晓钢		
	土默特右旗	土默特右旗疾病预防控制中心	贾卫军	王 峰	田晓丽	邬燕慧 刘茂林
	赤峰市红山区	赤峰市红山区疾病预防控制中心	何 丽			
	赤峰市元宝山区	赤峰市元宝山区疾病预防控制中心	韩小玉	孟晓东		
	赤峰市松山区	赤峰市松山区疾病预防控制中心	王梦元	许建斌	夏丽红	
	巴林左旗	巴林左旗疾病预防控制中心	凌海杰	宫 明		
	敖汉旗	敖汉旗疾病预防控制中心	耿文飞	崔海华		
	通辽市科尔沁区	通辽市科尔沁区疾病预防控制中心	周婷婷	高 晶		
	科尔沁左翼中旗	科尔沁左翼中旗疾病预防控制中心	李伟杰	刘艳玲		
	开鲁县	开鲁县疾病预防控制中心	吴艳伟	丁秀鸿	曹 亮	
	库伦旗	库伦旗疾病预防控制中心	于鑫刚	王朝民		
	奈曼旗	奈曼旗疾病预防控制中心	李丽媛	倪志华	张永红	
	扎鲁特旗	扎鲁特旗疾病预防控制中心	王晓琪	婷 婷		
	呼伦贝尔市海拉尔区	呼伦贝尔市海拉尔区疾病预防控制中心	孔程程	孙溯苑		

省(自治区、直辖市) Province (autonomous region, municipality)	肿瘤登记处 Cancer Registry	登记处所在单位 Affiliation	主要工作人员 Staff
	呼伦贝尔市扎赉诺尔区	呼伦贝尔市扎赉诺尔区疾病预防控制中心	刘杰峰 过 亮
	阿荣旗	阿荣旗疾病预防控制中心	郭天骅 高 智 林鸿鸣 张银华
	莫力达瓦达斡尔族自治旗	莫力达瓦达斡尔族自治旗疾病预防控制中心	赵占峰
	鄂温克族自治旗	鄂温克族自治旗疾病预防控制中心	张艺杰 田伟伟
	陈巴尔虎旗	陈巴尔虎旗疾病预防控制中心	永 梅
	满洲里市	满洲里市疾病预防控制中心	刘 伟 张欣越 张美燕
	牙克石市	牙克石市疾病预防控制中心	苏 燕 李覆男 夏 宇
	扎兰屯市	扎兰屯市疾病预防控制中心	李 静 陈 丽
	额尔古纳市	额尔古纳市疾病预防控制中心	张 欢
	根河市	根河市疾病预防控制中心	谷寒峰
	巴彦淖尔市临河区	巴彦淖尔市临河区疾病预防控制中心	马 萍 安 静 刘美丽 丁建平
	锡林浩特市	锡林浩特市疾病预防控制中心	刘福生 闫永峰 李智鹏 樊翠玲
辽宁省	辽宁省	辽宁省疾病预防控制中心	穆慧娟
	沈阳市	沈阳市疾病预防控制中心	吕 艺 白 杉 刘 岩 许秀莹 刘欣雨
	康平县	康平县疾病预防控制中心	彭红伟 白宇南
	法库县	法库县疾病预防控制中心	马云丽 张宝桐 曹海洋 白鹤楠
	大连市	大连市疾病预防控制中心	王晓锋 梅 丹 林 红 张新慧
	庄河市	庄河市疾病预防控制中心	王丽娜 姜金宏
	鞍山市	鞍山市疾病预防控制中心	徐绍和 王丽娟 邹青春 尹 晔 张微微 王肖琳 林立强 李绯璇 刘美玲 陈康境 张 颖 洪圣茹
	本溪市	本溪市疾病预防控制中心	安晓霞 李海娜
	丹东市	丹东市疾病预防控制中心	孙继绪 邹晓琳 盛禹萌
	东港市	东港市疾病预防控制中心	张武武 程笛珈
	营口市	营口市疾病预防控制中心	白明宇 刘 洋 陈丽莉 李 颖
	阜新市	阜新市疾病预防控制中心	代晓泽 刘 辉 徐 飒
	彰武县	彰武县疾病预防控制中心	王静艳 王 楠
	辽阳县	辽阳县疾病预防控制中心	何秀玲 李迎秋 李修竹
	盘锦市大洼区	盘锦市大洼区疾病预防控制中心	吕建峰 陆 阳
	建平县	建平县疾病预防控制中心	杨晓光 朱靖怡 熊丽杰 吕广艳

省（自治区、直辖市） Province （autonomous region, municipality）	肿瘤登记处 Cancer Registry	登记处所在单位 Affiliation	主要工作人员 Staff				
吉林省	吉林省	吉林省疾病预防控制中心慢病所	朱颖俐	侯筑林	贾淯媛		
	德惠市	德惠市疾病预防控制中心	程志芳	凌命新	邢 健		
	吉林市	吉林市疾病预防控制中心	张 迪	孙殿伟	刘 晔	王丽宇	王 刚
	吉林市昌邑区	吉林市昌邑区疾病预防控制中心	闫 双	何 冰	徐 翠	靳程程	
	吉林市龙潭区	吉林市龙潭区疾病预防控制中心	代肖瑶				
	吉林市船营区	吉林市船营区疾病预防控制中心	刘亚卓				
	吉林市丰满区	吉林市丰满区疾病预防控制中心	周兴超	周 岩			
	永吉县	永吉县疾病预防控制中心	王晓妍	何晓峰			
	蛟河市	蛟河市疾病预防控制中心	张黎黎				
	桦甸市	桦甸市疾病预防控制中心	王晓丽	李忠诚	于彩霞		
	磐石市	磐石市疾病预防控制中心	冀 鹏	步 颖			
	通化市	通化市疾病预防控制中心	何 柳	张 琳	魏 霞	王晓雪	
	柳河县	柳河县疾病预防控制中心	季洪伟				
	梅河口市	梅河口市疾病预防控制中心	王 彬	刘 宏	潘培丰	李红云	
	大安市	大安市疾病预防控制中心	王 越	王 威	李晓秋	刘艳萍	
	延吉市	延吉市疾病预防控制中心	方学哲	孙铭徽	谢 瑶		
	图们市	图们市疾病预防控制中心	宋立军	王嘉玉	郑玉凤		
	敦化市	敦化市疾病预防控制中心	李秀英	朱晓梅	马桂君		
	珲春市	珲春市疾病预防控制中心	任爱芳	李美子			
	龙井市	龙井市疾病预防控制中心	罗艳丽	金秀颖			
	和龙市	和龙市疾病预防控制中心	张春英	马晓宇	徐桐欣		
	汪清县	汪清县疾病预防控制中心	李美娜	刘 宇			
	安图县	安图县疾病预防控制中心	朴顺姬	段丽雪	方立强		
黑龙江省	黑龙江省	黑龙江省癌症中心	宋冰冰	孙惠昕	张茂祥	王婉莹	贾海晗
	哈尔滨市道里	哈尔滨市道里区疾病预防控制中心	王 欣	康 娟	杨媛媛	那 倩	张希羽
	哈尔滨市南岗	哈尔滨市南岗区疾病预防控制中心	王 驰	于 波	单晓丽	王威娜	
	哈尔滨市香坊区	哈尔滨市香坊区疾病预防控制中心	曲 洋	高艳丽			
	尚志市	尚志市疾病预防控制中心	姜 欣				
	五常市	五常市疾病预防控制中心	周 锐	田伟成			
	勃利县	勃利县疾病预防控制中心	石旭蕾	胡 月			
	牡丹江市东安区	牡丹江市东安区疾病预防控制中心	常 蓉				
	牡丹江市阳明区	牡丹江市阳明区疾病预防控制中心	姚 琳				
	牡丹江市爱民区	牡丹江市爱民区疾病预防控制中心	郝庆华				

省(自治区、直辖市) Province (autonomous region, municipality)	肿瘤登记处 Cancer Registry	登记处所在单位 Affiliation	主要工作人员 Staff				
	牡丹江市西安区	牡丹江市西安区疾病预防控制中心	邱　红	严海莹	付　饶		
	海林市	海林市疾病预防控制中心	余　斌	龙　江	牛春英		
上海市	上海市	上海市疾病预防控制中心	付　晨	施　燕	顾　凯	吴春晓	庞　怡
			王春芳	施　亮	向咏梅	龚杨明	窦剑明
			吴梦吟				
江苏省	江苏省	江苏省疾病预防控制中心（江苏省公共卫生研究院）	武　鸣	韩仁强	周金意	罗鹏飞	俞　浩
			缪伟刚				
	无锡市	无锡市疾病预防控制中心	王　璐	钱　云	杨志杰	董昀球	陈　海
			刘　佳	申　倩	刘雅琦		
	无锡市锡山区	无锡市锡山区疾病预防控制中心	徐红艳	顾　月	邹丽艳	薛文涛	姚吕航
			夏　焱	华　芬	浦佳林	张　丹	徐　芳
	无锡市惠山区	无锡市惠山区疾病预防控制中心	陈顺平	曹　军	蒋金彪	茹　炯	李心意
			赵　悦				
	无锡市滨湖区	无锡市滨湖区疾病预防控制中心	徐汉顺	刘俊华	杜　明	许丽佳	肖静燕
			叶文斌	许　敏	王　菁	顾　飞	朱　漪
			陶燕君				
	无锡市梁溪区	无锡市梁溪区疾病预防控制中心	沈晓文	陈　鑫	王　琳	包海明	徐凌云
	无锡市新吴区	无锡市新吴区疾病预防控制中心	陆绍琦	胡　磊	李　纯	吴晓慧	颜锁芳
			张　芳	殷锡琴	钱　郁	钱嘉红	华　怡
			朱明玉				
	无锡市经开区	无锡市经开区疾病预防控制中心	王礼华	高敏国	陈善辉	邹志红	王　景
			周梦迪	姚成帅	陈汉哲	段春晓	
	江阴市	江阴市疾病预防控制中心	章　剑	朱爱萍	李　莹	刘　娟	王敏洁
			汤海波	张燕茹			
	宜兴市	宜兴市疾病预防控制中心	胡　静	任露露	闵艺璇		
	徐州市	徐州市疾病预防控制中心	娄培安	常桂秋	张　盼	董宗美	陈培培
			张　宁	乔　程	李　婷		
	徐州市	徐州市鼓楼区疾病预防控制中心	刘娅娴	祁艳秋			
	徐州市	徐州市云龙区疾病预防控制中心	李玉波	宋兆芬	渠漫漫	刘　云	
	徐州市	徐州市贾汪区疾病预防控制中心	宗　华	张　迪	李金宇		
	徐州市	徐州市泉山区疾病预防控制中心	吴海宏	李　念	王艳梅	张　培	赵梦晨
	徐州市	徐州市铜山区疾病预防控制中心	唐士涛	侯书莹			

省（自治区、直辖市）Province（autonomous region，municipality）	肿瘤登记处 Cancer Registry	登记处所在单位 Affiliation	主要工作人员 Staff				
	丰县	丰县疾病预防控制中心	王友林	韩红芳	李爽爽		
	沛县	沛县疾病预防控制中心	独梅芝 倪 萌	陈 峰 魏文静	徐 丽	梁艳静	赵欲辉
	睢宁县	睢宁县疾病预防控制中心	仲崇义	张申亮	赵梦洁	姚建英	
	新沂市	新沂市疾病预防控制中心	王 志	张 奇			
	邳州市	邳州市疾病预防控制中心	温之花	刘 杰	李军政		
	常州市	常州市疾病预防控制中心	徐文超	骆文书	李贵英	周孟孟	
	常州市新北区	常州市新北区疾病预防控制中心	张 友	郑蜀贞	何 怡		
	常州市天宁区	常州市天宁区疾病预防控制中心	陈燕芬	施鸿飞			
	常州市武进区	常州市武进区疾病预防控制中心	强德仁 闫于飘	宗 菁	石素逸	杨佳成	孔晓玲
	常州市钟楼区	常州市钟楼区疾病预防控制中心	崔艳丽	吴振霞	陈志华	戴安迪	
	常州市金坛区	常州市金坛区疾病预防控制中心	周 鑫	程 鑫			
	溧阳市	溧阳市疾病预防控制中心	刘建平	狄 静	曹 磊	石一辰	朱阿仙
	苏州市	苏州市疾病预防控制中心	陆 艳	王临池	黄春妍	华钰洁	
	苏州市高新区	苏州市高新区疾病预防控制中心	王从菊	归国平	季 文	顾 晴	
	苏州市吴中区	苏州市吴中区疾病预防控制中心	顾建芬	周 游	刘景超	马菊萍	
	苏州市相城区	苏州市相城区疾病预防控制中心	古娜利	吴向青	张 群	任玮叶	
	苏州市姑苏区	苏州市姑苏区疾病预防控制中心	张 秋	孔芳芳	吴新凡	徐 焱	陈 丽
	苏州市吴江区	苏州市吴江区疾病预防控制中心	沈建新 杨 梅	沈红梅 沈 霞	张荣艳 俞哲宇	姚小燕	彭晓楚
	苏州市工业园区	苏州市工业园区疾病预防控制中心	周 慧	周靓玥	翟 静	景 阳	
	常熟市	常熟市疾病预防控制中心	陈冰霞 顾亦斌	盛红艳 叶映丹	吴 叶	薛雨星	陈丽枫
	张家港市	张家港市疾病预防控制中心	杜国明 王洵之	邱 晶 朱晓炜	秦敏晔	赵丽霞	王夏冬
	昆山市	昆山市疾病预防控制中心	张 婷 仝 岚	秦 威 邱和泉	金亦徐 贺方荣	陆吕霖 朱琴花	周 杰

省（自治区、直辖市） Province （autonomous region，municipality）	肿瘤登记处 Cancer Registry	登记处所在单位 Affiliation	主要工作人员 Staff				
	太仓市	太仓市疾病预防控制中心	张建安	高玲琳	颜小銮	陆鸿滋	
	南通市	南通市疾病预防控制中心	徐 红	王 秦	韩颖颖	潘少聪	梁潇静
	南通市崇川区	南通市崇川区疾病预防控制中心	刘海峰	郑会燕			
	南通市通州区	南通市通州区疾病预防控制中心	赵 培	刘 玉			
	海安市	海安市疾病预防控制中心	王小健	童海燕	孙 静		
	如东县	如东县疾病预防控制中心	张爱红 季佳慧	纪桂勤 周晓云	张红星	孙艳丽	吴双玲
	启东市	启东肝癌防治研究所	朱 健 陈建国	陈永胜	王 军	张永辉	丁璐璐
	如皋市	如皋市疾病预防控制中心	吕家爱	王书兰	徐周洲	吴 坚	
	南通市海门区	南通市海门区疾病预防控制中心	杨艳蕾	唐锦高	倪倬健	邱 敏	施 华
	连云港市	连云港市疾病预防控制中心	董建梅 柴丽丽	张春道	李伟伟	马昭君	秦绪成
	连云港市	连云港市海州区疾病预防控制中心	李炎炎	李佳雨	邓鑫鑫		
	连云港市	连云港市连云区疾病预防控制中心	付艳云	刘 敏	张 琦	李绪磊	惠康琴
	连云港市	连云港市经济技术开发区疾病预防控制中心	李存禄	宋家胜			
	连云港市	连云港市赣榆区疾病预防控制中心	张晓峰	金 凤	顾绍生		
	东海县	东海县疾病预防控制中心	吴同浩 陈 晓	仲 进	王 勇	马 进	吉园园
	灌云县	灌云县疾病预防控制中心	马士化	宋 靖	严春华		
	灌南县	灌南县疾病预防控制中心	张源生	陈学琴	丁梦秋	孟忆宁	
	淮安市	淮安市疾病预防控制中心	沈 欢 缪丹丹	潘恩春 王 璐	孙中明 唐 勇	张 芹	文进博
	淮安市淮安区	淮安市淮安区疾病预防控制中心	宋 光 开海涛	王 昕 马建玲	苏 明 顾忠祥	颜庆洋	朱丽萍
	淮安市淮阴区	淮安市淮阴区疾病预防控制中心	罗国良 高晓清	袁 瑛 李 敏	刘 丹	徐 静	滕笑雨
	淮安市清江浦区	淮安市清江浦区疾病预防控制中心	曹慷慷	万福萍			
	淮安市洪泽区	淮安市洪泽区疾病预防控制中心	李 栋 曹巧力	陈思红	张举巧	袁翠莲	王庶安

省（自治区、直辖市） Province （autonomous region，municipality）	肿瘤登记处 Cancer Registry	登记处所在单位 Affiliation	主要工作人员 Staff				
	涟水县	涟水县疾病预防控制中心	叶建玲	孙维新	浦继尹		
	盱眙县	盱眙县疾病预防控制中心	王　裕	姜其家	袁守国		
	金湖县	金湖县疾病预防控制中心	陈茂勇	何士林	吴　婷	雷茵子	
	盐城市	盐城市疾病预防控制中心	刘付东	吴玲玲	梁　季	郑春早	祁朝霞
	盐城市亭湖区	盐城市亭湖区疾病预防控制中心	严莉丽	开志琴	王　静		
	盐城市盐都区	盐城市盐都区疾病预防控制中心	何　飞	王建康	黄海涌		
	响水县	响水县疾病预防控制中心	潘永富	陈玥华	王　超	徐红云	刘宇春
	滨海县	滨海县疾病预防控制中心	蔡　伟 胡　裕	赵　鹏 樊明静	李　明	陈希冀	王　瑞
	阜宁县	阜宁县疾病预防控制中心	梁从凯	杨尚波	支　杰		
	射阳县	射阳县疾病预防控制中心	戴曙光	戴春云	王颖莹	陈星宇	戴　利
	建湖县	建湖县疾病预防控制中心	王　剑	肖　丽	孔文娟		
	东台市	东台市疾病预防控制中心	郑小祥	赵建华	丁海健	史春兰	
	盐城市大丰区	盐城市大丰区疾病预防控制中心	顾晓平	顾　昕	盛　凤	王银存	智恒奎
	扬州市	扬州市疾病预防控制中心	解　晔 蒋　萌	李秋梅 胡乃元	杨文彬	时巧梅	赵　培
	宝应县	宝应县疾病预防控制中心	梁永春	朱立文	任　涛	王元霞	潘艳玉
	镇江市	镇江市疾病预防控制中心	姜方平	徐　璐	王宏宇	古孝勇	何佳佳
	丹阳市	丹阳市疾病预防控制中心	应洪琰	周　超	陈丽黎	胡佳慧	王佳烨
	扬中市	扬中市肿瘤防治研究所	朱进华 宋统球	华召来	周　琴	施爱武	冯　祥
	泰州市	泰州市疾病预防控制中心	赵小兰 周　永	卢海燕 浦　栋	张德坤	杨玉雪	张慧琴
	泰兴市	泰兴市市疾病预防控制中心	黄素勤 刘静琦	范　敏 蒋　慧	徐　兴	封军莉	丁华萍
	宿迁市	宿迁市疾病预防控制中心	卢道山	于　蕾	邱玉保	高　歌	
	宿迁市宿城区	宿迁市宿城区疾病预防控制中心	漆苏洋	陈　英	张恋恋	朱　敏	于蒙蒙
	宿迁市宿豫区	宿迁市宿豫区疾病预防控制中心	朱　雷 胡彩红	郭鑫雨	陶　欣	孙绪远	王松梅
	泗阳县	泗阳县疾病预防控制中心	韩　奎	李红霞	符地宝	陈淑婷	
浙江省	浙江省	浙江省肿瘤防治办公室	程向东 裘燕飞 王悠清	俞　敏 钟节鸣 王　乐	杜灵彬 龚巍巍 陈雯冰	李辉章 周慧娟 陈　刚	陈瑶瑶 朱　陈

省（自治区、直辖市）Province（autonomous region，municipality）	肿瘤登记处 Cancer Registry	登记处所在单位 Affiliation	主要工作人员 Staff				
	杭州市	杭州市疾病预防控制中心	徐　珏　姜彩霞　姜　鹏　任艳军　张　艳 刘　冰				
	宁波市鄞州区	宁波市鄞州区疾病预防控制中心	林鸿波　沈　鹏　陈　奇　赵　磊				
	慈溪市	慈溪市疾病预防控制中心	吴逸平　马　旭　罗　丹　刘　琼　黄振宇 罗央努　黄　文　王利君　胡　吉　岑　鑫				
	温州市鹿城区	温州市鹿城区疾病预防控制中心	朱海深　谢海斌　陈　茜　陈　捷　张沛绮 徐晓旭　郑茹茹				
	嘉兴市	嘉兴市疾病预防控制中心	李雪琴　陈中文　顾伟玲　谢　亮　陈文燕 金　鎏　王　林　周夏芳　金泽彬				
	嘉善县	嘉善县肿瘤防治所	沈飞琼　杨金华　李其龙　吕洁萍　张小红				
	海宁市	海宁市中医院	朱云峰　祝丽娟　杨　靖　封　琳　白卿长				
	长兴县	长兴县疾病预防控制中心	施长苗　秦家胜　陈　蓉　臧宇凡　陈　芸 顾建萍　叶　萍				
	绍兴市上虞区	绍兴市上虞区疾病预防控制中心	王家开　章　军　丁萍飞　杨晓静　赵之青 龚月江　阮建江　王少华				
	永康市	永康市疾病预防控制中心	潘中伟　胡云卿　吴忠顶　胡　浩　朱洪挺 胡春生　徐玲巧　陈　璐　沈锦绣　周美儿				
	开化县	开化县疾病预防控制中心	严传富　汪德兵　项彩英　吴芝兰　应武群 万红建　叶　青　王贵平　余　虹				
	岱山县	岱山县疾病预防控制中心	李琼燕　虞吉寅　张彤杰　何存弘　赵剑刚 王坤炎　王志平　王建军　徐　妮　俞秀华				
	仙居县	仙居县疾病预防控制中心	蔡红卫　应江伟　吴武军　周立新　王丽君 王宇多　郑　红　王敏华　陈海仙　王丹枫				
	龙泉市	龙泉市疾病预防控制中心	钟伟文　梅盛华　万春松　刘卫红　潘伟文 叶水菊　尹丽梅　谢泽久　张美锦　吴国庆				
安徽省	安徽省	安徽省疾病预防控制中心	刘志荣　王华东　查震球　陈叶纪　戴　丹				
	合肥市	合肥市疾病预防控制中心	孙　锋　张小鹏　李佳佳　唐　伦　陈晓园 穆永春　屈跃斌　胡玉莹　张　欢　何丽芳				
	长丰县	长丰县疾病预防控制中心	孙多壮　郑　军　陈　春　吴海燕				
	肥东县	肥东县疾病预防控制中心	张全寿　徐　旭　陈海涛				
	肥西县	肥西县疾病预防控制中心	胡晓先　汪　飞　魏九丹				
	庐江县	庐江县疾病预防控制中心	黄国士　吴　骅				
	巢湖市	巢湖市疾病预防控制中心	宋玉华　叶正文　王义江　刘　涛				
	芜湖市	芜湖市疾病预防控制中心	朱君君　崔晓娟　陈佳瑶　盛　娟　鲍慧芬 王力炜　丁卫群　赵丽华　王秀丽　吴瑞萍 冯花平				

省（自治区、直辖市） Province （autonomous region, municipality）	肿瘤登记处 Cancer Registry	登记处所在单位 Affiliation	主要工作人员 Staff
	蚌埠市	蚌埠市疾病预防控制中心	陈　军　张威振　周国华　白　雪　陈　艳 尚晓静　苏一兰
	五河县	五河县疾病预防控制中心	夏立环　郭茂蕴　纪　琼　许美菱
	淮南市大通区	大通区疾病预防控制中心	王艳霞　张　娇　陈邦齐
	淮南市田家庵区	淮南市田家庵区卫生防疫和食品药品安全服务中心	周　蕾　李娜娜　崔　越
	淮南市谢家集区	淮南市谢家集区卫生防疫和食品药品安全服务中心	辛家魁　吕　娟
	淮南市八公山区	淮南市八公山区卫生防疫和食品药品安全服务中心	吴　婷　叶亚萍
	淮南市潘集区	潘集区卫生防疫和食品药品安全服务中心	左廷杰　孙海防　姚　媛
	凤台县	凤台县疾病预防控制中心	秦克波　郭　克　李　涛　陈志强
	淮南市毛集区	淮南市毛集区防疫保健计划生育服务中心	孙红霞
	马鞍山市	马鞍山市疾病预防控制中心	王　春　叶敏仕　张　燕　蔡华英　秦其荣
	当涂县	当涂县疾病预防控制中心	徐　薇　李代平　卜维霞
	濉溪县	濉溪县疾病预防控制中心	贾　林　周鹏程　杨　珂　朱　英　张贵然
	铜陵市	铜陵市疾病预防控制中心	吴　刚　钱　丹　刘　睿　汪　蕊
	铜陵市义安区	铜陵市义安疾病预防控制中心	张　标　丁　媛　高红霞
	安庆市宜秀区	安庆市宜秀区疾病预防控制中心	郝润华　鲍克彪
	岳西县	岳西县疾病预防控制中心	范莉莉　储琼瑛　亓志强
	黄山市屯溪区	黄山市屯溪区疾病预防控制中心	叶雯雯　裴　勇
	天长市	天长市疾病预防控制中心	胡　彪　赵培甫　张　浩
	阜阳市颍州区	阜阳市颍州区疾病预防控制中心	张海峰　郭　青　刘俊辉　王福军　王明玉 韦冰之　韩　梅
	阜阳市颍东区	阜阳市颍东区疾病预防控制中心	马朝阳　孙　涛　郭海昊　陈　雷　徐晓晴 张静静
	太和县	太和县疾病预防控制中心	张怡楠　李诗童　张西才　王允田　谭霈源 范　鑫
	阜南县	阜南县疾病预防控制中心	杨晓波　张永红　田　侠　单文华　张家棒
	颍上县	颍上县疾病预防控制中心	王　政　吴　昊　明　超　彭姝婷
	宿州市埇桥区	宿州市埇桥区疾病预防控制中心	刘中华　刘　森　张　鹏　张圆圆　黄　磊

省（自治区、直辖市） Province （autonomous region， municipality）	肿瘤登记处 Cancer Registry	登记处所在单位 Affiliation	主要工作人员 Staff				
	灵璧县	灵璧县疾病预防控制中心	郭启高	赵 辉	汤雅丽		
	寿县	寿县疾病预防控制中心	杨茂敏	蔡传毓	徐海军	黄 奎	霍圣菊
			唐晶晶	周 颖	王正友	周玉雪	陶俊婷
	霍邱县	霍邱县疾病预防控制中心	吴礼娟	周明琴			
	金寨县	金寨县疾病预防控制中心	俞 亮	廖家胜	张礼兵	王玉文	童 亮
	蒙城县	蒙城县疾病预防控制中心	刘珊珊	刘 翔	李银梅	张爱东	
	东至县	东至县疾病预防控制中心	景燕平	张 瑶	吴泽宁		
	泾县	泾县疾病预防控制中心	刘安阜	吴 鹏	程莉莉	周 伟	杨露露
			马雄梅				
	宁国市	宁国市疾病预防控制中心	胡倩华	付 超	唐 雯	朱韦辰	
福建省	福建省	福建省肿瘤医院	周 衍	马晶昱	相智声		
	福清市	福清市疾病预防控制中心	何道逢	钟女娟	翁瑜瑶	王小阳	
	福州市长乐区	福州市长乐区肿瘤防治研究所	陈建顺	陈礼慈	陈 英	陈心聪	陈聪明
			张祖霞				
	厦门市	厦门市疾病预防控制中心	伍啸青	许连升	林艺兰	陈月珍	连真忠
			陈 沁	张卓平	陈丽燕	张琼花	易艺鹏
			谭林华	谢丽珊			
	厦门市同安区	厦门市同安区疾病预防控制中心	陈仁忠	陈上清	陈珊瑚		
	厦门市翔安区	厦门市翔安区疾病预防控制中心	柯金练	林雅秀			
	莆田市涵江区	莆田市涵江区疾病预防控制中心	林玉成	方晓滨			
	永安市	永安市疾病预防控制中心	范 光	李杭生	李丽丽		
	惠安县	惠安县疾病预防控制中心	刘庆烟	张冬雪			
	漳州市长泰区	漳州市长泰区疾病预防控制中心	郑冬柏	张碧花			
	建瓯市	建瓯市疾病预防控制中心	官文婷	裴振义	徐肖健		
	龙岩市新罗区	龙岩市新罗区疾病预防控制中心	廖凌玲				
	龙岩市永定区	龙岩市永定区疾病预防控制中心	黄远田	张海丽			
江西省	江西省	江西省疾病预防控制中心	刘 杰	颜 玮	陈小娜		
	南昌市青云谱区	南昌市青云谱区疾病预防控制中心	章文华	李培松	邓云兰		
	南昌市青山湖区	南昌市青山湖区疾病预防控制中心	黄 静	杨盈华	蔡丹桃	陈昔梅	
	南昌市新建区	南昌市新建区疾病预防控制中心	万 信	熊 炜	周孔香	陶永军	

省（自治区、直辖市） Province （autonomous region，municipality）	肿瘤登记处 Cancer Registry	登记处所在单位 Affiliation	主要工作人员 Staff			
	芦溪县	芦溪县疾病预防控制中心	张 莉	张庆红	刘裕坤	李益球
	九江市浔阳区	九江市浔阳区疾病预防控制中心	涂波涌	郑 坤	田绍进	邓如蕙
	武宁县	武宁县疾病预防控制中心	潘盛林	邹德政	张赣湘	熊彩云 段红政
	新余市渝水区	新余市渝水区疾病预防控制中心	周 林 毛 麒	杨 竹	晏琳春	何志勇 宋 艳
	鹰潭市余江区	鹰潭市余江区疾病预防控制中心	曾串莲	陈紫云	危安安	
	赣州市章贡区	赣州市章贡区疾病预防控制中心	廖 顺	苏德云	任学纳	
	赣州市赣县区	赣州市赣县区疾病预防控制中心	罗文云	黄文姬		
	信丰县	信丰县疾病预防控制中心	王昱云	何光伟		
	大余县	大余县疾病预防控制中心	黄飞平	张祥金		
	上犹县	上犹县疾病预防控制中心	田玉平	李舒敏		
	崇义县	崇义县疾病预防控制中心	冯云洪	肖耳目	卢致强	
	龙南市	龙南市疾病预防控制中心	赖永赣	彭旻微	曾志斌	
	于都县	于都县疾病预防控制中心	刘冬秀	陈 军		
	吉安市吉州区	吉安市吉州区疾病预防控制中心	张艳玲	刘 琦		
	峡江县	峡江县疾病预防控制中心	陈志虹	袁怿飞	陈九英	
	安福县	安福县疾病预防控制中心	王 剑	胡水斌	王钟舟	刘忠明 王玉婷
	万载县	万载县疾病预防控制中心	郭巧红	卢 萍		
	上高县	上高县疾病预防控制中心	左 程	周 演		
	靖安县	靖安县疾病预防控制中心	赵朝强	舒小裕	刘志英	
	乐安县	乐安县疾病预防控制中心	戴招文			
	宜黄县	宜黄县疾病预防控制中心	徐媛锋			
	抚州市东乡区	抚州市东乡区疾病预防控制中心	陈 霞	艾欢欢		
	上饶市信州区	上饶市信州区疾病预防控制中心	叶栩艺	叶梦颖	陈婉婷	
	上饶市广丰区	上饶市广丰区疾病预防控制中心	胡翠芳	姚信飞	姚佳丽	严爱丽
	铅山县	铅山县疾病预防控制中心	黄永进	李振雄	暨丽敏	吴永丽
	横峰县	横峰县疾病预防控制中心	程立平	涂永海	毛术霞	杨 帆
	弋阳县	弋阳县疾病预防控制中心	曾雄文	林水旺	胡素华	方荣霞
	余干县	余干县疾病预防控制中心	徐建强	汤彩兰	付美玲	段 叠
	万年县	万年县疾病预防控制中心	盛根英	应 萍		

省（自治区、直辖市） Province (autonomous region, municipality)	肿瘤登记处 Cancer Registry	登记处所在单位 Affiliation	主要工作人员 Staff
	婺源县	婺源县疾病预防控制中心	叶鹏华
	德兴市	德兴市疾病预防控制中心	李彬明　许晓丹
山东省	山东省	山东省疾病预防控制中心	郭晓雷　付振涛　姜　帆
	济南市	济南市疾病预防控制中心	宫舒萍　张先慧　周　林　刘　冰　姜　超 王玉恒　李瑛鑫　李荣华　丁春明
	济南市章丘区	济南市章丘区疾病预防控制中心	刘庆皆　辛　佳　颛孙宁宁
	济南市莱芜区	济南市莱芜区疾病预防控制中心	丁丽平　常　安
	青岛市	青岛市疾病预防控制中心	张增智　宁　锋　王　康　郑晓艳
	青岛市黄岛区	青岛市黄岛区疾病预防控制中心	廖　倩　张金太
	淄博市临淄区	淄博市临淄区疾病预防控制中心	卢　斌　韦　洁　张城倩
	沂源县	沂源县疾病预防控制中心	李东芝　孙　璞　陈义菊　王　慧
	滕州市	滕州市疾病预防控制中心	徐玉銮　于雪静　李玉春　龚　理
	广饶县	广饶县疾病预防控制中心	徐海霞
	烟台市	烟台市疾病预防控制中心	于绍轶　刘海韵　曲淑娜
	烟台市芝罘区	烟台市芝罘区疾病预防控制中心	赵　冲
	烟台市福山区	烟台市福山区疾病预防控制中心	孙　昕
	烟台市莱山区	烟台市莱山区疾病预防控制中心	赵万里
	烟台市牟平区	烟台市牟平区疾病预防控制中心	李东洪
	烟台市开发区	烟台市开发区疾病预防控制中心	厉　程
	招远市	招远市疾病预防控制中心	翟玉庭　宁巍巍　李　玮
	临朐县	临朐县疾病预防控制中心	郭　超　刘卫东　张兰福　井　斌
	高密市	高密市疾病预防控制中心	黄一峰　冷冠群　马瑞花　谢　珍　宋　娟 刘　晓
	济宁市任城区	济宁市任城区疾病预防控制中心	郗帅帅　段世彬　唐　琪
	汶上县	汶上县疾病预防控制中心	李　岩　张　燕
	梁山县	梁山县疾病预防控制中心	张建鲁　冯昌红　谢书丹　王春秀　孔甜甜

省（自治区、直辖市） Province （autonomous region，municipality）	肿瘤登记处 Cancer Registry	登记处所在单位 Affiliation	主要工作人员 Staff				
	曲阜市	曲阜市疾病预防控制中心	孔　超 乔　乔	侯爱平	颜　俊	孔　晖	王　蕊
	邹城市	邹城市疾病预防控制中心	骆秀美 李　娜	张廷番	杨建宁	刘亚琪	王　薇
	宁阳县	宁阳县疾病预防控制中心	刘婷婷	马学成	董芙蓉	张丽杰	
	肥城市	肥城市人民医院	李琰琰 郑春娟	尹晓燕	姜　敏	张婷婷	王　青
	乳山市	乳山市疾病预防控制中心	邹跃威	李立科	张玉佳	李小菲	
	日照市东港区	日照市东港区疾病预防控制中心	尚明风	韩志军			
	沂南县	沂南县疾病预防控制中心	华国梁	王家倩			
	沂水县	沂水县疾病预防控制中心	王维霞 王翠翠	杨登强	马夔玲	伏祥浩	张江宝
	莒南县	莒南县疾病预防控制中心	文章军	张斌磊	李学刚	邓　花	
	德州市德城区	德州市德城区疾病预防控制中心	屠永梓	马莉莉	安德峰		
	高唐县	高唐县疾病预防控制中心	刘淑梅	王秀珍	尹　红	杨亮亮	穆守常
	滨州市滨城区	滨州市滨城区疾病预防控制中心	范美霞	赵贝贝	付立平		
	菏泽市牡丹区	菏泽市牡丹区疾病预防控制中心	秦　舒	国　锦	仇翠梅	刘洋洋	
	单县	单县疾病预防控制中心	赵海洲	李　锦	赵　娥		
	巨野县	巨野县疾病预防控制中心	高杨波	张　晋			
河南省	河南省	河南省肿瘤医院	张韶凯 徐慧芳	陈　琼 郑黎阳	刘曙正 刘　茵	孙喜斌	郭兰伟
	郑州市	郑州市疾病预防控制中心	李建彬	宋彩娟	郭向娇	武恩平	
	巩义市	巩义市疾病预防控制中心	蒋蔚林	王燕青	张文君		
	开封市祥符区	开封市祥符区疾病预防控制中心	马　师	李慎榜	田艳玲	朱方敏	
	洛阳市	洛阳市疾病预防控制中心	闫云燕 刘培培 齐虹飞	常　颖 马昊翔 刘青青	李爱红 魏冰燕 张菲菲	马　凯 石晓红 陈家琦	邢建乐 陈亚楠 李　博
	洛阳市孟津区	洛阳市孟津区疾病预防控制中心	许瑞瑞	张琰琰			
	新安县	新安县疾病预防控制中心	付文莉	翟亚楠	李　辉		
	栾川县	栾川县疾病预防控制中心	刘爱坡	孙亚琦	周园园	刘杏杏	

省（自治区、直辖市） Province （autonomous region, municipality）	肿瘤登记处 Cancer Registry	登记处所在单位 Affiliation	主要工作人员 Staff				
	嵩县	嵩县疾病预防控制中心	杨欣欣 梁秋娟	乔 幸	石梦瑶	杨静媛	姜开霞
	汝阳县	汝阳县疾病预防控制中心	李白鸟	耿振强			
	宜阳县	宜阳县疾病预防控制中心	楚玉梅	李若男	陈 培		
	洛宁县	洛宁县疾病预防控制中心	段乐永	刘龙安			
	伊川县	伊川县疾病预防控制中心	王蜓蜓	董 芳	刘 峰		
	洛阳市偃师区	洛阳市偃师区疾病预防控制中心	秦延锦				
	平顶山市	平顶山市疾病预防控制中心	吕锐利 彭 浩	宋 波 李智伟	颜欣颖 郑红云	张泽华 仲晓伟	许艺苑 温红旭
	鲁山县	鲁山县疾病预防控制中心	王一博	郭启民	田广恩	许姗姗	
	郏县	郏县疾病预防控制中心	孙 颖	王晓艳	昝 哲	宁海燕	董人阁
	舞钢市	舞钢市疾病预防控制中心	刘青兰	刘亚红	尹馨可	段慧娟	
	安阳市	安阳市肿瘤医院	张金文 张晓星	王能超 秦永超	方 岩	张媛媛	闫焕勤
	林州市	林州市肿瘤医院	郭贵周 侯 凯	付方现 王 丽	王振海 刘 畅	李变云	于晓东
	鹤壁市	鹤壁市人民医院	钞利娜 任红勤	王冰冰 郭雪琴	王梦媛	胡凤琴	裴树英
	新乡市	新乡市中心医院	朱智玲	曹河璐			
	辉县市	辉县市疾病预防控制中心	孙花荣	赵小聪	李 颖		
	焦作市	焦作市疾病预防控制中心	孟春辉 周琳菲	田 珍	路娜娜	韩晓宁	高丽利
	孟州市	孟州市疾病预防控制中心	武晓华	潘小燕			
	濮阳市华龙区	濮阳市华龙区疾病预防控制中心	王培贤	齐庆荣	胡利娟		
	范县	范县疾病预防控制中心	田军艳	邢秀娟	薛 辉	王静芳	周瑞敏
	濮阳县	濮阳县疾病预防控制中心	郭秋献	穆晓红	刘 军		
	禹州市	禹州市疾病预防控制中心	王全新	郭 影	李 蔚	杨宗慧	张亚楠
	漯河市	漯河市疾病预防控制中心	代 莹	孙路平	孟 蕾	胡 昕	代君君
	漯河市郾城区	漯河市郾城区疾病预防控制中心	李爱会 邓 婕	袁兵翔 张 楠	庞 静	常帅奇	何怡聪
	舞阳县	舞阳县疾病预防控制中心	何 洁 杨艳芳	马永晓	周小佳	谷来君	张艳丽
	临颍县	临颍县疾病预防控制中心	吴 真	罗 婷	秦苏丹	马玉智	

省（自治区、直辖市）Province（autonomous region，municipality）	肿瘤登记处 Cancer Registry	登记处所在单位 Affiliation	主要工作人员 Staff				
	三门峡市湖滨区	三门峡市湖滨区疾病预防控制中心	李粉妮	刘润娣	罗　丹		
	南阳市卧龙区	南阳市卧龙区疾病预防控制中心	刘　凯	周　静	张　爽		
	南召县	南召县疾病预防控制中心	靳万春 宋　峰	王青勤 樊　璞	陈立明	朱广博	张　营
	方城县	方城县疾病预防控制中心	马建民 张禄军	马璟颖	李　谱	仝成杰	倪林静
	内乡县	内乡县疾病预防控制中心	李亚波	金　花	代　阳		
	睢县	睢县疾病预防控制中心	袁　帅	刘　艳			
	虞城县	虞城县疾病预防控制中心	张亚威 江　培	冯金洪	马　宁	毕兴华	刘　威
	信阳市浉河区	信阳市浉河区疾病预防控制中心	兰宏旺	楚尚兰	耿祎祎	周　娣	李　刚
	罗山县	罗山县疾病预防控制中心	江　坤	徐蔚静	王明阳		
	固始县	固始县疾病预防控制中心	张　柯	沈　玉			
	沈丘县	沈丘县疾病预防控制中心	徐　玲	李庆文	郭丽花	李旭东	孙梦洋
	郸城县	郸城县疾病预防控制中心	张吉志 李慧珍	孙　忠	郭德银	陈　静	马　慧
	太康县	太康县疾病预防控制中心	董　洪	魏国成	李　昂		
	西平县	西平县疾病预防控制中心	毛小辉	邵天堂	王中梅	赵春玲	刘彩霞
	济源市	济源市疾病预防控制中心	马璐瑶 郑莹茹	刘　磊	黄艳芳	郑飞飞	张雷锋
	漯河市源汇区	漯河市源汇区疾病预防控制中心	张　祥	王宏博	牛艳丽	叶　静	
	漯河市召陵区	漯河市召陵区疾病预防控制中心	王军奇	陶　哲	樊永立	鞠晨云	
湖北省	湖北省	湖北省肿瘤医院	庹吉好 夏雅芬	姚　霜	张　敏	秦　宇	孟繁地
	武汉市	武汉市疾病预防控制中心	杨念念 张晓霞	严亚琼	金琦曼	代　娟	赵原原
	大冶市	大冶市疾病预防控制中心	徐　鹏 曹群芳	黄泽华 袁雪冰	徐新建 冯　辉	陈旭东	曹宏利
	十堰市郧阳区	十堰市郧阳区疾病预防控制中心	柯　华	左顺彦	曹　琳	贺　锐	
	宜昌市	宜昌市疾病预防控制中心	胡　池 吴　婵	杨佳娟 邓亚玲	刘　军	张　培	朱　婕

省（自治区、直辖市） Province （autonomous region, municipality）	肿瘤登记处 Cancer Registry	登记处所在单位 Affiliation	主要工作人员 Staff				
	五峰土家族自治县	五峰土家族自治县疾病预防控制中心	熊　斌	邹晓丹	王仁兴		
	襄阳市	襄阳市疾病预防控制中心	陈小慧	龚文胜	鲲　鹏	刘　杰	
	宜城市	宜城市疾病预防控制中心	龚新洪 胡艳芳	朱　波 曾卓璇	王吉国 陈晓霞	李　勇	杨　波
	京山市	京山市疾病预防控制中心	李　宏	代　建	杨　丹		
	钟祥市	钟祥市疾病预防控制中心	赵　丽	霍军荣	廖金凤	高雅玲	
	云梦县	云梦县疾病预防控制中心	周　浩	李纯波	潘雨晴	徐敏莉	
	荆州市	荆州市疾病预防控制中心	毛安禄	江　鸿			
	公安县	公安县疾病预防控制中心	洪　杰 张　丹	申立琼	文良军	龚　春	胡长贵
	洪湖市	洪湖市疾病预防控制中心	廖　涛	向代成	徐海涛	刘登洪	
	麻城市	麻城市疾病预防控制中心	柳以泽 王金荣	丁　成	徐胜平	项维红	库守能
	嘉鱼县	嘉鱼县疾病预防控制中心	刘晓玲 曾　晶 唐　文	刘　庆 肖德顺 姚智敏	黄忠文 杜清华 殷　珊	范锡芳 李小红 魏　雯	陈圆圆 李　燕
	通城县	通城县疾病预防控制中心	刘加军	杨　劲	熊新征	熊子鹏	
	恩施市	恩施市疾病预防控制中心	王　斌	胡燕琳	刘迪军	廖荣芳	
	天门市	天门市疾病预防控制中心	刘　积 李　锐 黄红艳	罗　芬 方　亮 胡　嶙	王义华 邹红艳 胡珍贵	何明辉 彭菊萍 郭　芳	倪亚敏 董君华
湖南省	湖南省	湖南省肿瘤防治研究办公室	肖亚洲 邹艳花 李　娜	王　静 石朝晖 王石玉	颜仕鹏 肖海帆 郭　佳	廖先珍 曹世钰	许可葵 李　灿
	长沙市芙蓉区	长沙市芙蓉区疾病预防控制中心	张运秋	胡辉伍	杨　丽	罗霜艳	
	长沙市天心区	长沙市天心区疾病预防控制中心	许超伦	兰泽龙	王红江		
	长沙市岳麓区	长沙市岳麓区疾病预防控制中心	苏威武	陈继怀	杨思进		
	长沙市开福区	长沙市开福区疾病预防控制中心	林　玲	陈腊梅	刘　阳	刘　玲	
	长沙市雨花区	长沙市雨花区疾病预防控制中心	周建湘 段利霞	何　韬 廖丽艳	黄　芬	胡　蓉	邓谦成
	长沙市望城区	长沙市望城区疾病预防控制中心	程新和 胡利英	王华良	赵劲良	熊　浩	邹思伟

省(自治区、直辖市) Province (autonomous region, municipality)	肿瘤登记处 Cancer Registry	登记处所在单位 Affiliation	主要工作人员 Staff				
	长沙县	长沙县疾病预防控制中心	罗辉琴	黄 云	彭 敏	刘 丹	刘遂怡
	浏阳市	浏阳市疾病预防控制中心	许 欣 谭诗花	陈建伟 李光辉	李 跳	龙花君	王 群
	株洲市芦淞区	株洲市芦淞区疾病预防控制中心	何 礼 彭 彬	唐 晶 陈 慧	卞晓嘉	刘慧颖	鲍 芳
	株洲市石峰区	株洲市石峰区疾病预防控制中心	袁 湘 袁 敏	刘 杰 齐佳锐	黄 平	刘 宏	彭玉梅
	攸县	攸县疾病预防控制中心	符三乃	欧阳四新	刘擎雄	杨华艳	
	湘潭市雨湖区	湘潭市雨湖区疾病预防控制中心	邓莉芳	杨玉环	马超颖	马子涵	蔡文迪
	衡东县	衡东县疾病预防控制中心	尹 炜 刘银月	单健生 周 玲	刘早红 丁 莉	肖静娴	李俊华
	常宁市	常宁市疾病预防控制中心	曹诗鹏 郭 兰	郭秀连	欧 琦	滕德伟	吴良元
	邵东市	邵东市疾病预防控制中心	曾 平 谢清玲	田 丽 谭辉路	陈文伟 刘冬梅	谢 玉	金海燕
	新宁县	新宁县疾病预防控制中心	邓海名	周前富	陈 富	刘倩文	
	岳阳市岳阳楼区	岳阳市岳阳楼区疾病预防控制中心	陈艳芳 鲁小霞	黄 平 宋 婷	罗江洪	罗 莎	李 盛
	常德市武陵区	常德市武陵区疾病预防控制中心	管元平 朱晓辉	涂林立 周宏惠	张志刚	彭学文	唐志敏
	慈利县	慈利县疾病预防控制中心	朱从喜 寇渝东	向 英	吴 双	陈华云	刘 波
	益阳市资阳区	益阳市资阳区疾病预防控制中心	龚建华 范朝彪	王迪军 张丽情	鲁 容	陈 晶	王玲玲
	桃江县	桃江县人民医院	刘 军 邹朝霞	廖亚男 郭 纯	薛媚娟	邹 平	黄 德
	临武县	临武县疾病预防控制中心	周贤文 曹玲芳	李伟生	李国斌	谭林林	刘 冰
	资兴市	资兴市疾病预防控制中心	徐贤雄	李雄豹	黎利文	夏云磊	王英籍
	道县	道县疾病预防控制中心	肖拥军 胡雨华	胡建湘 刘海萍	郑 平 蒋忠葵	何林秀 许洪平	何英俊
	宁远县	宁远县疾病预防控制中心	李万忠	李万清	欧阳小芳	陈颖香	李 玮
	新田县	新田县疾病预防控制中心	欧阳乐 刘君红	谢众麟 刘 波	黄 锋	何忠勇	段良祥
	麻阳苗族自治县	麻阳县疾病预防控制中心	陈 琳	赵 辉	陈启佳	张春玉	滕 瑶
	洪江市	洪江市疾病预防控制中心	向湘林 林嘉兴	易思连	寻英姿	杨小琴	向丽琼

省(自治区、直辖市) Province (autonomous region, municipality)	肿瘤登记处 Cancer Registry	登记处所在单位 Affiliation	主要工作人员 Staff				
	冷水江市	冷水江市疾病预防控制中心	方吉贤	宾远忠	张彬彬	罗三峰	杨　娟
	涟源市	涟源市疾病预防控制中心	文申根 张晓勇	李秀兰 肖艳慎	周红大 李　清	龙爱梅	黄　靖
广东省	广东省	广东省疾病预防控制中心	夏　亮 许晓君	林立丰	许燕君	孟瑞琳	王　晔
	广州市	广州市疾病预防控制中心	王穗湘 陈远源	李　科 董　航	许　欢	秦鹏哲	梁伯衡
	广州市郊区	广州市疾病预防控制中心	梁伯衡 陈远源	王穗湘 董　航	李　科	许　欢	秦鹏哲
	佛山市顺德区	佛山市顺德区慢性病防治中心	杨俊杰	罗洁莹	王谦可	陈　榕	吴　焜
	佛山市南海区	佛山市南海区疾病预防控制中心	谢威龙				
	江门市	江门市疾病预防控制中心	莫兆波	于雪芳			
	梅州市梅江区	梅州市疾病预防控制中心	刘雅姬	古彩红	胡艳红	林文渊	
	梅州市梅县区	梅州市梅县区疾病预防控制中心	杨　慧	李加宁			
	东莞市	东莞市疾病预防控制中心	陈妙嫦	钟洁莹	姚旭芳	黄雅卿	
	南雄市	南雄市疾病预防控制中心	张艳艳	邬香华			
	揭西县	揭西县疾病预防控制中心	贝晶利				
	惠州市惠阳区	惠州市惠阳区疾病预防控制中心	黄惠玲	陈　萍			
	中山市	中山市人民医院(中山市肿瘤研究所)	魏矿荣	梁智恒	李柱明		
	深圳市	深圳市慢性病防治中心	彭　绩	赵志广	雷　林	刘芳江	
	阳山县	阳山县疾病预防控制中心	毛智趣	丘银霞	梁时力	黄永杰	
	罗定市	罗定市疾病预防控制中心	陈红艳	张乔珍	梁惠玲		
	阳江市阳东区	阳江市阳东区疾病预防控制中心	谭家伟	关　设	李海凤	雷玉燕	
	四会市	四会市惠民平价门诊部(四会市肿瘤研究所)	卢玉强	姚继洲	李晓翌	乡一萍	丁惠玲
	珠海市	珠海市慢性病防治中心	郭红革	滕勇勇	陈美婷	谢水仙	
	肇庆市	肇庆市疾病预防控制中心	方艺娟	陆素颖	冼国佳	梁大艳	
广西壮族自治区	广西壮族自治区	广西医科大学附属肿瘤医院	李秋林 容敏华	余家华 周子寒	余红平	葛莲英	曹　骥
	南宁市兴宁区	南宁市兴宁区疾病预防控制中心	梁翠敏	欧阳丽华	黄礼庆		
	南宁市青秀区	南宁市青秀区疾病预防控制中心	李　颖	黄绍旎	卢志玲	黄中学	

省(自治区、直辖市) Province (autonomous region, municipality)	肿瘤登记处 Cancer Registry	登记处所在单位 Affiliation	主要工作人员 Staff				
	南宁市江南区	南宁市江南区疾病预防控制中心	戴姮	卢珠	曾俊		
	南宁经济技术开发区	南宁经济技术开发区疾病预防控制中心	覃燕红				
	南宁市西乡塘区	南宁市西乡塘区疾病预防控制中心	苏升灿	唐盛志	韦鹏	何雨澄	
	南宁市良庆区	南宁市良庆区疾病预防控制中心	唐英花				
	南宁东盟经济开发区	广西-东盟经济技术开发区疾病预防控制中心	宁栈				
	隆安县	隆安县疾病预防控制中心	陈珍莲	黄建云	方孔雄		
	宾阳县	宾阳县疾病预防控制中心	陈伟强 龚冰冰	甘晓琴 莫少梅	韦柳青 张华	李秀霞	陈源珍
	柳州市	柳州市疾病预防控制中心	覃忠书 陈宁钰	蓝剑 刘芸	王晓伟 欧蕾	孟繁文 朱庭萍	覃宇禄 谭晓萍
	桂林市	桂林市疾病预防控制中心	潘定权	蒋富生	汤杰	石瑀	
	梧州市	梧州市红十字会医院	郑裕明 苏阳红	汤伟文 陈骐炜	苏韶华	谢红英	黄金菊
	苍梧县	苍梧县疾病预防控制中心	李汉福 苏石汉	杨敏生 林冰	谭夏敏 余思洁	麦新苗	李北金
	北海市	北海市疾病预防控制中心	梁耀洁	谢平			
	合浦县	合浦县疾病预防控制中心	苏福康 陈鑫祖	曹松 谢贤缤	张强	秦晓丽	罗世琼
	钦州市钦南区	钦州市钦南区疾病预防控制中心	陆玉培	黄红英			
	贵港市港北区	贵港市港北区疾病预防控制中心	韦坚峥				
	贵港市港南区	贵港市港南区疾病预防控制中心	莫桂琼	谭金贤	黎兆华		
	贵港市覃塘区	贵港市覃塘区疾病预防控制中心	熊维				
	平南县	平南县疾病预防控制中心	冯翠				
	玉林市	玉林市疾病预防控制中心	陈立锐	周阳洋	吴定康	黄胜	
	陆川县	陆川县疾病预防控制中心	黄文宁				
	北流市	北流市疾病预防控制中心	唐美玲 黄胜	陈金武	李鸿玲	黎丹	陈雪
	百色市右江区	百色市右江区疾病预防控制中心	吴美秀				

省（自治区、直辖市） Province （autonomous region, municipality）	肿瘤登记处 Cancer Registry	登记处所在单位 Affiliation	主要工作人员 Staff
	百色市田阳区	百色市田阳区疾病预防控制中心	李洁玲　黄志刚　何少松
	罗城仫佬族自治县	罗城仫佬族自治县疾病预防控制中心	韦政兴　梁玉春　卢永钧　罗黎霞　韦愿
	合山市	合山市疾病预防控制中心	黄海浪
	扶绥县	扶绥县人民医院	李海华　梁威丽　李云西　韦忠亮　黄志斌 陶哲艺
海南省	海南省	海南省肿瘤防治中心	董华　范康琼　华婧　王定彬
	三亚市	三亚市疾病预防控制中心	陈莲芬　黄炯媚　潘超
	五指山市	五指山市疾病预防控制中心	符美艳　卢耿慧
	琼海市	琼海市疾病预防控制中心	符芳敏　颜李丽
	定安县	定安县疾病预防控制中心	李建斌　黎才刚　郭芳华
	昌江黎族自治县	昌江黎族自治县疾病预防控制中心	符为巨　王灵珍　钟玲慧
	陵水黎族自治县	陵水黎族自治县疾病预防控制中心	许声文　林仕栋
重庆市	重庆市	重庆市疾病预防控制中心	吕晓燕　丁贤彬
	重庆市万州区	重庆市万州区疾病预防控制中心	彭瑾　吴波　唐亮
	重庆市涪陵区	重庆市涪陵区疾病预防控制中心	周义芬　陈晓明　王杨凤　王琪
	重庆市渝中区	重庆市渝中区疾病预防控制中心	周琦　凌瑜双
	重庆市大渡口区	重庆市大渡口区疾病预防控制中心	赵璨　刘勇言
	重庆市江北区	重庆市江北区疾病预防控制中心	郭梅　刘静
	重庆市沙坪坝区	重庆市沙坪坝区疾病预防控制中心	邓丽君　支倩　蒙怡
	重庆市九龙坡区	重庆市九龙坡区疾病预防控制中心	汤成　贺明　陶然　肖伦
	重庆市南岸区	重庆市南岸区疾病预防控制中心	何英淑　黄治兰　廖晓澄
	重庆市北碚区	重庆市北碚区疾病预防控制中心	李大兵　邓小霞
	重庆市綦江区	重庆市綦江区疾病预防控制中心	罗春亮　周梦雪

省（自治区、直辖市） Province （autonomous region，municipality）	肿瘤登记处 Cancer Registry	登记处所在单位 Affiliation	主要工作人员 Staff
	重庆市大足区	重庆市大足区疾病预防控制中心	李万华　任香勇　杨　颖
	重庆市渝北区	重庆市渝北区疾病预防控制中心	郭昌融　张晓慧
	重庆市巴南区	重庆市巴南区疾病预防控制中心	陶小红　刘成果
	重庆市黔江区	重庆市黔江区疾病预防控制中心	吴　畅　吴彩霞　李　卫　王　敏
	重庆市长寿区	重庆市长寿区疾病预防控制中心	马周俊　邓　静
	重庆市江津区	重庆市江津区疾病预防控制中心	杨　媚　孟秋雨　李西同
	重庆市合川区	重庆市合川区疾病预防控制中心	贺　玲　王绍梅
	重庆市永川区	重庆市永川区疾病预防控制中心	吴　欢　程莉莎　刘　琳
	重庆市南川区	重庆市南川区疾病预防控制中心	钟　静
	重庆市万盛经济开发区	重庆市万盛经济开发区疾病预防控制中心	杨　琴　田　哲
	重庆市潼南区	重庆市潼南区疾病预防控制中心	龙　凤　陈雪莲　郝真强
	重庆市铜梁区	重庆市铜梁区疾病预防控制中心	周昇杰
	重庆市荣昌区	重庆市荣昌区疾病预防控制中心	舒　强　于均梅　熊华利
	重庆市璧山区	重庆市璧山区疾病预防控制中心	陈　静　张　瑜
	重庆市梁平区	重庆市梁平区疾病预防控制中心	游茂林　邱虹蛟
	丰都县	丰都县疾病预防控制中心	熊　薇　曾正英　刘　琳
	垫江县	垫江县疾病预防控制中心	杨世亚　谭　格
	重庆市武隆区	重庆市武隆区疾病预防控制中心	万　泉　刘浩然　李婷婷
	忠县	忠县疾病预防控制中心	熊晓世　袁　英　方　君
	重庆市开州区	重庆市开州区疾病预防控制中心	肖幸平　崔喜闻

省（自治区、直辖市） Province (autonomous region, municipality)	肿瘤登记处 Cancer Registry	登记处所在单位 Affiliation	主要工作人员 Staff
	云阳县	云阳县疾病预防控制中心	张 星　张 林　王 芳
	奉节县	奉节县疾病预防控制中心	向 嫱　张克燕　罗 宇　姜孝凤
	巫山县	巫山县疾病预防控制中心	何成丹　曾 蓉　梁 辉
	巫溪县	巫溪县疾病预防控制中心	吕文宾　王发辉　任兴荣
	石柱土家族自治县	石柱土家族自治县疾病预防控制中心	汤剑峰
	秀山土家族苗族自治县	秀山土家族苗族自治县疾病预防控制中心	郭 敏
	酉阳土家族苗族自治县	酉阳土家族苗族自治县疾病预防控制中心	冉悦函
	彭水苗族土家族自治县	彭水苗族土家族自治县疾病预防控制中心	陈 节　郭 超　杨 璇　胡元红
四川省	四川省	四川省疾病预防控制中心	成姝雯　邓 颖　胥馨尹　董 婷　曾 晶 张 新　乔 良　刘潇霞
	成都市青羊区	成都市青羊区疾病预防控制中心	韩湘意　彭长燕　蔡 鹏　刘 嘉
	成都市成华区	成都市成华区疾病预防控制中心	胡 莹　许 凌　王 超　周 静　赵子君
	成都市龙泉驿区	成都市龙泉驿区疾病预防控制中心	卢清平　江 柯　张群英　阮红海
	成都市新都区	成都市新都区疾病预防控制中心	文婧唯　焦 娇　刘 芳　赵子贺　刘 燕
	金堂县	金堂县疾病预防控制中心	李林容　叶立力
	成都市双流区	成都市双流区疾病预防控制中心	王照华　胡 容　黄先志　唐 爽　裴宗琴
	成都市天府新区	成都市天府新区疾病预防控制中心	袁晓宇　罗 刚　袁 伟　姚菲菲　罗 杰
	成都市郫都区	成都市郫都区疾病预防控制中心	林超兰　江 秀　黄小芳　余 林
	成都市新津区	成都市新津区疾病预防控制中心	刘凤容　杨 杰　苟念秋
	彭州市	彭州市疾病预防控制中心	蒋 微　罗国金　李建国　陈小芳　刘佳秋 孙 强　王建娜
	自贡市自流井区	自贡市自流井区疾病预防控制中心	熊端萍　冯小伟　李 刚　刘筱颖　商 静
	自贡市贡井区	自贡市贡井区疾病预防控制中心	邱玉琼　江 超　毛喜艳

省(自治区、直辖市) Province (autonomous region, municipality)	肿瘤登记处 Cancer Registry	登记处所在单位 Affiliation	主要工作人员 Staff				
	自贡市大安区	自贡市大安区疾病预防控制中心	徐 爽	倪 嘉	张小林	李蕾思	
	自贡市沿滩区	自贡市沿滩区疾病预防控制中心	陈 燕	郑尚红			
	荣县	荣县疾病预防控制中心	陈 莉	刘 莉	夏和珍	胡 杰	杨 玲
	富顺县	富顺县疾病预防控制中心	刘兴莉	黄帮雨	关晓旭	徐小丽	吴 帆
	攀枝花市东区	攀枝花市东区疾病预防控制中心	陈 莹				
	攀枝花市西区	攀枝花市西区疾病预防控制中心	贺绍琼	李 英	关绍婷		
	攀枝花市仁和区	攀枝花市仁和区疾病预防控制中心	毛 鹏	赫永新	汪 杰	周玉萍	
	米易县	米易县疾病预防控制中心	甘 泉 董家君	曾文海 刘天慧	罗 欢	廖长春	曹 珊
	盐边县	盐边县疾病预防控制中心	程 平	任宗良			
	泸州市江阳区	泸州市江阳区疾病预防控制中心	邵 红	李 奕	杨廷婷	李娅凌	林叶清
	泸州市纳溪区	泸州市纳溪区疾病预防控制中心	林 利	虞旭东	曾世林		
	泸州市龙马潭区	泸州市龙马潭区疾病预防控制中心	唐 伟	韦汉淬	雷启云	李春艳	曾 瑜
	泸县	泸县疾病预防控制中心	谢 婧	余 军	熊 君	汪正刚	陈平平
	合江县	合江县疾病预防控制中心	胡 东	王 蓉	黎 溢	邓艳艳	刘明海
	叙永县	叙永县疾病预防控制中心	郭庆洁	魏策进	黄 嵩	罗 刚	李玉开
	古蔺县	古蔺县疾病预防控制中心	邓 波	文 兵	姜春霞	冯华强	龙巧林
	德阳市旌阳区	德阳市旌阳区疾病预防控制中心	叶先太	苏小波	于 进	陈 思	周小华
	中江县	中江县疾病预防控制中心	邹 红 邓 庆	蒋文斌	邓绍清	秦国胜	谢 伟
	德阳市罗江区	德阳市罗江区疾病预防控制中心	管小琴	彭 茹	刘怀淑		
	广汉市	广汉市疾病预防控制中心	肖昌华	刘丹丹	王 玲	龙小刚	何 柳
	什邡市	什邡市疾病预防控制中心	蒋 丽	郑小军	钟雪飞	肖家慧	邢婷婷
	绵竹市	绵竹市疾病预防控制中心	张 桃 廖伯勇	周道兴	周 平	何启明	周义健
	绵阳市涪城区	绵阳市涪城区疾病预防控制中心	李 洁	王蒙杰	周晓凤		

省（自治区、直辖市） Province （autonomous region，municipality）	肿瘤登记处 Cancer Registry	登记处所在单位 Affiliation	主要工作人员 Staff
	绵阳市游仙区	绵阳市游仙区疾病预防控制中心	安水玲　王　慧
	绵阳市安州区	绵阳市安州区疾病预防控制中心	季洪兵　许　强　李艳梅　周海英　滕　椤
	三台县	三台县疾病预防控制中心	黄　丽　周　欢
	盐亭县	盐亭县肿瘤防治研究所(肿瘤医院)	李　军　李　林　黄　政
	梓潼县	梓潼县疾病预防控制中心	帖映伟　赵金华
	北川羌族自治县	北川羌族自治县疾病预防控制中心	蒋素红　韩　丽
	平武县	平武县疾病预防控制中心	严松林　焦　剑　罗　健　刘严娇　黄莉蓉
	江油市	江油市疾病预防控制中心	夏丽莉　竹晓琴　王定邦　李　宁　李春梅　薛　莉
	广元市利州区	广元市利州区疾病预防控制中心	张小玲　王　平　谢晓莉
	广元市昭化区	广元市昭化区疾病预防控制中心	曹　智　漆志军　李小建
	广元市朝天区	广元市朝天区疾病预防控制中心	何　磊　解明成　张玉芬
	旺苍县	旺苍县疾病预防控制中心	陈晓红　米家君　贾正常
	青川县	青川县疾病预防控制中心	张淑兰　袁正华　袁伟贤　柳青蓉　王桂花
	剑阁县	剑阁县疾病预防控制中心	田　辉　吴　婷　赵　彬
	苍溪县	苍溪县疾病预防控制中心	张　娟　吴德明　何　楠　朱友德
	遂宁市船山区	遂宁市船山区疾病预防控制中心	王　婧　刘　淼
	遂宁市安居区	遂宁市安居区疾病预防控制中心	李　谦　吴　高　冯裕如　陈胜春
	蓬溪县	蓬溪县疾病预防控制中心	邱　林　杨建红　梁　波　陈　恒
	射洪市	射洪市疾病预防控制中心	石晓柳　刘　扬　杜思豪
	大英县	大英县疾病预防控制中心	夏　冰　唐　霞　韦　伊
	内江市市中区	内江市市中区疾病预防控制中心	董永年　唐纯丽　尤　霄　达　希　刘小波
	内江市东兴区	内江市东兴区疾病预防控制中心	黄　艳　冷江涛
	威远县	威远县疾病预防控制中心	陈秀兰　陈　娜　杨卉玲
	资中县	资中县疾病预防控制中心	崔红刚　钟　鸣　李　静　陈　璐　孙于茹
	隆昌市	隆昌市疾病预防控制中心	罗　睿　高雪娅　代　敬

省（自治区、直辖市） Province （autonomous region，municipality）	肿瘤登记处 Cancer Registry	登记处所在单位 Affiliation	主要工作人员 Staff
	乐山市市中区	乐山市市中区疾病预防控制中心	赵彬茜　钟　钰　岑晓喻　冯　亮
	乐山市沙湾区	乐山市沙湾区疾病预防控制中心	张春霞　苟　伟　朱　攀
	乐山市五通桥区	乐山市五通桥区疾病预防控制中心	侯　亮
	乐山市金口河区	乐山市金口河区疾病预防控制中心	吕伟华　刘海燕　江旭婷
	犍为县	犍为县疾病预防控制中心	谯　宇　余美帆　童　宇
	井研县	井研县疾病预防控制中心	税智群　李泳梅　何　芳　吕中林
	夹江县	夹江县疾病预防控制中心	晏　荧　龙建坤　干晓辉
	沐川县	沐川县疾病预防控制中心	刘　焱　周玉萍　郑　玲
	峨边彝族自治县	峨边彝族自治县疾病预防控制中心	黄代骥　李忠林
	马边彝族自治县	马边彝族自治县疾病预防控制中心	立机妹美
	峨眉山市	峨眉山市疾病预防控制中心	吴　洁　伍毕英　吴凌燕　周　敏
	南充市顺庆区	南充市顺庆区疾病预防控制中心	杨　欢　徐　捷　梁　熙　肖　强
	南充市高坪区	南充市高坪区人民医院	邢　丽　岳小林　廖　波
	南充市嘉陵区	南充市嘉陵区疾病预防控制中心	黄　维　祝　倩　陈洪春
	南部县	南部县疾病预防控制中心	陈　进　杨晓萍　张燕军
	营山县	营山县疾病预防控制中心	苟军平　彭　勇
	蓬安县	蓬安县疾病预防控制中心	林　波　罗　容　蒲泓兵
	仪陇县	仪陇县疾病预防控制中心	曹　成　曹秋菊　何　倩　吴相遇　刘　燕
	西充县	西充县疾病预防控制中心	赵　辉　孙青青
	阆中市	阆中市疾病预防控制中心	游宁静　任　焱　刘　刚　许　华
	眉山市东坡区	眉山市东坡区疾病预防控制中心	陈兰芬
	眉山市彭山区	眉山市彭山区疾病预防控制中心	周建容　潘　耀　余志祥
	仁寿县	仁寿县疾病预防控制中心	宋良文　瞿遥来　黄佳玲　宁　芳　杨　红
	洪雅县	洪雅县疾病预防控制中心	赖　兵　吴　莹　杨利琴
	丹棱县	丹棱县疾病预防控制中心	罗　源　梁学祥

省（自治区、直辖市） Province （autonomous region, municipality）	肿瘤登记处 Cancer Registry	登记处所在单位 Affiliation	主要工作人员 Staff
	青神县	青神县疾病预防控制中心	徐琴 张邻 黄彬鑫
	宜宾市翠屏区	宜宾市翠屏区疾病预防控制中心	马坤容 刘如葵 戴自强 陈志富 应元玲 黄昌学 朱德琴
	宜宾市叙州区	宜宾市叙州区疾病预防控制中心	陈小芳 周刘
	江安县	江安县疾病预防控制中心	王芳 李军 李必容 杨晴 程彦
	长宁县	长宁县疾病预防控制中心	王宇
	高县	高县疾病预防控制中心	黄小清 任燃
	筠连县	筠连县疾病预防控制中心	张迪
	屏山县	屏山县疾病预防控制中心	程伟 徐江红
	广安市广安区	广安市广安区疾病预防控制中心	李国辉 杜承彬 李荣川
	广安市前锋区	广安市前锋区疾病预防控制中心	王维 黄春凤 叶正明 李川
	岳池县	岳池县疾病预防控制中心	邓平 聂勇
	武胜县	武胜县疾病预防控制中心	王文婷 张泽军 张建东 米惠琼 王惊秋
	邻水县	邻水县疾病预防控制中心	廖冬娟 刘健 钟晓辉
	华蓥市	华蓥市疾病预防控制中心	何阳 李建川 韩小月
	达州市达川区	达州市达川区疾病预防控制中心	段凯岚 罗玲 周莉 熊舒书
	宣汉县	宣汉县疾病预防控制中心	赵鹏飞 李波 桂国尧 张冬梅
	开江县	开江县疾病预防控制中心	卢有见 舒进川 陈红
	大竹县	大竹县疾病预防控制中心	袁东娅 王大骞 叶明兰 赵红艳 师小林
	渠县	渠县疾病预防控制中心	李平 王秀瑛
	万源市	万源市疾病预防控制中心	何莉 黄明锋 徐洁
	雅安市雨城区	雅安市雨城区疾病预防控制中心	王登琪 吴波 朱春明 李雅苹 刘杰 范娟
	雅安市名山区	雅安市名山区疾病预防控制中心	王修华 胡启源
	荥经县	荥经县疾病预防控制中心	李明远
	汉源县	汉源县疾病预防控制中心	廖卓航 王新 杜涓 辜豪
	石棉县	石棉县疾病预防控制中心	李桂芬 王琴 廖艳萍
	天全县	天全县疾病预防控制中心	高鸿敏
	芦山县	芦山县疾病预防控制中心	李唐芳 王鸿 熊欣

省（自治区、直辖市）Province（autonomous region，municipality）	肿瘤登记处 Cancer Registry	登记处所在单位 Affiliation	主要工作人员 Staff				
	宝兴县	宝兴县疾病预防控制中心	徐新红	姜　亚			
	巴中市巴州区	巴中市巴州区疾病预防控制中心	叶南宁	李俊杰			
	巴中市恩阳区	巴中市恩阳区疾病预防控制中心	罗　斌	张　翼	谢明芳	谯　健	
	通江县	通江县疾病预防控制中心	刘德泉　岳秀凤　李　鑫	赵廷明　王　丽　徐　畅	张　劲　李　骁　杨　清	陈　静　王清华	谢东柏　何开莉
	南江县	南江县疾病预防控制中心	赵正强	郭春燕	王光秀	谢　蓉	刘　兰
	平昌县	平昌县疾病预防控制中心	邹晓兰　钟　鑫	谢　凯　杨晓莉	涂亚平	李健生	何　勇
	资阳市雁江区	资阳市雁江区疾病预防控制中心	李仕海	王红艳	李成维		
	安岳县	安岳县疾病预防控制中心	杨　建	谢益琼	江　霁	唐承美	
	乐至县	乐至县疾病预防控制中心	吴志敏	李　光	雷方君	沈　莎	肖　洋
	马尔康市	马尔康市疾病预防控制中心	陈跃文	任跃文	马武胜		
	汶川县	汶川县疾病预防控制中心	余小芳	张　胜	姚　云	张诗卓	
	理县	理县疾病预防控制中心	余石花	班玉萍	杨敏菲	晏名辉	
	茂县	茂县疾病预防控制中心	黄德亮	夏　明	文德强	付　琴	
	松潘县	松潘县疾病预防控制中心	马静瑶	罗金磋	如妹磋		
	金川县	金川县疾病预防控制中心	马华美	熊　云			
	小金县	小金县疾病预防控制中心	张测铭	王术琼			
	黑水县	黑水县疾病预防控制中心	江友林				
	若尔盖县	若尔盖县疾病预防控制中心	欧志婷	邓　斌			
	红原县	红原县疾病预防控制中心	尕尔姆				
贵州省	贵州省	贵州省疾病预防控制中心	刘　涛	李　凌	周　婕		
	贵阳市花溪区	贵阳市花溪区疾病预防控制中心	刘　靖				
	开阳县	开阳县疾病预防控制中心	颜克梅				
	息烽县	息烽县疾病预防控制中心	吴　会				
	清镇市	清镇市疾病预防控制中心	付　敏				
	六盘水钟山区	六盘水市钟山区疾病预防控制中心	朱　娟				
	六盘水市六枝特区	六盘水市六枝特区疾病预防控制中心	张徐巾				

省（自治区、直辖市） Province （autonomous region, municipality）	肿瘤登记处 Cancer Registry	登记处所在单位 Affiliation	主要工作人员 Staff
	六盘水市水城区	六盘水市水城区疾病预防控制中心	刘作英
	盘州市	盘州市疾病预防控制中心	章有建
	遵义市红花岗区	遵义市红花岗区疾病预防控制中心	陈艳娟
	遵义市汇川区	遵义市汇川区疾病预防控制中心	杨　敏
	习水县	习水县疾病预防控制中心	杨存焜
	赤水市	赤水市疾病预防控制中心	邓金勇
	安顺市西秀区	安顺市西秀区疾病预防控制中心	鲁玲亚
	镇宁布依族苗族自治县	安顺市镇宁县疾病预防控制中心	杨　琳
	毕节市七星关区	毕节市七星关区疾病预防控制中心	李　琴
	金沙县	金沙县疾病预防控制中心	王天赐
	铜仁市碧江区	铜仁市碧江区疾病预防控制中心	杨江艳
	玉屏侗族自治县	玉屏侗族自治县疾病预防控制中心	陆承凯
	思南县	思南县疾病预防控制中心	王伟忠
	普安县	普安县疾病预防控制中心	顾凤莉
	册亨县	册亨县疾病预防控制中心	覃明江
	黄平县	黄平县疾病预防控制中心	杨　玲
	镇远县	镇远县疾病预防控制中心	顾先桃
	榕江县	榕江县疾病预防控制中心	吴永莲
	雷山县	雷山县疾病预防控制中心	毛　海
	麻江县	麻江县疾病预防控制中心	吴晓云
	都匀市	都匀市疾病预防控制中心	李国叶
	福泉市	福泉市疾病预防控制中心	唐秋红
	荔波县	荔波县疾病预防控制中心	周雪梅
	独山县	独山县疾病预防控制中心	马清兰
	龙里县	龙里县疾病预防控制中心	杜月清
云南省	云南省	云南省疾病预防控制中心	文洪梅　陈　杨　石青萍
	昆明市	昆明市疾病预防控制中心	李　吉　杨　昭

省（自治区、 直辖市） Province （autonomous region， municipality）	肿瘤登记处 Cancer Registry	登记处所在单位 Affiliation	主要工作人员 Staff				
	昆明市五华区	昆明市五华区疾病预防控制中心	周　丽 王紫玉	张　洁	许秋婧	曾成琴	高柏强
	昆明市盘龙区	昆明市盘龙区疾病预防控制中心	何丽明	王睿翊	马琳玲	何开浚	
	昆明市官渡区	昆明市官渡区疾病预防控制中心	张　龙 段培华	詹　恒 佘旭敏	王晓珺	张慧萍	王　丽
	昆明市西山区	昆明市西山区疾病预防控制中心	李　杰 张艺嘉	周欣霞 袁寂州	龚　林 高俊楠	李赛云 李绍叶	李子美
	昆明市东川区	昆明市东川区疾病预防控制中心	赵亚楠	韩贵卫			
	昆明市晋宁区	昆明市晋宁区疾病预防控制中心	张美莲	李明珠			
	昆明市呈贡区	昆明市呈贡区疾病预防控制中心	张永丽				
	富民县	富民县疾病预防控制中心	李俊兴				
	嵩明县	嵩明县疾病预防控制中心	郭树岚	保　尚			
	禄劝彝族苗族自治县	禄劝彝族苗族自治县疾病预防控制中心	钟玉美 耿天顺	王　鑫 李锡军	潘庆葵	杨祖宏	李泽蕊
	安宁市	安宁市疾病预防控制中心	杨宝学	赵会联			
	曲靖市	曲靖市疾病预防控制中心	李继华	李　云	牛文倩		
	曲靖市麒麟区	曲靖市麒麟区疾病预防控制中心	雷芸华	关秋艳	施红娟	丁鹏俊	吴林凤
	曲靖市沾益区	曲靖市沾益区疾病预防控制中心	雷宝琼	付　进			
	曲靖市马龙区	曲靖市马龙区疾病预防控制中心	王慈蓉	万正文			
	陆良县	陆良县疾病预防控制中心	钱康林	朱　姗			
	富源县	富源县疾病预防控制中心	王　云				
	宣威市	宣威市疾病预防控制中心	宁伯福				
	玉溪市	玉溪市疾病预防控制中心	李六九	马真飞	李　吉		
	玉溪市红塔区	玉溪市红塔区疾病预防控制中心	瞿　媛 陶　然 孟源珂	杜春华 邹　容	张　莉 白光宝	刘　蕊 管　颖	林　蕾 赵明洪
	玉溪市江川区	玉溪市江川区疾病预防控制中心	史伊冉	陈艺丹	赵媛丽		
	澄江市	澄江市疾病预防控制中心	马重义	周红云	董志鹏		

省(自治区、直辖市) Province (autonomous region, municipality)	肿瘤登记处 Cancer Registry	登记处所在单位 Affiliation	主要工作人员 Staff				
	通海县	通海县疾病预防控制中心	高瑞芳	李德雄	杨春琼	李 艳	
	华宁县	华宁县疾病预防控制中心	施云丽	王志鹏	杨 蓉	杨忠卫	
	易门县	易门县疾病预防控制中心	樊学琼	吕 宏	许 葵	阮 伟	王冬梅
	峨山彝族自治县	峨山彝族自治县疾病预防控制中心	李晓燕				
	新平彝族傣族自治县	新平彝族傣族自治县疾病预防控制中心	殷文学				
	元江哈尼族彝族傣族自治县	元江哈尼族彝族傣族自治县疾病预防控制中心	张坤平 陆拾妹	杨太专	卫 芳	杨忠强	杨生宝
	保山市	保山市疾病预防控制中心	徐仙会	李明松	邓 丽	褚钊颖	
	保山市隆阳区	保山市隆阳区疾病预防控制中心	杨璐竹 王 伟	杨善华	董全玉	杨保国	陈 浩
	施甸县	施甸县疾病预防控制中心	吴新会	朱海燕	杨丝丝	杨继虎	杨进水
	腾冲市	腾冲市疾病预防控制中心	刘晓丽 李相妹	李亚丹	杨艳芳	封占益	段立敏
	龙陵县	龙陵县疾病预防控制中心	杨福娣	寸勐震	李菊云	王云春	
	昌宁县	昌宁县疾病预防控制中心	曾映竹	杨绍杰	宋金阳	黄丽琼	
	昭通市	昭通市疾病预防控制中心	马东琼				
	昭通市昭阳区	昭通市昭阳区疾病预防控制中心	刘 卫	刘红英	陈 会		
	巧家县	巧家县疾病预防控制中心	王开芳				
	绥江县	绥江县疾病预防控制中心	刘晓静				
	水富县	水富县疾病预防控制中心	朱晓蕾				
	丽江市	丽江市疾病预防控制中心	杨丽梅	冉钦玉			
	丽江市古城区	丽江市古城区疾病预防控制中心	和臣慧	王艳红	崔舒静		
	玉龙纳西族自治县	玉龙纳西族自治县疾病预防控制中心	杨翠香	杨 俊	和致祥		
	华坪县	华坪县疾病预防控制中心	王正英	黄同琼	卢国春		
	普洱市	普洱市疾病预防控制中心	周锦涛	唐 颖	段义军		
	景东彝族自治县	景东彝族自治县疾病预防控制中心	祝章美	龚 晨	陶 梅	周晓波	
	景谷傣族彝族自治县	景谷傣族彝族自治县疾病预防控制中心	周新玉	王丽娇	李 健		
	镇沅彝族哈尼族拉祜族自治县	镇沅彝族哈尼族拉祜族自治县疾病预防控制中心	自家梅	罗开萍	吴容容		

省（自治区、直辖市） Province （autonomous region，municipality）	肿瘤登记处 Cancer Registry	登记处所在单位 Affiliation	主要工作人员 Staff				
	江城哈尼族彝族自治县	江城哈尼族彝族自治县疾病预防控制中心	鲍月月	刘红兵	罗　路		
	临沧市	临沧市疾病预防控制中心	李秋圆				
	临沧市临翔区	临沧市临翔区疾病预防控制中心	罗忠芳	王新梅	董秀玲	施正仙	李天玺
	镇康县	镇康县疾病预防控制中心	杨　凤	刘志梅			
	沧源倪族自治县	沧源倪族自治县疾病预防控制中心	赵福芳	李　瑶	李　波		
	楚雄彝族自治州	楚雄彝族自治州疾病预防控制中心	赵会勇				
	楚雄市	楚雄市疾病预防控制中心	刘家早	仇剑芝			
	双柏县	双柏县疾病预防控制中心	张雅薇				
	牟定县	牟定县疾病预防控制中心	何　磊	杨　芳			
	南华县	南华县疾病预防控制中心	吕美英	费建琼			
	姚安县	姚安县疾病预防控制中心	苏菊芬	刘洪文			
	大姚县	大姚县疾病预防控制中心	班琼珍	赵宗和			
	永仁县	永仁县疾病预防控制中心	肖甫仁	孙丽华			
	元谋县	元谋县疾病预防控制中心	仲丽红				
	武定县	武定县疾病预防控制中心	赵学敏				
	禄丰市	禄丰市疾病预防控制中心	刘雪丽	毕志梅			
	红河哈尼族彝族自治州	红河州第三人民医院	潘龙海				
	个旧市	个旧市肿瘤防治工作领导小组办公室	王建宁				
	开远市	开远市疾病预防控制中心	杜晓芳	顾春芳	陈亚苏	闫友芸	
	蒙自市	蒙自市疾病预防控制中心	杨　涛				
	弥勒市	弥勒市疾病预防控制中心	徐建华	杨晓静			
	屏边苗族自治县	屏边苗族自治县疾病预防控制中心	吴　娅				
	建水县	建水县疾病预防控制中心	周艳梅	张艳芳	刘　怡	白玉仙	白　琼
	石屏县	石屏县疾病预防控制中心	王昌钰	高　霞			
	泸西县	泸西县疾病预防控制中心	戴　丽	王秋婷			
	河口县	河口县疾病预防控制中心	王海波	刘　源	姚　倩		
	文山壮族苗族自治州	文山壮族苗族自治州疾病预防控制中心	程　艳				
	砚山县	砚山县疾病预防控制中心	祁红芬				

省（自治区、直辖市） Province （autonomous region，municipality）	肿瘤登记处 Cancer Registry	登记处所在单位 Affiliation	主要工作人员 Staff
	西畴县	西畴县疾病预防控制中心	袁 丽
	丘北县	丘北县疾病预防控制中心	杨燕琼
	富宁县	富宁县疾病预防控制中心	何利华
	西双版纳傣族自治州	西双版纳傣族自治州疾病预防控制中心	陈 萍　范芸苑
	景洪市	景洪市疾病预防控制中心	石保英　杨舒寒
	大理市	大理市疾病预防控制中心	何俊涵　杨 清　张 莹　杜雅素　魏朝晖 赵庆平
	祥云县	祥云县疾病预防控制中心	周亚娟　张建荣　丁雪琴
	弥渡县	弥渡县疾病预防控制中心	孙海欧　姚绍梅　张美华
	永平县	永平县疾病预防控制中心	马迎春　李亚芳
	鹤庆县	鹤庆县疾病预防控制中心	洪 梅　吴玉蓉　董 垚
	德宏傣族景颇族自治州	德宏傣族景颇族自治州疾病预防控制中心	李家才　高右东
	梁河县	梁河县疾病预防控制中心	李素一　方永兴
	盈江县	盈江县疾病预防控制中心	刘永艳　杨 洁　毕 锐
	怒江傈僳族自治州	怒江傈僳族自治州疾病预防控制中心	杨卫美
	兰坪白族普米族自治县	兰坪白族普米族自治县疾病预防控制中心	李晓燕　和绍梅　杨红玉
西藏自治区	西藏自治区	西藏自治区疾病预防控制中心	扎西宗吉
	拉萨市城关区	拉萨市疾病预防控制中心	袁 静
	林芝市巴宜区	林芝市疾病预防控制中心	王 英
	昌都市卡若区	昌都市疾病预防控制中心	卓 玛
	日喀则市	日喀则市疾病预防控制中心	晋 扎　格 吉
陕西省	陕西省	陕西省疾病预防控制中心	刘 峰　程永兵　邱 琳　王艳平
	西安市碑林区	西安市碑林区疾病预防控制中心	范 颖　周 鼎　李福强　朱 倩　郑君茹
	西安市莲湖区	西安市莲湖区疾病预防控制中心	李 凡　孙婷婷
	西安市未央区	西安市未央区疾病预防控制中心	李 倩　杨 梦
	西安市雁塔区	西安市雁塔区疾病预防控制中心	王 宁　薛静怡

省（自治区、直辖市） Province （autonomous region，municipality）	肿瘤登记处 Cancer Registry	登记处所在单位 Affiliation	主要工作人员 Staff
	西安市高陵区	西安市高陵区疾病预防控制中心	黄维娜　汪　洋
	西安市鄠邑区	西安市鄠邑区疾病预防控制中心慢病科	张　莹　丁　珍
	铜川市王益区	铜川市王益区疾病预防控制中心	赵旭东
	铜川市耀州区	铜川市耀州区疾病预防控制中心	陈雯雯
	宝鸡市金台区	宝鸡市金台区疾病预防控制中心	李　倩
	宝鸡市陈仓区	宝鸡市陈仓区疾病预防控制中心	王新梅
	宝鸡市凤翔区	宝鸡市凤翔区疾病预防控制中心	周晓梅
	岐山县	岐山县疾病预防控制中心	袁小红
	眉县	眉县疾病预防控制中心	赵　云
	陇县	陇县疾病预防控制中心	郭小兰
	千阳县	千阳县疾病预防控制中心	茹夏丽　赵　倩　尚　博
	麟游县	麟游县疾病预防控制中心	马方伟
	泾阳县	泾阳县疾病预防控制中心	闫阿妮
	渭南市临渭区	渭南市临渭区疾病预防控制中心	权巧玲
	渭南市华州区	渭南市华州区疾病预防控制中心	张亚莹
	潼关县	潼关县疾病预防控制中心	亢　静
	大荔县	大荔县疾病预防控制中心	陈艳萍　高卫丽
	合阳县	合阳县疾病预防控制中心	雷艳玲　梁忠义
	澄城县	澄城县疾病预防控制中心	王　鹏　雷晓利　楚　莹
	蒲城县	蒲城县疾病预防控制中心	赵　莹
	富平县	富平县疾病预防控制中心	苏木兰　简　琳
	华阴市	华阴市疾病预防控制中心	张济德　郝青青
	延安市宝塔区	延安市宝塔区疾病预防控制中心	刘　鑫　贺军宏　尹明萍　孙　婧
	富县	富县疾病预防控制中心	冯　超　王忠学　吕亚军　罗英利
	黄陵县	黄陵县疾病预防控制中心	雷云云　王　曼　杨明霞

省（自治区、直辖市）Province（autonomous region，municipality）	肿瘤登记处 Cancer Registry	登记处所在单位 Affiliation	主要工作人员 Staff
	汉中市汉台区	汉中市汉台区疾病预防控制中心	杨宝亮　刘轩岐
	城固县	城固县疾病预防控制中心	尹　勇　高智平　李　罡
	宁强县	宁强县疾病预防控制中心	向凤义
	绥德县	绥德县疾病预防控制中心	刘　成
	安康市汉滨区	安康市汉滨区疾病预防控制中心	单林涛　刘卫军　王大锋　柯　娴
	汉阴县	汉阴县疾病预防控制中心	王　鹏
	石泉县	石泉县疾病预防控制中心	冯如月　陈梨花
	宁陕县	宁陕县疾病预防控制中心	代　鹏　易秉涛
	紫阳县	紫阳县疾病预防控制中心	许金华　陈　涛
	镇坪县	镇坪县疾病预防控制中心	杜誉淇
	旬阳市	旬阳市疾病预防控制中心	沈　龙　杜小菊
	商洛市商州区	商洛市商州区疾病预防控制中心	王天军　张　琪
	镇安县	镇安县疾病预防控制中心	刘家政　王　雯
甘肃省	甘肃省	甘肃省肿瘤医院/甘肃省癌症中心	刘玉琴　丁高恒
	兰州市	兰州市疾病预防控制中心	史危安　陆署元
	兰州市城关区	兰州市城关区疾病预防控制中心	杨海峰　韩　霞　杨　菁
	兰州市七里河区	兰州市七里河区疾病预防控制中心	陶　涛　王志龙
	兰州市西固区	兰州市西固区疾病预防控制中心	苟丽萍　徐　梅　徐　洁
	兰州市安宁区	兰州市安宁区疾病预防控制中心	何秀芬　殷　行
	兰州市红古区	兰州市红古区疾病预防控制中心	齐国怀　张　青
	白银市	白银市疾病预防控制中心	马骥雄　鲁朝霞
	白银市白银区	白银市白银区疾病预防控制中心	李顺翠　张小琴
	白银市平川区	白银市平川区疾病预防控制中心	李　霞　胡晓俊
	靖远县	靖远县疾病预防控制中心	高跟霞　欧志秀
	会宁县	会宁县疾病预防控制中心	程永莲　党丽琴

省（自治区、直辖市） Province （autonomous region, municipality）	肿瘤登记处 Cancer Registry	登记处所在单位 Affiliation	主要工作人员 Staff
	景泰县	景泰县疾病预防控制中心	梁志龙　周福新　王生芸
	天水市	天水市疾病预防控制中心	张　庆　杨　婧
	天水市秦州区	天水市秦州区疾病预防控制中心	马　明　安珊珊
	天水市麦积区	天水市麦积区疾病预防控制中心	杨　慧　王　芳
	武威市	甘肃省武威肿瘤医院	叶延程　胡军国　高彩云
	武威市凉州区	武威市凉州区疾病预防控制中心	刘海峰　李玉霞
	民勤县	民勤县疾病预防控制中心	姜玉平
	古浪县	古浪县疾病预防控制中心	严艳玲　高娟娟
	天祝藏族自治县	天祝藏族自治县疾病预防控制中心	石福娟　王生玲
	张掖市	张掖市疾病预防控制中心	银万栋　王　清
	张掖市甘州区	张掖市甘州区疾病预防控制中心	王金金　陈国辉
	高台县	高台县疾病预防控制中心	黄充盈　闫述凯
	静宁县	静宁县疾病预防控制中心	闫润芳　杨　娟　师　慧
	敦煌市	敦煌市疾病预防控制中心	淳志明　殷海燕　杜文倩
	庆城县	庆城县疾病预防控制中心	慕杰民　项霞霞
	临洮县	临洮县疾病预防控制中心	汪生虎　康玉霞
	临潭县	临潭县疾病预防控制中心	姚文林　祁少华
青海省	青海省	青海省疾病预防控制中心	周素霞
	西宁市	西宁市疾病预防控制中心	汤海霞　年晓亮　马丽娟　张丁鑫乐　郝广洪
	大通回族土族自治县	大通回族土族自治县疾病预防控制中心	张　莹
	西宁市湟中区	西宁市湟中区疾病预防控制中心	汪有库
	海东市	海东市疾病预防控制中心	魏　青
	海东市乐都区	海东市乐都区疾病预防控制中心	谢淑雯
	民和回族土族自治县	民和县疾病预防控制中心	张学强
	互助土族自治县	互助土族自治县疾病预防控制中心	王小庆

省(自治区、直辖市) Province (autonomous region,municipality)	肿瘤登记处 Cancer Registry	登记处所在单位 Affiliation	主要工作人员 Staff
	循化撒拉族自治县	循化撒拉族自治县疾病预防控制中心	陕国清
	海南藏族自治州	海南藏族自治州疾病预防控制中心	拉毛才让　齐迎兰　贺永庆　张　琼　石君红　拉先太
宁夏回族自治区	宁夏回族自治区	宁夏疾病预防控制中心	马　芳　杨　艺　魏　嵘
	银川市兴庆区	银川市兴庆区疾病预防控制中心	王洪丽　王　晶　侯静娅
	银川市西夏区	银川市西夏区疾病预防控制中心	张　婷　仇婷婷
	银川市金凤区	银川市金凤区疾病预防控制中心	保红莉　王海霞
	贺兰县	贺兰县疾病预防控制中心	盛春宁　陈海荣　姜旭红　董　威　陈　娥　马美娜
	石嘴山市大武口区	石嘴山市疾病预防控制中心	马　洁　张平稳　任海丽　刘　英　吴永军　张　悦
	石嘴山市惠农区	石嘴山市惠农区疾病预防控制中心	叶　璐　李冬梅　冯　羽
	平罗县	平罗县疾病预防控制中心	刘凤香
	青铜峡市	青铜峡市疾病预防控制中心	哈艳茹　赵仲刚　马　丽
	固原市原州区	固原市原州区疾病预防控制中心	南　艳
	中卫市沙坡头区	中卫市疾病预防控制中心	姚永红
	中宁县	中宁县疾病预防控制中心	赵寿桃
新疆维吾尔自治区	新疆维吾尔自治区	新疆维吾尔自治区疾病预防控制中心	董　言　张　荣　者　炜　王雯雷　张　俊　方　萍
	乌鲁木齐市天山区	乌鲁木齐市天山区疾病预防控制中心	郭颖贞　古丽努尔
	乌鲁木齐市米东区	乌鲁木齐市米东区疾病预防控制中心	刘　馨　马　芳
	克拉玛依市	克拉玛依市疾病预防控制中心	陈志萍　陈雪莹
	新源县	新源县疾病预防控制中心	田鹏昊　杨贺霞
	库尔勒市	库尔勒市疾病预防控制中心	
	和田市	和田市疾病预防控制中心	
	和田县	和田县疾病预防控制中心	
新疆生产建设兵团	新疆生产建设兵团	兵团疾病预防控制中心	申嘉丛　李凡卡　张宏伟　敬　雯

省（自治区、直辖市） Province (autonomous region, municipality)	肿瘤登记处 Cancer Registry	登记处所在单位 Affiliation	主要工作人员 Staff
	第二师	第二师疾病预防控制中心	文　静　周喜元　丁宏达　闫　澈
	第七师	第七师疾病预防控制中心	周　倩　杨海东　龚　耀　刘长龙
	第八师	石河子大学	李　锋　崔晓宾　李述刚　胡云华　刘春霞 刘成刚　陈　瑜　王　蓉　牛　强　闫贻忠 卢香云